CRC HANDBOOK SERIES IN CLINICAL LABORATORY SCIENCE

David Seligson, M.D., Sc.D.
Editor-in-Chief

SECTIONS AND SECTION EDITORS

Section A: Nuclear Medicine
Volumes I and II
Richard P. Spencer, M.D., Ph.D.

Section B: Toxicology
Volume I
Irving Sunshine, Ph.D.

Section C: Pathology
Volume I
Raymond Yesner, M.D.

Section D: Blood Banking
Volumes I—III
Tibor J. Greenwalt, M.D.
Edwin A. Steane, Ph.D.

Section E: Clinical Microbiology
Volumes I and II
Alexander von Graevenitz, M.D.

Section F: Immunology
Volume I: Parts 1 and 2
Alexander Baumgarten, M.D.
Frank F. Richards, M.D.

Section G: Clinical Chemistry
Volumes I—III
Mario Werner, M.D.

Section H: Virology and Ricksettsiology
Volume I: Parts 1 and 2
Guen-Djen Hsiung, Ph.D.
Robert H. Green, M.D.

Section I: Hematology
Volumes I—IV
Robert M. Schmidt, M.D., M.P.H., Ph.D.

CRC Handbook Series in Clinical Laboratory Science

Section I: Hematology
Volume IV

Section Editor
Robert M. Schmidt, M.D., M.P.H., Ph.D.
Professor of Hematology
San Francisco State University
Director, Preventive Medicine and Health Research
Pacific Presbyterian Medical Center
San Francisco, California

Volume Co-Editor
Virgil F. Fairbanks, M.D.
Professor of Laboratory Medicine
Mayo Clinic
Rochester, Minnesota

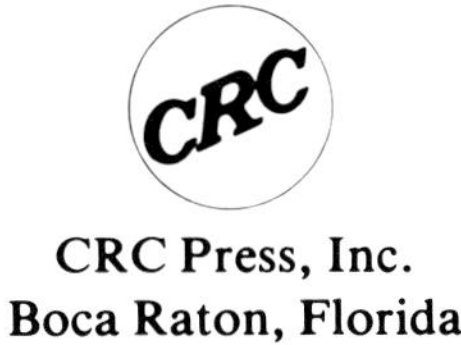

CRC Press, Inc.
Boca Raton, Florida

Library of Congress Cataloging-in-Publication Data
(Revised for section I, volume 4)

CRC handbook series in clinical laboratory science.

Spine title: Handbook series in clinical laboratory science.
Vols. for 1978 published in West Palm Beach, Fla.; vols. for 1979- published in Boca Raton, Fla.
Includes bibliographies and indexes.
Contents: Section A. Nuclear medicine.—Section B. Toxicology.—[etc.]—Section I. Hematology.
1. Diagnosis, Laboratory—Handbooks, manuals, etc.—Collected works. I. Seligson, David. II. Chemical Rubber Company. III. Title: Handbook series in clinical laboratory science.
RB37.C18 616.07'56 76-27688

This book represents information obtained from authentic and highly regarded sources. Reprinted material is quoted with permission, and sources are indicated. A wide variety of references are listed. Every reasonable effort has been made to give reliable data and information, but the author and the publisher cannot assume responsibility for the validity of all materials or for the consequences of their use.

Direct all inquiries to CRC Press, Inc., 2000 Corporate Blvd., N.W., Boca Raton, Florida, 33431.

International Standard Book Number 0-8493-7094-9

Library of Congress Card Number 76-27688
Printed in the United States

PREFACE

SECTION I: HEMATOLOGY

VOLUME IV

This is the fourth and final volume of the Hematology section of the *CRC Handbook Series in Clinical Laboratory Science*. The section was organized to provide a single ready reference for information on hematology which is found in a wide variety of textbooks, laboratory manuals, monographs and journal articles written to reach specialized audiences. Organization of the section was performed with the assistance of an Editorial Advisory Board whose members represent the major hematologic disciplines including internal medicine, pathology, pediatrics, laboratory medicine, and basic research. Advisory Board members who served varying terms between 1976 and 1986 include Drs. Kenneth M. Brinkhous, Robin W. Carrell, Lemuel W. Diggs, Virgil F. Fairbanks, Harvey R. Gralnick, Robert W. Kellermeyer, John A. Koepke, John B. Miale, Thomas F. Necheles, Walter A. Schroeder, Douglas A. Triplett, Frank E. Trobaugh, Jr., Onno W. vanAssendelft, and Maxwell M. Wintrobe.

Three volumes were published in 1979-1980:

—Volume I: Blood Collection, Blood Volume, Hemoglobin, Platelets
—Volume II: Blood Cell Morphology, Quality Control in Hematology, The White Cell
—Volume III: Thrombosis and Hemostasis

Volume IV contains chapters on the red cell and an update of important chapters on hemoglobin, reflecting the rapid advances in this area of hematology during the past 6 years.

Publication of the Hematology Section would not have been possible without the enthusiastic support of the Editorial Advisory Board and the efforts of our 110 contributors. Dr. Virgil F. Fairbanks served as the Board member who edited chapters in the fourth volume.

Robert M. Schmidt
Section Editor

THE EDITOR-IN-CHIEF

David Seligson, M.D., Sc.D., is Professor in the Department of Laboratory Medicine, Yale University and past Vice Chairman of the Medical Board and Director of the Department of Clinical Laboratories, Yale-New Haven Hospital, New Haven, Connecticut. Dr. Seligson received his Sc.D. degree from Johns Hopkins University and M.D. degree from the University of Utah. He is a member of numerous organizations and has received the John G. Reinhold Award and the Donald D. Van Slyke Award in 1966 and the Ames Award in 1971 from the AACC. Dr. Seligson has published several articles on laboratory medicine, renal and hepatic failure, and bilirubin bound to albumin.

THE EDITOR

Robert M. Schmidt, M.D., M.P.H., Ph.D., is Professor of Hematology, Center for Advanced Medical Technology, San Francisco State University and Director of Preventive Medicine and Health Research, Medical Research Institute of San Francisco, Pacific Presbyterian Medical Center, San Francisco. He has an A.B. from Northwestern University (1966), an M.D. from the Columbia University College of Physicians and Surgeons (1970), an M.P.H. from Harvard University (1975), and a Ph.D. from Emory University (1982.)

Previous positions include Director, Hematology Division, Centers for Disease Control, Atlanta and Medical Director, International Health Resource Center of Hawaii. He is a member of numerous scientific and professional associations, has served on editorial boards and national and international hematology committees and is the author of numerous publications including 15 books and manuals.

THE CO-EDITOR

Virgil F. Fairbanks, M.D., is Professor of Laboratory Medicine and Internal Medicine (Hematology), Mayo Medical School and Mayo Clinic, Rochester, Minn. He is a native of Ann Arbor, Michigan and a graduate of the Universities of Utah (B.A.) and Michigan (M.D.) He has served in laboratories of the University of Utah Medical Center, Scripps Clinic, City of Hope Medical Center, and Mayo Clinic.

Dr. Fairbanks is author of approximately 150 articles relating to iron metabolism, iron deficiency, iron overload, erythrocyte enzymopathies, hemoglobinopathies and thalassemias, and he is co-author or editor of eight books in the field of hematology, including the annual review *Current Hematology and Oncology*. He directs a laboratory concerned with the investigation of abnormalities of erythrocytes.

ADVISORY BOARD

CONTRIBUTORS

Solomon Adler, M.D.
Associate Professor
Department of Medicine
Rush Presbyterian-St. Luke's Medical Center
Chicago, Illinois

Stylianos E. Antonarakis, M.D.
Associate Professor
Department of Pediatrics
The Johns Hopkins University School of Medicine
Baltimore, Maryland

Ronald C. Barwick, Ph.D.
Associate Director
Paternity Evaluation
Roche Biochemical Laboratories
Burlington, North Carolina

Joel Anne Chasis, M.D.
Assistant Professor
Department of Medicine
University of California
San Francisco, California

Walter Fried, M.D.
Professor
Department of Medicine
Rush Presbyterian-St. Luke's Medical Center
Chicago, Illinois

Hisaichi Fujii, M.D.
Lecturer
Department of Internal Medicine
Institute of Medical Science
University of Tokyo
Tokyo, Japan

Chaim Hershko, M.D.
Chief, Department of Medicine
Shaare Zedek Medical Center
Professor of Medicine
Hebrew University Hadassah Medical School
Jerusalem, Israel

Gabriel Izak
Deceased
Formerly, Professor of Medicine
Department of Hematology
Hadassah University Hospital
Jerusalem, Israel

Richard T. Jones, M.D., Ph.D.
Professor and Chairman
Department of Biochemistry
School of Medicine
Oregon Health Sciences University
Portland, Oregon

Haig H. Kazazian, Jr., M.D.
Professor of Pediatrics
Director, Pediatric Genetics Unit
The Johns Hopkins University
Baltimore, Maryland

Robert D. Koler, M.D.
Professor and Chairman
Department of Medical Genetics
Oregon Health Science University
Portland, Oregon

Avraham M. Konijn
Senior Lecturer
Department of Medicine
Shaare Zedek Medical Center
Departments of Hematology and Nutrition
Hebrew University Hadassah Medical School
Jerusalem, Israel

Shira Miwa, M.D.
Professor
Department of Internal Medicine
Institute of Medical Science
University of Tokyo
Tokyo, Japan

Kenneth W. Olsen, Ph.D.
Associate Professor
Department of Chemistry
Loyola University
Chicago, Illinois

Rose G. Schneider, Ph.D.
Research Professor
Department of Pediatrics
Department of Human Biological
Chemistry and Genetics
University of Texas Medical Branch
Galveston, Texas

Walter A. Schroeder, Ph.D.
Senior Research Associate
Division of Chemistry and Chemical
Engineering
California Institute of Technology
Pasadena, California

Stephen B. Shohet, M.D.
Professor of Medicine and Laboratory
Medicine
University of California
San Francisco, California

William P. Winter, Ph.D.
Senior Biochemist
Center for Sickle Cell Disease
Associate Professor of Genetics and
Human Genetics
Associate Professor of Medicine
Howard University
Washington, D.C.

Ruth N. Wrightstone, D.P.A.
Assistant Research Scientist
Sickle Cell Center
Medical College of Georgia
Augusta, Georgia

TABLE OF CONTENTS

RED CELL PRODUCTION/DESTRUCTION

Solomon Adler and Walter Fried

EARLY EVENTS IN ERYTHROPOIESIS (HEMATOPOIETIC STEM CELLS AND THE HEMATOPOIETIC MICROENVIRONMENT)

Introduction To Hemopoietic Precursor Cells

Red blood cell production, or erythropoiesis, occurs as a result of a complex set of cellular events regulated by multiple but still incompletely understood mechanisms. Erythropoiesis may be divided, albeit somewhat artifically, into two phases. The first involves the progression from the primitive, pluripotent, hemopoietic stem cell to the erythroid colony-forming unit (CFU-E). This phase has as its primary objective the maintenance of an intact population of erythroid precursors capable of replenishing the CFU-E population as these cells mature into end stage erythrocytes. Noteworthy is the fact that none of the cells in this sequence is morphologically identifiable as a red cell precursor. The second phase is initiated by the interactions of the CFU-E with erythropoietin which results in CFU-E proliferation and also triggers the CFU-E to mature into the earliest morphologically identifiable red blood cell precursor, the proerythroblast, which in turn continues to mature into the circulating end stage cell, the erythrocyte.

The hierarchial structure of the hemopoietic precursor cell population is depicted in Figure 1. The most primitive hemopoietic precursor cell is one capable of selfrenewal throughout the lifespan of the organism and of commitment to any one of the myeloid (erythrocytic, granulocytic-monocytic, and megakaryocytic) or lymphoid cell lines, i.e., it possesses the characteristic of totipotency.[1] An immediate progeny of this cell is the pluripotent myeloid stem cell. Traditionally, primitive myeloid stem cells have been assayed by their capacity to form colonies on the spleens of irradiated mice[2] and because of this capacity they are referred to as CFU-S, an acronym which stands for colony forming unit-spleen. It is now fairly clear that the CFU-S population is a heterogenous one since, in addition to multipotent stem cells,[3] it also is comprised of cells with more restricted differentiation potentials,[4] i.e., progenitor cells lacking the capacity to give rise to progeny of one or more of the hemopoietic cell lines; some CFU-S may even be unipotent.[4,5] However, in keeping with tradition and the overwhelming bulk of literature, we will use the term CFU-S to refer to the primitive population of hemopoietic stem cells capable of giving rise to trilineal hemopoiesis. As this section deals with erythropoiesis, the discussion of CFU-S will be limited to their role as progenitors of red blood cells.

Control of Pluripotent Stem Cell Differentiation

Restriction of CFU-S pluripotency occurs early in stem cell development though not necessarily abruptly; the latter is suggested by the existence of various bipotent precursors[6-9] in addition to tripotent and unipotent stem cells. Along with restriction of pluripotency, and temporally closely related to it, hemopoietic precursor cells also become restricted in their proliferative capacity;[10-12] thus, the most primitive stem cells have the capacity to undergo many more divisions than do the more committed ones; nevertheless, during steady state conditions a larger percentage of committed precursors than CFU-S are in cell cycle.

What regulates commitment of pluripotent stem cells to a specific cell line? This is one of the major questions which still confronts experimental hematologists. At least three major theories have been forwarded to answer this question: (1) the hemopoietic inductive microenvironmental theory, (2) the humoral factor theory, and (3) the theory of intrinsically mediated differentition.

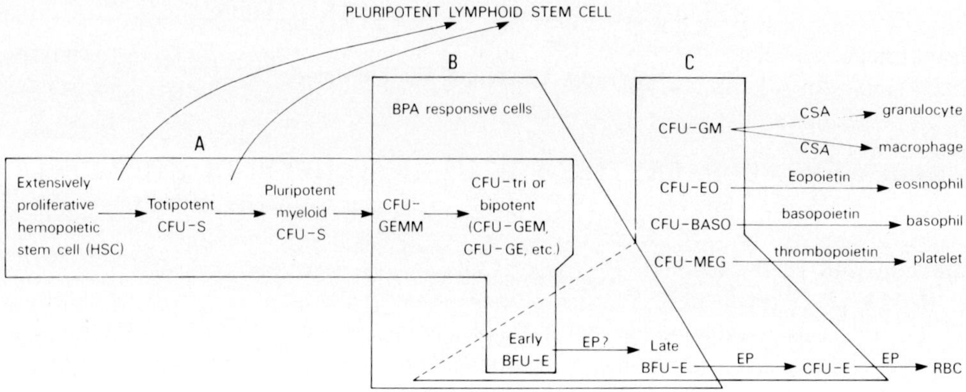

FIGURE 1. Hemopoietic stem cell hierarchy.

The first of these suggests that local, more or less, fixed factors are present in the environment of hemopoietic tissue which induce CFU-S differentiation. Accordingly, the type of differentiation which any individual CFU-S undergoes is determined by cells in its immediate microenvironment. Evidence for this theory has been derived primarily from in vivo studies of hemopoiesis in marrow and spleens of mice.[13,22] However, with information gained from in vitro culture systems, this theory has become somewhat less attractive than it once was,[12,23] although some environmental control may well play a role in hemopoiesis.

Goldwasser and colleagues have suggested that pluripotent stem cells are responsive to various hemopoietic growth factors (poietins) such as erythropoietin and granulopoietin.*[24-28] They postulate that pluripotent hemopoietic stem cells possess specific receptors for the various humoral factors. It may be that densities of the receptors for these factors vary with the phase of the cell cycle or perhaps with other yet undefined phenomena. Hence, it may be that the absolute or relative concentration of a given hemopoietic factor on the cell surface at a critical time regulates commitment. This theory predicts that, when present simultaneously, different hemopoietic growth factors should create competition for commitment. Although several investigators have reported that excess erythropoietin results in decreased myelopoiesis, and an increased concentration of granulopoietin reduces the response to erythropoietin both in vivo and in vitro,[23-32] there is substantial doubt as to whether these studies definitively support the humoral factor theory of differentiation.

Other investigators believe that commitment of pluripotent cells is not regulated by external factors, but rather by mechanisms intrinsic to the stem cell itself. Early proponents of this theory were Till and colleagues[33] and major support for this theory may be adduced from recent in vitro experiments of Eaves et al.[12] and Johnson.[34] The former investigators postulate that commitment is a stochiastic process, i.e., a random event. Johnson has performed elegant investigations in which he separately subcultured the progeny of single multipotent hemopoietic stem cells after one or two cell divisions and studied the resulting colonies. He found that multipotent stem cells in vitro undergo commitment to the erythropoietic cell line even in the absence of erythropoietin. Moreover, regardless of the culture milieu, he could not identify mixed colonies (colonies formed from stem cells with at least bipotent capacity) devoid of erythropoietic elements. These findings suggest that multipotent stem cells possess as a universal part of their program the capacity to generate erythroid-committed cells. Johnson has postulated that as pluripotent hemopoietic precursors undergo differentiation they lose their capacity to form the entire gamut of myeloid elements in a stepwise fashion

* Granulopoietin is a glycoprotein, or group of glycoproteins, which are required for the maintenance of and proliferation of granulocyte/macrophage precursors in vitro. It has no effect on erythroid precursor growth. These substances are also called CSFs or CSAs (colony-stimulating factors or activities).

but always retain their erythropoietic capacity.[34] This theory implies that at least a subset of pluripotent myeloid stem cells differentiate in a nonstochiastic fashion. In addition to these studies of Johnson, which suggest that erythropoietin plays little role in CFU-S differentiation, there are no conclusive studies which suggest that this hormone plays a role in control of CFU-S proliferation.

Although, as discussed above, a number of in vitro studies mitigate against exogenous control of commitment, it must be recognized that in vitro systems are artificial and there may well be factors in vivo which modulate the commitment process; for instance, in studies using irradiated mice, Chervenick and Boggs[35] have demonstrated that following depletion of the pluripotent stem cell compartment in mice, differentiation of committed RBC precursors is not detectable until the CFU-S population has become repleted to about 10% of normal and, as cited previously, there are studies which suggest that the in vivo microenvironment plays a role in hemopoietic regulation.[13-21]

Immature Committed Erythropoietic Precursor Cells

Situated in the linear sequence of erythropoiesis (Figure 1) between the CFU-S and the late-committed erythroid precursors (CFU-E) is a series of closely related yet heterogenous[8,36] in vitro clonable stem cells belonging to the CFU-GEMM/BFU-E complex. The most primitive of these is a multipotent cell which is closely related to the CFU-S[36-39] and is capable of generating macroscopic colonies which contain up to 10,000 cells,[12] trilineal hematopoiesis, and even CFU-S;[38] this cell is known as a CFU-GEMM (colony forming unit granulocytes/erythrocytes/monocytes/megakaryocytes),[39-41] CFU-mix,[42] or mixed-erythroid precursor.[8] Although only a small percentage of the CFU-GEMM/BFU-E complex is tripotent, 50% or more seem to be bipotent[8,43] and these may be labeled by the cells they generate (e.g., CFU-E meg, CFU-EG, etc.). Bipotent colonies apparently always contain erythroid elements, i.e., mixed granulocyte megakaryocytes or macrophage megakaryocyte colonies are rare or nonexistent.[8]

The primitive unipotent erythroid precursors, burst-forming unit erythroids (BFU-E) are so-called because in culture they give rise to very large erythroid colonies or to multiple small colonies in close proximity to each other. Early (immature) BFU-E give rise to large bursts after prolonged culture periods (about 10 days in mice and 10 to 14 days in man), whereas "late" BFU-E give rise to smaller bursts (50 to 200 erythroblasts) at earlier times (e.g., 3 days in mice or 8 to 10 days in man).[44]

The primitive erythroid-mixed erythroid precursors (i.e., CFU-GEMM through BFU-E) do not require erythropoietin for survival or proliferation in culture.[8,12,45-47] The primary stimulatory factors for these precursors are known as "burst-promoting factors" or activities* (BPAs or BFAs); they are glycoproteins generally derived from tissue containing activated lymphocytes.[45,48] The very early proliferation (up to five divisions) of these cells can also be fostered by a purified glycoprotein with essentially only granulopoietic qualities (CSA). BPA has the capacity not only to maintain and stimulate proliferation of BFU-E, but, when present in large amounts, also to enhance hemoglobin synthesis by the mature cells in the colonies; BPA in large amounts can also augment proliferation of precursors committed to produce fetal hemoglobin.[49] Although proliferation of the early BFU-E does not require erythropoietin, and erythropoietin is not required for differentiation of the immature BFU-E into "late" BFU-E, "late" BFU-E proliferation does seem to be influenced by erythropoietin.[12] In addition, at least one study suggests that cycling of early BFU-E may be transiently influenced by hypertransfusion (low erythropoietin levels). Thus, the possibility exists that even immature BFU-E respond to erythropoietin even though they do not require this hormone to flourish.[12]

* Recently, the lymphokine, IL-3, has been found to have full burst-promoting activity and the capacity to support growth of multilineage colonies in murine systems.[188]

In addition to the humoral stimulators of erythropoiesis, there is evidence that cellular interactions play a role in the control of erythropoiesis. Although not universally accepted, evidence has been adduced for a role of thymocytes in this process.[50-55] Sawada and Adler[50] have shown that murine BFU-E growth is modestly enhanced by adding thymocytes to the cultures, and Nathan and co-workers[51,52] have suggested that T-lymphocytes (thymic-processed lymphocytes) enhance the growth of human BFU-E derived from blood, but not marrow.[51,52] In the presence of T-lymphocytes and high doses of erythropoietin, a larger proportion of primitive BFU-E gives rise to fetal hemoglobin-containing colonies than would otherwise be expected.[52] Recently, Sharkis et al. have reported that thymocytes, when cocultured with normal mouse marrow cells, stimulate or suppress CFU-E and BFU-E proliferation depending on the ratio of the lymphoid elements to marrow cells.[53] Erythropoiesis in diffusion chambers implanted into mice may also be enhanced by coculture with T lymphocytes.[54] Other investigators suggest that it is the monocyte[56-60] rather than the T lymphocyte[59,60] which influences erythropoiesis. It has been suggested by Rinehart et al.[56] and Gordon[58] that monocytes at low concentrations stimulate BFU-E proliferation, but if concentration of monocytes approaches or exceed 15%, BFU-E proliferation is suppressed. The possibility exists that there are T lymphocyte/monocyte interactions which in turn act as the stimuli for erythropoiesis either by direct cell-cell interaction or via short-range-acting humoral stimulators.[59] Additional evidence for cell-cell interaction in hemopoieses emanates from studies using a system for maintaining hemopoiesis in vitro for long periods of time.[61] In this system, hemopoiesis is supported in a liquid phase in flasks in which an adherent layer of bone marrow-derived cells has been permitted to form. The adherent layer provides a milieu conducive to pluripotent and committed stem cell survival and proliferation. Although mature granulocytic elements regularly form in this culture system, mature erythropoietic elements (CFU-E and beyond) do not develop even in the presence of added erythropoietin.[62-64] However, if the flasks are gently rocked during the culture period, full erythropoietic differentiation does take place.[63] It has been postulated that the rocking action affects or facilitates certain cell-cell interactions required for terminal red cell differentiation.

The immediate progeny of the most mature BFU-E are the CFU-E, cells which give rise to terminally differentiated red cell colonies. CFU-E derived colonies of human origin develop after 6 to 7 days in culture and rarely contain more than 128 cells. The CFU-E are considered the major target for erythropoietin, which induces them both to proliferate and to mature after one or two divisions into morphologically identifiable red cell precursors, the proerythroblasts, which then go on to mature into erythrocytes. The proliferation of CFU-E may also be facilitated[50,53] or suppressed[53] by normal thymocytes and possibly also by macrophages.

LATE EVENTS IN ERYTHROPOIESIS

Erythropoietin

Day by day adjustments in the rate of erythropoiesis as well as the response to major changes in tissue oxygen requirements are determined by the interaction of the glycoprotein, erythropoietin, with putative receptors on the CFU-E. Accordingly, increases in the number of CFU-E, or the amount of erythropoietin, or both will result in an increase in the rate of erythropoiesis; the opposite would obtain for decreases in these constituents.

The existence of a humoral mediator of erythropoiesis was postulated by Carnot and DeFlandre in 1906.[65] However, convincing experimental evidence to support this hypothesis was first reported by Reissmann et al.,[66] who showed that exposure of one of a pair of parabiotic rats to a hypoxic environment resulted in an increase in the rate of erythropoiesis in both rats even though only one rat had a reduced pO_2 in the arterial blood. In 1954, Erslev[67] showed that plasma of anemic rabbits contains a substance that increases the rate of erythropoiesis in normal rabbits. Since that time, considerable progress has been made in the purification and characterization of this substance, erythropoietin,[68-71] and in understanding its role in the regulation of erythropoiesis in health and in disease.[72-78]

Erythropoietin is a glycoprotein with a molecular weight of about 39,000, 20% of which consists of carbohydrates.[71] It has now been concentrated from human urine (and purified to apparent homogeneity). The amino acid sequences of the erythropoietin molecule have been determined. However, its carbohydrate components have not yet been totally characterized. Half of the carbohydrate content of biologically active erythropoietin is sialic acid.[71] However, a small amount of asialated erythropoietin is normally presented in the bloodstream. Although asialated erythropoietin is biologically active in vitro, it is not active in vivo because of its very rapid plasma clearance rate.[79]

Site of Erythropoietin Production

In adult mammals, the major site of erythropoietin production is the kidney. Accordingly, removal of the kidneys (with the inevitable development of uremia) results in a rise in the plasma erythropoietin titer during exposure to hypoxia which is only a fraction of that observed either in rats with intact kidneys, or in rats made comparably uremic by ureteral ligation.[80,84] Furthermore, in rats exposed to hypoxia, extracts of renal tissue but not of other organs, contain high erythropoietin titers[85-87] even before the plasma erythropoietin titer becomes detectably elevated.[85,87] The specific cell in the kidney responsible for erythropoietin production is not yet known, although several lines of evidence point to a cell within the cortex.[88,89] A few early studies suggest that the kidneys do not produce biologically active erythropoietin, but rather that they produce either a proerythropoietin which must be converted by a plasmaborne substance to biologically active erythropoietin[90] or an enzyme that acts on a plasma protein to generate the biologically active hormone.[91] More recently published observations, however, tend to favor the concept that biologically active erythropoietin is produced in the kidney.[86-88,92]

Extrarenal sites produce a small amount of erythropoietin in anephric adult rats,[84,93] rabbits,[94] and humans.[95-97] It is estimated that the amounts of erythropoietin produced by these sites is approximately 10% of that produced by the kidneys in normal adult rats.[84] On the other hand, the majority of the erythropoietin produced in fetal and neonatal mammals is of extrarenal origin;[98-100] the kidneys become active sites of erythropoietin production only after the 4th week of life.[98-100] The major site of extrarenal erythropoietin production is the liver[99-103] and circumstantial evidence favors the Kupffer cells[104,105] rather than the hepatocytes as the responsible cells, but this requires more direct confirmation.

Assays for Erythropoietin

The following three general types of assays for erythropoietin are available: (1) in vivo bioassays, (2) in vitro bioassays, and (3) immunoassays. The first assays to be developed, and still the most reliable for measuring biologically active erythropoietin, are the in vivo bioassays.[106-110] These are based on the phenomenon that animals with decreased levels of endogenous erythropoietin are exceptionally sensitive to injection of erythropoietin. Thus, mice are made plethoric either by transfusion of RBCs or by chronic exposure to hypoxia. Some 3 or 4 days later the substance to be assayed is injected and 2 days later ^{59}Fe is injected. The percentage of injected ^{59}Fe which has been incorporated into the circulating RBCs after 2 or 3 days is then determined and compared to a dose-response curve based on the assay of several doses of a standardized erythropoietin preparation. In most laboratories this assay is linear between amounts of 0.03 and 1.0 unit when plotted on semilog paper.[111] The disadavantages of this assay are (1) its costliness in terms of mice and technician time, (2) its slowness (at least 1 week is required to complete an assay), and (3) its insensitivity (titers of less than 0.03 μ/mℓ are not detectable, whereas normal circulating titers in humans are estimated to be 0.009 to 0.018 μ/mℓ).

In vitro bioassays are based on incorporation of radioactive iron or carbon into newly produced hemoglobin, either in short-term suspension cultures or in erythroid colonies grown in a semisolid medium.[112-115] In vitro bioassays are more sensitive than the in vivo assays as they can even detect subnormal erythropoietin titers. Moreover, they are less time-consuming and less expensive than in vivo tests. The drawbacks of the in vitro bioassays include (1) a lack of specifity (a variety of factors in plasma, urine, and in tissue extracts nonspecifically inhibit or promote the growth of hemopoietic cells in culture) and (2) difficulty with standardization (batches of commercially available fetal calf serum or bovine serum albumin, ingredients of the in vitro system, vary widely in their capacity to support erythropoiesis).

A variety of immunoassays for erythropoietin have been developed. These are based on immunodiffusion,[116] hemagglutination-inhibition,[117] or radioimmunoassay[118,119] techniques. Radioimmunoassays are based on the competitive binding of erythropoietin in the unknown sample and of radioiodinated erythropoietin with antierythropoietin antibodies (produced in rabbits against human urinary erythropoietin). Of the currently available immunoassays, only the radioimmunoassays using purified radioiodinated erythropoietin are reliable. Others, which depend for specificity on antibodies produced against impure erythropoietin preparations or on radioiodinated impure erythropoietin preparations, correlate poorly with results obtained using in vivo bioassays. Unfortunately, purified erythropoietin is in extremely small supply and only available in a few laboratories. The radioimmunoassay is the most sensitive, reproducible, and practical assay currently available; however, because it detects an antigenic site on erythropoietin which is not necessarily essential to the biologic action of the molecule, it will be necessary to obtain more comparative data on the results of bioassays and radioimmunoassays in a variety of pathologic states before the results of the radioimmunoassays can be accurately interpreted.

Regulation of Erythropoietin Production

Renal erythropoietin production is regulated principally by renal oxygen requirements relative to oxygen supply. Conditions which decrease the supply of oxygen to the kidneys and those which increase the oxygen requirements of the kidneys increase erythropoietin production and vice versa.[120] Erythropoietin production is sensitive to small and very transient stimuli,[121] and such changes alter the production of red blood cells which survive over 100 days. Consequently, if the sole regulator of erythropoietin production were the ratio of oxygen demand to oxygen supply, one would expect the size of the red cell mass to oscillate widely about a mean value rather than being quite constant as it actually is. Hence, other factors must modulate the rate of erythropoietin production and/or the response of erythroid precursors to erythropoietin. Several such factors have been identified and are listed in Table 1; other important regulatory mechanisms remain to be discovered. An example of our ignorance of some important mechanisms which regulate erythropoiesis is our inability to explain the phenomenon of the compensated hemolytic state. This is a condition most commonly seen in patients with hereditary spherocytosis in which sustained supranormal red cell production compensates for persistent shortening of the red cell lifespan, resulting in a constant normal, or near normal, hematocrit. Because the oxygen supply to the kidneys of these patients is normal, there is no obvious stimulus for the increased rate of red cell production. It is not even clear whether the increase in erythropoiesis is due to an increase in the level of erythropoietin or to an increased response to erythropoietin; the latter explanation is favored by the observations of Erslev et al.[141]

Of the factors listed in Table 1 that cause either an increase or a decrease in erythropoietin production by mechanisms other than through changes in the oxygen demand to supply ratio, we will discuss two, sex hormones and protein deprivation, in greater detail.

The observation that males have higher red blood cell counts than females was first made

Table 1
FACTORS THAT INFLUENCE THE ERYTHROPOIETIN TITER IN PLASMA AND THE RESPONSIVENESS TO ERYTHROPOIETIN

Condition	Effect	Postulated mechanism of action	Ref.
Factors that Influence Erythropoietin Titer in Plasma			
O_2 demand:O_2 supply	↑	Relative renal hypoxia	120
Hormones			
Calorigenic	↑	Relative renal hypoxia	122
Androgenic anabolic	↑	Renal hypertrophy	123
Prolactin	↑	?	124
Aldosterone	↑	Increase renal O_2 requirements	125
Estrogens	↓	?	126
Prostaglandins	↑	Redistribute intrarenal blood flow	127
Protein calorie malnutrition	↓	↓ In nutrients to kidney or in O_2 utilization	120 128
Protein deprivation	↓	↓ Availability of amino acids for erythropoietin synthesis	129 130
Vasoconstriction	↑	↓ In renal blood flow	131
Decrease in responsiveness to erythropoietin (due to decrease in erythropoietin responsive cells)		Either due to ↓ "consumption" of erythropoietin or to negative feedback by erythropoietin responsive cells on erythropoietin production	132
Metabolic poisons			
Dinitrophenol	↑	Increases O_2 requirements by	120
	↑	impairment of oxidative	
Cobaltous chloride		phosphorylation	133
Factors that Influence the Responsiveness to Erythropoietin			
Nutritional deficiency			
Protein-calorie	↓ (only when deficiency is severe	↓ Hemopoietic stem cells	120
Iron	↓		
Folic acid or B_{12}	↓	Defective erythrocyte maturation	
Spermine	↓	May be effective in vitro only	132
Uremic plasma	↓	May be effective in vitro only	135,136
5β H androstanes	↑	Increase proliferation of CFU-E	137
Androgenic-anabolic steroids	↑ ?	Increases sensitivity to erythropoietin	138
Parathormone	↓	Changes hematopoietic microenvironment in marrow	139
cAMP	↑	?	140
Estrogens	↓	Damages hematopoietic microenvironment in marrow	

in chickens more than 50 years ago[142] and, subsequently, this was observed to pertain to various species of mammals, including humans.[143-145] Castration of males reduces their red blood cell counts to levels observed in females[144] and injection of androgenic steroids into castrated males restores their red blood cell counts to the normal male level.[144] Similarly, injection of androgenic steroids into females raises their red blood cell counts to supranormal levels.[143,145] Injection of pharmacologic doses of either androgenic steroids or androstanes

Table 2
CONDITIONS KNOWN TO AFFECT BOTH RENAL AND EXTRARENAL ERYTHROPOIETIN PRODUCTION

Condition	Effect on renal erythropoietin		Extrarenal erythropoietin	Ref.
Hypoxic hypoxia	↑		↑	84
Anemic hypoxia	↑		↑	84
Cobaltous chloride	↑		↑	159
Protein deprivation	↓		0	160
Protein calorie malnutrition	↓		↓ ?	128
Liver regeneration	0		↑	161,162
Androgenic-anabolic steroids	↑	>	±[a]	159
Angiotensin II	↑	<	↑	163
Renin	↑	<	↑	164,165

[a] May cause a slight increase in extrarenal erythropoietin.

with predominantly anabolic properties into females increases plasma erythropoietin levels to supranormal levels and increases the rate of erythropoiesis[146-152] (male rats are insensitive to the effects of androgens on erythropoiesis).[152] The effects of androgens on hematopoiesis may not be only via their effects on erythropoietin production since androgens in vitro have been shown to increase the sensitivity of erythroid precursors to erythropoietin[137,138,153] and to trigger the cycling of resting multipotential stem cells.[138,154]

Both protein deprivation[129,130,155-157] and protein-calorie deprivation reduce erythropoietin production and erythropoiesis in experimental animals and humans.[120,128] The mechanism by which protein deprivation reduces erythropoietin production is thought to be related directly to an acute decrease in the availability of amino acids essential for erythropoietin synthesis.[130,160]

Extrarenal erythropoietin production, as renal erythropoietin production, is responsive to the oxygen supply to demand ratio.[84] There are, however, several conditions which affect renal and extrarenal erythropoietin production differently (Table 2). Of particular interest is the observation that extrarenal erythropoietin production is substantially increased during the recovery period following either partial hepatectomy[161,162] or injection of the hepatotoxic compound CCl_4.[166] Extrarenal erythropoietin production also increases in response to injection of renin[164,165] or to infusion of angiotensin.[163] Indeed, it has been hypothesized that angiotensin II is involved in the physiologic regulation of extrarenal erythropoietin production and perhaps also in the regulation of renal erythropoietin production.[163]

Mechanism by Which Erythropoietin Acts on its Target Cell

Erythropoietin does not have to enter its target cell[167] and, therefore, is believed to act on membrane-borne receptors as is the case for most polypeptide hormones.[167] The erythropoietin receptor has, however, not yet been identified or purified. The earliest change observed in cultured murine bone marrow cells after exposure to erythropoietin is the appearance of a protein in the cytosol which, in addition to isolated nuclei, causes the production of a large, short-lived species of RNA.[168-170] This RNA species is postulated to be a transcriptional unit, which is involved in the translation of a specific essential protein; the identity of this protein remains unknown. Exposure to erythropoietin irreversibly triggers erythroid progenitors (CFU-E) into mature erythrocytes[171] and causes CFU-E to multiply.[172] Erythropoietin may also promote early release of reticulocytes from the marrow;[173] however, it is not clear whether this effect is caused by erythropoietin or by other substances in the plasma of hypoxic rats.

Maturation of the CFU-E progresses to the proerythroblast, basophilic, polychromatic, orthochromatic erythroblast, and finally, after extrusion of the nucleus, to the reticulocyte. During this maturation process, the cell acquires specific membrane receptors such as those for transferrin and the enzymes essential for the synthesis and maintenance of hemoglobin as a functional molecule. Also, during their maturation process, erythroid precursors continue to divide; they undergo an average of four divisions before the orthochromatic erythroblast stage is reached, at which time cell division ceases. It has been postulated that cell division is terminated as the mean cell homoglobin concentration reaches a critical level.[174,175] Shortly after this time, the nucleus is extruded and the polyribosomes gradually disperse. A correlate of this postulate is that cells that produce hemoglobin slowly will undergo at least one extra division and will be microcytic, whereas those that undergo mitosis slowly will undergo one fewer division during the process of maturation and will be macrocytic. Although this explanation of the pathogenesis of microcytic and macrocytic anemias is not based on firm scientific evidence, it is generally correct that conditions which impair DNA synthesis result in macrocytic anemias, whereas those that impair hemoglobin synthesis result in microcytic anemias.

Hemoglobin synthesis is dependent on an adequate supply of iron to erythroid progenitors.[176] Iron is transported to the maturing erythroid precursors by transferrin. Saturated transferrin has a high affinity for receptor sites on the erythroid cell. At the cell membrane, iron is either transferred to ferritin, which is internalized by a process of pinocytosis to form a ferritin-containing vacuole, or internalized by pinocytosis of the iron transferrin complex.[177-181] From these ferritin or transferrin-containing vacuoles, iron is delivered to the mitochondria where the heme molecule is synthesized. Globin chains are in turn produced on the ribosomes. Four globin chains, each containing one heme molecule, then combine in the cytosol to form hemoglobin. Regulation of heme and globin synthesis is linked through a variety of reactions to prevent production of an excess of either molecule.[182-184]

The orthochromatic erythroblast, after extrusion of its nucleus, is called a reticulocyte. Because reticulocytes retain transferrin receptors, mitochondria, and polyribosomes, they normally can continue to synthesize hemoglobin for approximately 72 hr. During the first 48 hr of its lifespan, the reticulocyte resides in the bone marrow; thereafter it changes physically in a manner which permits it to migrate through the sinusoidal endothelium into the circulation, at which time its polyribosomes disperse, its transferrin receptors become nonfunctional, and its mitochondria are removed. In addition, the cell becomes smaller because of loss of membrane lipids.[185] This cell, which is no longer capable of synthesizing hemoglobin, is called an erythrocyte. When the erythropoietin titer is very high, as occurs during severe anemia or hypoxia, the reticulocyte may enter the circulation after only 1 day, and circulate for 2 days before maturing into an erythrocyte.[173] These cells are called ''shift'' reticulocytes. When the stimulus for erythropoiesis is exceptionally strong, the maturation process is accelerated and the final cell division of the polychromatic erythroblast is skipped. The resulting cell, called ''stress reticulocytes'', are exceptionally macrocytic and have a shortened lifespan.[175]

Mature erythrocytes are capable of sustaining energy-utilizing reactions which are essential for the maintenance of their cell membranes and hemoglobin. Mature erythrocytes generate energy-rich phosphates (ATP) by the metabolism of glucose, utilizing the Embden Myerhoff pathway. The pentose-phosphate shunt enzymes, on the other hand, result in the production of NADPH which functions as a hydrogen donor in reactions that reduce glutathionine; the latter is essential for the prevention of the oxidation of hemoglobin to a nonfunctional form. Since several of the enzymes in the Embden-Myerhoff and pentose phosphate shunt pathways decay as the erythrocyte ages, the cell has a finite lifespan (approximately 120 days) after which it is removed from the circulation by splenic or hepatic macrophages. The iron is recycled for use in erythropoiesis and the remainder of the heme molecule is converted to bilirubin, which is glycosylated in the liver and excreted in the bile.

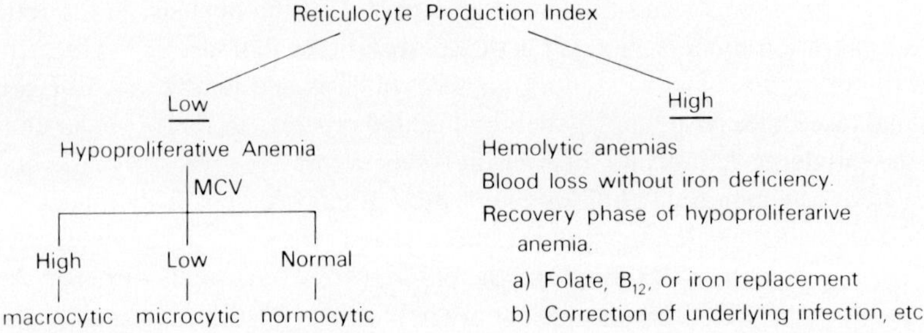

FIGURE 2. Reticulocyte production index.

The normal steady state, therefore, is a compensated hemolytic state in which approximately 0.8% of the circulating red blood cells are destroyed and produced each day.

ABNORMAL STAGES OF ERYTHROPOIESIS

Anemia

Anemia occurs when either the rate of erythropoiesis declines to a level which results in fewer erythrocytes being delivered to the circulating blood than are normally destroyed or the rate of red blood cell destruction or loss increases to a level that exceeds the capacity of the eythron to generate new red blood cells. The former is known as a hypoproliferative or nonregenerative anemia, and the latter as a hemolytic anemia or the anemia of blood loss. When the rate of red blood cell destruction exceeds normal but does not exceed the capacity of the erythron to accelerate its rate of erythropoiesis, a compensated hemolytic state, without anemia, results. It should be noted that, with an adequate supply of iron and cofactors, a well-functioning erythron can accelerate to ten times the normal rate of erythropoiesis or more.

The rate of red blood cell production is most easily estimated by the corrected reticulocyte count.[187]

$$\text{Corrected reticulocyte count} = \%\ \text{reticulocytes} \times \frac{45}{\text{hematocrit}} \left(\begin{matrix}\text{normal}\\ \text{range}\end{matrix} = 0.5\text{—}1.5\right)$$

The corrected reticulocyte count may be modified as the hematocrit declines to account for the early release of reticulocytes which results in the presence of circulating reticulocytes whch circulate in the bloodstream for more than 1 day; the value obtained by this correction is the reticulocyte production index (RPI). Figure 2 shows a scheme for using the patient's RPI to discriminate between hypoproliferative and hemolytic anemias.

Hypoproliferative Anemia

Hypoproliferative anemias are always associated with an inappropriately low reticulocyte production index. It is important to remember that a normally functioning erythron is capable of increasing the rate of erythropoiesis several-fold in response to anemia. Accordingly, a normal rate of erythropoiesis (RPI of 1) in association with severe anemia inidcates a defective erythropoietic response. The amount of erythropoietic activity in the marrow usually varies proportionally with the RPI in hypoproliferative states. On the other hand, under certain circumstances there may be evidence of substantial erythropoietic activity in the marrow without release of a proportional number of red cells into the peripheral blood as reflected in the reticulocyte index. This is a characteristic of ineffective erythropoiesis which results from red blood cells that are so abnormal that they are destroyed shortly after being produced

Table 3
CLASSIFICATION OF HYPOPROLIFERATIVE ANEMIAS

- A. Normocytic
  - 1. CFU-S defects
    - a. CFU-S dysfunction or depletion — aplastic anemia
    - b. CFU-S mutation — leukemias — some refractory anemias
  - 2. Defect in microenvironment — myelophthisic
    - a. Metastatic disease
    - b. Neoplasms of lymphoid or plasma cells
    - c. Myelofibrosis — osteosclerosis, etc.
      - 1. Primary
      - 2. Secondary
  - 3. Diseases of BFU-E or CFU-E
    - a. Red cell aplasia
  - 4. Diseases affecting erythropoietin production
    - 1. Renal disease
    - b. Endocrine disease
    - c. Protein deprivation
    - d. Anemia of chronic illness
  - 5. Others
    - a. Mild disorders of hemoglobin synthesis
    - b. Combined disorders of hemoglobin synthesis and DNA synthesis
- B. Microcytic (disorders of hemoglobin synthesis)
  - 1. Heme synthesis
    - a. Iron deficiency
    - b. Chronic disease
    - c. Sideroblastic anemia
  - 2. Globin synthesis
    - a. Thalassemia
- C. Macrocytic anemias (disorders of DNA synthesis)
  - 1. B12 deficiency
  - 2. Folate deficiency
  - 3. Others (MCV — rarely over 115 μm)
    - a. Liver disease
    - b. Miscellaneous primary marrow dyscrasias
    - c. Secondary to chemotherapeutic agents
    - d. Rare inherited disorders of purine metabolism
    - e. Reticulocytosis

before they can be delivered into the circulating blood. Ineffective erythropoiesis occurs commonly in conditions caused by abnormalities in erythrocyte maturation such as megaloblastic anemias and severe iron deficiency. Also, ineffective erythropoiesis is characteristically present in dyserythropoietic conditions such as sideroblastic and nonsideroblastic refractory anemias and in agnogenic myeloid metaplasia. Hypoproliferative anemias may result from defects in any stage of erythropoiesis. The MCV of the erythrocytes often provides a clue to the nature of the disorder in erythropoiesis. Table 3 lists the various types of anemia associated with normocytic, microcytic, or macrocytic indices.

Disorders of Shortened Red Cell Survival

Red cells that are not able to survive normally in the peripheral blood may be more fragile or less able to handle stresses which occur during circulation. Such is the case in the inherited red cell membrane disorders (hereditary spherocytosis, hereditary stomatocytosis, hereditary ovalocytosis, etc.), red cell enzyme disturbances, and hemoglobinopathies (Table 4). In the above disorders, erythropoiesis increases in response to the anemia but abnormal red cells are produced.

In contrast to the aforementioned disorders, decreased red cell survival may occur in

Table 4
ANEMIAS CAUSED PRIMARILY BY SHORTENED RED BLOOD CELL SURVIVAL

- I. Intrinsic (corpuscular) red cell abnormalities
  - A. Red cell membrane-related disorders
    - 1. Disorders of red cell shape, e.g., spherocytosis, elliptocytosis, xeroxytosis, stomatocytosis, pyropoikilocytosis
    - 2. Inherited disorders of membrane lipids: acanthocytosis (abetalipoprotinemia), lecithin cholesterol acyltransferase (LCAT) deficiency
    - 3. Paroxysmal nocturnal hemoglobinuria
  - 3. Inherited enzyme deficiencies
    - 1. Glycolytic enzyme deficiencies: pyruvate kinase, glucose-phosphate isomerase, hexokinase, phosphofructokinase, aldolase, 2,3-diphosphoglyceromutase, phosphoglycerate kinase, triose isomerase, glyceraldehyde-3-phosphate dehydrogenase
    - 2. Pentose phosphate pathway and glutathione-related enzyme deficiences; glucose-6-phosphate dehydrogenase, glutathione reductase, glutathione peroxidase, glutathione synthetase, glutamyl-cysteine synthesase, 6 phosphogluconic dehydrogenase
    - 3. Miscellaneous enzyme deficiencies: adenylate kinase, pyrimidine 5′ nucleotides
  - C. Defective globin structure and synthesis
    - 1. Hemoglobinopathies
      - a. Homozygous disorders, e.g., SS, CC, DD, EE
      - b. Double heterozygous disorders, e.g. SC, SD, S-thalassemia etc.
      - c. Thalassemias: β-chain, e.g., β, $\gamma\beta$, $\gamma\beta$, Lepore: α-chain, e.g., α, Hgb Constant Spring Koza Dora, Seal Rock, Q, H, etc.
      - d. Unstable hemoglobins, e.g., Hb Zurich
- II. Extrinsic (extracorpuscular) abnormalities
  - A. Immunologically mediated hemolysis
    - 1. Transfusion reactions
    - 2. Hemolytic disease of the newborn
    - 3. Autoimmune
      - a. Warm-antibody related
        - i. Idiopathic
        - ii. Secondary to other diseases, e.g., infections, malignancies, autoimmune and immunodeficiency disorders
      - b. Cold-antibody related
        - i. Idiopathic
        - ii. Secondary
    - 4. Drug related
  - B. Mechanical and physical factors
    - 1. External mechanical trauma, e.g., March hemoglobinuria, hemolysis related to Conga drumming or Karate practice, etc.
    - 2. Internal mechanical trauma, e.g., severely damaged heart valves, prosthetic heart valves, ? malignancies
    - 3. Fibrin-mesh-mediated red cell fragmentation, e.g., disseminated intravascular coagulation, thrombotic thrombocytopenic purpura, hemolytic-uremic syndrome, renal-vascular hypertension, vasculitides, ? malignancies
    - 4. Immunologically related, e.g., organ graft rejection, immune complex disease related
    - 5. Miscellaneous, e.g., thermal injury, radiation injury
  - C. Infection-related (nonimmune)
    - 1. Bacterial, e.g., bartonellosis, cholera, typhoid fever, tuberculosis, other infections, e.g., *Escherichia coli,* recurrentis
    - 2. Protozoal, e.g., malaria, toxoplasmosis, leishmaniasis, babesiosis
    - 3. Viral
  - D. Chemical drug and toxin mediated
    - 1. Oxidants, e.g., antimalarials, sulfones, sulfonamides, nitrofurans, aspirin, acetanilid, aminopyrene, naphthalene, vitamin K
    - 2. Other substances, e.g., arsine, copper (? hemolytic anemia related to Wilson's Disease), water etc.
    - 3. Toxins
        - i. Venoms, e.g., snake, wasp
        - ii. Toxins, e.g., clostridial phospholipase C
    - 4. Others, e.g., hypophosphatemia

Table 4 (continued)
ANEMIAS CAUSED PRIMARILY BY SHORTENED RED BLOOD CELL SURVIVAL

E. Plasma lipid related disorders, not inherited
  1. Spur cell anemia secondary to liver disease
  2. ? Zieve's Syndrome related to alcoholism

patients with normally formed red blood cells as a result of extracellular factors such as immunological mechanisms (autoimmune or drug induced, etc.), abnormal serum lipoproteins, mechanical destruction (disseminated intravascular coagulation, thrombotic thrombocytopenic purpura, hemolytic uremic syndrome, March hemoglobinuria, etc.), or toxins and venoms, and hypersplenism.

Historically, whether a given disorder of shortened red cell lifespan was due to an abnormality of the red cell or due to an extracellular cause was determined by measuring the survival of transfused red cells. Hence, if shortened survival is due to an intrinsic cell abnormality, such red cells have curtailed lifespans even when transfused into the unaffected person whose red cells have normal lifespans. In cases of extrinsic hemolytic anemias, the reverse is the case (see Table 4). Today, there are more sophisticated methods of separating intrinsic or corpuscular red cell defects from extracorpuscular defects and these methods also circumvent the ethical problems on nontherapeutic transfusions. Such methods include the antiglobulin tests for immune-mediated problems, enzyme analyses for the enzymopathies, etc.

Erythrocytosis

When the rate of erythropoiesis increases without a decrease in the red blood cell survival, the red cell mass increases, resulting in erythrocytosis. Erythrocytosis should be suspected in persons with a hematocrit that exceeds the 95% confidence limits for normal in any given geographical location. It should be noted that the normal levels in cities situated at high altitudes may be higher than those at sea level.

High hematocrits or a high blood hemoglobin concentration may result from either an increase in the red cell mass or a decrease in the plasma volume. An increased hematocrit caused by decreased plasma volume has been called "spurious polycythemia" and may be distinguished from true erythrocytosis by direct measurement of the red cell mass and plasma volume.

Erythrocytosis may occur as a result of an increase in the plasma erythropoietin titer or a change in the responsiveness of CFU-E to erythropoietin. The former is referred to as secondary erythrocytosis and the latter primary erythrocytosis. Table 5 shows a scheme for classification of the secondary and primary erythrocytoses.

Table 5
CLASSIFICATION OF ERYTHROCYTOSIS

- A. Spurious polycythemia
  - 1. Decreased plasma volume — normal red cell mass by ^{51}Cr method
- B. Secondary erythrocytosis (high plasma erythropoietin level)
  - 1. Generalized hypoxia
    - a. Residence at high altitude
    - b. Chronic lung disease with saturation of hemoglobin < 92%
    - c. Chronic congestive failure
    - d. Cigarette or cigar smoking
      - 1. Normal pO_2
      - 2. Normal O_2 saturation by indirect method
      - 3. Decreased O_2 saturation by direct measurement of amount of oxyhemoglobin
      - 4. Increased carboxyhemoglobin
      - 5. Occasionally normal red cell mass with increased plasma volume
    - e. Abnormal hemoglobin with high O_2 affinity
  - 2. Intermittent hypoxia
    - a. Modified Pickwickian syndrome
      - 1. Decreased O_2 only while reclining
    - b. Congestive heart failure
      - 1. Decreased O_2 only while exercising
  - 3. Localized hypoxia
    - a. Renal blood flow
      - 1. Renovascular hypertension
      - 2. Essential hypertension (rare)
      - 3. Renal cysts (unilateral or polycystic)
      - 4. Miscellaneous renal diseases (rare)
        - a. Hydronephrosis
        - b. Glomerulonephritis
        - c. Pyelonephritis
  - 4. Neoplastic
    - a. Hypernephroma
    - b. Hepatoma
    - c. Cerebellar tumors
    - d. Leiomyoma of uterus
    - e. Pheochromocytoma
    - f. Androgen-producing tumor
  - 5. Others
    - a. Androgen therapy
    - b. Cushing's disease
    - c. Bartter's syndrome
  - 6. Congenital causes
    - a. Abnormal hemoglobin with high O_2 affinity (see above)
    - b. Familial polycythemia secondary to high Ep with normal pO_2 saturation and O_2 affinity
- C. Primary polycythemia (increase in responsiveness to erythropoietin)
  - 1. Polycythemia rubra vera[a]
  - 2. Familial erythrocytosis with increased numbers of CFU-E but normal or low erythropoietin levels

[a] This is a primary change in the multipotential hematopoietic stem cell. Whether they are unresponsive to erythropoietin or intensely responsive to small doses remains to be definitively determined.

REFERENCES

1. **Boggs, D. R., Bogg, S. S., Saxe, D. F., Gress, L. A., and Canfield, D. R.,** Hematopoietic stem cells with high proliferative potential. Assay of their concentration in marrow by the frequency and duration of cure of W/W^v mice, *J. Clin. Invest.*, 70, 242, 1982.
2. **Till, J. E. and McCulloch, E. A.,** A direct measurement of the radiation sensitivity of normal mouse bone marrow cells, *Radiat. Res.*, 14, 213, 1961.
3. **McCulloch, E. A. and Till, J. E.,** Regulatory mechanisms acting on hemopoietic stem cells, *Am. J. Pathol.*, 65, 601, 1971.
4. **Magli, M. C., Iscove, N. N., and Odartchenko, N.,** Transient nature of early haematopoietic spleen colonies, *Nature (London)*, 295, 527, 1982.
5. **Gregory, C. J., McCulloch, E. A., and Till, J. E.,** The cellular basis for the defect in haemopoiesis in flexed-tailed mice. III. Restriction of the defect to erythropoietic progenitors capable of transient colony formation *in vivo*, *Br. J. Haematol.*, 30, 401, 1975.
6. **Dexter, T. M., Allen, T. D., and Scott, D.,** Isolation and characterization of a bipotential haematopoietic cell line, *Nature (London)*, 277, 471, 1979.
7. **Nakahata, T. and Ogawa, M.,** Clinical origin of murine hemopoietic colonies with apparent restriction to granulocyte-macrophage-megakaryocyte (GMM) differentiation, *J. Cell. Physiol.*, 111, 239, 1982.
8. **Johnson, G. R.,** Clonal erythroid differentiation from multipotential hemopoietic stem cell in vitro, in *Hemoglobins in Development and Differentiation*, Stomatoyannopoulos, G. and Niehaus, A. W., Eds., Alan R. Liss, New York, 1981, 23.
9. **McLeod, D. L., Shreeve, M. M., and Axelrad, A. A.,** Chromosome marker evidence for the bipotentiality of BFU-E, *Blood*, 56, 318, 1980.
10. **Gregory, C. J. and Kenkelman, R. M.,** Relationships between early hemopoietic progenitor cells determined by correlation analysis of their numbers in individual spleen colonies, in *Experimental Hematology Today*, Baum, S. J. and Ledney, G. D., Eds., Springer-Verlag, Basel, 1977, 93.
11. **Eaves, C. J., Humphries, R. K., and Eaves, A. C.,** In vitro characterization of erythroid precursor cells and the erythropoietic differentiation process, in *Cellular and Molecular Hemoglobin Switching*, Stamatoyannopoulos, G. and Nienhuis, A. W., Eds., Grune & Stratton, New York, 1979, 251.
12. **Eaves, C. J., Humphries, R. K., and Eaves, A. C.,** Self-renewal of hemopoietic stem cells: evidence for stochastic regulatory processes, in *Hemoglobins in Development and Differentiation*, Stamatoyannopoulos, G. and Nienhuis, A. W., Eds., Alan R. Liss, New York, 1981, 35.
13. **Curry, J. L. and Trentin, J. J.,** Hemopoietic spleen colony studies. I. Growth and differentiation, *Dev. Biol.*, 15, 395, 1967.
14. **Trentin, J. J., Curry, J. L., Wolf, N., and Cheng, V.,** Factors controlling stem cell differentiation and proliferation: the hemopoietic inductive microenvironment (HIM), in *Proliferation and Spread of Neoplastic Cells*, A collection of papers, M.D. Anderson Hospital and Tumor Institute, Williams & Wilkins, Baltimore, 1968, 713.
15. **Trentin, J. J.,** Influence of hematopoietic organ stroma (hemopoietic inductive microenvironments) on stem cell differentiation, in *Regulation of Hematopoiesis*, Gordon, A., Ed., Appleton-Century-Crofts, New York, 1970, 161.
16. **Trentin, J. J.,** Determination of bone marrow stem cell differentiation by stromal hemopoietic inductive microenvironments (HIM), *Am. J. Pathol.*, 65, 621, 1971.
17. **Trentin, J. J., Rauchwerger, J. M., and Gallagher, M. T.,** Regulation of hemopoietic inductive microenvironments, in *Control of Proliferation in Animals Cells*, Clarkson, B. and Baserga, R., Eds., Cold Spring Harbor Publ., Cold Spring Harbor, N.Y., 1974, 927.
18. **Wolf, N. S.,** Dissecting the hematopoietic microenvironment. I. Stem cell lodgment and commitment, and the proliferation and differentiation of erythropoietic descendants in the Sl/Sl^d mouse, *Cell Tissue Kinet.*, 7, 89, 1974.
19. **Jaley, J. E., Tjio, J. H., Smith, W. W., and Brecher, G.,** Hematopoietic differentiation properties of murine spleen implanted in the omenta of irradiated and nonirradiated hosts, *Exp. Hematol.*, 3, 187, 1975.
20. **LaPushin, R. W. and Trentin, J. J.,** Identification of distinctive stromal elements in erythroid and neutrophil granuloid spleen colonies: light and electron microscopic study, *Exp. Hematol.*, 5, 505, 1977.
21. **Wolf, N. S.,** Dissecting the hematopoietic microenvironment. III. Evidence for a positive short range stimulus for cellular proliferation, *Cell Tissue Kinet.*, 11, 335, 1978.
22. **Nordegraaf, E. M., Erkens-Versluis, M., and Ploemacher, R. E.,** Studies of the haematopoietic microenvironments. IV. Changes in glycosaminoglycan content of murine spleen in relation to haematological parameters following induction of anaemia or polycythaemia, *Haematologica*, 66, 409, 1981.
23. **Humphries, R. K., Eaves, A. C., and Eaves, C. J.,** Expression of stem cell behavior during macroscopic burst formation in vitro, in *Experimental Hematology Today*, Baum, S. J., Ledney, G. D., and van Bekkum, D. W., Eds., S. Karger, Basel, 1980, 39.

24. **Goldwasser, E.,** Erythropoietin and the differentiation of red blood cells, *Fed. Proc.*, 34, 2285, 1975.
25. **Van Zant, G. and Goldwasser, E.,** The effects of erythropoietin in vitro on spleen colony forming cells, *J. Cell. Physiol.*, 90, 241, 1977.
26. **Van Zant, G. and Goldwasser, E.,** The simultaneous effects of erythropoietin and colony stimulating factor on bone marrow cells, *Science*, 198, 733, 1977.
27. **Van Zant, G. and Goldwasser, E.,** Suppression of erythroid differentiation by colony-stimulating factor, in *Experimental Hematology Today*, Baum, S. J. and Ledney, G. D., Eds., Springer-Verlag, New York, 1979, 63.
28. **Van Zant, G. and Goldwasser, E.,** Competition between erythropoietin and colony-stimulating factor for target cells in mouse marrow, *Blood*, 53, 946, 1979.
29. **Bradley, T. R., Robinson, W., and Metcalf, D.,** Colony production in vitro by normal polycythaemic and anaemic bone marrow, *Nature (London)*, 214, 511, 1967.
30. **Harris, P. F., Harris, R. S., and Kugler, J. H.,** Studies of the leukocyte compartment of guinea pig bone marrow after acute haemorrhage and severe hypoxia. Evidence for a common stem cell, *Br. J. Haematol.*, 12, 219, 1966.
31. **Hellman, S. and Grate, H. E.,** Haemopietic stem cells: evidence for competing proliferative demands, *Nature (London)*, 216, 65, 1967.
32. **Morley, A. D., Howard, D., Bennett, B., and Stohlman, F.,** Studies on the regulation of granulopoiesis. II. Relationship to other differentiation pathways, *Br. J. Haematol.*, 19, 523, 1970.
33. **Till, J. E., McCulloch, E. A., and Siminovitch, L.,** A stochastic model of stem cell proliferation, based on the growth of spleen colony-forming cells, *Proc. Natl. Acad. Sci. U.S.A.*, 51, 29, 1974.
34. **Johnson, G. R.,** Is erythropoiesis an obligatory step in the commitment of multipotential hematopoietic stem cells?, in *Experimental Hematology Today*, Baum, S. J., Ledney, G. D., and Kahn, A., Eds., S., Karger, Basel, 1981, 13.
35. **Chervenick, P. A. and Boggs, D. R.,** Patterns of proliferation and differentiation of hematopoietic stem cells after compartment depletion, *Blood*, 37, 568, 1971.
36. **Gregory, C. J. and Eaves, A. C.,** Three stages of erythropoietin progenitor cell differentiation distinguished by a number of physical and biologic properties, *Blood*, 51, 527, 1978.
37. **Humphries, R. K., Eaves, A. C., and Eaves, C. J.,** Characterization of a primitive erythropoietic progenitor found in mouse marrow before and after several weeks in culture, *Blood*, 53, 746, 1979.
38. **Humphries, R. K., Jacky, P. B., Dill, F. J., Eaves, A. C., and Eaves, C. J.,** CFU-S in individual erythroid colonies derived in vitro from adult mouse marrow, *Nature (London)*, 279, 718, 1979.
39. **Fauser, A. A. and Messner, H. A.,** Identification of megakaryocytes, macrophages and eosinophils in colonies of human bone marrow containing neutrophilic granulocytes and erythroblasts, *Blood*, 53, 1023, 1979.
40. **Neumann, H. A., Lohn, G. W., and Fauser, A. A.,** Radiation sensitivity of pluripotent hemopoietic progenitors (CFU_{GEMM}) derived from human bone marrow, *Exp. Hematol.*, 9, 742, 1981.
41. **Ash, R. C., Detrick, R. A., and Zanjani, E. D.,** Studies of human pluripotential hemopoietic stem cells (CFU-GEMM) in vitro, *Blood*, 58, 309, 1981.
42. **Johnson, G. R. and Metcalf, D.,** Multipotential hemopoietic colony formation in agar cultures stimulated by spleen-conditioned medium, in *Experimental Hematology Today*, Baum, S. J. and Ledney, G. D., Eds., Springer-Verlag, Basel, 1980, 29.
43. **Hara, H. and Noguchi, K.,** Clonal nature of pluripotential hemopoietic precursors in vitro (CFU-mix), *Stem Cells*, 1, 53, 1981.
44. **Eaves, C. J., Humphries, R. K., Krystal, G., and Eaves, A. C.,** Erythropoietin action: models, data, and speculation, *Hemoglobins in Development and Differentiation*, Stamatoyannopoulos, G. and Nienhuis, A. W., Eds., Alan R. Liss, New York, 1981, 63.
45. **Wagemaker, G.,** Cellular and soluble factors influencing the differentiation of primitive erythroid progenitor cells (BFU-e) in vitro, in *In Vitro Aspects of Erythropoiesis*, Murphy, M. J., Jr., Ed., Springer-Verlag, Basel, 1978, 44.
46. **Wagemaker, G.,** Hemopoietic factors required for differentiation of multipotential cells in vitro, in *Hemoglobins in Development and Differentiation*, Stomatoyannopoulos, G. and Neinhuis, A. W., Eds., Alan R. Liss, New York, 1981.
47. **Wagemaker, G.,** Early erythropoietin-independent stage of in vitro erythropoiesis: relevance to stem cell differentiation, in *Experimental Hematology Today*, Baum, S. J. and Ledney, G. D., Eds., S. Karger, Basel, 1980, 47.
48. **Lusis, A. J. and Golde, D. W.,** Human T-lymphocyte-derived erythroid-potentiating activity: partial purification and characterization, in *Hemoglobins in Development and Differentiation*, Stomatoyannopoulos, G. and Nienhuis, A. W., Eds., Alan R. Liss, New York, 1981, 93.
49. **Ogawa, M., Porter, P. N., Terasawa, T., and Brockbank, K. G. M.,** Effects of burst-promoting activity (BPA) on hemoglobin biosynthesis in culture, *Exp. Hematol.*, 8, 90, 1980.

50. **Sawada, U. and Adler, S. S.,** In vitro interactions between thymocytes and hemopoietic precursor cells, *Blut,* 42, 1, 1981.
51. **Nathan, D. G., Chess, L., Hillman, D. G., Clarke, B., Breard, J., Merler, E., and Housman, D. E.,** Human erythroid burst-forming unit: T-cell requirement for proliferation in vitro, *J. Exp. Med.,* 147, 324, 1978.
52. **Nathan, D. G. and Lipton, J. M.,** The role of T lymphocytes in erythropoiesis, in *Hemoglobins in Development and Differentiation,* Stomatoyannopoulos, G. and Nienhuis, A. W., Eds., Alan, R. Liss, New York, 1981, 111.
53. **Sharkis, S. J., Spivak, J. L., Ahmed, A., Misiti, J., Stuart, R. K., Wiktor-Jedrzejczak, W., Sell, K. W., and Sensenbrenner, L. L.,** Regulation of hematopoiesis: helper and suppressor influences of the thymus, *Blood,* 55, 524, 1980.
54. **Niskanen, E., Ashman, R., and Cline, M. J.,** Enhancement of murine erythroid colony formation in the presence of activated T lymphocytes, *J. Lab. Clin. Med.,* 95, 934, 1980.
55. **Goodman, J. W. and Shinpock, S. G.,** Interaction between T lymphocytes and hemopoietic stem cells. A critical min-review, in *Biology of Bone Marrow Transplantation,* ICN-UCLA Symposia on Molecular and Cellular Biology, Vol. 17, Academic Press, New York, 1980.
56. **Rinehart, J. J., Zanjani, E. D., Nomdedeu, B., Gormus, B. J., and Kaplan, M. E.,** Cell-cell interactions in erythropoiesis. Role of human monocytes, *J. Clin. Invest.,* 62, 979, 1978.
57. **Grilli, G. and Carbonell, F.,** Effect of blood derived monocytes on the promotion of in vitro erythropoietic colony growth in human bone marrow cultures, *Scand. J. Haematol.,* 29, 345, 1982.
58. **Gordon, L. I., Branda, R. F., Zanjani, E. D., and Jacob, H. S.,** Regulation of erythroid colony (EC) formation by bone marrow (BM) macrophages, *Clin. Res.,* 26, 667A, 1978.
59. **Zuckerman, K. S.,** Human erythroid burst-forming units. Growth in vitro is dependent on monocytes, but not lymphocytes, *J. Clin. Invest.,* 67, 702, 1980.
60. **Nomdedeu, B., Gormus, B. J., Banisadre, M., Rinhart, J. J., Kaplan, M. E., and Zanjani, E. D.,** Human peripheral blood erythroid burst forming unit (BFU-E): evidence against T-lymphocyte requirement for proliferation in vitro, *Exp. Hematol.,* 8, 845, 1980.
61. **Moore, M. A. S., Sheridan, A. P. C., Allen, T. D., and Dexter, T. M.,** Prolonged hematopoiesis in a primate bone marrow culture system: characteristics of stem cell production and hematopoietic microenvironment, *Blood,* 54, 775, 1979.
62. **Dexter, T. M.,** Differentiating cell lines and factors controlling proliferation, in *Hemoglobins in Development and Differentiation,* Stamatoyannopoulos, G. and Nienhuis, A. W., Eds., Alan R. Liss, New York, 1981, 15.
63. **Dexter, T. M.,** Stromal cell associated haemopoiesis, *J. Cell Physiol. Suppl.,* 1, 87, 1982.
64. **Eliason, J. F., Testa, N. G., and Dexter, T. M.,** Erythropoietin stimulated erythropoiesis in long-term bone marrow culture, *Nature (London),* 281, 382, 1979.
65. **Carnot, P. and Deflandre, C.,** Sur l'activite hemopoietique des differents organes au cours de la regeneration due sang, *C.R. Acad. Sci.,* 143, 432, 1906.
66. **Reissman, K. R.,** Studies on the mechanism of erythropoietic stimulation in parabiotic rats during hypoxia, *Blood,* 5, 372, 1950.
67. **Erslev, A. M.,** Humoral regulation of red cell production, *Blood,* 5, 372, 1950.
68. **Gordon, A. S., Piliero, S. J., Kleinberg, W., and Freedman, H. H.,** A plasma extract with erythropoietic activity, *Proc. Soc. Exp. Biol. Med.,* 86, 255, 1954.
69. **Borsook, H. A., Graybiel, A., Keighley, G., and Windsor, E.,** Polycythemic response in normal adult rats to a nonprotein plasma extract from anemic rabbits, *Blood,* 9, 734, 1954.
70. **Slaunwhite, W. R., Mirand, E. A., and Prentice, T. C.,** Probable polypeptide nature of erythropoietin, *Proc. Soc. Exp. Biol. Med.,* 96, 61, 1957.
71. **Miyake, T., Kung, C. K. H., and Goldwasser, E.,** Purification of human erythropoietin, *J. Biol. Chem.,* 252, 5558, 1977.
72. **Koeffler, H. P. and Goldwasser, E.,** Erythropoietin radioimmunoassay in evaluating patients with polycythemia, *Ann. Int. Med.,* 94, 44, 1981.
73. **Rege, A. B., Brookins, J., and Fisher, J. W.,** A radioimmunoassay for erythropoietin in serum levels in normal human subjects and patients with hemopoietic disorders, *J. Lab. Clin. Med.,* 10, 829, 1982.
74. **Krystal, G., Eaves, A. C., and Eaves, C. J.,** Determination of normal human serum erythropoietin levels, using mouse bone marrow, *J. Lab. Clin. Med.,* 97, 158, 1981.
75. **Caro, J., Brown, S., Miller, O., Murphy, T., and Erslev, A. J.,** Erythropoietin levels in uremic nephric and anephric patients, *J. Lab. Clin. Med.,* 93, 449, 1979.
76. **Gurney, C. W., Goldwasser, E., and Pan, E.,** Studies on erythropoiesis. IV. Erythropoietin in human plasma, *J. Lab. Clin. Med.,* 50, 534, 1957.
77. **Cotes, P. M., Brozovic, B., Mansell, M., and Sauson, D. M.,** Radioimmunoassay of erythropoietin in human serum: validation and application of an assay system, *Exp. Hematol.,* 8, 292, 1980.

78. **Garcia, J. F., Ebbe, S. N., Hollander, L., Cutting, H. O., Miller, M. E., and Cronkit, E. P.,** Radioimmunoassay of erythropoietin circulating levels in normal and polycythemic human being, *J. Lab. Clin. Med.*, 99, 624, 1982.
79. **Goldwasser, E., Kung, C. K. H., and Eliason, J. F.,** On the mechanism of erythropoietin-induced-differentiation. VIII. The role of sialic acid in erythropoietin action, *J. Biol. Chem.*, 249, 4202, 1974.
80. **Jacobson, L. O., Goldwasser, E., Fried, W., and Plzak, L. F.,** Studies on erythropoiesis. VII. The role of the kidneys in the production of erythropoietin, *Trans. Assoc. Am. Physicians*, 70, 305, 1957.
81. **Naets, J. P.,** Erythropoiesis in nephrectomized dogs, *Nature (London)*, 181, 1134, 1958.
82. **Kuratowska, Z., Lewartowski, B., and Michalak, E.,** Studies on the production of erythropoietin by isolated perfused organs, *Blood*, 18, 527, 1961.
83. **Fisher, J. W. and Birdwell, B. J.,** The production of erythropoietic factor by the *in situ* perfused kidney, *Acta Haematol.*, 26, 224, 1961.
84. **Fried, W., Kilbridge, T., Krantz, S., MacDonald, T. Y., and Lange, R. D.,** Studies on extrarenal erythropoietin, *J. Lab. Clin. Med.*, 73, 244, 1969.
85. **Fried, W., Barone-Varelas, J., and Berman, M.,** Detection of high erythropoietin titers in renal extracts of hypoxic rats, *J. Lab. Clin. Med.*, 97, 82, 1981.
86. **Erslev, A. J., Caro, J., Birgegard, G., Silver, R., and Miller, O.,** The biogenesis of erythropoietin, *Exp. Hematol.*, 8, 1, 1980.
87. **Jelkmann, W.,** Temporal pattern of erythropoietin titers in kidney tissue during hypoxic hypoxia, *Pflugers Arch.*, 393, 88, 1982.
88. **Fried, W., Barone-Varelas, J., and Barone, T.,** The influence of age and sex on erythropoietin titers in the plasma and tissue homogenates of hypoxic rats, *Exp. Hematol.*, 10, 472, 1982.
89. **Busuttil, R. W., Roh, B. L., and Fisher, J. W.,** The cytological localization of erythropoietin in the human kidney using the fluorescent antibody technique, *Proc. Soc. Exp. Biol. Med.*, 137, 327, 1971.
90. **Peschle, C. and Condorelli, M.,** Biogenesis of erythropoietin: evidence for pro-erythropoietin in a sub-cellular fraction of kidney, *Science*, 190, 910, 1975.
91. **Gordon, A. S., Cooper, G. W., and Zanjani, E. D.,** The kidney and erythropoiesis, *Semin. Hematol.*, 4, 337, 1967.
92. **Erslev, A. J.,** In vitro production of erythropoietin by kidneys perfused with a serum-free solution, *Blood*, 44, 77, 1974.
93. **Mirand, E. A. and Prentice, T. C.,** Presence of plasma erythropoietin in hypoxic rats with or without kidneys and/or spleen, *Proc. Soc. Exp. Biol. Med.*, 96, 49, 1957.
94. **Erslev, A. J.,** Erythropoietin function in uremic rabbits, *Arch. Int. Med.*, 101, 407, 1958.
95. **Nathan, D. G., Schupak, E., and Stohlman, F.,** Erythropoiesis in anephric man, *Clin. Invest.*, 43, 2158, 1964.
96. **Naets, J. P. and Wittek, M.,** Presence of erythropoietin in the plasma of one anephric patient, *Blood*, 31, 249, 1968.
97. **Mirand, E. A., Murphy, G. P., Steever, R. A., Weber, H. W., and Retief, F. P.,** Extrarenal production of erythropoietin in man, *Acta Haematol.*, 39, 359, 1968.
98. **Carmena, A. O., Howard, D., and Stohlman, F.,** Regulation of erythropoietin. XXII. Production in the newborn animal, *Blood*, 32, 376, 1968.
99. **Zanjani, E. D., Foster, J., Burlington, H., Mann, L. J., and Wasserman, R. L.,** Liver as a primary site of erythropoietin formation in the fetus, *J. Lab. Clin. Med.*, 89, 640, 1977.
100. **Zanjani, E. D., Ascensao, J. L., McGlave, P. B., and Ash, R. C.,** Studies on the liver to kidney switch of erythropoietin production, *J. Clin. Invest.*, 67, 1183, 1981.
101. **Schooley, J. C. and Mahlmann, L. J.,** Extrarenal erythropoietin production by the liver in the weaning rat, *Proc. Soc. Exp. Biol. Med.*, 143, 310, 1973.
102. **Fried, W.,** The liver as a source of extrarenal erythropoietin, *Blood*, 40, 671, 1972.
103. **Gruber, D. F., Zucali, J. R., and Mirand, E. A.,** Identification of erythropoietin producing cells in fetal mouse liver cultures, *Exp. Hematol.*, 5, 392, 1977.
104. **Dornfest, B. S., Naughton, B. A., Johnson, R., and Gordon, A. S.,** Hepatic production of erythropoietin in a phenylhydrazine-induced compensated hemolytic state in the rat, *J. Lab. Clin. Med.*, 102, 274, 1983.
105. **Rich, I. N., Heit, W., and Kubanek, B.,** Extrarenal erythropoietin production by macrophages, *Blood*, 60, 1007, 1982.
106. **Jacobson, L. O., Goldwasser, E., Plzak, L., and Fried, W.,** Studies on erythropoiesis. IV. Reticulocyte response of hypophysectomized and polycythemic rodents to erythropoietin, *Proc. Soc. Exp. Biol. Med.*, 94, 243, 1957.
107. **DeGowin, R. L., Hofstra, D., and Gurney, C. W.,** The mouse with hypoxia-induced erythemia, an erythropoietin bioassay animal, *J. Lab. Clin. Med.*, 60, 846, 1962.
108. **Fogh, J. A.,** A sensitive erythropoietic assay on mice exposed to CO-hypoxia, *Scand. J. Clin. Lab. Invest.*, 18, 33, 1966.

109. **Weintraub, A. H., Gordon, A. S., and Camiscoli, J. F.**, Use of the hypoxia induced polycythemic mouse in the assay and standardization of erythropoietin, *J. Lab. Clin. Med.*, 67, 743, 1966.
110. **Lange, R. D., Simmons, M. L., and Dibelius, N. R.**, Polycythemic mice produced by hypoxia in silicone rubber membrane enclosures: a new technique, *Proc. Soc. Exp. Biol. Med.*, 122, 761, 1966.
111. **Keighley, G., Lowy, P. H., Borsook, H., Goldwasser, E., Gordon, A. S., Prentice, T. C., Rambach, W. A., Stohlman, F., Jr., and Van Dyke, D. S.**, A cooperative assay of a sample with erythropoietic stimulating activity, *Blood*, 16, 1424, 1960.
112. **Dunn, C. F. R., Jarvis, J. H., and Greenman, J. M.**, A quantitative bioassay for erythropoietin using mouse fetal liver cells, *Exp. Hematol.*, 3, 65, 1975.
113. **Goldwasser, E., Eliason, J. F., Sikkema. D.**, An assay for erythropoietin in-vitro at the milliunit level, *Endocrinology*, 97, 315, 1975.
114. **Krantz, S. B., Gallien-Lartique, O., and Goldwasser, E.**, The effect of erythropoietin on heme synthesis by marrow cells in-vitro, *J. Biol. Chem.*, 238, 4085, 1963.
115. **Adamson, J. W., Dale, D. C., and Elin, R. J.**, Hematopoiesis in the gray collie dog, *J. Clin. Invest.*, 54, 965, 1974.
116. **Goudsmit, R., Kruger, P. G., Dagneaux, L. C., and Krijnen, H. W.**, Oorspronkelijke stukken. Een immunochemische bepaling van erythropoietine, *Folia Med. Neerl.*, 10, 39, 1967.
117. **Lange, R. D., Jordon, T. A., Ichiki, A. T., and Chernoff, A. E.**, Hemagglutination-inhibition assay for erythropoietin, in *Regulation of Erythropoiesis*, Gordon, A. S., Condorelli, M., and Peschle, C., Eds., Il Ponte, Milano, 1971, 107.
118. **Sherwood, J. B. and Goldwasser, E.**, A radioimmunoassay for erythropoietin, *Blood*, 54, 885, 1979.
119. **Garcia, J. F., Sherwood, J. B., and Goldwasser, E.**, Radioimmunoassay of erythropoietin, *Blood Cells*, 5, 405, 1979.
120. **Fried, W., Plzak, L. E., Jacobsen, L. O., and Goldwasser, E.**, Studies on erythropoiesis. III. Factors controlling erythropoietin production, *Proc. Soc. Exp. Biol. Med.*, 94, 237, 1957.
121. **Gurney, C. W., Munt, P., Brazell, I., and Hofstra, D.**, Quantitation of the eythropoietic stimulus produced by hypoxia in the plethoric mouse, *Acta Haematol.*, 33, 246, 1965.
122. **Evans, E. S., Rosenerg, L. L., and Simpson, M. E.**, Erythropoietic response to calorigenic hormones, *Endocrinology*, 68, 517, 1961.
123. **Fried, W. and Gurney, C. W.**, Erythropoietic effect of plasma from mice receiving testosterone, *Nature (London)*, 206, 1160, 1965.
124. **Jepson, J. H. and Lowenstein L.**, Effect of prolactin on erythropoiesis in the mouse, *Blood*, 24, 726, 1964.
125. **Zivny, J., Neuwirt, J., and Borova, J.**, The effect of aldosterone on erythropoietin production and erythropoiesis, *J. Lab. Clin. Med.*, 80, 217, 1972.
126. **Mirand, E. A., and Gordon, A. S.**, Mechanism of estrogen action in erythropoiesis, *Endocrinology*, 29, 817, 1941.
127. **Schooley, J. C. and Mahlmann, L. J.**, Stimulation of erythropoiesis in plethoric mice by prostaglandins and their inhibition by antierythropoietin, *Proc. Soc. Exp. Biol. Med.*, 137, 1289, 1971.
128. **Caro, J., Silver, R., Erslev, A. J., Miller, O. P., and Biregegard, G.**, Erythropoietin production in fasted rats. Effects of thyroid hormones and glucose supplementation, *J. Lab. Clin. Med.*, 98, 860, 1981.
129. **Reissmann, K. R.**, Protein metabolism and erythropoiesis. II. Erythropoietin formation and erythroid responsiveness in protein deprived rats, *Blood*, 23, 146, 1964.
130. **Anagnostou, A., Schade, S., Ashkinaz, M., Barone, J., and Fried, W.**, Effect of protein deprivation on erythropoiesis, *Blood*, 50, 1093, 1977.
131. **Fisher, J. W., Samuels, A. I., and Langston, J.**, Effects of angiotensin, norepinephrine and renal artery constriction on erythropoietin production, *Ann. N.Y. Acad. Sci.*, 149, 308, 1968.
132. **Fried, W., Gregory, S. A., and Knospe, W. H.**, Regulation of plasma erythropoietin levels in mice with impaired responsiveness to erythropoietin, *J. Lab. Clin. Med.*, 87, 449, 1971.
133. **Jacobson, L. O., Goldwasser, E., Fried, W., and Plzak, L.**, The role of the kidney in erythropoiesis, *Nature (London)*, 179, 633, 1957.
134. **Radtke, H. W., Rege, A. B., LaMarche, M. B., Bartos, D., Bartos, F., Campbell, R. A., and Fisher, J. W.**, Identification of spermine as an inhibitor of erythropoiesis in patients with chronic renal failure, *J. Clin. Invest.*, 67, 1623, 1981.
135. **Moriyama, Y., Rege, A., and Fisher, J. W.**, Studies on an inhibitor of erythropoiesis. II. Inhibitory effect of serum from uremic rabbits on heme synthesis in rabbit bone marrow cultures, *Proc. Soc. Exp. Biol. Med.*, 148, 94, 1975.
136. **Wallner, S. F., Vautrin, R., Kornick, J. E., and Ward, H. P.**, The effect of serum from patients with chronic renal failure on erythroid colony growth in-vitro, *J. Lab. Clin. Med.*, 92, 370, 1978.
137. **Necheles, T. F., and Rai, U. S.**, Studies on the control of hemoglobin synthesis: the in vitro effect of 5 beta H-steroid metabolites on hematopoiesis in vitro, *Blood*, 34, 380, 1969.

138. **Jepson, J. H., Leonard, R. A., Gorshein, D., Gardner, F. H., and Besa, E.,** Review of the induction of cycling of ESC by androgens and their 5 H-metabolites, *Biomedicine,* 20, 262, 1974.
139. **Meytes, D., Bogin, E., Andrew, M., Dukes, P., and Massry, S. G.,** Effect of parathyroid hormone on erythropoiesis, *J. Clin. Invest.,* 67, 1263, 1981.
140. **Schooley, J. C. and Mahlmann, L. J.,** Stimulation of erythropoiesis in the plethoric mouse by cyclic AMP and its inhibition by antierythropoietin, *Proc. Soc. Exp. Biol. Med.,* 137, 1289, 1971.
141. **Erslev, A. J.,** Compensated anemia caused by overwork hyperplasia of the stem cell pool, *XII Congr. Int. Soc. Hematol.,* Buenos Aires, 1968, 152.
142. **Blacher, L. J.,** On the influence of sexual hormones upon the number of erythrocytes and percentage quantity of hemoglobin in fowl, *Biol. Gen.,* 2, 435, 1926.
143. **Steinglass, P., Gordon, A. S., and Charipper, H. A.,** Effect of castration and sex hormones on blood of the rat, *Proc. Soc. Exp. Biol. Med.,* 48, 169, 1941.
144. **McCullogh, E. P. and Jones, R.,** Effect of androgens on the blood count of men, *J. Clin. Endocrinol. Metab.,* 2, 243, 1942.
145. **Kennedy, B. J. and Gilbertsen, A. S.,** Increased erythropoiesis induced by androgenic hormone therapy, *N. Engl. J. Med.,* 256, 719, 1957.
146. **Eschbach, J. W. and Adamson, J. W.,** Improvement in the anemia of chronic renal failure with fluoxymesterone, *Ann. Intern. Med.,* 72, 913, 1973.
147. **Rishpon Myerstein, N., Kilbridge, T., Simone, J., and Fried, W.,** The effect of testosterone on erythropoietin levels in anemic patients, *Blood,* 31, 453, 1968.
148. **Alexanian, R.,** Erythropoietin excretion in man following androgens, *Blood,* 28, 1007, 1966.
149. **Gordon, A. S., Mirand, E. A., Wemig, J., Katz, R., and Zanjani, E. D.,** Androgen action on erythropoiesis, *Ann. N.Y. Acad. Sci.,* 149, 318, 1968.
150. **DeGowin, R. L., Lavender, A. R., Forland, M., Charleston, D., and Gottschalk, A.,** Erythropoiesis and erythropoietin in patients with chronic renal failure treated with hemodialysis and testosterone, *Ann. Intern. Med.,* 72, 913, 1970.
151. **Fried, W., Jonasson, O., Lang, G., and Schwartz, F.,** The hematologic effect of androgens in uremic patients, *Ann. Intern. Med.,* 79, 823, 1978.
152. **Fried, W. and Gurney, C. W.,** The erythropoietic stimulating effects of androgens, *Ann. N.Y. Acad. Sci.,* 149, 356, 1968.
153. **Mizoguchi, H. and Levere, R. D.,** Enhancement of heme and globin synthesis in cultured human marrow by certain 5 H steroid metabolites, *J. Exp. Med.,* 134, 1501, 1971.
154. **Byron, J. W.,** Comparison of the action of H^3-thymidine and hydroxyurea on testosterone-treated hemopoietic stem cells, *Blood,* 40, 198, 1972.
155. **Whipple, G. H.,** *The Dynamic Equilibrium of Body Proteins,* Charles C Thomas, Springfield, Ill., 1956.
156. **Bethard, W. F., Wissler, R. W., Thompson, J. S., Schroeder, M. A., and Robsen, M. J.,** The effect of acute protein deprivation upon erythropoiesis in rats, *Blood,* 13, 216, 1958.
157. **Catchatourian, R., Eckerling, G., and Fried, W.,** Effect of short-term protein deprivation on hemopoietic functions of healthy volunteers, *Blood,* 55, 625, 1980.
158. **Anagnostou, A., Schade, S., and Fried, W.,** Stimulation of erythropoietin secretion by single amino acids, *Proc. Soc. Exp. Biol. Med.,* 159, 139, 1978.
159. **Fried, W. and Kilbridge, T.,** Effect of testosterone and of cobalt on erythropoietin production by anephric rats, *J. Lab. Clin. Med.,* 74, 623, 1968.
160. **Anagnostou, A., Schade, S., Barone, J., and Fried, W.,** Effect of protein deprivation on extrarenal erythropoietin production, *Blood,* 51, 549, 1978.
161. **Anagnostou, A., Schade, S., Barone, J., and Fried, W.,** Effects of partial hepatectomy on extrarenal erythropoietin production in rats, *Blood,* 50, 457, 1977.
162. **Naughton, B. A., Kaplan, S. M., Burdowski, R. M., Gordon, A. S., and Piliero, S. J.,** Hepatic regeneration and erythropoietin production in the rat, *Science,* 197, 301, 1977.
163. **Fried, W., Barone-Varelas, J., Barone, T., and Anagnostou, A.,** Effect of angiotensin infusion on extrarenal erythropoietin production, *J. Lab. Clin. Med.,* 99, 520, 1982.
164. **Gould, A. B., Goodman, S. A., and Green, D.,** Effect of renin on erythropoietin formation in normal and anephric rats, *Lab. Invest.,* 28, 719, 1973.
165. **Fried, W.,** Effect of renin on extrarenal erythropoietin production, *J. Lab. Clin. Med.,* 88, 707, 1976.
166. **Fried, W., Barone, J., Schade, S., and Anagnostou, A.,** Effect of carbon tetrachloride on extrarenal erythropoietin production, *J. Lab. Clin. Med.,* 93, 700, 1979.
167. **Roodman, G. D., Spivak, J. L., and Zanjani, E. D.,** Stimulation of erythroid colony formation by erythropoietin immobilized on agarose-bound lectin, *J. Lab. Clin. Med.,* 98, 684, 1981.
168. **Chang, C. S. and Goldwasser, E.,** On the mechanism of erythropoietin induced differentiation. XII. A cytoplasmic protein mediating-induced nuclear RNA synthesis, *Dev. Biol.,* 34, 246, 1973.

169. **Gross, M. and Goldwasser, E.,** On the mechanism of erythropoietin-induced differentiation. V. Characterization of the ribonucleic acid formed as a result of erythropoietin action, *Biochemistry,* 8, 1795, 1969.
170. **Gross, M. and Goldwasser, E.,** On the mechanism of erythropoietin-induced differentiation. IX. Induced synthesis of 9S ribonucleic acid and of hemoglobin, *J. Biol. Chem.,* 246, 2480, 1971.
171. **Schooley, J. C., Garcia, J. F., Cantor, L. N., and Havens, V. W.,** A summary of some studies on erythropoiesis using anti-erythropoietin immune serum, *Ann. N.Y. Acad. Sci.,* 149, 266, 1968.
172. **Iscove, N. N.,** The role of erythropoietin in regulation of population size and cell cycling of early and late erythroid precursors in mouse bone marrow, *Cell Tissue Kinet.,* 10, 323, 1977.
173. **Chamberlain, J. K., Leblond, P. E., and Wee, R. I.,** Reduction of adventitial cell cover, an early effect of erythropoietin on bone marrow ultrastructure, *Blood Cells,* 1, 655, 1975.
174. **Stohlman, F., Jr.,** Humoral regulation of erythropoiesis. XIV. A model for abnormal erythropoiesis in thalassemia, *Ann. N.Y. Acad. Sci.,* 117, 578, 1964.
175. **Stohlman, F., Jr.,** Erythropoietin and erythroid cell kinetics, in *Kidney Hormones,* Fisher, J. W., Ed., Academic Press, New York, 1971, 331.
176. **Hillman, R. S. and Henderson, P. A.,** Control of marrow production by the level of iron supply, *J. Clin. Invest.,* 48, 454, 1969.
177. **Sly, D. A., Grohlich, D., and Bezkorvainy, A.,** Transferrin in the reticulocyte cytosol, *Biochim. Biophys. Acta,* 385, 36, 1975.
178. **Jandl, J. H., Inman, J. K., Simmons, R. L., and Allen, D. W.,** Transfer of iron from serum iron-binding protein to human reticulocytes, *J. Clin. Invest.,* 38, 161, 1959.
179. **Katz, J. H.,** The delivery of iron to the immature red cell: a critical review, *Semin. Haematol.,* 6, 15, 1965.
180. **Sullivan, A. L., Grasso, J. A., and Weintraub, L. R.,** Micropinocytosis of transferrin by developing red cells, *Blood,* 47, 133, 1976.
181. **Tanaka, Y. and Brecher, G.,** Effect of surface digestion and metabolic inhibitors on the appearance of ferritin in guinea pig erythroblasts in vitro, *Blood,* 37, 211, 1971.
182. **Waxman, H. S. and Rabinovit, M.,** Control of reticulocyte polyribosome content and hemoglobin synthesis by heme, *Biochim. Biophys. Acta,* 129, 369, 1966.
183. **Bruns, G. P. and London, I. M.,** The effect of hemin on the synthesis of globin, *Biochim. Biophys. Res. Commun.,* 18, 236, 1965.
184. **Burnham, B. F. and Lascelles, J.,** Control of prophyrin biosynthesis through a negative feedback mechanism, *Biochem. J.,* 87, 462, 1963.
185. **Song, S. H. and Groom, A. C.,** Sequestration and possible maturation of reticulocytes in the normal spleen, *Can. J. Physiol. Pharmacol.,* 50, 400, 1972.
186. **Crosby, W. H.,** The limits of erythropoiesis: how much can the marrow produce with total recruitment, *Blood Cells,* 1, 497, 1975.
187. **Hillman, R. S. and Finch, C. A.,** Erythropoiesis: normal and abnormal, *Semin. Hematol.,* 4, 327, 1967.
188. **Suda, T., Junko, S., Ogawa, M., and Ihle, J. N.,** Permissive role of interleukin 3 (IL-3) in proliferation and differentiation of multipotential hemopoietic progenitors in culture, *J. Cell. Physiol.,* 124, 182, 1985.

HEMOGLOBIN

Walter A. Schroeder

INTRODUCTION

Hemoglobin has probably been subjected to more experiments and probably more is known about it than about any other protein. These few pages give a broad background for the detailed information of many kinds that will be provided in the following sections. The emphasis is on human hemoglobins.

The information about hemoglobin is far more extensive than could possibly be included in this chapter. Of the many books and reviews on the topic of hemoglobin, the following are cited as sources of additional information: Antonini and Brunori,[1] Bunn and Forget,[2] Fairbanks,[3] Huisman and Jonxis,[4] Lehmann and Huntsman,[5] Ranney,[6] Schneider et al.,[7] Weatherall,[8,9] and Weatherall and Clegg.[10]

GENERAL PROPERTIES OF HEMOGLOBIN

Nomenclature

The function of hemoglobin is to combine with oxygen in the lungs and to release that oxygen in the tissues. In this process, oxygen combines with (but does not oxidize in the chemical sense) the ferrous iron of the heme group. In this form it is commonly called "oxyhemoglobin". Many other ligands, such as carbon monoxide, will also combine. When the ligand is carbon monoxide, the proper name is carbonmonoxyhemoglobin, although it is commonly incorrectly called carboxyhemoglobin in the literature. When oxygen is released, deoxyhemoglobin results; the incorrect designation "reduced" hemoglobin appears in the older literature. When oxidation to the ferric form occurs either spontaneously or by chemical means, the product is methemoglobin. Oxygen no longer combines, but many ions such as cyanide, fluoride, etc. will combine.

Molecular Weight and Subunit Status

Human and other mammalian hemoglobins have molecular weights of the order of 64,500. The actual molecular weight does not vary more than a few hundred units from hemoglobin to hemoglobin and depends on the actual amino acid composition and the state of liganding.

Normally, hemoglobins are composed of two pairs of different subunits. These subunits are designated α- and non-α-chains. This distinction is made because in any one species the α-chains are combined with various non-α (β,γ,δ, etc.) chains. Thus, for normal adult human hemoglobin A (Hb A), the subunit structural formula is $\alpha_2\beta^A{}_2$, where the subscripts have the usual chemical significance and the superscript identifies the hemoglobin. Variant hemoglobins such as Hb S are designated as $\alpha_2\beta^S{}_2$ because the aberration is in the β-chain, or as $\alpha^X{}_2\beta_2$ if it is in the α-chain. Human fetal hemoglobin (Hb F) is $\alpha_2\gamma_2$, and a minor component called hemoglobin A_2 (Hb A_2) is $\alpha_2\delta_2$. α-Chains are usually five residues shorter than non-α-chains and have a molecular weight that is 700 to 800 less than that of non-α-chains.

Functional Properties

Because of the pickup and release of oxygen by hemoglobin, its functional properties can be described in terms of certain parameters of the "oxygen dissociation" or "oxygen equilibrium" curve. It has long been known that this curve has the sigmoid shape shown in Figure 1 whether the determination is done with blood or hemoglobin solution. The curve

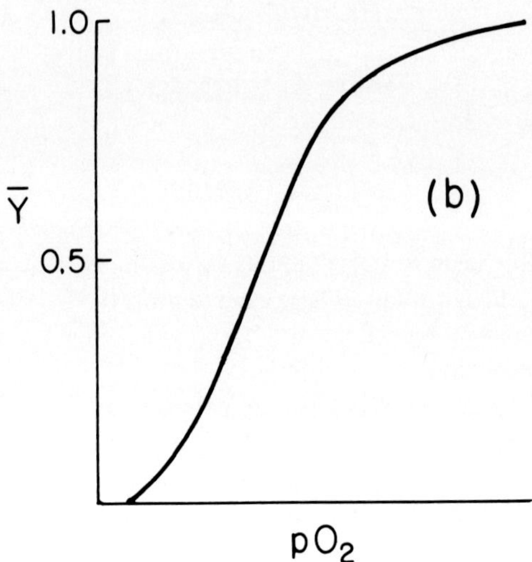

FIGURE 1. Schematic representation of the oxygen association-dissociation curve of hemoglobin. $\overline{Y}$ is the fractional saturation of the protein with oxygen, and pO_2 is the partial pressure of oxygen.

is usually plotted with percent saturation or fractional saturation on the ordinate and partial pressure or log of the partial pressure of oxygen on the abscissa.

One parameter of function is termed "p_{50}", "$p_{1/2}$", "log p_{50}", or "log $p_{1/2}$". All of these are merely different forms of defining the pressure at 50% or half saturation. Thus, in studying a hemoglobin variant, a comparison of its p_{50} with that of Hb A under identical conditions would determine whether the oxygen affinity is normal, increased, or decreased. The smaller the p_{50}, the greater the affinity of oxygen and vice versa.

Another parameter of function is the so-called "n of the Hill equation". Hill considered the reaction of oxygen with hemoglobin in terms of the equation:

$$Hb_n + nO_2 \rightleftharpoons (HbO_2)_n$$

and converted this by the mass law to:

$$\overline{Y}/(1 - \overline{Y}) = Kp^n$$

where $\overline{Y}$ is the fractional saturation, p is the partial pressure of oxygen, and K is the equilibrium constant. Although n does not yield the information about mechanism or order of reaction that Hill had hoped to obtain, it is a convenient means of representing the shape of the curve or, more precisely, its slope at p_{50}. Normally, n is 2.7 ± 0.2. It does not rise above this value, but a decrease below it is a measure of abnormality.

The abscissa in Figure 1 has been given no values because p_{50} and therefore, the position of the curve along this axis, is dependent on pH, temperature, ion concentration, and cofactors. However, n (the shape of the curve) is independent of these variables.

The effect of pH, or the Bohr effect, is another parameter of function and is reported as $\Delta p_{50}/\Delta pH$. The maximum value of p_{50} (minimum affinity) occurs at approximately pH 6.2 and decreases at pH above or below. Below the maximum, this is termed the "acid" Bohr effect and above the maximum the "alkaline" Bohr effect. Only the latter is of any physiological significance.

Because the p_{50} is dependent on several factors, it is important that the exact conditions of pH, temperature, and ion concentration be stated. Since 1967, another factor, the concentration of 2,3-diphosphoglyceric acid (2,3-DPG), has had to be considered. Chanutin and Curnish[11] and Benesch and Benesch[12] discovered that the presence of 2,3-DPG decreases the oxygen affinity (increases p_{50}) of hemoglobin and that the n does not change. 2,3-DPG is a glycolytic intermediate that normally approximately equals hemoglobin in millimolar concentration in the red cell. In any determination of p_{50}, the concentration of 2,3-DPG cannot be ignored. Either it must be removed ("stripped") or its concentration must be known. Consequently, data on oxygen equilibrium curves published before the effect of 2,3-DPG was discovered in 1967 must be examined with caution because its concentration in such studies is unknown (see Huisman and Schroeder[13] for a review of this topic).

Time Course of Hemoglobins in the Individual

Hemoglobins appear and disappear in sequence from the first production of hemoglobin in the developing fetus until the infant is 6 months to 1 year old, at which time it has attained the hematological status of an adult. Toward the middle of the first trimester of gestation, when sufficient blood for study can be obtained, four chains make up most of the hemoglobin; they are the α-, γ-, ϵ- and ζ-chains in the combinations $\alpha_2\gamma_2$ (Hb F), $\alpha_2\epsilon_2$ (Hb-Gower-2), $\zeta_2\epsilon_2$ (Hb-Gower-1), and $\zeta_2\gamma_2$ (Hb-Portland-1). Although Hb-Gower-1 was first thought to be ϵ_4, it is, in fact, $\zeta_2\epsilon_2$, and the ζ-chain is a type of α-chain. The ϵ- and ζ-chains are not detectable after the end of the first trimester.

The β-chains (hence, $\alpha_2\beta_2$ or Hb A) may be detected early in pregnancy, and during the second trimester Hb A makes up 5 to 10% and Hb F the remainder of the hemoglobin. During the last trimester, Hb A production increases and that of Hb F decreases so that at birth Hb A approximates 25% (with considerable variation) and Hb F the remainder of the hemoglobin, except for 0.2 to 0.5% of Hb A_2.

Postnatally, the reciprocal rise of Hb A and Hb A_2 and the fall of Hb F continue. By the time an infant is approximately 6 months old, the Hb F has decreased to a few percent, Hb A is the preponderant hemoglobin, and HbA_2 makes up to 2 to 3% of the total hemoglobin.

AMINO ACID SEQUENCES IN THE HUMAN HEMOGLOBIN CHAINS

The amino acid sequences of the α-, β-, γ-, δ-, ϵ-, and ζ-chains follow below.

Human α-Chain

```
                   5                   10                  15
Val-Leu-Ser-Pro-Ala-Asp-Lys-Thr-Asn-Val-Lys-Ala-Ala-Trp-Gly-

                  20                   25                  30
Lys-Val-Gly-Ala-His-Ala-Gly-Glu-Tyr-Gly-Ala-Glu-Ala-Leu-Glu-

                  35                   40                  45
Arg-Met-Phe-Leu-Ser-Phe-Pro-Thr-Thr-Lys-Thr-Tyr-Phe-Pro-His-

                  50                   55                  60
Phe-Asp-Leu-Ser-His-Gly-Ser-Ala-Gln-Val-Lys-Gly-His-Gly-Lys-

                  65                   70                  75
Lys-Val-Ala-Asp-Ala-Leu-Thr-Asn-Ala-Val-Ala-His-Val-Asp-Asp-

                  80                   85                  90
Met-Pro-Asn-Ala-Leu-Ser-Ala-Leu-Ser-Asp-Leu-His-Ala-His-Lys-

                  95                  100                 105
Leu-Arg-Val-Asp-Pro-Val-Asn-Phe-Lys-Leu-Leu-Ser-His-Cys-Leu-
```

110 115 120
Leu-Val-Thr-Leu-Ala-Ala-His-Leu-Pro-Ala-Glu-Phe-Thr-Pro-Ala-

125 130 135
Val-His-Ala-Ser-Leu-Asp-Lys-Phe-Leu-Ala-Ser-Val-Ser-Thr-Val-

140
Leu-Thr-Ser-Lys-Tyr-Arg

Human β-Chain

5 10 15
Val-His-Leu-Thr-Pro-Glu-Glu-Lys-Ser-Ala-Val-Thr-Ala-Leu-Trp-

20 25 30
Gly-Lys-Val-Asn-Val-Asp-Glu-Val-Gly-Gly-Glu-Ala-Leu-Gly-Arg-

35 40 45
Leu-Leu-Val-Val-Tyr-Pro-Trp-Thr-Gln-Arg-Phe-Phe-Glu-Ser-Phe-

50 55 60
Gly-Asp-Leu-Ser-Thr-Pro-Asp-Ala-Val-Met-Gly-Asn-Pro-Lys-Val-

65 70 75
Lys-Ala-His-Gly-Lys-Lys-Val-Leu-Gly-Ala-Phe-Ser-Asp-Gly-Leu-

80 85 90
Ala-His-Leu-Asp-Asn-Leu-Lys-Gly-Thr-Phe-Ala-Thr-Leu-Ser-Glu-

95 100 105
Leu-His-Cys-Asp-Lys-Leu-His-Val-Asp-Pro-Glu-Asn-Phe-Arg-Leu-

110 115 120
Leu-Gly-Asn-Val-Leu-Val-Cys-Val-Leu-Ala-His-His-Phe-Gly-Lys-

125 130 135
Glu-Phe-Thr-Pro-Pro-Val-Gln-Ala-Ala-Tyr-Gln-Lys-Val-Val-Ala-

140 145
Gly-Val-Ala-Asn-Ala-Leu-Ala-His-Lys-Tyr-His

Human γ-Chain

5 10 15
Gly-His-Phe-Thr-Glu-Glu-Asp-Lys-Ala-Thr-Ile-Thr-Ser-Leu-Trp-

20 25 30
Gly-Lys-Val-Asn-Val-Glu-Asp-Ala-Gly-Gly-Glu-Thr-Leu-Gly-Arg-

35 40 45
Leu-Leu-Val-Val-Tyr-Pro-Trp-Thr-Gln-Arg-Phe-Phe-Asp-Ser-Phe-

50 55 60
Gly-Asn-Leu-Ser-Ser-Ala-Ser-Ala-Ile-Met-Gly-Asn-Pro-Lys-Val-

65 70 75
Lys-Ala-His-Gly-Lys-Lys-Val-Leu-Thr-Ser-Leu-Gly-Asp-Ala-Ile-

80 85 90
Lys-His-Leu-Asp-Asp-Leu-Lys-Gly-Thr-Phe-Ala-Gln-Leu-Ser-Glu-

95 100 105
Leu-His-Cys-Asp-Lys-Leu-His-Val-Asp-Pro-Glu-Asn-Phe-Lys-Leu-

```
                       110                           115                           120
Leu-Gly-Asn-Val-Leu-Val-Thr-Val-Leu-Ala-Ile-His-Phe-Gly-Lys-

                       125                           130                           135
Glu-Phe-Thr-Pro-Glu-Val-Gln-Ala-Ser-Trp-Gln-Lys-Met-Val-Thr-

                       140                           145
Gly-Val-Ala-Ser-Ala-Leu-Ser-Ser-Arg-Tyr-His
```

Normally, Hb F has a mixture of γ-chains which are the products of nonallelic genes. Thus, position 136 may have either glycine or alanine.[14] In some instances isoleucine at position 75 may be replaced by threonine[15] in the chain that has alanine at position 136.[16]

Human δ-Chain

```
                         5                            10                            15
Val-His-Leu-Thr-Pro-Glu-Glu-Lys-Thr-Ala-Val-Asn-Ala-Leu-Trp-

                        20                            25                            30
Gly-Lys-Val-Asn-Val-Asp-Ala-Val-Gly-Gly-Glu-Ala-Leu-Gly-Arg-

                        35                            40                            45
Leu-Leu-Val-Val-Tyr-Pro-Trp-Thr-Gln-Arg-Phe-Phe-Glu-Ser-Phe-

                        50                            55                            60
Gly-Asp-Leu-Ser-Ser-Pro-Asp-Ala-Val-Met-Gly-Asn-Pro-Lys-Val-

                        65                            70                            75
Lys-Ala-His-Gly-Lys-Lys-Val-Leu-Gly-Ala-Phe-Ser-Asp-Gly-Leu-

                        80                            85                            90
Ala-His-Leu-Asp-Asn-Leu-Lys-Gly-Thr-Phe-Ser-Gln-Leu-Ser-Glu-

                        95                           100                           105
Leu-His-Cys-Asp-Lys-Leu-His-Val-Asp-Pro-Glu-Asn-Phe-Arg-Leu-

                       110                           115                           120
Leu-Gly-Asn-Val-Leu-Val-Cys-Val-Leu-Ala-Arg-Asn-Phe-Gly-Lys-

                       125                           130                           135
Glu-Phe-Thr-Pro-Gln-Met-Gln-Ala-Ala-Tyr-Gln-Lys-Val-Val-Ala-

                       140                           145
Gly-Val-Ala-Asn-Ala-Leu-Ala-His-Lys-Tyr-His
```

Human ϵ-Chain

Although this sequence was partly determined by amino acid sequencing, [17] it was completed by DNA sequencing.[18]

```
                         5                            10                            15
Val-His-Phe-Thr-Ala-Glu-Glu-Lys-Ala-Ala-Val-Thr-Ser-Leu-Trp-

                        20                            25                            30
Ser-Lys-Met-Asn-Val-Glu-Glu-Ala-Gly-Gly-Glu-Ala-Leu-Gly-Arg-

                        35                            40                            45
Leu-Leu-Val-Val-Tyr-Pro-Trp-Thr-Gln-Arg-Phe-Phe-Asp-Ser-Phe-

                        50                            55                            60
Gly-Asn-Leu-Ser-Ser-Pro-Ser-Ala-Ile-Leu-Gly-Asn-Pro-Lys-Val-
```

```
                65                  70                  75
Lys-Ala-His-Gly-Lys-Lys-Val-Leu-Thr-Ser-Phe-Gly-Asp-Ala-Ile-

                80                  85                  90
Lys-Asn-Met-Asp-Asn-Leu-Lys-Pro-Ala-Phe-Ala-Lys-Leu-Ser-Glu-

                95                  100                 105
Leu-His-Cys-Asp-Lys-Leu-His-Val-Asp-Pro-Glu-Asn-Phe-Lys-Leu-

                110                 115                 120
Leu-Gly-Asn-Val-Met-Val-Ile-Ile-Leu-Ala-Thr-His-Phe-Gly-Lys-

                125                 130                 135
Glu-Phe-Thr-Pro-Glu-Val-Gln-Ala-Ala-Trp-Gln-Lys-Leu-Val-Ser-

                140                 145
Ala-Val-Ala-Ile-Ala-Leu-Ala-His-Lys-Tyr-His
```

Human ζ-Chain

The amino acid sequence of the ζ-chain was determined by amino acid sequencing.[19] The ζ-chain has a blocked N-terminal residue.

```
                5                   10                  15
Ser-Leu-Thr-Lys-Thr-Glu-Arg-Thr-Ile-Ile-Val-Ser-Met-Trp-Ala-

                20                  25                  30
Lys-Ile-Ser-Thr-Gln-Ala-Asp-Thr-Ile-Gly-Thr-Glu-Thr-Leu-Glu-

                35                  40                  45
Arg-Leu-Phe-Leu-Ser-His-Pro-Gln-Thr-Lys-Pro-Tyr-Phe-Pro-His-

                50                  55                  60
Phe-Asp-Leu-His-Pro-Gly-Ser-Ala-Gln-Leu-Arg-Ala-His-Gly-Ser-

                65                  70                  75
Lys-Val-Val-Ala-Ala-Val-Gly-Asp-Ala-Val-Lys-Ser-Ile-Asp-Asp-

                80                  85                  90
Ile-Gly-Gly-Ala-Leu-Ser-Lys-Leu-Ser-Glu-Leu-His-Ala-Tyr-Ile-

                95                  100                 105
Leu-Arg-Val-Asp-Pro-Val-Asn-Phe-Lys-Leu-Leu-Ser-His-Cys-Leu-

                110                 115                 120
Leu-Val-Thr-Leu-Ala-Ala-Arg-Phe-Pro-Ala-Asp-Phe-Thr-Ala-Glu-

                125                 130                 135
Ala-His-Ala-Ala-Trp-Asp-Lys-Phe-Leu-Ser-Val-Val-Ser-Ser-Val-

                140
Leu-Thr-Glu-Lys-Tyr-Arg
```

POSTSYNTHETIC CHANGES

A portion of the β- and γ- chains is modified after the biosynthesis is complete. In the hemoglobin designated as Hb A_{1c}, which accounts for 5 to 6% of the total hemoglobin in the normal adult, the β-chains have a carbohydrate in Schiff's base linkage to the N-terminal valyl residue.[20,21]

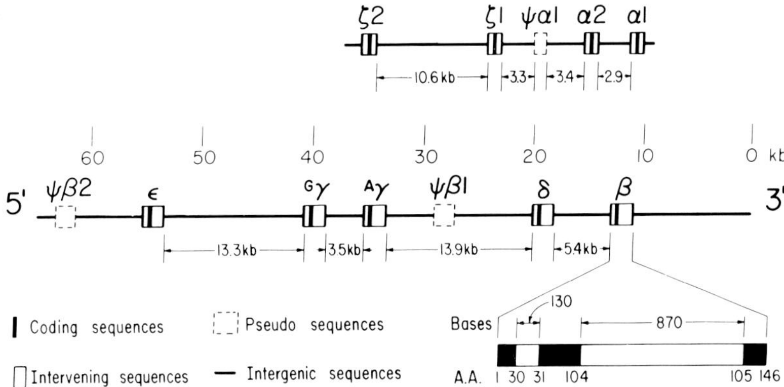

FIGURE 2. Arrangement of genes and pseudogenes in the cluster of α-type genes on human chromosome 16 and in the cluster of non-α-type genes on the short arm of human chromosome 11.

The hemoglobin known as Hb F_1 or Hb F_I has γ-chains that are acetylated (and glycosylated) on the N-terminal glycyl residue.[22,23] The ratio of Hb F_I to Hb F is approximately 1:4.

CHROMOSOMAL ARRANGEMENT OF THE GLOBIN GENES

Recent studies of DNA have provided detailed information about the arrangement of the globin genes. This topic, which is presented only in broad outline here, is described more fully in the chapter by Antonarakis and Kazazian.

The α-type genes (α and ζ) are located on chromosome 16, whereas the non-α-types (β, γ, δ, and ϵ) are clustered on the short arm of chromosome 11. Figure 2 shows the arrangement of the α- and non-α-gene clusters to scale. Prior to the DNA studies, the basic arrangement of the β-, γ-, and δ-genes was known and evidence for two α-genes was convincing, but little was known about the ϵ and ζ-chains or genes. In addition to the active genes, pseudogenes (Ψα1,Ψβ1, and Ψβ2) have a relationship to the respective active gene, but are of unknown function. The genes in each cluster are separated by intergenic segments which are longer than an individual gene. However, the genes themselves have about three times the bases that are needed to code for the particular chain. This excess DNA forms the so-called "intervening sequences". The structure of the β-gene has been magnified in Figure 2 to show these details. Thus, between the codons for residues 30 and 31 are 130 base pairs (bp) of intervening sequence 1 (IVS 1) whereas IVS 2 with 870 bp lies between codons for residues 104 and 105. IVS 1 and IVS 2 differ slightly in length in the non-α-genes but are always between residues 30 and 31 and 104 and 105. In the α- and ζ-genes, IVS 2 is about 150 bp in length, but the α- and ζ-IVSs are in analogous position to those in non-α-type genes. During transcription to mRNA, the IVSs are transcribed as well as some DNA both 5′ and 3′ to a gene. Further processing then removes the IVSs to produce the final mRNA.

REFERENCES

1. **Antonini, E. and Brunori, M.,** *Hemoglobin and Myoglobin in Their Reactions with Ligands,* Elsevier, New York, 1971.
2. **Bunn, H. F. and Forget, B. G.,** *Hemoglobin: Molecular, Genetic and Clinical Aspects,* W. B. Saunders, Philadelphia, 1986.

3. **Fairbanks, V. F.,** *Hemoglobinopathies and Thalassemias,* Thieme-Stratton, New York, 1980.
4. **Huisman, T. H. J. and Jonxis, J. H. P.,** *The Hemoglobinopathies. Techniques of Identification,* Marcel Dekker, New York, 1977.
5. **Lehmann, H. and Huntsman, R. G.,** *Man's Hemoglobins,* 2nd ed., North-Holland, Amsterdam, 1974.
6. **Ranney, H. M., Ed.,** Hemoglobinopathies, *Semin. Hematol.,* 11, 383, 1974.
7. **Schneider, R. G., Charache, S., and Schroeder, W. A., Eds.,** Human hemoglobins and hemoglobinopathies: a review to 1981, *Tex. Rep. Biol. Med.,* 40, 1—504, 1980—81.
8. **Weatherall, D. J., Ed.,** Abnormal hemoglobins, *Clin. Haematol.,* 3, 215, 1974.
9. **Weatherall, D. J., Ed.,** Hemoglobin: structure, function, and synthesis, *Br. Med. Bull.,* 32, 193, 1976.
10. **Weatherall, D. J. and Clegg, J. B.,** *The Thalassaemia Syndromes,* 3rd ed., Blackwell Scientific, Oxford, 1981.
11. **Chanutin, A. and Curnish, R. R.,** Effect of organic and inorganic phosphates on the oxygen equilibrium of human erythrocytes, *Arch. Biochem. Biophys.,* 121, 96, 1967.
12. **Benesch, R. and Benesch, R. E.,** The effect of organic phosphates from the human erythrocyte on the allosteric properties of hemoglobin, *Biochem. Biophys. Res. Commun.,* 26, 162, 1967.
13. **Huisman, T. H. J. and Schroeder, W. A.,** New aspects of the structure, function, and synthesis of hemoglobins, *CRC Crit. Rev. Clin. Lab. Sci.,* 1, 490, 1970.
14. **Schroeder, W. A., Huisman, T. H. J., Shelton, J. R., Shelton, J. B., Kleihauer, E. F., Dozy, A. M., and Robberson, B.,** Evidence for mutiple structural genes for the γ chain of human fetal hemoglobin, *Proc. Natl. Acad. Sci. U.S.A.,* 60, 537, 1968.
15. **Ricco, G., Mazza, U., Turi, R. M., Pich, P. G., Camaschella, C., Saglio, G., and Bernini, L. F.,** Significance of a new type of human fetal hemoglobin carrying a replacement isoleucine $\rightarrow$ threonine at position 75 (E19) of the γ chain, *Hum. Genet.,* 32, 305, 1976.
16. **Saglio, G., Ricco, G., Mazza, U., Camaschella, C., Pich, P. G., Gianni, A. M., Gianazza, E., Righetti, P. G., Giglioni, B., Comi, P., Gusmeroli, M., and Ottolenghi, S.,** Human $^{T}\gamma$ globin chain is a variant of the $^{A}\gamma$ chain ($^{A}\gamma$ Sardinia), *Proc. Natl. Acad. Sci. U.S.A.,* 76, 3420, 1979.
17. **Gale, R. E., Clegg, J. B., and Huehns, E. R.,** Human embryonic haemoglobins Gower 1 and Gower 2, *Nature (London),* 280, 162, 1979.
18. **Barelle, F. E., Shoulders, C. C., and Proudfoot, N. J.,** The primary structure of the human ϵ-globin gene, *Cell,* 21, 621, 1980.
19. **Clegg, J. B. and Gagnon, J.,** Structure of the ζ chain of human embryonic hemoglobin, *Proc. Natl. Acad. Sci. U.S.A.,* 78, 6076, 1981.
20. **Holmquist, W. R. and Schroeder, W. A.,** A new N-terminal blocking group involving a Schiff base in hemoglobin A, *Biochemistry,* 5, 2489, 1966.
21. **Koenig, R. J., Blobstein, S. H., and Cerami, A.,** Structure of carbohydrate of hemoglobin A_{Ic}, *J. Biol. Chem.,* 252, 2992, 1977.
22. **Schroeder, W. A., Cua, J. T., Matsuda, G., and Fenninger, W. D.,** Hemoglobin F_I, an acetyl-containing hemoglobin, *Biochim. Biophys. Acta,* 63, 532, 1962.
23. **Stegink, L. D., Meyer, P. D., and Brummel, M. C.,** Human fetal hemoglobin F_I — acetylation status, *J. Biol. Chem.,* 246, 3001, 1971.

GENETICS OF HEMOGLOBINS

Robert D. Koler

PHYLOGENY

One or more globin gene products are found in all vertebrates as well as in mollusks, annelids, and some plants. All globins share the same homologous structure; they all provide a pocket for the binding of heme and have the common property of reversible combination with oxygen. Comparative biochemistry of globins has been reviewed by Fitch,[1] Dayhoff et al.,[2] Goodman et al.,[3] and Coates[4] in the era before genomic DNA structure was known, and by Efstratiadis et al.[5] and by Jeffreys,[6] who used actual globin nucleotide sequences. The phylogeny based on these recent determinations of the DNA structures has confirmed conclusions based on amino acid sequence results, and has raised new opportunities for investigating not only evolution, but the molecular basis of genetic control.

Comparison of the amino acid sequences of globins first led to the construction of an evolutionary tree such as that found in Figure 1. It is based on the maximum parsimony method, which ascribes the descent or related protein amino acid sequences to the fewest number of mutational changes. The result is in general agreement with paleontologic dating of the divergence from common ancestors. The primitive gene that gave rise to all existing globin genes may be as ancient as the time plant life diverged from animal lineages about 1 billion years ago. In agreement with this model, an evolutionary tree based on comparisons of human β-like globin gene nucleotide sequences[5] places the common vertebrate ancestral gene at 500 million years ago. Comparisons of nucleotide sequences of mammalian γ-globin[7] and α-globin[8] genes show striking retentions of homology which are interpreted as evidence for self-correcting gene conversion or gene duplication events. These will be discussed later.

A schematic model of the formation of the earth and its atmosphere is shown in Figure 2. A predominantly reducing environment was present until about 3 billion years ago when the earliest living forms appeared. Organic evolution resulted in organisms that were able to trap energy from sunlight by photosynthesis. One product of photosynthesis — oxygen — then accumulated and reached its present atmospheric concentration about 1 billion years ago. This chronology is consistent with the known function of all hemoglobins, i.e., to transport oxygen in those metazoans in which it occurs. The absence of a globin counterpart in more primitive protozoans is also in keeping with an age of less than 3 billion but more than 1 billion years. This chapter will review what has happened to that common ancestral globin gene.

Change in Function

There are species differences among vertebrates in the hemoglobin-oxygen equilibrium and the kinetics that describe the basic reaction:

$$Hb + nO_2 \rightleftharpoons Hb(O_2)n$$

Coates[4] has proposed a model (Figure 3) suggesting that a sequence of minor modifications of globin structure will account for the evolutionary differences among species. His model begins with a primitive monomer that successively becomes:

1. A dimer in the deoxy form, thus acquiring a Bohr effect and cooperative rather than hyperbolic binding of oxygen (hagfish → lamprey)
2. A tetramer with a greater Bohr effect, greater cooperativity, and further reduction in oxygen affinity (cyclostoma → elasmobranchii)

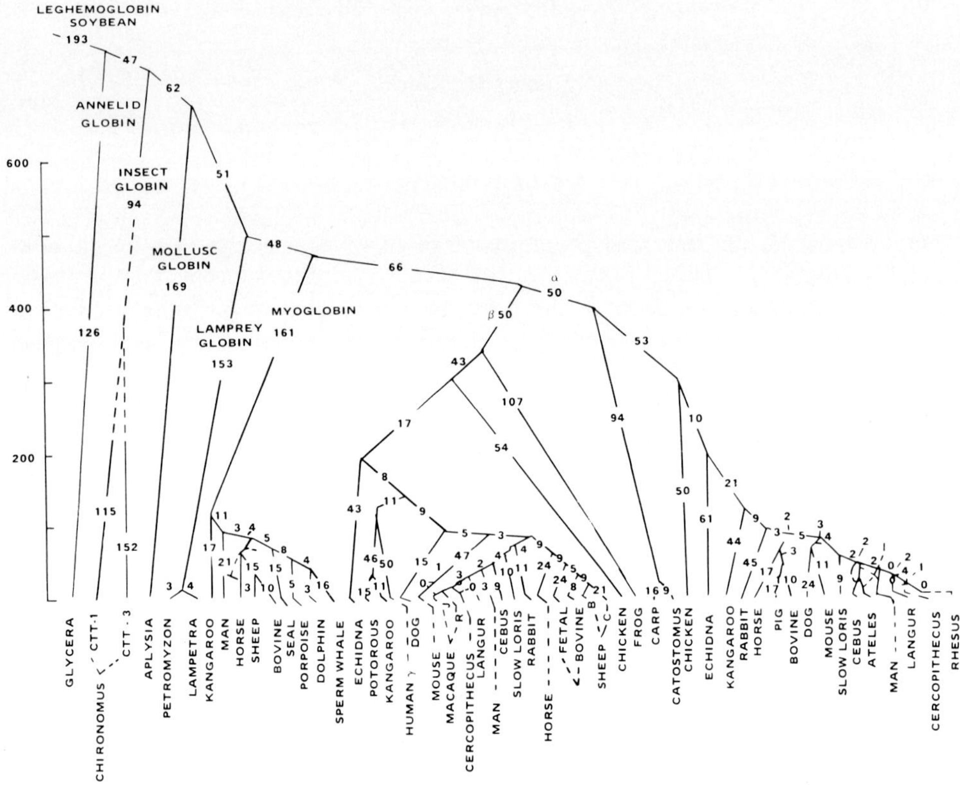

FIGURE 1. Maximum parsimony tree of 55 more adequately sequenced globins. (From Goodman, M., Moore, G. W., and Matsuda, G., *Isozymes. IV. Genetics and Evolution*, Markert, C. L., Ed., Academic Press, New York, 1975, 181. With permission.)

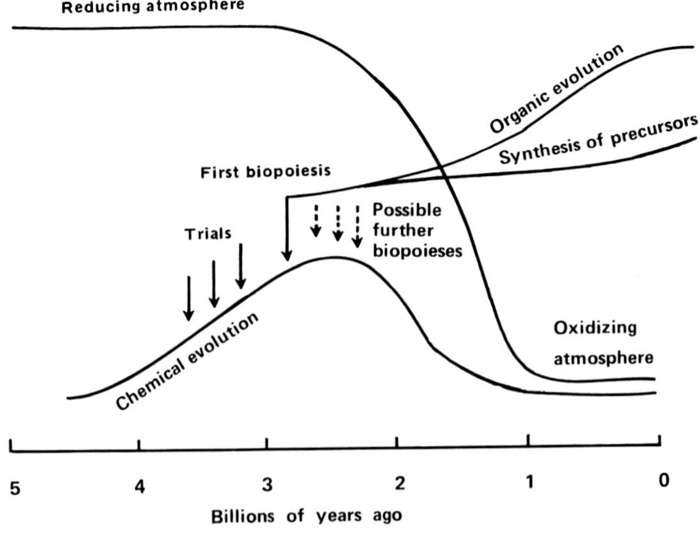

FIGURE 2. Probable origin of life and course of evolutionary events. (From Michael, I., Lerner, M. I., and Libby, W. J., *Heredity, Evolution, and Society*, 2nd ed., W. M. Freeman, San Francisco, 1976. With permission.)

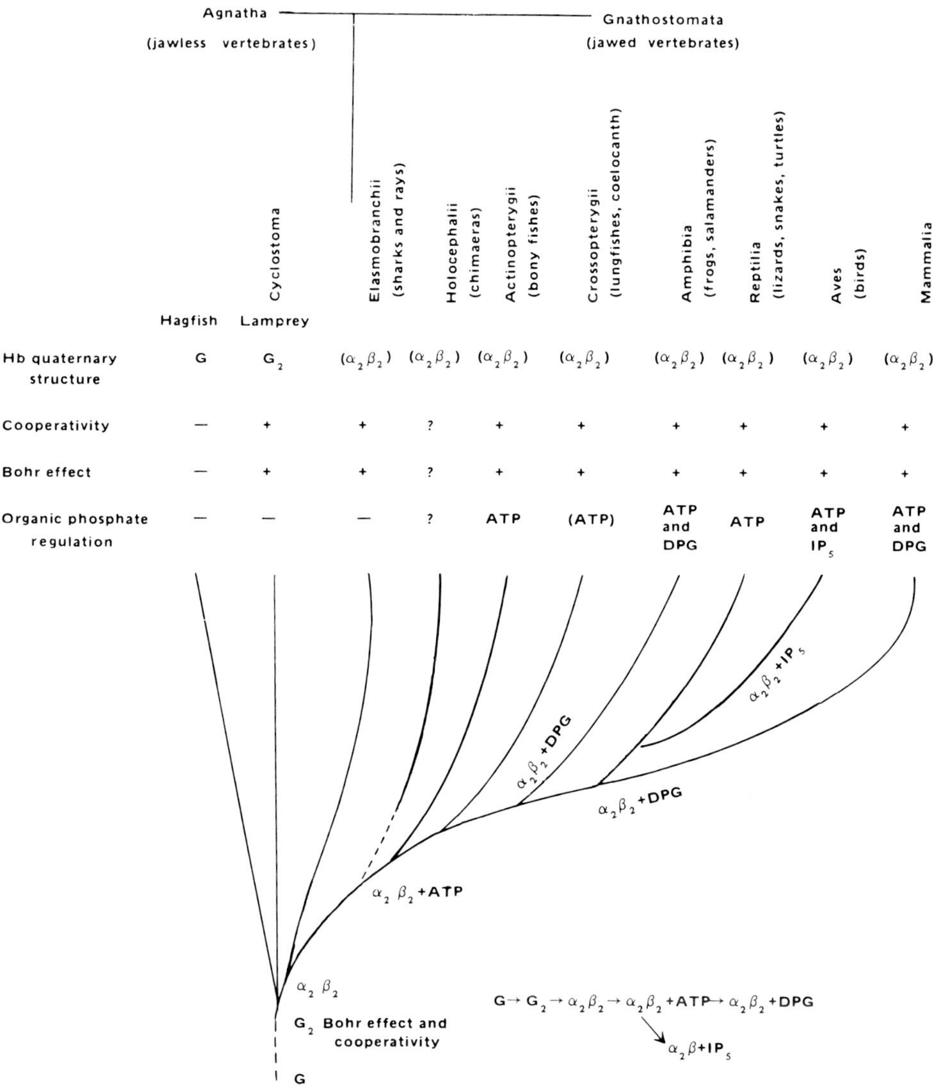

FIGURE 3. Evolution of hemoglobin function in vertebrates. (From Coates, M., *J. Mol. Evol.*, 6, 285, 1975. With permission.)

3. A tetramer that acquires a phosphate-binding site leading to a further increase in Bohr effect and a decrease in oxygen affinity (elasmobranchii → bony fishes and all higher forms)

There has also been a progression in the type of organic phosphate bound. More primitive forms use only ATP. Amphibia, birds, and mammals use 2,3-diphosphoglyceric (2,3-DPG); after hatching, birds use myoinositol pentaphosphate.[10]

Change in Number and in Structure

Duplication of the ancestral globin gene has resulted in two classes and six different types of globin genes found in the human haploid complement. Ohno[11] has reviewed both the teleologic reasons for gene duplication and the evidence that it has happened. Comparative studies of both phylogenetic and ontogenic development are in keeping with a progressive

Table 1
HUMAN GLOBIN GENES

Class	Type	Subtype	Ontogeny	Tetramer	Name
α	ζ	ζ	Embryo	$\zeta_2\epsilon_2$	Gower I
	α	α_1		$\alpha_2\epsilon_2$	Gower II
		α_2		$\zeta_2\gamma_2$	Portland
Nonα		ϵ	Fetus	$\alpha_2\gamma_2$	Fetal
	γ	$^A\gamma$		$\alpha_2\gamma_2$	Fetal
		$^G\gamma$	Adult	$\alpha_2\beta_2$	Hb A
	β	β		$\alpha_2\delta_2$	Hb A_2
	δ	δ			

Note: Two classes of globin genes with the presently known types and subtypes within each class, the names assigned to tetramers, and the time during development that they appear.

adaptation of hemoglobins[4-6,11,12] by both gene duplication and amino acid substitutions. Human globin genes and their active period during development are listed in Table 1.

α and non-α classes of globin genes are found in all vertebrates beyond the agnatha or jawless forms. They probably resulted from polyploidization or doubling of the entire chromosome complement early in the evolution of vertebrates. Tandem duplication then resulted in multiple subtypes at both cistrons.

At the non-α-cistron, a minimum of three tandem duplications would account for the human subtypes $^A\gamma$, $^G\gamma$, δ, and β. Duplication of the non-α-locus is also found in other species. A δ-globin is present in a number of primate species[13] but not in other mammals. A fetal α-globin analogous to that in humans has been structurally characterized in cattle, sheep, goats,[14] and mice,[15] and may occur in elephants and rats;[16] none has been found in dogs[16] and pigs.[17]

Human fetal hemoglobin consists of tetramers with two α-globins that differ only at the 136th amino acid position. One contains glycine and is termed $^G\gamma$; the other contains alanine and is termed $^A\gamma$.[18-23] In addition, Ricco et al.[24] have reported further heterogeneity due to the presence of threonine or isoleucine at the 75th amino acid position. The substitution of threonine for isoleucine was found in about one third of cord blood samples from a variety of ethnic groups. It represents a polymorphism with two different alleles at the $^G\gamma$ locus.

Embryonic globins from rabbit and mouse embryos[25] and from chickens[26] contain a ζ-like chain based on partial amino acid sequences. The time of divergence and classification of embryonic hemoglobins is still tentative, however, because these gene products have not been sought systematically in other species.

ORGANIZATION OF GLOBIN GENES

The arrangement of globin genes on two different human chromosomes has been unambiguously demonstrated using both somatic cell hybrids[27-29] and *in situ* hybridization with cDNA probes.[30,31] The α-globin loci have been placed on the short arm of chromosome 16, and the non-α-loci on the short arm of chromosome 11.

Absence of Linkage Between α- and Non-α-Cistrons

Independent segregation of allelic genes at the α- and β-loci has been found in all families in which structural variants of both globins occur. Interestingly, Jeffreys et al.[32] have found in *Xenopus* that the α- and β-globin genes are closely linked.

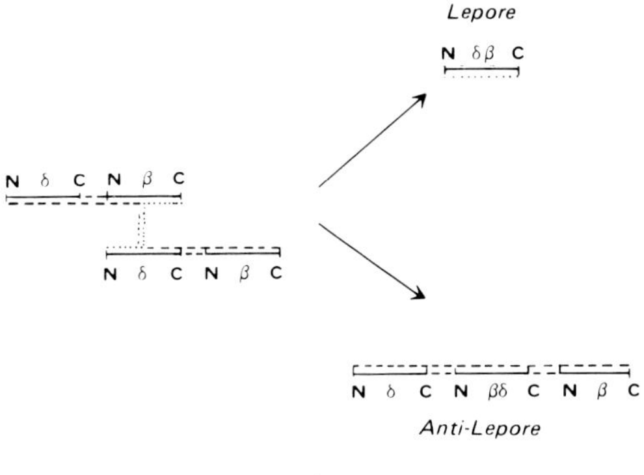

A

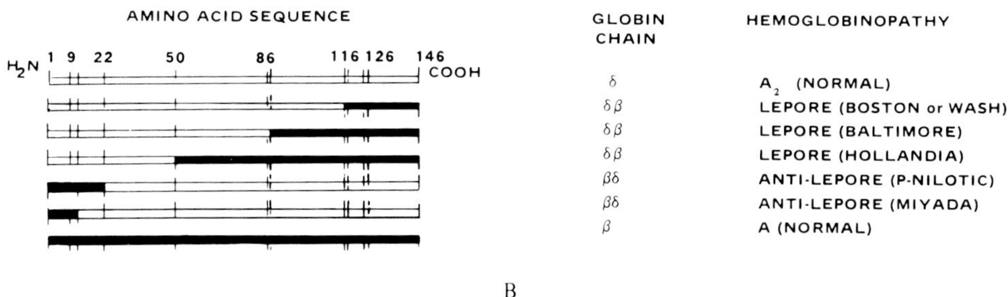

B

FIGURE 4. (A) Origin of the Lepore and anti-Lepore globin chains by crossing over between misaligned δ- and β-globin genes. N and C refer to the extremities of the gene coding for the amino- and carboxy-terminal ends of the globin chains. (B) Different types of Lepore and anti-Lepore globin chains. (From Benz, E. J. and Forget, B. G., *Progress in Hematology*, Vol. 9, Brown, E. B., Ed., Grune & Stratton, New York, 1975, 107. With permission.)

Polarity of Linked Globin Genes in the Non-α-Cistron

The alignment of non-α-globin genes was based initially on the study of rare fusion gene products. The first was found in members of a family who had a thalassemia-like phenotype, and it was designated Hb Lepore.[33] This abnormal hemoglobin was chemically characterized by Baglioni.[34] who found the N-terminal amino acid sequence to be identical with that of the normal δ-chain and the C-terminal sequence identical to that of the normal β-chain. The mechanism he proposed to explain this finding proved to be consistent with all of the fusion globin genes since discovered. It involves mispairing during meiosis and crossing over* at a region in the DNA sequence that codes for amino acid sequence, as illustrated in Figure 4. Four different Lepore hemoglobins with differing points of crossover have been reported, as have four different anti-Lepore variants. The recombinant chromosomes differ in that the normal δ- and β-globin loci are absent from the chromosome carrying the Lepore fusion gene and are retained on the chromosome with the anti-Lepore δβ fusion gene (see chapter by Wrightstone for list of all reported variants).

Another abnormal hemoglobin, Hb Kenya, has an N-terminal amino acid sequence identical to the $^{A}\gamma$ globin and a C-terminal sequence identical to the normal β-chain.[36,37] This

* Use of the adjective "nonhomologous" to describe the crossover is ambiguous. The parental chromosomes involved are homologs. The tandemly duplicated globin loci are homologous because of common evolutionary ancestry. The retention of homology, in fact, probably accounts for the similarity in DNA sequence that permits the mispairing. To the extent that they represent separate replicates of the common ancestral globin gene, the pairing is out of register and abnormal, but it is between homologous DNA sequences. Thus it is incestuous, perhaps, but not nonhomologous.

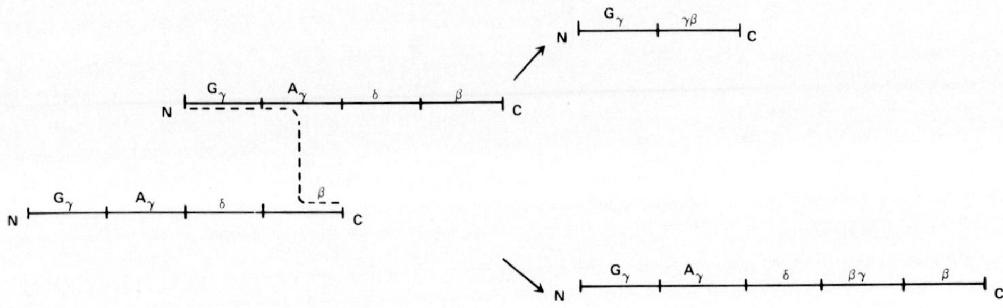

FIGURE 5. Origin of the Kenya globin chain by crossing over between misaligned $^{A}\gamma$- and β-globin genes.

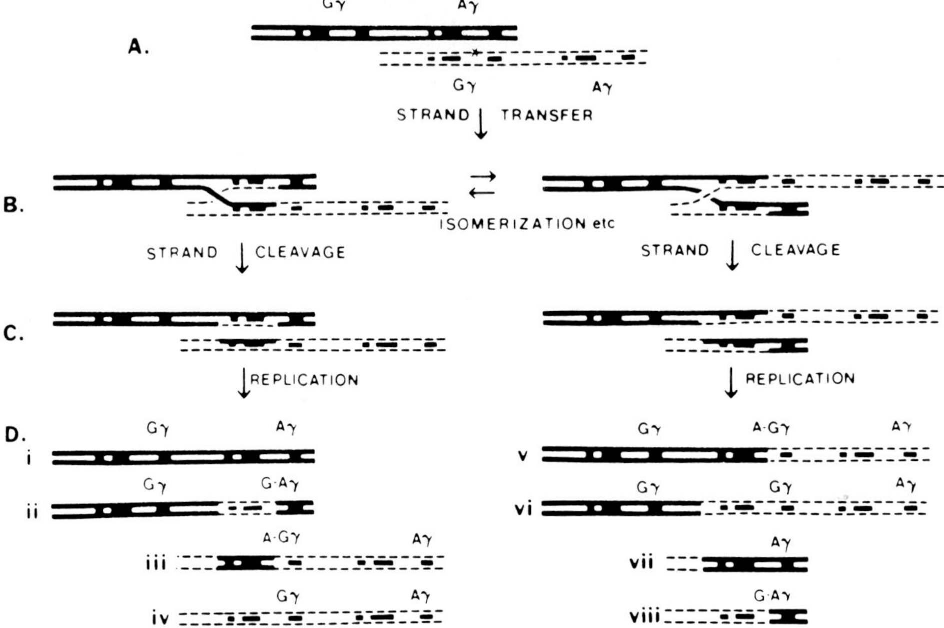

FIGURE 6. Diagrammatic model for gene conversion between $^{G}\gamma 0$ and $^{A}\gamma$-globin genes. Two misaligned chromosomes are shown as continuous and dashed lines containing black bars to indicate coding sequences. (A) Recombination is initiated at the simple sequence hotspot (X) in the second intervening sequence. (B) Strand transfer, isomerization, branch migration, and ligation yield the isomers. (C) Strand cleavage leads to the intermediate heteroduplex products. (D) DNA replication then leads to the final products. The products ii and iii, vi and vii show conversion. (From Slightom et al., *Cell,* 21, 627, 1980. With permission.)

fusion gene product, like that for Hb Lepore, is thought to result from a crossover product of mispaired $^{A}\gamma$ and β-loci. Figure 5 illustrates the two theoretical products, of which the Hb Kenya chromosome lacks the genetic loci for $^{A}\gamma$-, and δ-, and β-globins. This interpretation is in keeping with the phenotypes of subjects heterozygous for Hb Kenya and one individual doubly heterozygous for Hb Kenya and Hb S.

In addition to structural characterization of the fusion gene products, the key information supporting the polarity as diagrammed is that the individual homozygous for Hb Lepore produces no Hb A or Hb A_2,[38] and the individual doubly heterozygous for Hb Kenya and HbS produces no Hb A and half-normal amounts of Hb A_2.[37] These observations predicted that the polarity of globin structure genes within the non-α-cistron would be as diagrammed in Figure 6. Flavell et al.[39] have now demonstrated that the Lepore genomic DNA is indeed rearranged as Baglioni suggested from amino acid sequences in 1962.

In fact, as shown in Figure 2 of the Schroeder chapter, the two globin cistrons are much larger than anticipated now that the DNA sequences are known. In addition, the coding regions (exons) are separated by intervening sequences both flanking and within (introns) each gene. Individual globin genes are about 1.5 kilobases (kb) in length, including the transcribed introns. They are separated by more than 3 kb from each other, and pseudogenes occur at both the α- and non-α-cistron.

The same pattern of genomic arrangement of globin genes, including the position of the two introns, is found in all vertebrates thus far studied. This is presumed to reflect a similar arrangement in the ancestral gene that diverged into separate classes about 500 million years ago. The structural information at the DNA level has been well reviewed by Efstratiadis et al.,[5] Jeffreys,[6] and Dahl et al.[40] Gilbert[41] first suggested that the separate exons may reflect functional protein domains and that new proteins with different functions may have evolved by recombination between two genes within their introns. Craik et al.[42] have recently pointed out that intron-exon junctions for a number of proteins, including globins, map to amino acid residues located at the protein surface, suggesting a restriction on the permitted position of introns within a gene.

Pseudogenes

The occurrence of additional gene sequences, ψβ and ψα, that retain homology with globin genes but are no longer functional, was another unexpected finding when genomic DNA was studied. These are presumed to represent ancient gene duplications followed by mutations that result in premature termination or failure of normal processing of the pseudogene transcript.

Concerted Evolution

Within the globin gene family, there has been less divergence of certain pairs of genes than would be expected from the time interval since the ancestral gene underwent duplication. This is true of the two γ-globin loci and of the two α-globin loci. The tendency of a family of genes to evolve in unison was termed "concerted evolution" by Zimmer et al.[43] to imply that a causal relation accounts for this process. Two mechanisms have been proposed. The first involves mispairing of homologous duplicated genes followed by unequal crossover to give daughter chromosomes with one fewer and one extra globin locus. There is good evidence to believe that such a process can occur, since individuals with one, two, or three α-globin genes have been found. (See also chapter by Antonarakis and Kazazian.) In addition, Lauer et al.[44] derived genomic clones from the human gene library in which the same deletion of one of the two α-globin genes that is observed in α-thalassemia 2 occurred during propagation in phage. Multiple rounds of unequal crossing over between α-globin genes that had diverged, followed by fixation in the population of chromosomes carrying identical genes, could account for concerted evolution.

A second mechanism to account for concerted evolution is termed "gene conversion". Slightom et al.[7] propose this explanation for retention of homology between the $^{G}\gamma$ and $^{A}\gamma$ loci. They compared DNA nucleotide sequences for these two loci from one chromosome, and of the $^{A}\gamma$ locus of the other chromosome of the same individual. No differences were present in the coding regions other than one expected at residue 36. Near the middle of the large intervening sequence all three have a long series of TG dinucleotide repeats. Other parts of the silent regions sequenced showed striking shared homology of the smaller intervening sequence and of the regions at the 5′ and 3′ ends of the larger intervening sequence. There was also a greater homology in comparisons of the nonallelic $^{G}\gamma$ vs. $^{A}\gamma$ at the 5′ two thirds of these genes, and of the allelic $^{A}\gamma$ loci at the 3′ one third. Figure 6, from their paper, illustrates a model for gene conversion in which mispairing and recombination at the middle of the second intervening sequence was followed by strand transfer, isomerization, branch migration and ligation, strand cleavage to give intermediate heteroduplexes, and DNA replication to produce the final products, of which ii and iii, vi and vii show the conversion outcomes. This more complicated intergenic exchange could occur between sister chromatids or between homologs, and need not alter the copy number of a family of genes.

The lack of evidence for gene conversion between the δ- and β-loci may relate to divergence of both coding and noncoding regions. Nonetheless, Petes[45] has recently suggested that δ-chain variants affecting residues known to differ from the β-chain in two of three examples reverted to the β-chain sequence. They could represent back mutations, or intrachromosomal gene conversion.

GENETIC CONTROL

The normal switch from embryonic to fetal to adult types of globin chain production has been of interest for many years. Newer techniques are providing some insights to the underlying genetic mechanisms. In a series of papers, Weintraub et al.[46-50] have demonstrated that the chromatin structure is altered at the transcriptional site. They used mild digestion of chick red cell nuclei with DNAase-I and obtained fragments that correspond to a DNA domain which spans the active globin gene and extends 7 kb from the 5′ end. This "hypersensitive" DNA is single stranded and is unmethylated as compared with chromatin outside the active domain. These changes are specific for erythrocytes. When cells from 5- and 14-day-old chicks were compared, the embryonic globin genes had these chromatin changes at 5 days, and the adult globin genes at 14 days. Other tissues, including brain, liver, fibroblasts, and oviduct, did not contain hypersensitive sites at the globin gene regions.

Comparisons of the nucleotide sequences of the 5′ flanking region for a number of eukaryotic genes, including globins, show consensus homologies that include a CCAAT sequence about 80 nucleotides and an ATA sequence about 30 nucleotides upstream from the mRNA capping site. These constant sequences are thought to be necessary for proper initiation of transcription. There is also considerable retention of homology for other nucleotide positions in the 5′ flanking region in all globin genes in addition to the ATA and CCAAT boxes. That for δ-globin shows the greatest divergence from other non-α-loci.[5]

This is in keeping with recent reports of the expression of globin genes in transfected monkey kidney cells. Humphries et al.[51] prepared SV 40 vectors containing the 5′ flanking regions and genes for human α-, β-, and δ-globin. The α-globin gene was expressed as measured by production of mRNA whether or not the SV 40 vector contained a 72 base pair (bp) repeat, which enhances the expression of genetic material in this system. The δ- and β-genes were expressed only if the vector contained the enhancing sequence and the amount of β-mRNA was approximately 50 times greater than that of δ-mRNA. This is what would be predicted if the amounts of δ(2 to 3%) and β(97 to 98%) containing tetramers in normal red cells is controlled at the level of transcription.

Comparisons of noncoding genomic sequences from subjects with a variety of thalassemias as discussed in the chapter by Antonarakis and Kazazian also suggests that information contained in the nucleotide sequences of these silent regions is essential for the control of normal sequential globin gene expression.

The α_2- and α_1-globin genes are identical from the 5′ capping site through the UAA termination codon. They differ in the 110-nucleotide long sequence at the 3′ end of the mRNA by 18 substitutions.[53] It is of interest that while transcription is three-fold greater for α_2 mRNA, translation of α_1 mRNA is more efficient.[54] The net result in normal subjects is the production of the same amount of gene product from each locus.

GENETIC MECHANISMS ACCOUNTING FOR ABNORMAL GLOBIN SYNTHESIS

Abnormalities in globin synthesis may be in amount (resulting in an imbalance of chain production) or in structure.

Imbalance of Chain Production

Shortly after the subunits of hemoglobin were identified, it became apparent that normally the biosynthesis of globin chains and their assembly into tetramers is balanced. The progression of hemoglobin types from embryonic to adult life (Table 1) presupposes equal rates of production of α- and non-α-subunits. This balance could theoretically be upset if an increase or decrease in production differentially affected either class of globin genes.

Decreased or absent production of α-chains results in a spectrum of phenotypes designated α-thalassemia. These range in severity from a "silent carrier" to a lethal form, the hydrops fetalis phenotype in which no α-chain is produced. At the non-α-cistron, defects in biosynthesis of β- and/or δ-chains have been recognized and the corresponding phenotypes designated β- or δ-thalassemia, or hereditary persistence of fetal hemoglobin. The molecular basis of thalassemias has proven to be a productive model for studying the control of human genes. This information has been collected in several recent reviews, including those by Bunn et al.[52] and Weatherall and Clegg[38] and is covered in the chapter by Antonarakis and Kazazian.

Altered Globin Structure

The structure of human globin chains, both normal and abnormal, is well known. It encompasses a large literature beginning with the classic papers by Pauling et al.[55] and Ingram.[56] Since 1976, the International Hemoglobin Information Center has provided periodically updated lists of hemoglobin variants.[57] (See chapter by Wrightstone) At this writing, the total includes 116 different alleles at the α-globin loci and 198 different alleles at the β-globin locus that differ from the wild type by a single amino acid substitution.

The agreement of the codon changes that account for hemoglobin variants with the genetic code has been reviewed by Perutz and Lehmann,[58] Bunn et al.,[52] and Wilson et al.[59] With rare exceptions, all amino acid substitutions can be accounted for as a single base change, and the autosomal inheritance of these variants indicates a change in the DNA of the structural gene. As might be expected, a number of mutations that result in marked instability of the globin chain and severe hemolytic anemia have occurred as sporadic cases.[52,60]

In addition to the single base change and the fusion gene products discussed above, two other types of variant have been found. Deletions of one or more adjacent amino acid residues have thus far been detected in 11 β-chain variants and 1 α-chain variant. These are believed to result from meiotic errors in synapsis of the homologous genes with crossing over similar to that described for fusion gene products. Efstratiadis et al.[5] have noted the presence of short, direct repeats of nucleotides flanking such deleted residues in the β-chain. This is not the case for the only α-chain deletion. One variant, Hb McKees Rock,[61] lacks the last two C-terminal amino acids, Tyr-His. This could have resulted from a frame shift during synapsis, or it could represent a "nonsense" mutation or termination (UAU→UAA/G) mutation at the 145th codon.

Additions of amino acids to the normal globin sequence have also been discovered. Most of these represent elongations beyond the normal C-terminal residue due either to a frameshift mutation or a base change in the normal termination codon to a triplet that permits translation. Hb Constant Spring[62] was the first such example. The final mechanism, illustrated by Hb Grady,[63] represents an insertion of three repeating residues, Glu-Phe-Thr, between the 118th and 119th position in the normal β-globin sequence.

ADDENDUM

Since this chapter was prepared, two extensive and authoritative reviews of the literature on hemoglobin have been published.[64,65] Even more recently, the pattern of ancestral, non-α globin gene loci has been reinterpreted, based on new genomic DNA comparisons.[66,68] Primate 4β genes are now thought to be orthologous to a common ancestral gene, called η, such that the cluster of tandem duplicates 5′-ε-γ-η-δ-β-3′ is dated to 200 to 100 M year. Finally, a new class of human globin mutants with N-terminal extensions of the β-chain has been identified.[69-73] In the three examples, the methionine residue at the initiation site is not cleaved off of the completed chain, which is thus 147 instead of 146 amino acids in length. This process is thought to be enzymic due to a methionyl aminopeptidase and is prevented in Hb Long Island because the normal histidine at residue two is replaced by proline.[69-71] In Hb South Florida the N-terminal value is substituted by methionine,[72] and in Hb Doha the N-terminal value is replaced by glutamic acid.[73] It is of interest that substitution of the histidine at residue two by glutamine in Hb Okayama[74] does not prevent removal of the initiating methionine residue.

REFERENCES

1. **Fitch, W. M.,** Evolutionary variability in hemoglobins, *Haematol. Bluttransfus.*, 10, 199, 1972.
2. **Dayhoff, M. O., Hunt, L. T., McLaughlin, P. J., and Jones, D. D.,** Gene duplications in evolution: the globins, in *Atlas of Protein Sequence and Structure 1972*, Dayhoff, M. O., Ed., National Biomedical Research Foundation, Washington, D.C., 1972, 17.
3. **Goodman, M., Moore, G. W., and Matsuda, G.,** Evolution of vertebrate hemoglobin amino acid sequences, in *Isozymes. IV. Genetics and Evolution*, Markert, C. L., Ed., Academic Press, New York, 1975, 181.
4. **Coates, M.,** Hemoglobin function in the vertebrates: an evolutionary model, *Aust. J. Biol. Sci.*, 28, 367, 1975.
5. **Efstratiadis, A., Posakony, J. W., Maniatis, T., Lawn, R. W., O'Connell, C., Spritz, R. A., DeRiel, J. K., Forget, B. G., Weissman, S. M., Slightom, J. L., Blechl, A. E., Smithies, O., Baralle, F. E., Shoulders, C. C., and Proudfoot, N. J.,** The structure and evolution of the human β-globin gene family, *Cell*, 21, 653, 1980.
6. **Jeffreys, A. J.,** Recent studies of gene evolution using recombinant DNA, in *Genetic Engineering 2*, Williamson, R., Ed., Academic Press, New York, 1981, 1.
7. **Slightom, J. L., Blechl, A. E., and Smithies, O.,** Human fetal $^{G}\gamma$- and $^{A}\gamma$-globin genes: complete nucleotide sequences suggest that DNA can be exchanged between these duplicated genes, *Cell*, 21, 627, 1980.
8. **Liebhaber, S. A., Goossens, M., and Kan, Y. W.,** Homology and concerted evolution at the α1 and α2 loci of human α-globin, *Nature (London)*, 290, 26, 1981.
9. **Lerner, I. M.,** *Heredity, Evolution and Society*, W. H. Freeman, San Francisco, 1968, 22.
10. **Isaacks, R. E., Harkness, D. R., Goldman, P. H., Adler, J. L., and Kim, C. Y.,** Studies on avian erythrocyte metabolism. VII. Effect of inositol pentaphosphate and other organic phosphates on oxygen affinity of the embryonic and adult-type hemoglobins of the turkey embryo, *Hemoglobin*, 1, 577, 1977.
11. **Ohno, S.,** *Evolution by Gene Duplication*, Springer-Verlag, Basel, 1970, 59.
12. **Czelusniak, J., Goodman, M., Hewett-Emmett, D., Weiss, M. L., Venta, P. J., and Tashian, R. E.,** Phylogenetic origins and adaptive evolution of avian and mammalian haemoglobin genes, *Nature (London)*, 298, 297, 1982.
13. **Boyer, S. H., Crosby, E. F., Noyes, A. N., Fuller, G. F., Leslie, S. E., Donaldson, L. J., Vrablik, G. R., Shaefer, E. W., Jr., and Thurman, L. F.,** Evolution of primate hemoglobin β and δ chains, *Biochem. Genet.*, 5, 405, 1971.
14. **Huisman, T. H. J.,** Structural aspects of fetal and adult hemoglobins from nonanemic ruminants, *Ann. N. Y. Acad. Sci.*, 241, 392, 1974.
15. **Gilman, J. G.,** Rodent hemoglobin structure: a comparison of several species of mice, *Ann. N.Y. Acad. Sci.*, 241, 416, 1974.

16. **Dhindsa, D. S., Hoversland, A. S., and Templeton, J. W.,** Postnatal changes in oxygen affinity and concentrations of 2,3-diphosphoglycerate in dog blood, *Biol. Neonat.*, 20, 226, 1972.
17. **Novy, M. J., Hoversland, A. S., Koler, R. D., and Metcalfe, J.,** A comparison of oxygen affinity and hemoglobin type in the adult and fetal miniature pig, *Fed. Proc.*, 26, 485, 1967.
18. **Schroeder, W. A., Huisman, T. H. J., Shelton, J. R., Shelton, J. B., Kleihauer, E. F., Dozy, A. M., and Robberson, B.,** Evidence for multiple structural genes for the γ chain of human fetal hemoglobin, *Proc. Natl. Acad. Sci. U.S.A.*, 60, 537, 1968.
19. **Huisman, T. H. J., Schroeder, W. A., Dozy, A. M., Shelton, J. R., Shelton, J. B., Boyd, E. M., and Apell, G.,** Evidence for multiple structural genes for the gamma chain of human fetal hemoglobin in hereditary persistence of fetal hemoglobin, *Ann. N.Y. Acad. Sci.*, 165, 320, 1969.
20. **Schroeder, W. A., Huisman, T. H. J., Shelton, J. R., Shelton, J. B., Apell, G., and Bouver, N.,** Heterogeneity of fetal hemoglobin in β-thalassemia of the Negro, *Am. J. Hum. Genet.*, 22, 505, 1970.
21. **Huisman, T. H. J., Schroeder, W. A., Stamatoyannopoulos, G., Bouver, N., Shelton, J. R., Shelton, J. B., and Apell, G.,** Nature of fetal hemoglobin in the Greek type of hereditary persistence of fetal hemoglobin with and without concurrent β-thalassemia, *J. Clin. Invest.*, 49, 1035, 1970.
22. **Stamatoyannopoulos, G., Schroeder, W. A., Huisman, T. H. J., Shelton, J. R., Shelton, J. B., Apell, G., and Bouver, N.,** Nature of foetal haemoglobin in F-thalassemia, *Br. J. Haematol.*, 21, 633, 1971.
23. **Schroeder, W. A., Shelton, J. R., Shelton, J. B., Apell, G., Huisman, T. H. J., and Bouver, N. G.,** World-wide occurrence of nonallelic genes for the γ chain of human foetal haemoglobin in newborns, *Nature (New Biol.)*, 240, 273, 1972.
24. **Ricco, G., Mazza, U., Turi, R. M., Pich, P. G., Camaschella, C., Saglio, G., and Bernini, L. F.,** Significance of a new type of human fetal hemoglobin carrying a replacement isoleucine → threonine at position 75 (E19) of the γ chain, *Hum. Genet.*, 32, 305, 1976.
25. **Melderis, H., Steinheider, G., and Ostertag, W.,** Evidence for a unique kind of α-type globin chain in early mammalian embryos, *Nature (London)*, 250, 774, 1974.
26. **Chapman, B. S., Tobin, A. J., and Hood, L. E.,** Complete amino acid sequences of the major early embryonic α-like globins of the chiken, *J. Biol. Chem.*, 255, 9051, 1980.
27. **Deisseroth, A., Nienhuis, A., Turner, P., Velez, R., and Anderson, W. F.,** Localization of the human α-globin structural gene to chromosome 16 in somatic cell hybrids by molecular hybridization assay, *Cell*, 12, 205, 1977.
28. **Deisseroth, A., Nienhuis, A., Ruddle, F., Lawrence, J., and Turner, P.,** Chromosomal localization of the human β globin gene to human chromosome 11, *Blood*, 50 (Suppl. 1), 105, 1977.
29. **Gusella, J., Varsanyi-Breiner, A., Kao, F., Jones, C., Puck, T. T., Keys, C., Orkin, S., and Housman, D.,** Precise localization of human β-globin gene complex on chromosome 11, *Proc. Natl. Acad. Sci. U.S.A.*, 76, 5239, 1979.
30. **Gerhard, D. S., Kawasaki, E. S., Bancroft, F. C., and Szabo, P.,** Localization of a unique gene by direct hybridization *in situ*, *Proc. Natl. Acad. Sci. U.S.A.*, 78, 3755, 1981.
31. **Malcolm, S., Barton, P., Murphy, C., and Ferguson-Smith, M. A.,** Chromosomal localization of a single copy gene by in situ hybridization — human β-globin genes on the short arm of chromosome 11, *Ann. Hum. Genet.*, 45, 135, 1981.
32. **Jeffreys, A. J., Wilson, V., Wood, D., and Simons, J. P.,** Linkage of adult α- and β-globin genes in *X. laevis* and gene duplication by tetraploidization, *Cell*, 21, 555, 1980.
33. **Gerald, P. S. and Diamond, L. K.,** The diagnosis of thalassemia trait by starch block electrophoresis of the hemoglobin, *Blood*, 13, 61, 1958.
34. **Baglioni, C.,** The fusion of two peptide chains in hemoglobin Lepore and its interpretation as a genetic deletion, *Proc. Natl. Acad. Sci. U.S.A.*, 48, 1880, 1962.
35. **Benz, E. J. and Forget, B. G.,** The molecular genetics of the thalassemia syndromes, in *Progress in Hematology*, Vol. 9, Brown, E. B., Ed., Grune & Stratton, New York, 1975, 107.
36. **Huisman, T. H. J., Wrightstone, R. N., Wilson, J. B., and Schroeder, W. A.,** Hemoglobin Kenya, the product of fusion of γ and β polypeptide chains, *Arch. Biochem. Biophys.*, 153, 850, 1972.
37. **Kendall, A. G., Ojwang, P. J., Schroeder, W. A., and Huisman, T. H. J.,** Hemoglobin Kenya, the product of a γ-β fusion gene: studies of the family, *Am. J. Hum. Genet.*, 25, 548, 1973.
38. **Weatherall, D. J. and Clegg, J. B.,** *The Thalassemia Syndromes*, 3rd ed., Blackwell Scientific, Oxford, 1981.
39. **Flavell, R. A., Kooter, J. M., DeBoer, E., Little, P. F. R., and Williamson, R.,** Analysis of the β-δ-globin gene loci in normal and Hb Lepore DNA: direct determination of gene linkage and intergene distance, *Cell*, 15, 25, 1978.
40. **Dahl, H. H., Flavell, R. A., and Grosveld, F. G.,** The use of genomic libraries for the isolation and study of eukaryotic genes, *Genetic Engineering 2*, Williamson, R., Ed., Academic Press, New York, 1981, 49.

41. **Gilbert, W.,** Why genes in pieces?, *Nature (London),* 271, 501, 1978.
42. **Craik, C. S., Sprang, S., Fletterick, R., and Rutter, W. J.,** Intron-exon splice junctions map at protein surfaces, *Nature (London),* 299, 180, 1982.
43. **Zimmer, E. A., Martin, S. L., Beverly, S. M., Kan, Y. W., and Wilson, A. C.,** Rapid duplication and loss of genes coding for the α chains of hemoglobin, *Proc. Natl. Acad. Sci. U.S.A.,* 77, 2158, 1980.
44. **Lauer, J., Che-Kun, J. S., and Maniatis, T.,** The chromosomal arrangement of human α-like globin genes: sequence homology and α-globin gene deletions, *Cell,* 20, 119, 1980.
45. **Petes, T. D.,** Evidence that structural variants within the human δ-globin protein may reflect genetic interactions between the δ- and β-globin genes, *Am. J. Hum. Genet.,* 34, 820, 1982.
46. **Alberts, B., Worcel, A., and Weintraub, H.,** On the biological implications of chromatin structure, in *Proceedings of the International Symposium on the Eukaryotic Genome,* Bradbury, M., Ed., Academic Press, New York, 1977, 165.
47. **Stalder, J., Groudine, M., Dodgson, J. B., Engel, J. D., and Weintraub, H.,** Hb switching in chickens, *Cell,* 19, 973, 1980.
48. **Stalder, J., Larsen, A., Engel, J. D., Dolan, M., Groudine, M., and Weintraub, H.,** Tissue specific DNA cleavages in the globin chromatin domain induced by DNAse I, *Cell,* 20, 451, 1980.
49. **Weintraub, H., Larsen, A., and Groudine, M.,** α-Globin gene switching during the development of chicken embryos: expression and chromosome structure, *Cell,* 24, 333, 1981.
50. **Groudine, M. and Weintraub, H.,** Propagation of globin DNAase I — hypersensitive sites in absence of factors required for induction: a possible mechanism for determination, *Cell,* 30, 131, 1982.
51. **Humphries, R. K., Ley, T., Turner, P., Moulton, A. D., and Nienhuis, A. W.,** Differences in human α-, β- and δ-globin gene expression in monkey kidney cells, *Cell,* 30, 173, 1982.
52. **Bunn, H. F., Forget, B. G., and Ranney, H. M.,** *Human Hemoglobins,* W. B. Saunders, Philadelphia, 1977, 101.
53. **Michelson, A. M. and Orkin, S. H.,** The 3′ untranslated regions of the duplicated human α-globin genes are unexpectedly divergent, *Cell,* 22, 371, 1980.
54. **Liebhaber, S. A. and Kan, Y. W.,** Different rates of mRNA translation balance the expression of the two human α-globin loci, *J. Biol. Chem.,* 257, 11852, 1982.
55. **Pauling, L., Itano, H. A., Singer, S. J., and Wells, I. C.,** Sickle-cell anemia, a molecular disease, *Science,* 110, 543, 1949.
56. **Ingram, V. M.,** Abnormal human haemoglobins. II. The chemical difference between normal and sickle cell haemoglobins, *Biochim. Biophys. Acta,* 36, 402, 1959.
57. **Wrightstone, R. N.,** International hemoglobin information center, *Hemoglobin,* 6, 258, 1982.
58. **Perutz, M. F.,** Stereochemistry of cooperative effects in haemoglobin, *Nature (London),* 228, 726, 1970.
59. **Wilson, J. T., Marotta, C. A., Forget, B. G., and Weissman, S. M.,** Structure of human hemoglobin messenger RNA and its relation to hemoglobinopathies, *Trans. Am. Assoc. Phys.,* 90, 117, 1977.
60. **Jones, R. T., Koler, R. D., Duerst, M., and Stocklen, Z.,** Hemoglobin Casper, G8 β106 Leu → Pro: further evidence that hemoglobin mutations are not random, in *Hemoglobin and Red Cell Structure and Function,* Brewer, G., Ed., Plenum Press, New York, 1972, 79.
61. **Winslow, R. M., Swenberg, M. L., and Gross, E.,** Hemoglobin McKees Rock (α_2 β_2 145 Tyr → Term). A human "nonsense" mutation leading to a shortened β-chain, *J. Clin. Invest.,* 57, 772, 1976.
62. **Clegg, J. B., Weatherall, D. J., and Milner, P. F.,** Haemoglobin Constant Spring. A chain termination mutant?, *Nature (London),* 234, 337, 1971.
63. **Huisman, T. H. J., Wilson, J. B., Gravely, M., and Hubbard, M.,** Hemoglobin Grady: the first example of a variant with elongated chains due to an insertion of residues, *Proc. Natl. Acad. Sci. U.S.A.,* 71, 3270, 1974.
64. **Collins, F. S. and Weissman, S. M.,** The molecular genetics of human hemoglobin, *Prog. Nucleic Acid Res. Mol. Biol.,* 31, 317, 1984.
65. **Bunn, H. F. and Forget, B. G.,** *Hemoglobin: Molecular Genetic and Clinical Aspects,* W. B. Saunders, Philadelphia, 1986.
66. **Goodman, M., Koop, B. F., Czelusniak, J., Weiss, M. L., and Slightom, J. L.,** The η-globin gene. Its long evolutionary history in the β-globin gene family of mammals, *J. Mol. Biol.,* 180, 803, 1984.
67. **Harris, S., Barrie, P., Weiss, M. L., and Jeffreys, A. J.,** The primate $\chi\beta^1$ gene. An ancient β-globin pseudogene, *J. Mol. Biol.,* 180, 785, 1984.
68. **Koop, B. F., Goodman, M., Xu, P., Chan, K., and Slightom, J. L.,** Primate η-globin DNA sequences and man's place among the great apes, *Nature (London),* 319, 234, 1986.
69. **Barwick, R. C., Jones, R. T., Head, C. G., Shih, M., Prchal, J. T., and Shih, D.,** Hb-Long Island: a hemoglobin variant with a methionyl extension at the NH_2 terminus and a prolyl substitution for the normal histidyl residue 2 of the β chain, *Proc. Natl. Acad. Sci. U.S.A.,* 82, 4602, 1985.
70. **Blouquit, Y., Arous, N., Lena, D., Delanoe-Garin, J., Lacombe, C., Bardakdjian, J., Vovan, L., Orsini, A., Rosa, J., and Galacteros, F.,** Hb Marseille [$\alpha_2\beta_2$ N methionyl-2(NA_2) his→pro]: a new β chain variant having an extended N-terminus, *FEBS Lett.,* 178, 315, 1984.

71. **Prchal, J. T., Cashman, D. P., and Kan, Y. W.,** Hb Long Island [β-1(NA-1) met; β(NA2) his→pro] is caused by a single mutation (A to C) resulting in a failure to cleave N-terminal methionine, *Proc. Natl. Acad. Sci. U.S.A.*, 83, 24, 1986.
72. **Boissel, J., Kasper, T., Shah, S. C., Malone, J. I., and Bunn, H. F.,** NH_2-terminal processing of proteins — Hemoglobin South Florida, a new variant with retention of initiator methionine and N-α acetylation, *Proc. Natl. Acad. Sci., U.S.A.*, 82, 8448, 1985.
73. **Kamel, K., El-Najjar, A., Webber, B. B., Chen, S. S., Wilson, J. B., Kutlar, A., and Huisman, T. H. J.,** Hb Doha or $\alpha_2\beta_2$[X-N-met-1(NA1) val→glu]; a new β chain abnormal hemoglobin observed in a Qatari female, *Biochim. Biophys. Acta*, 831, 257, 1985.
74. **Harano, T., Harano, K., Shibata, S., Veda, S., Mori, H., and Arimsa, N.,** Hemoglobin Okayama [β2 (NA2) his→gln]; a new 'silent' hemoglobin variant with substituted amino acid residue at the 2,3-diphosphoglycerate site, *FEBS Lett.*, 156, 20, 1983.

THE THREE-DIMENSIONAL STRUCTURE OF HEMOGLOBIN*

K. W. Olsen

The determination of the three-dimensional structure of hemoglobin by Perutz and coworkers is a major milestone in the progress of biochemistry. This work makes possible the study of the stereochemical role of each amino acid residue in the function of hemoglobin. As a result, many physiologically and chemically important aspects of hematology, such as the Bohr effect, the allosteric mechanism of oxygen binding, and the nature of abnormal hemoglobins, can be explained by the three-dimensional structure of this protein. The subject has been reviewed numerous times[1-5,147-151] and is discussed in every modern biochemistry text.[6-10] In this chapter, the structure of hemoglobin will be briefly described and related to its function. The three-dimensional data will be tabulated, so that they can be applied to future problems involving hemoglobin.

THE GLOBIN FOLD

The globin fold is the characteristic tertiary structure of the oxygen-binding hemoproteins. It has been demonstrated by X-ray crystallography (Tables 1 and 2), not only in hemoglobins and myoglobins[11-36] of several different species, but also in the globins of the sea lamprey,[23] the midge larva,[19,20] and the bloodworm.[21,22] Although the sequences of these proteins differ by as much as 87%,[37] the tertiary structure is maintained, as can be seen in the stereo-pair drawings of Figure 1.** There are over 50 known globin sequences that have internal gaps when compared with each other. Thus, it is necessary to have a residue numbering system based on the three-dimensional structure. The globin fold (Figure 2) consists of eight helical segments, labeled A through H, which are connected by nonhelical regions and are named for the helices that they connect. For example, the region between helices A and B is the AB section. The region from amino terminus to the start of the first helical is named NA, while that from the end of the H helix to the carboxyl terminus is called HC. The first residue of the A helix is designated as A1, the second as A2, and so forth. The sequences of the human myoglobin[38] and hemoglobin[39-42] chains are given in Table 3 with these designations. The advantage of this numbering system is that homologous residues will always have the same designation. Thus the proximal histidine that binds the iron of the heme is at position F8, although it is residue 87 in the α-chain and 92 in the β-chain. Since the horse methemoglobin is the most accurately determined of these crystal structures, it will be described first, and the other proteins will be related to it.

The globin fold (Figure 2) is a compact structure with dimensions of 45 × 35 × 25 Å.[11] The eight helical segments of the globin fold account for about 75% of the residues. It should be noted, however, that the X-ray structures of the various globins do differ from each other. Even two closely related proteins, such as seal and sperm whale myoglobin that differ at only 26 of their 153 residues, have a root mean-square distance of 1.5 Å between equivalent pairs of α-carbons.[171]

The differences between myoglobin and the α- and β-chains of hemoglobin are summarized in Table 4. Helix D is not present in the α-chain, and the AB connecting segment is absent in the β-chain. Most of the segments are α-helices, but segment C is a 3_{10} helix in both hemoglobin chains, and segment F is followed by one turn of π-helix,[4,29] as shown in Figures

* All figures and tables for this chapter follow text.

** Stereoviewers are available from Edmond Scientific Company, Barrington, N.J. 08007; Taylor-Merchant Corporation, 25 West 45th Street, New York, N.Y. 10036; Lansing Instrument Corporation, Lansing, Mich. A pair of enlarging lenses with 85-mm focal lengths, mounted 70 mm apart in cardboard, is also adequate.

6 and 7. The conformational parameters for the three types of helices are given in Table 5, and they are illustrated in Figures 3 to 5. Some of the globin helices have irregular hydrogen bonds. This is particularly true of the heme-linked helices E and F and of the FG corner (Figures 6 to 10). These helices contain few linear hydrogen bonds, and several bifurcated hydrogen bonds are formed. Helix E is more regular in the α-subunit than in the β-subunit (Figures 8 and 9). The π-helix involving F7 to FG3 is stabilized by a hydrogen bond, from the side chain of Arg FG4(92) α to the main chain carbonyl of Lys (FG2(90)α (Figure 6) in the α-subunit, and by a hydrogen bond from the imidazole of His FG4(97)β to the carbonyl of Cys F9(93)β in the β-chain. The entire hydrogen bonding network for the horse methemoglobin molecule is given in Figures 11 and 12.* The secondary and tertiary structures of the α- and β-chains of methemoglobin are shown in Figures 13 and 14.

FORCES STABILIZING THE GLOBIN FOLD

The major forces that determine the tertiary structures of proteins are thought to be hydrophobic interactions.[47,48] The strength of these interactions depends on the increase in the entropy of the solution, when the nonpolar side chains are packed together on the interior of the protein. Thus the hydrophobic residues are found on the interior of the globin fold, and the hydrophilic ones are on the exterior (Figure 15). Serine and threonine residues that are occasionally found on the interior form hydrogen bonds with other residues, but nonpolar residues are not generally found at internal positions, as shown in Table 6.[49] In contrast, only a few of the surface or surface-crevice residues are consistently nonpolar (Table 7). The variation in the hydrophobicity of partially buried residues may be a source of species variation in the stability of the tertiary structure.[50] The residue variability due to species differences in myoglobins and hemoglobins is summarized in Table 8. These data emphasize the importance of having nonpolar residues at internal positions for the maintenance of the globin fold. Thus a mutation that introduces a charged residue into one of these positions will produce an unstable, abnormal hemoglobin.[51]

Calculations of the free energy contributions from individual pairs of charged residues in sperm whale metmyoglobin have shown that the native structure receives a net stabilization from intramolecular electrostatic interactions.[172,173] Much of this stabilization energy is provided by specific charge-pairs that are very highly conserved among 53 mammalian myoglobin species. The charge sites play a dual role in both stabilizing and solubilizing the protein. Examination of the primary stabilizing interactions of the charge pairs indicated a possible major role for these interactions in the nucleation and docking stages.

THE HEME ENVIRONMENT

The structure and environment of the heme groups is critically important to the function of hemoglobin. The porphyrin rings in methemoglobin appear to be planar, although small deformations may be present, since they would not be detectable in a 2.0-Å resolution electron density map. The distance that the iron atom is displaced from the plane of the porphyrin ring depends on both the ligands and the spin state of the iron. A detailed discussion of spin states can be found in Reference 3. The spin states of various hemoglobin derivatives

* The amino acid residues discussed in this chapter are abbreviated with the normal three-letter code, the segment name and number, the sequence position number in parentheses, and the chain designation. Figures 11 and 12 use the one-letter code for the amino acids. The codes are as follows: alanine, Ala, A; arginine, Arg, R; asparagine, Asn, N; aspartic acid, Asp, D; cysteine, Cys, C; glutamine, Gln, Q; Glutamic acid, Glu, E; glycine, Gly, G; histidine, His, H; isoleucine, Ile, I; leucine, Leu, L; lysine, Lys, K; methionine, Met, M; phenylalanine, Phe, F; proline, Pro, P; serine, Ser, S; threonine, Thr, T; tryptophan, Trp, W; tyrosine, Tyr, Y; and valine, Val, V. Asx refers to either aspartic acid or asparagine (not established).

are listed in Table 9. The high-spin iron atom in both deoxy- and methemoglobin should have a radius that is too large to fit into the plane of the porphyrin. This effect is seen only in deoxy- and metmyoglobin, deoxyhemoglobin, and the model compound 2-methylimidazole iron[11] tetraphenylporphin, and is not seen in methemoglobin (Table 10). The small displacement seen in the α-subunits of methemoglobin[29] could be most easily explained if the pyrrole rings were ruffled, so that the nitrogens would be either side of the iron. When the crystallographic studies of hemoglobin were begun, the significance of spin states was not apparent, and the methemoglobin was assumed to be very similar to oxyhemoglobin. In most respects this assumption still seems to be true. Thus the comparison of the deoxy- and methemoglobin structure should show us the changes that occur during oxygenation.

The environment of the hemes is shown in Figures 16 and 17 for horse methemoglobin and in Figures 18 and 19 for human deoxyhemoglobin. The hemes are bound to the globin by a covalent bond between the nitrogen atom of the proximal His F8 and the iron atom, and by a large number of nonpolar interactions between the prophyrin and the hydrophobic residues that form its binding pocket. A list of these interactions is given in Table 11. The propionic acid side chains of the α-heme form salt links with His CD3(45)α and Lys E10(61)α, but those of the β-heme do not. If methemoglobin is used as a model for oxyhemoglobin, the heme environments change upon deoxygenation. Table 12 compares the distances between various points on the hemes to the surrounding residues in horse methemoglobin and human deoxyhemoglobin. The relative movements of the hemes and the various helices are quite similar in the α- and β-subunits. Figure 20 shows the changes in the distance from the heme center to the surrounding residues between methemoglobin and deoxyhemoglobin for both subunits. Helix E is closer to the hemes in the deoxy state; however, this change is greater in the β- subunits than in the α-subunits. On the other hand, helix B and the CD segment have moved further away from the heme axis in all subunits of deoxyhemoglobin. One of the most significant movements that occurs during deoxygenation involves helix F, which contains the proximal histidine at position F8. This helix rotates clockwise, as seen from the FG corner. The imidazole groups of F8 moves approximately 0.4 Å away from the porphyrin in the deoxy structure. As a result of this rotation, Leu F7 moves away from the heme, but Leu F4 moves toward the heme. The FG segment also moves toward the heme, particularly Leu FG3. The movements of the tertiary structure are summarized in Figure 21. Obviously, the largest movements are those involving the FG corner and the HC segment. The carboxyl terminal residues appear to be free in solution in methemoglobin, but they make several interchain salt linkages in deoxyhemoglobin.[55,56] The changes in these salt bridges are an important aspect of the heme-heme interactions. Helix A, which is remote from the heme group, also moves; however, the importance of this movement is difficult to assess, since the position of this helix differs in human and horse deoxyhemoglobins.[25] Data showing the extent of this species difference in the three-dimensional structure of deoxyhemoglobin are presented in Table 13.

During deoxygenation both heme groups rotate slightly clockwise, as viewed from their propionic acid side chains. The β-heme moves toward the solvent, but the α-heme is held somewhat more rigidly, because of the interactions of His CD3(45)α and Lys E10(61)α with its propionate groups.

The oxygen molecule lies in a tight pocket, bounded by two hydrophobic groups (Phe CD1 and Val E11) and the distal histidine (His E7). The presence of the distal histidine causes steric hinderance to molecules that bind perpendicular to the heme plane, such as carbon monoxide, and favors the binding of "bent" ligands, such as oxygen. Neutron diffraction studies have shown that the distal histidine forms a hydrogen bond to bound oxygen.[186]

An important difference between the α- and β-subunits is the position of valine E11 relative to the heme-linked water. The distance between the water molecule and gamma carbon of Val E11 is 3.8 Å in the α-subunit, but only 3.3 Å in the β-subunit.[29] The resulting steric interference between the chains and the ligands explains why the β-hemes are more easily reduced than the α-hemes in the oxy quaternary structure. In the deoxy quaternary structure, the β-hemes are less readily autoxidized than the α-hemes for the same reason.[25]

THE QUATERNARY STRUCTURE OF HEMOGLOBIN

Many of the physiologically important properties of hemoglobin depend on the changes in its quaternary structure. The basic quaternary structure is shown in Figure 22. To form the quaternary structure, the subunits bury approximately one fifth of their surface area in the interfaces between them.[54] The $\alpha_1\beta_1$ contact accounts for 60% of that area, and the $\alpha_1\beta_2$ contact accounts for 33%. The other 7% is in $\alpha_1\alpha_2$ and $\beta_1\beta_2$ contacts. The stability of the tetramer comes largely from hydrophobic interactions in the subunit interfaces.[54] However, these interfaces are far more polar than earlier studies[57,58] indicated. In methemoglobin there are 15 bound water molecules in the $\alpha_1\beta_1$ contact and 4 bound water molecules in the $\alpha_1\beta_2$ contact.[29] There are 17 to 19 hydrogen bonds present in the $\alpha_1\beta_1$ interface, and 6 to 7 hydrogen bonds in the $\alpha_1\beta_2$ interface.[29] The amount of surface area buried in the subunit contacts, and the percentage of polar interactions in the contract regions, which was estimated from the number of nitrogen and oxygen atoms found there, is given in Table 14.

The $\alpha_1\beta_1$ dimer of methemoglobin is seen in Figure 23. More detailed views of this contact are given in Figures 24 and 25. The residues involved in this interface and their interactions are summarized in Table 15A for methemoglobin, and in Table 16A for deoxyhemoglobin. The α-carbon coordinates for this dimer in the deoxy- and methemoglobins can be superimposed on each other as a rigid body,[54] demonstrating that there are no major changes in the $\alpha_1\beta_1$ contact during the allosteric transition. The relative rotation of the α_1- and β_1-subunits by 3.7°, found in earlier reports,[59] appears to result from the changes in tertiary structure.

The $\alpha_1\beta_2$ dimer is shown in Figure 26. Two points are immediately obvious from this stereodiagram. First, the FG corner, which is subject to a large movement during the deoxygenation, is intimately involved in this subunit contact, which can be seen in detail in Figure 27. Second, the heme groups are closer and more directly connected through the protein structure in this dimer than in the $\alpha_1\beta_1$ dimer. The residues and interactions involved in this contact are summarized in Table 15B. The differences in the $\alpha_1\beta_2$ interfaces in deoxy- and methemoglobin can be seen by comparing Table 16B and Figures 28 to 30 with Table 15B and Figures 26 and 27. The contact region of deoxyhemoglobins is shown diagrammatically in Figure 31. The changes in this dimer are much more dramatic than in the $\alpha_1\beta_1$ dimer. The two subunits have turned 13° relative to each other. The contact is dovetailed, so that the C helix of one subunit fits into the FG segment of the other. Thus there are two C-FG interactions per $\alpha_1\beta_1$ interface, related to each other by the pseudo-dyad. In both met- and deoxyhemoglobin, Trp C3(37)β fits into a V-shaped groove formed by the α-carbon of Val FG5(93)α, but the two residues move slightly relative to one another. The other C-FG interaction, however, changes greatly during the transition of the quaternary structure. In methemoglobin, the side chain of Thr C3(38)α fits into the groove of Val FG5(98)β, but in deoxyhemoglobin this threonine is replaced by Thr C6(41)α. This change is shown diagrammatically in Figure 32. These two threonines are on successive turns of the C helix. Thus there is no intermediate residue that could fit into the groove at Val FG5(98)β. In addition, Asp G1(94)α forms a hydrogen bond with Asn G4(102)β in methemoglobin, while Tyr C7(42)α forms one with Asp G1(99)β in deoxyhemoglobin. No intermediate hydrogen bonding patterns are possible. Thus, the hemoglobin molecule is constrained to be in one of only two possible quaternary structures, by the dovetailing and the intersubunit hydrogen bonding.

The resulting two-state model provides a structural explanation for many of the physiological properties, including diphosphoglycerate binding, the Bohr effect, and heme-heme interaction.

DIPHOSPHOGLYCERATE BINDING

The binding of diphosphoglycerate (DPG) to deoxyhemoglobin has been studied by X-ray crystallography.[60] One molecule of DPG per tetramer binds in the central cavity between the β-subunits, which can be seen in Figure 22A. The phosphate groups form salt bridges to the cationic groups of Val NA1(1)β, His NA2(2)β, Lys EF6(82)β, and His H21(143)β, as shown in Figure 33. In methemoglobin the amino termini move further apart, while the EF segments move closer together. The complementarity of the binding site and DPG is lost, and the affinity for DPG drops 150-fold. Since DPG can bind only to the deoxy conformation of hemoglobin, it stabilizes this form, resulting in a lower oxygen affinity in the presence of DPG. This phenomenon explains the difference in the oxygen affinity of fetal and adult blood. In fetal hemoglobin, the γ-chain has serine rather than histidine at position H21, decreasing the affinity for DPG. In the presence of DPG, adult hemoglobin has a lower oxygen affinity than fetal hemoglobin, even though they have similar affinities when stripped of DPG. Inositol hexaphosphate can also occupy the DPG-binding site in deoxyhemoglobin[61] and in fluoromethemoglobin,[62] which has the same conformation as deoxyhemoglobin.

Comparison of mammalian hemoglobins that have intrinsically high oxygen affinity and high DPG sensitivity with those that have intrinsically low oxygen affinity and low DPG sensitivity showed the only consistent structural difference between the two groups involves position NA2β, which is a hydrophilic residue in the first group and a large hydrophobic residue in the second group.[186] Perutz and Imai suggest that the hydrophobic group in bovine, feline, and other low oxygen affinity hemoglobins points into the interior of the β-subunit locking helix A in position and thus mimicking the action of DPG in stabilizing the deoxy tertiary structure.[186] Electrostatic energy calculations of the stabilization of deoxy hemoglobin by DPG binding compare well with the experimental findings.[187]

The DPG binding site is also the binding site for the band 3 protein of the erythrocyte membrane.[206] The acidic amino terminal peptide binds deep into the central cavity between the β-chains and interacts with residues Arg G6(104)β_1 and Arg G6(104)β_2, as well as some of the basic residues of the DPG site.

THE BOHR EFFECT

The Bohr effect is the lowering of the oxygen affinity of hemoglobin with decreasing pH. At the present time, approximately 60% of the alkaline Bohr effect, which operates above pH 7, can be accounted for by structural explanations. Carbamylation of the α-amino groups of Val NA1(1) with cyanate demonstrated that this group accounted for about 20% of the Bohr effect.[63] The X-ray structure of this carbamylated deoxyhemoglobin shows that the anion normally bound between the α-amino group and the positively charged guanidinium of Arg HC3(141)α of the second α-chain (Figure 34) is missing.[64,157] In the oxy conformation, this salt bridge is not formed and the anion is released, causing the pK of the α-amino group to decrease by 0.8 units.[65] His HC3(146)β is also involved in the Bohr effect. The imidazole of this residue forms a salt linkage to the carboxyl group of Asp FG1(94)β in the deoxy structure only. When the pK of His HC3(146)β was measured by proton nuclear magnetic resonance, it was found to be 8.0 in deoxyhemoglobin and 7.1 in carboxyhemoglobin. This change in pK would account for 40% of the total Bohr effect. It has been suggested that His H5(122)α was responsible for the different interactions in deoxy- and methemoglobin.[55] However, more recent results at higher resolution show that this histidine has identical interactions in both structures.[25,29] Measurements of the Bohr effects of mutant and animal hemoglobins that lacked particular histidines could not attribute the remainder of the Bohr effect to any of these residues.[66] Thus the groups responsible for the last 40% are still unknown.

Recently, the role of His HC3(146)β in the Bohr effect has been questioned. Ho and co-workers have concluded from high-resolution proton nuclear magnetic resonance studies that these histidyl residues do not significantly change their electrostatic environments when carbon monoxide binds to deoxyhemoglobin and, therefore, do not make a large contribution to the Bohr effect.[177] These investigators examined normal, mutant, and modified hemoglobins in both the deoxy and carbonmonoxy forms and suggested that the detailed mechanism of Bohr effect depends on the solvent composition and other experimental conditions. Kilmartin et al., on the other hand, found that either removal of His HC3(146)β or modification of it by *N*-ethyl-succinimide results in the inhibition of 60% of the alkaline Bohr effect.[178] Measurement of the association and dissociation rate constants for the fourth carbon monoxide molecule have been determined as a function of pH for normal and des-(His 146β) hemoglobin A.[179] The results indicate that this hisitidine is a major participant in the Bohr effect.

Gurd and co-workers have calculated the titration behavior of individual groups in hemoglobin using a discrete charge electrostatic model.[180] They predicted that 10 groups per tetramer would contribute to the Bohr effect at 0.1 *M* ionic strength and 28 groups would be involved at 0.01 *M* ionic strength. The major contributions would be from Val 1α, Val 1β, His 117β, and His 146β, assuming that chloride ions are bound to Val 1α and His 117β in deoxyhemoglobin.

When the Bohr effect was measured for hemoglobins from different species and for various abnormal hemoglobins, several additional residues were implicated.[181] His H21(143)β seemed to be responsible for about half of the acid Bohr effect and Lys EF6(82)β for the missing part of the alkaline Bohr effect in stripped hemoglobin. Since Lys EF6(82)β is part of the diphosphoglycerate binding site, it probably does not contribute in vivo.

The Bohr group salt bridges are intimately involved in the cooperativity of hemoglobin (see below). Measurements of the first Adair constant for normal hemoglobin, hemoglobin reacted with cyanate at Val 1α and des-(His 146β) hemoglobin showed that the Bohr group salt bridges break on oxygen binding to the T (or deoxy) form and are partially responsible for the free energy of cooperativitiy.[182] The Bohr effect and its relationship to carbon dioxide and DPG binding has been reviewed by Kilmartin.[183]

Carbon dioxide can react reversibly with the α-amino groups of hemoglobin to form carbamino compounds.[67] Since the deoxy structure reacts more readily than does the oxy structure, CO_2 binding lowers oxygen affinity. The β-chain carbamate group probably forms a salt linkage with Lys EF6(82)β, but it does not appear that this interaction would differ between the oxy and deoxy conformations.[68] The α-chain carbamate group probably displaces the inorganic anion and interacts directly with Arg HC3(141) on the other α-subunit. Thus the deoxy structure is stabilized, but the oxy structure is not.

THE ALLOSTERIC MECHANISM

The heme-heme interaction of hemoglobin is the positive cooperativitity of oxygen binding to the tetramer. This type of allosteric binding behavior is often explained by the Monod-Wyman-Changeux[69] or by the Koshland-Nemethy-Filmer[70] models. Both of these models were developed by applying certain assumptions to the equilibrium equations for binding oxygen. The Monod-Wyman-Changeux model assumes that there are only two possible quaternary structures, which differ in oxygen affinity. Oxygen binding would affect the equilibrium between the two quaternary structures, but the binding to one subunit is not affected by the oxygenation state of the other subunits in the same molecule. The Koshland-

Nemethy-Filmer model differs, by assuming that binding of oxygen to one subunit increases the affinity of a neighboring subunit. Perutz,[55,56,71] on the other hand, has developed a stereochemical theory that explains heme-heme interactions on the basis of the known conformational differences between oxy- and deoxyhemoglobin. Figure 35 illustrates this theory. In this diagram, oxygen binds to the α-subunit first. While it is not necessary to assume this binding order, there is some evidence supporting a sequential order with the α-subunits reacting before the β-subunits.[72] The α-heme pocket is open enough to allow oxygen to enter and bind to the iron, whereas in the β-chain, the entrance is closed and must be opened by thermal energy. On the other hand, results of multidimensional spectroscopic studies indicate that β-subunits have a higher affinity for oxygen than α-subunits.[184] When the oxygen binds to the α_1-subunit, the iron changes from high spin to low spin with a simultaneous decrease in its radius, so that it can move into the plane of the porphyrin. This movement triggers a sequence of conformational changes, since the iron atom pulls the proximal histidine (F8) with it. As a result, helix F moves toward helix H, and Tyr HC2(140)α_1 is expelled from its position between these helices. This is illustrated diagrammatically in Figure 36. The movement of this tyrosine causes the displacement of the carboxyterminal Arg HC3(141)α_1. This, in turn, breaks the salt linkages to the α_2-chain shown in Figures 34 and 35. The dissolution of the salt bridges allows the release of a Bohr proton from the α-amino group of Val NA1(1)α_2. The α_1 chain now has an oxy tertiary structure, but the quaternary structure is still in the deoxy conformation. The process is essentially identical for the β-subunits, except for the changes in the intersubunit salt linkages, shown in Figure 34. The successive transitions of the subunits from the deoxy to the oxy tertiary structure, and the associated rupturing of the ionic bonds between subunits, increases the strain until a transition to the oxy quaternary structure occurs. In Figure 35 this transition happens between steps 3 and 4. The central idea of the stereochemical theory is that the positive cooperativity is directly linked to this change in the quaternary structure. Once the molecule is in the oxy quaternary conformation, the remaining deoxy subunits can more easily adopt the oxy tertiary structure, which means that oxygen can be bound more readily.

The stereochemical mechanism and the evidence for it has been reviewed by Perutz.[149-151] A detailed comparison of the human deoxy, horse met, and human carbonmonoxy hemoglobin supports this model.[188] Specific modification of the α chain carboxyl terminus by hydrazide results in the loss of the Arg-141α_1-Lys-127α_2 salt bridge in the X-ray structure of the deoxyhemoglobin.[158] Accurate oxygen equilibrium curves of this modified hemoglobin showed that removing this ionic bond raised the oxygen affinity of the T state without affecting that of the R state. The relationship of the spin state of the iron to the quarternary structure has been extensively investigated.[189,190] The results showed that the change in quaternary structure from R to T is associated with transition to higher spin state in solutions of methemoglobin derivatives.[189] Measurements of paramagnetic susceptibilities showed that the free energy differences between the six coordinate high- and low-spin states is approximately 1 kcal/mol heme lower in the T structure than in the R structure.[190] These data support the stereochemical mechanism proposed by Perutz.

Several investigators have discussed various problems with Perutz mechanism. Energy calculations have indicated that nonelectrostatic factors favoring deoxy dimer-tetramer assembly may be the major source of the cooperative energy.[175] The asymmetric oxygen binding curves of hemoglobin indicate that a more complex model may be needed.[191] When a statistical thermodynamic model is formulated from the stereochemical postulates of Perutz, it does not predict reasonable values for the Bohr effect without simultaneously predicting unreasonable values for the affinities of individual chains.[192] Finally, the stereochemical model has been modified to account for the kinetic, rather than equilibrium, properties of hemoglobin.[193] These studies showed that steric hindrance to ligand binding through nonbonded ligand-globin interactions is a significant factor in lowering ligand affinity of the T state by decreasing the association rate constants.[193] While the debate continues over the explanation for the allosteric properties of hemoglobin, Perutz's stereochemcial proposal remains as the model to which newer ideas must be compared.

ABNORMAL HEMOGLOBINS

The three-dimensional structure of hemoglobin also provides us with an understanding of the changes in the functional properties of abnormal hemoglobins.[73] Perutz, Lehmann, and co-workers have investigated the molecular pathology of human hemoglobin[51,74] and have concluded that there are four basic types of mutant proteins. First, there are mutations of the residues that are in contact with the heme group. These substitutions often have a direct effect on oxygen affinity and sometimes result in an unstable hemoglobin. In some cases, replacement of a nonpolar contact between the heme group and the globin will eliminate the heme-binding affinity of the protein. Other changes, characteristic of the hemoglobins M, stabilize the ferric form of the iron. The effects of some mutations of this type are summarized in Table 17.

The second type of mutation that causes major functional changes involves replacements in the subunit contacts. Some of these substitutions trap the molecule into either the oxy or deoxy quaternary structure, resulting in the loss of allosteric properties. Alterations in the subunit interfaces also promote dissociation of the tetramer into dimers and monomers. Examples of this type of abnormal hemoglobin are given in Table 18.

The other two types of mutation involve changes in the positions that are not directly involved in the heme pockets or the subunit interactions. In one class, an altered tertiary is the result of a substitution that prevents the polypeptide chain from folding into the normal tertiary structure. If a hydrophobic, internal residue is replaced by an ionic amino acid, the resulting hemoglobin is generally unstable, as illustrated by hemoglobin Wien in Table 19. The positions of mutations that lead to instability are shown in Figure 37. The second type of mutation in a general position is one that causes an alteration to the exterior of the tetramer. Nearly all of these substitutions are harmless, but hemoglobin S is an obvious exception. The conclusions obtained by examining the effect of several changes in general positions on the three-dimensional structure of hemoglobin are listed in Table 19.

The explanations of Perutz and Lehmann[51,74] for the altered functional properties of abnormal hemoglobins have proven to be generally correct. Investigations of these mutant proteins by X-ray crystallography, however, have provided additional details. In several cases, such as oxyhemoglobin Chesapeake[115] and deoxyhemoglobin Kansas,[119,120] the structural effects are not limited to the area surrounding the replacement, but are spread throughout the tetramer. Thus these diffraction studies not only provide a greater understanding of the abnormal physiological properties of the mutant hemoglobins, but also allow an investigation of the relationship between the amino acid sequence and the three-dimensional structure of a protein. The results of the X-ray determinations of abnormal hemoglobin structures are summarized in Table 20.

The best studied and most common abnormal hemoglobin is hemoglobin S, which causes sickle cell anemia. The X-ray structure of this variant hemoglobin showed that the mutation, Glu A3(6)$\beta \rightarrow$Val, does not affect the conformation of the hemoglobin molecule.[125] Deoxyhemoglobin S forms long fibers that group together into bundles that stiffen the erythrocyte and distort it into an elongated sickle shape. These deformed, rigid cells are trapped in the capillaries, blocking the microcirculation and causing pain and inflammation. Two models have been proposed for the fibers: a 14-strand model put forth by Edelstein and colleagues[194-198] and a 16-strand model from Josephs and co-workers.[199-201] There is evidence in favor of both models, and more experimental data will be needed to determine which one is best.

Magdoff-Fairchild and Chiu[202] have shown that the fiber can slowly convert to crystals having the same diffraction pattern as those studied by Love and co-workers.[125] Thus, the fiber and the crystal must be quite similar. In the crystal, the molecules form double strands running parallel to one of the crystallographic axes. Val A3(6)β is involved in side-to-side contacts between adjacent strands. In the deoxy structure, an acceptor pocket for the valine is formed by the EF corner of the β-chain. Phe F1(85)β and Leu F4(88)β interact with Val A3(6)β by hydrophobic bonding. In the oxy structure, these interactions are impossible because the F helix moves toward the FG corner upon oxygenations are impossible because the F helix moves toward the FG corner upon oxygenation, pulling Phe F1(85)β toward the center of the molecule and destroying the binding site for Val A 3(6)β.

Hybrid hemoglobins can be made from the β-chains of hemoglobin S and the α- or β-chains of other abnormal hemoglobins.[203-205] When these hybrid molecules are tested for their ability to gel, the results indicate the areas of the molecule that are involved in the intermolecular contacts of sickle fibers. The mutations that increased the solubility of hemoglobin S are listed in Table 21. In addition, the I Toulouse-S hybrid, in which one β-chain has the sickle cell mutation and the other one, a Lys E10(66)β→Glu mutation, is less soluble than hemoglobin S.[204] In general, these studies indicate that the interactions stabilizing fiber formation are the same ones found in the deoxyhemoglobin S crystal.

The structural studies have suggested several ways to cure sickle cell anemia, which have been summarized by Dickerson and Geis.[147] Perhaps the most interesting approach to this problem from both the structural and clinical perspectives is the use of bis(3,5-dibromosalicyl)fumarate.[160,161] Crystallographic studies have established that this reagent cross-links Lys EF6(82)β_1 to Lys EF6(82)β_2, spanning the DPG binding site. This modification causes Phe F1(85)β and Leu F4(88)β, which form the acceptor site for Val A3(6)β, to be pulled to the central cavity of the tetramer. Thus, the residues of the EF corner are constrained by the cross-link to the positions of the T state, but the rest of the molecule is free to shift as it normally would during the allosteric transition.[161] Since DPG cannot bind to this modified hemoglobin S, the oxygen affinities of the T and R states are almost the same as normal hemoglobin stripped of its DPG. The presence of the nonpolar bromine atoms increases the membrane solubility of this reagent and, therefore, it may be active in vivo.

ACKNOWLEDGMENT

The author wishes to thank Ms. Romie Brown for her secretarial assistance and the Division of Research Resources, National Institutes of Health, for providing access to the PROPHET Computer Network.

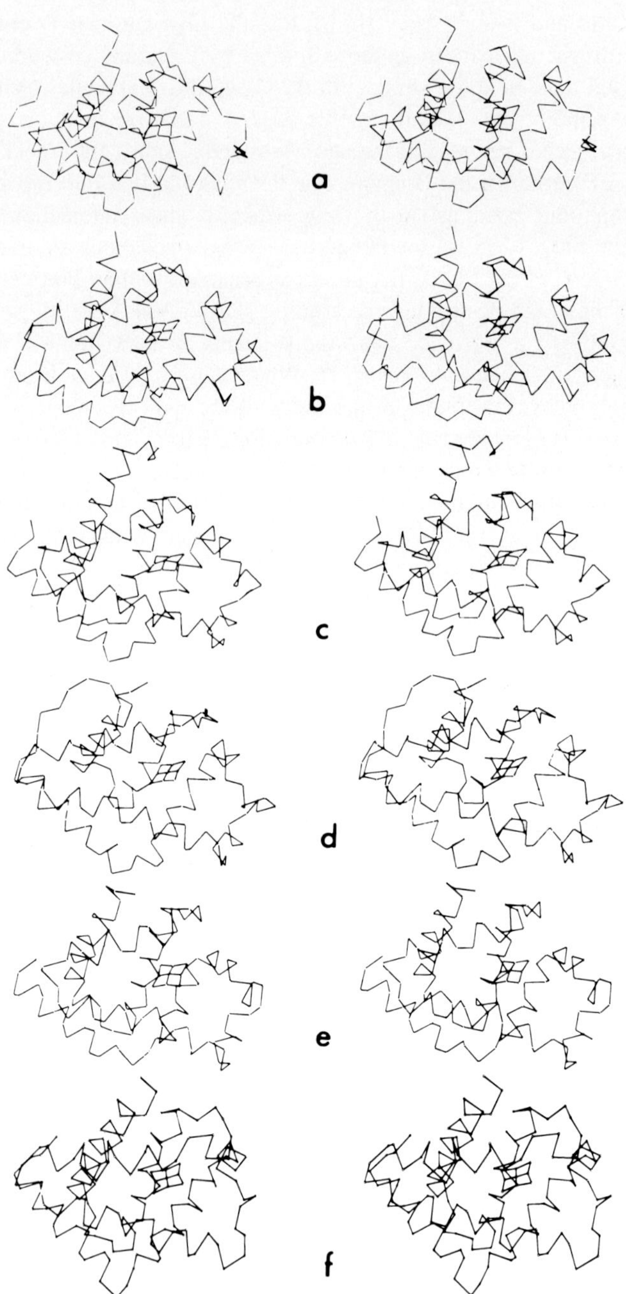

FIGURE 1. Stereo-pair drawings of the α-carbon backbones of six globins. All have the same orientation to demonstrate the conservation of the three-dimensional structure. (a) Horse hemoglobin α-chain, (b) horse hemoglobin β-chain, (c) sperm whale myoglobin, (d) sea lamprey globin V, (e) midge larva globin CTT-III (erythrocruorin), and (f) bloodworm major monomeric globin. (From Padlan, E. A. and Love, W. E., *J. Biol. Chem.*, 249, 4067, 1974. With permission.)

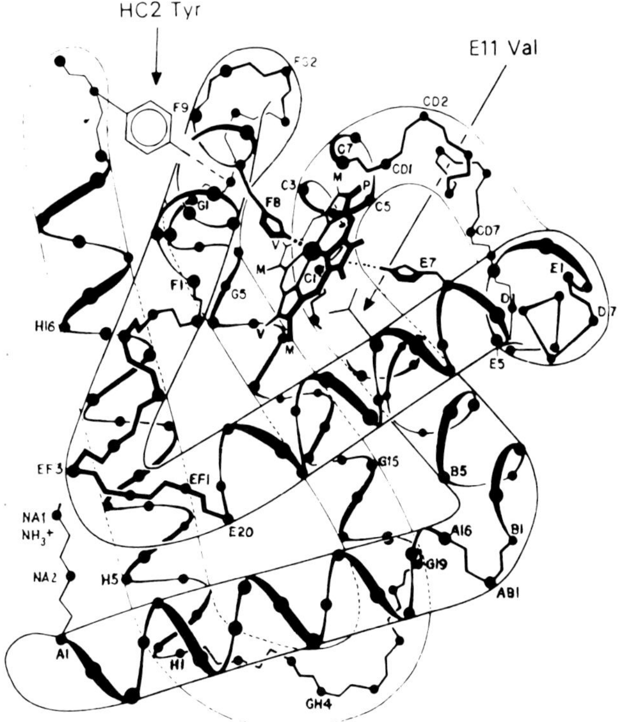

FIGURE 2. The globin fold. This diagram shows the secondary and tertiary structure that is common to all of the globins. Proximal His F8, distal His E7, Val E11, and Tyr HC2 are important residues in the mechanism of mammalian hemoglobins. The letters M, V, and P refer to the methyl, vinyl, and propionate side chains of the heme. (From Perutz, M. F., *Br. Med. Bull.*, 32, 195, 1976. Reproduced by permission of the Medical Department, The British Council.)

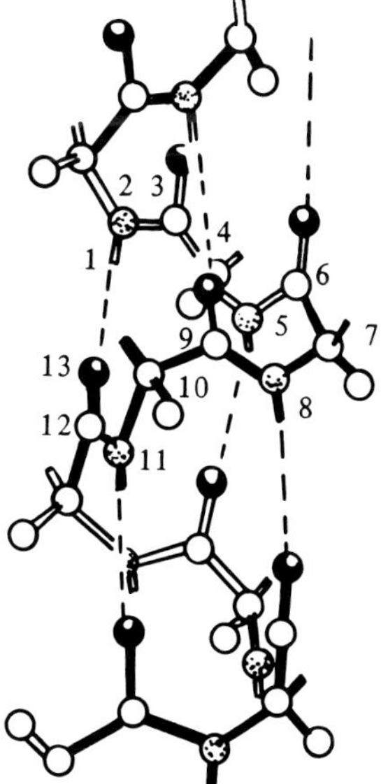

FIGURE 3. The right-handed 3.6_{13} or α-helix.

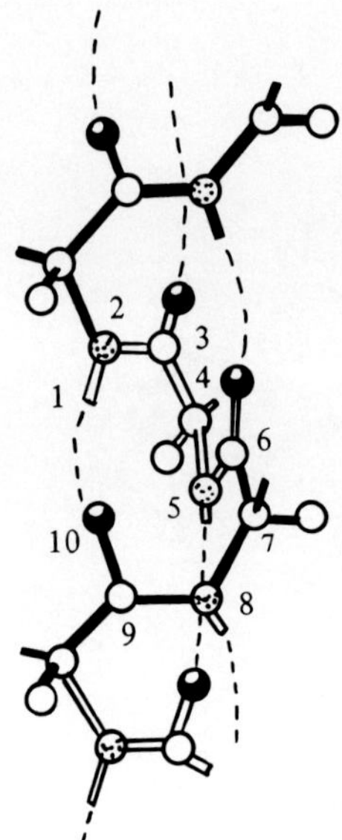

FIGURE 4. The right-handed 3_{10} helix.

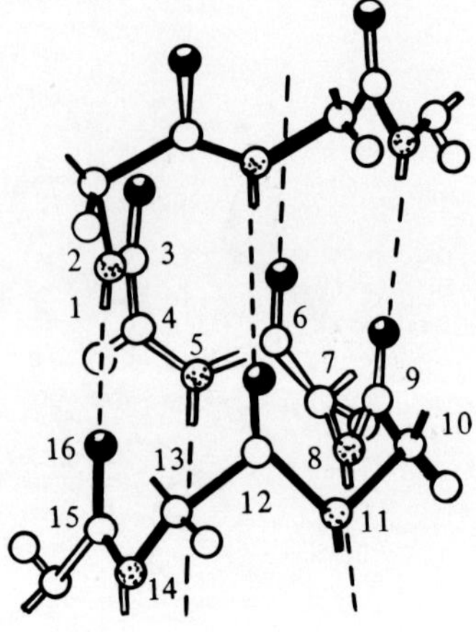

FIGURE 5. The right-handed 4.4_{16} or π-helix.

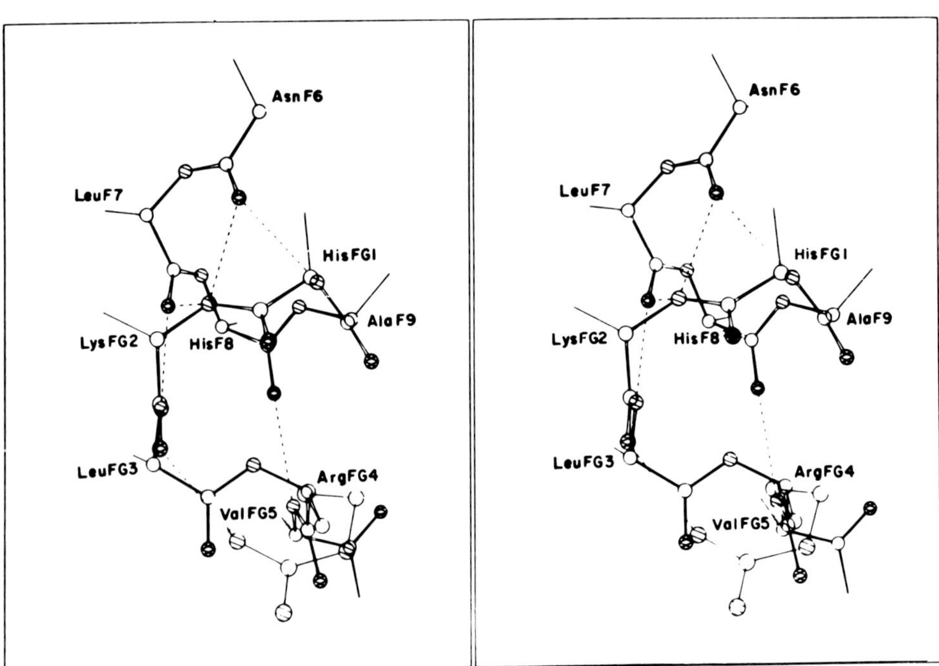

FIGURE 6. Stereo-pair drawing of the transition from α- to π-helix at the end of segment F in the α-subunit of horse methemoglobin. (From Ladner, R. C., Heidner, E. J., and Perutz, M. F., *J. Mol. Biol.*, 114, 385, 1977. Copyright by Academic Press, London. With permission.)

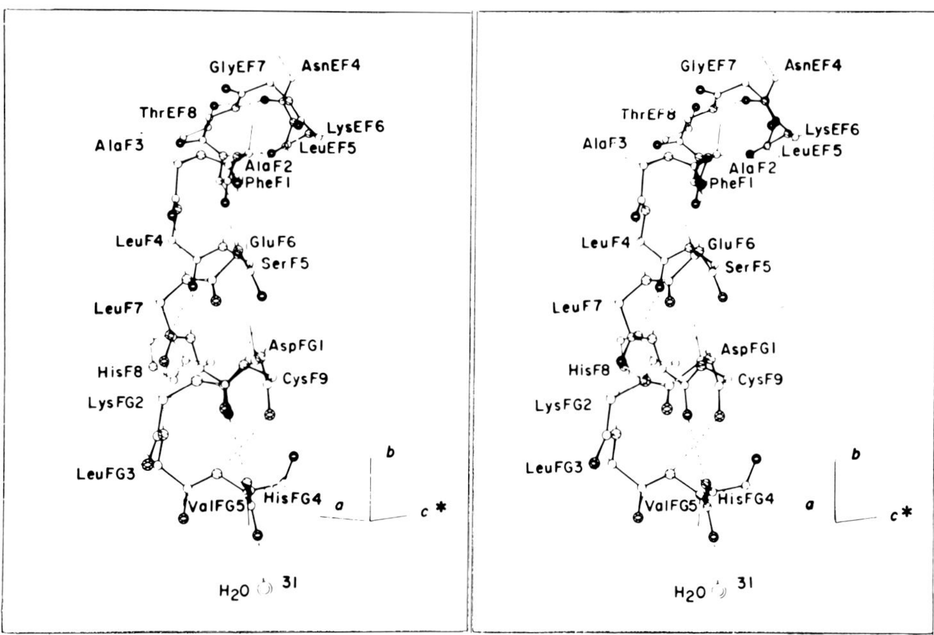

FIGURE 7. Stereo-pair drawing of helix F and segment FG in the β-subunit of horse methemoglobin. (From Ladner, R. C., Heidner, E. J., and Perutz, M. F., *J. Mol. Biol.*, 114, 385, 1977. Copyright by Academic Press, London. With permission.)

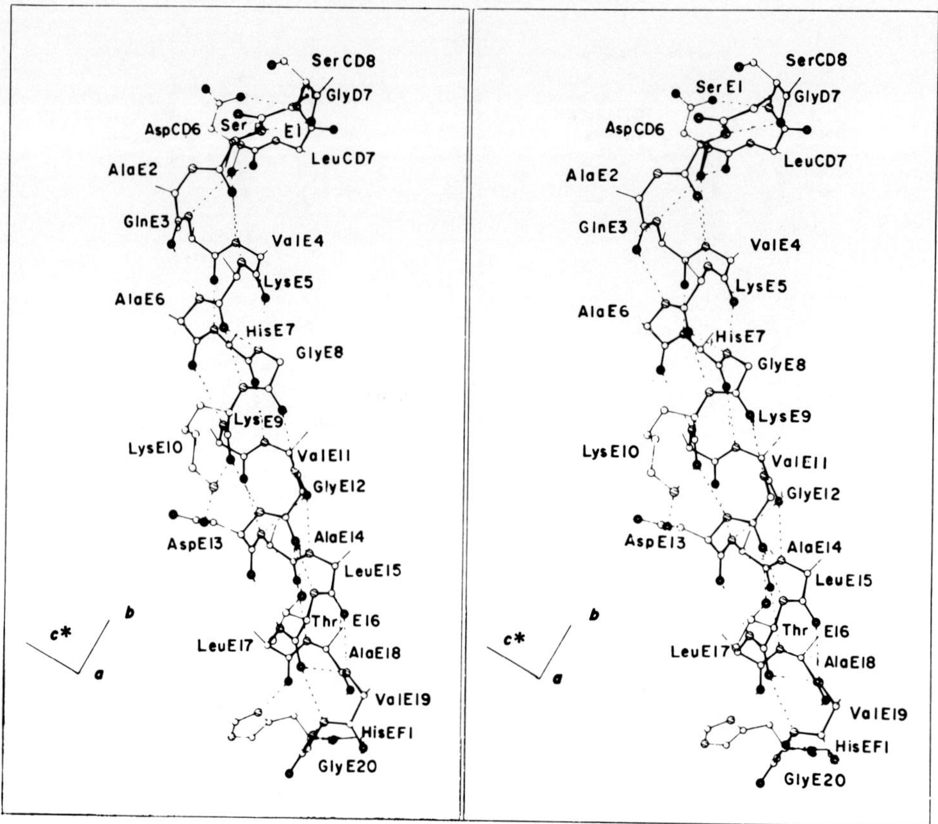

FIGURE 8. Stereo-pair drawing of the CD segment and the E helix in the α-subunit of horse methemoglobin. The hydroxyl group of Ser (E1(52)α accepts protons from the main-chain nitrogens of Gln E3(54)α and Val E4(55)α and donates a proton to the main-chain carbonyl group of Asp CD6(47)α. These hydrogen bonds help stabilize the corner between the CD segment and the E helix. (From Ladner, R. C., Heidner, E. J., and Perutz, M. F., *J. Mol. Biol.*, 114, 385, 1977. Copyright by Academic Press, London. With permission.)

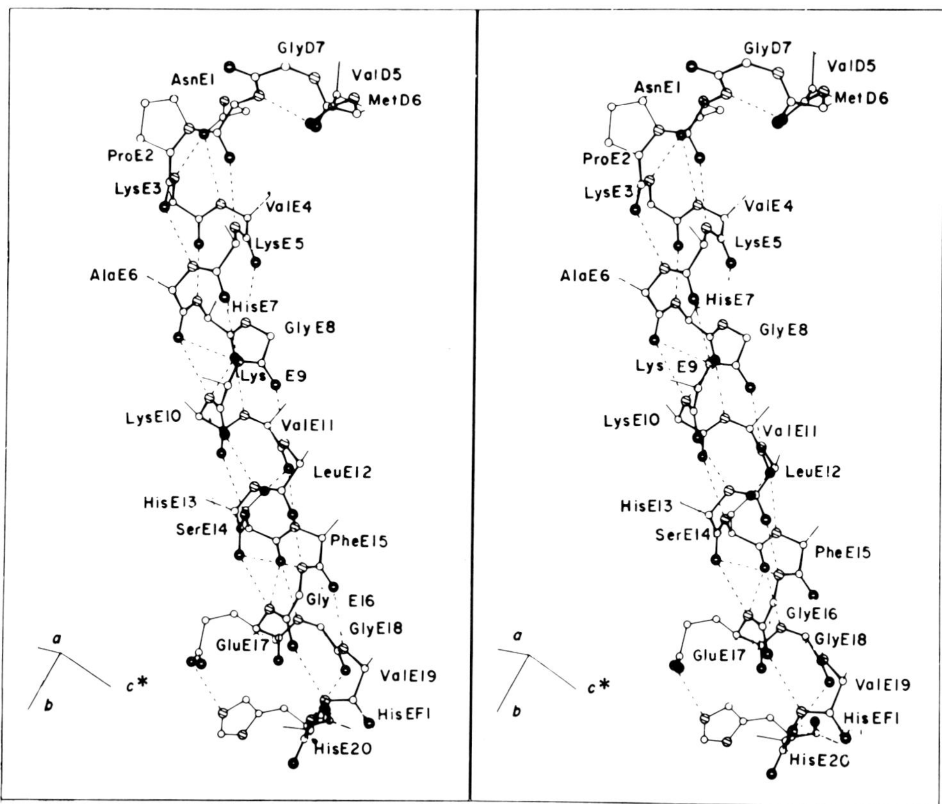

FIGURE 9. Stereo-pair drawing of the E-helix in the β-subunit of horse methemoglobin. The side-chain carbonyl group of Asn E1(57)β accepts protons from the main-chain nitrogens of Lys E3(59)β and Val E4(60)β, while the main-chain nitrogen of Asn E1(57)β denotes a proton to the main-chain carbonyl group of Val D5(54)β. These hydrogen bonds stabilize the start of the E-helix. (From Ladner, R. C., Heidner, E. J., and Perutz, M. F., *J. Mol. Biol.*, 114, 385, 1977. Copyright by Academic Press, London. With permission.)

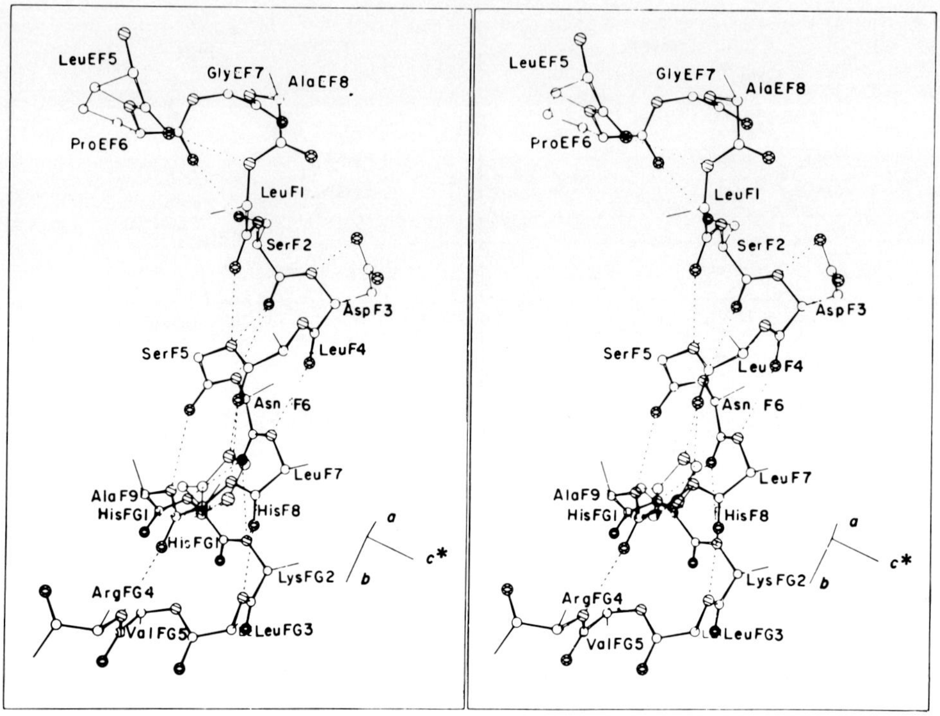

FIGURE 10. Stereo-pair drawing of the F-helix in the α subunit of horse methemoglobin. This helix is particularly irregular with several bifurcated hydrogen bonds and with additional hydrogen bonds involving the side chains of Ser F2(81)α, Asp F3(82)α, and His F8(87)α. (From Ladner, R. C., Heidner, E. J., and Perutz, M. F., *J. Mol. Biol.*, 114, 385, 1977. Copyright by Academic Press, London, With permission.)

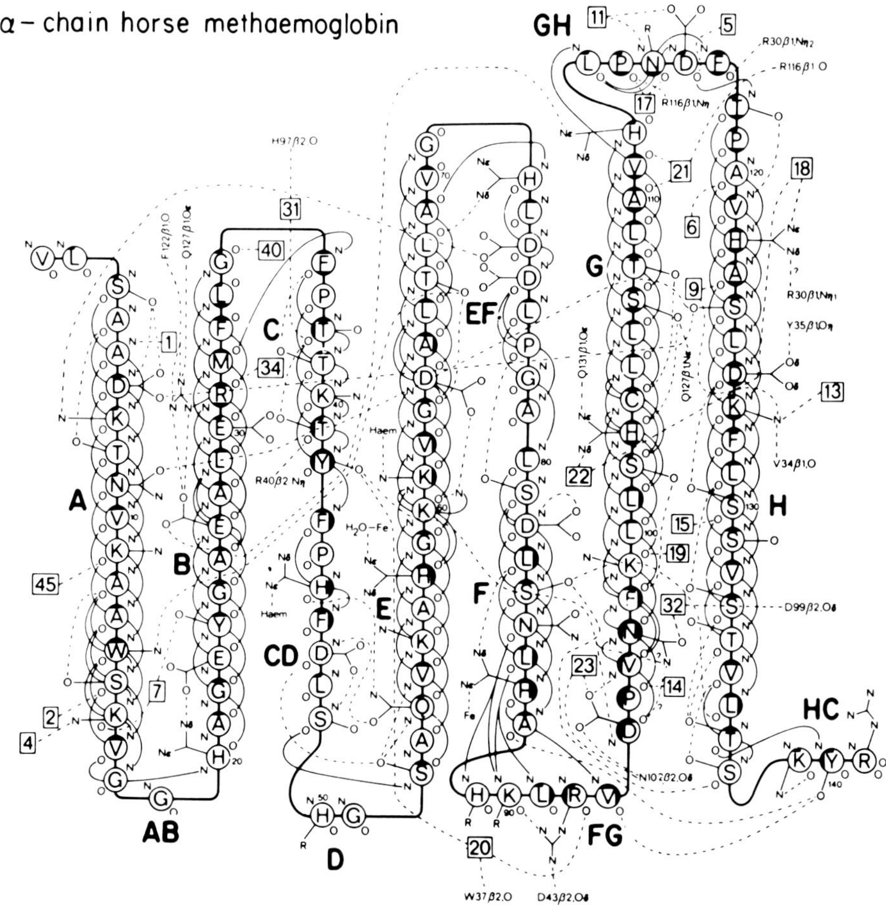

FIGURE 11. Network of hydrogen bonds stabilizing the α chain of horse methemoglobin. Full lines depict bonds between main-chain atoms and broken lines depict bonds involving side-chain atoms. The marks in the circles mean: ○, external residue; ◓, internal residue; ◔, residue in surface crevice; ◑, heme contact; ◒, $\alpha_1\beta_1$ contact; ◐, $\alpha_1\beta_2$ contact. The letters denote the amino acid residues as noted above. The numbers in squares refer to bound water molecules. Bold capitals denote the segments of secondary structure. (From Ladner, R. C., Heidner, E. J., and Perutz, M. F., *J. Mol. Biol.*, 114, 385, 1977. Copyright by Academic Press, London. With permission.)

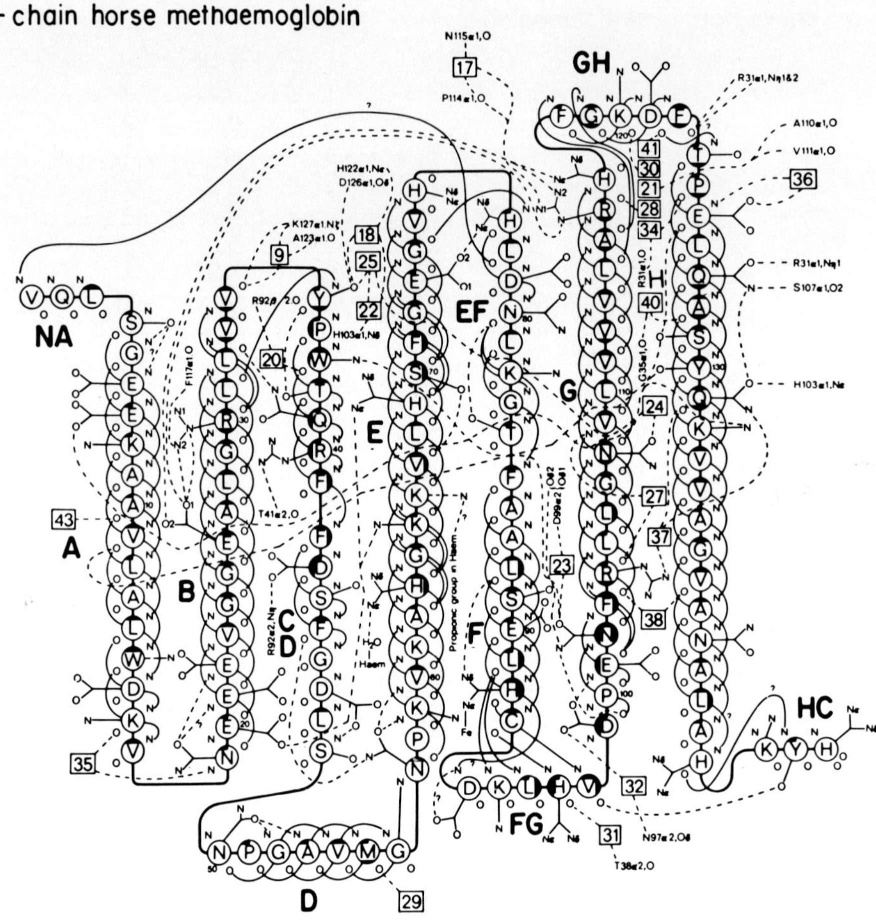

FIGURE 12. Network of hydrogen bonds stabilizing the β-chain of horse methemoglobin. The key is the same as in Figure 11. (From Ladner, R. C., Heidner, E. J., and Perutz, M. F., *J. Mol. Biol.*, 114, 385, 1977. Copyright by Academic Press, London. With permission.)

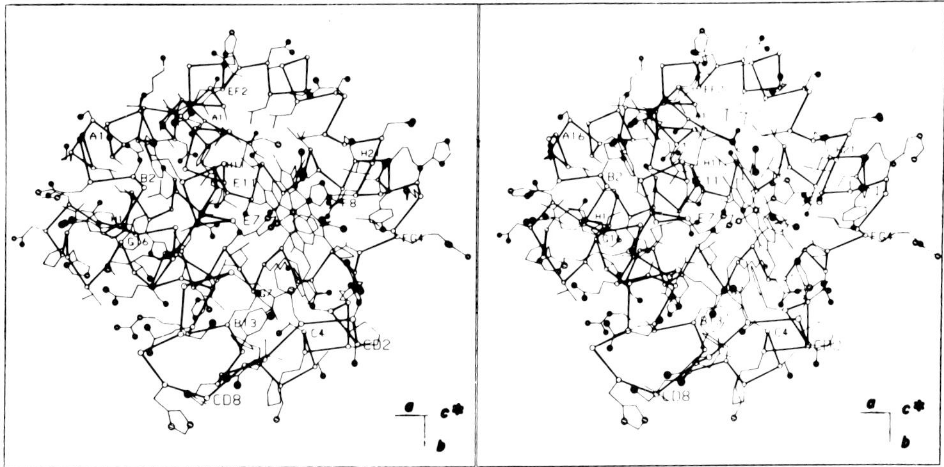

FIGURE 13. Stereo-pair drawing of the α-subunit of horse methemoglobin. Only the α-carbons and simplified side chains are shown. (From Ladner, R. C., Heidner, E. J., and Perutz, M. F., *J. Mol. Biol.*, 114, 385, 1977. Copyright by Academic Press, London. With permission.)

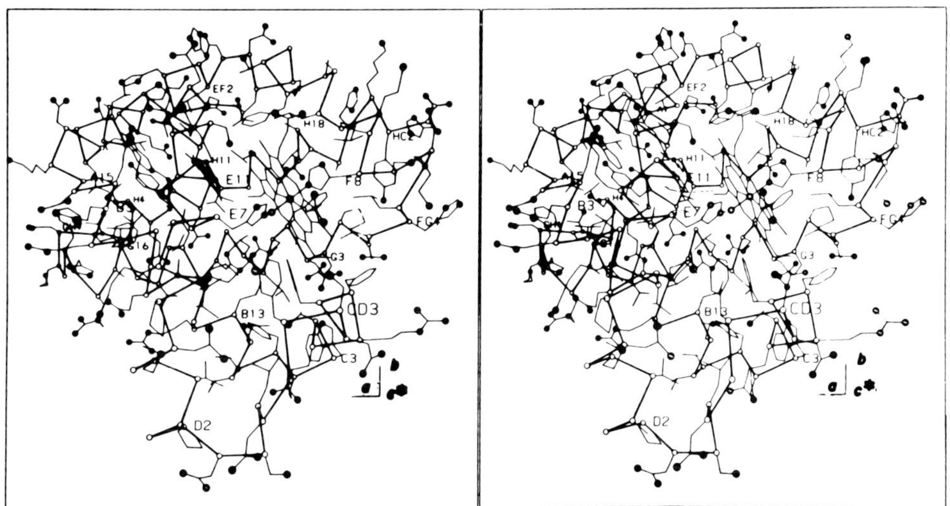

FIGURE 14. Stereo-pair drawing of the β-subunit of horse methemoglobin. Only the α-carbons and simplified side chains are shown. (From Ladner, R. C., Heidner, E. J., and Perutz, M. F., *J. Mol. Biol.*, 114, 385, 1977. Copyright by Academic Press, London. With permission.)

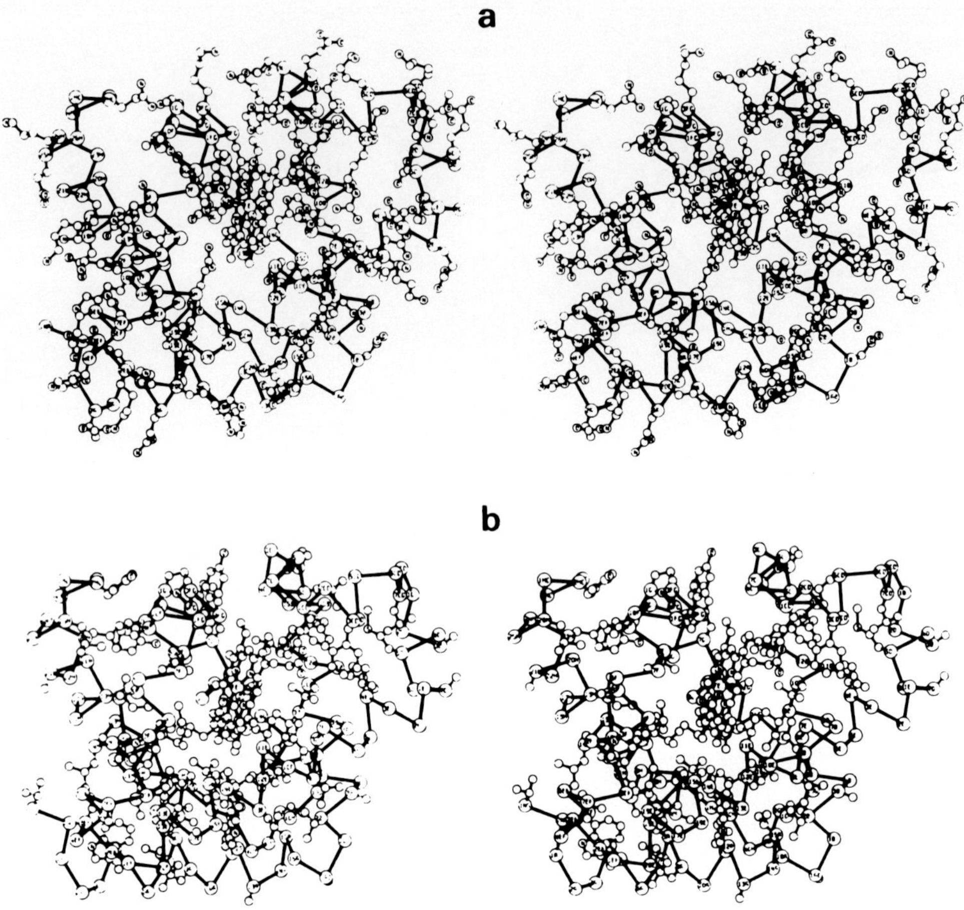

FIGURE 15. Stereo-pair drawing of sperm whale myoglobin. In Figure 15a the hydrophilic side chains are shown. All of these residues are external, except Thr C4, Ser G9, His B5, His E7, and His F8, which are hydrogen bonded internally. Phe CDl is included by mistake. In Figure 15b the hydrophobic side chains are shown. (From Takano, T., *J. Mol. Biol.*, 110, 569, 1976. Copyright by Academic Press, London. With permission.)

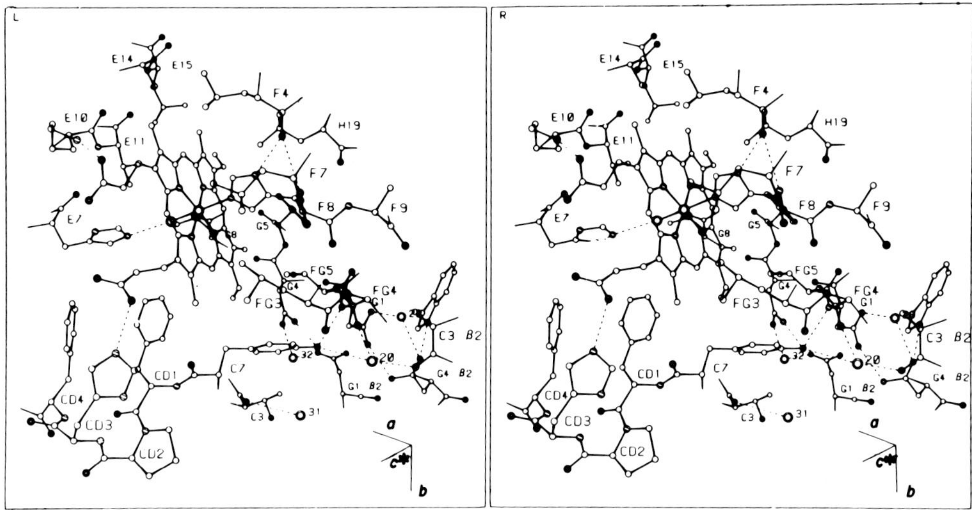

FIGURE 16. Stereo-pair drawing of the heme environment in the α-subunit of horse methemoglobin. (From Ladner, R. C., Heidner, E. J., and Perutz, M. F., *J. Mol. Biol.*, 114, 385, 1977. Copyright by Academic Press, London. With permission.)

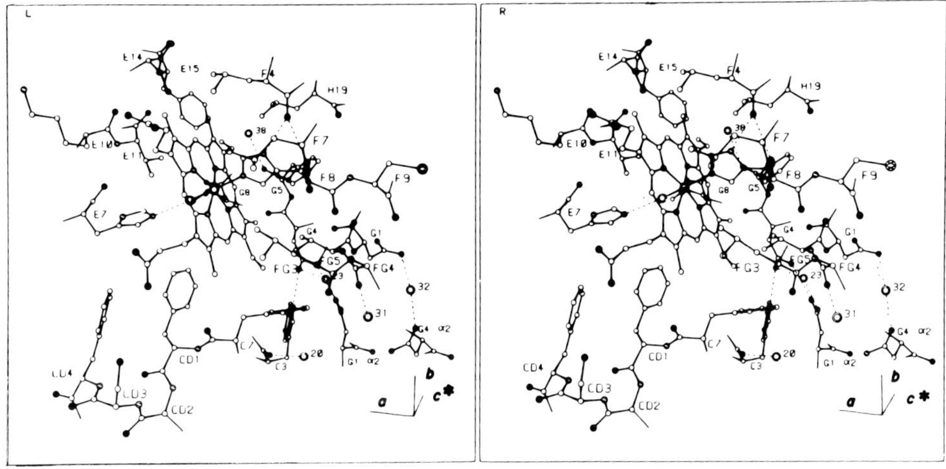

FIGURE 17. Stereo-pair drawing of the heme environment in the β-subunit of horse methemoglobin. (From Ladner, R. C., Heidner, E. J., and Perutz, M. F., *J. Mol. Biol.*, 114, 385, 1977. Copyright by Academic Press, London. With permission.)

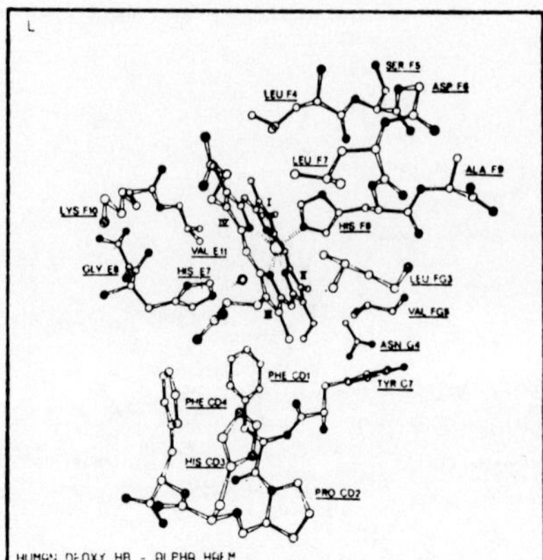

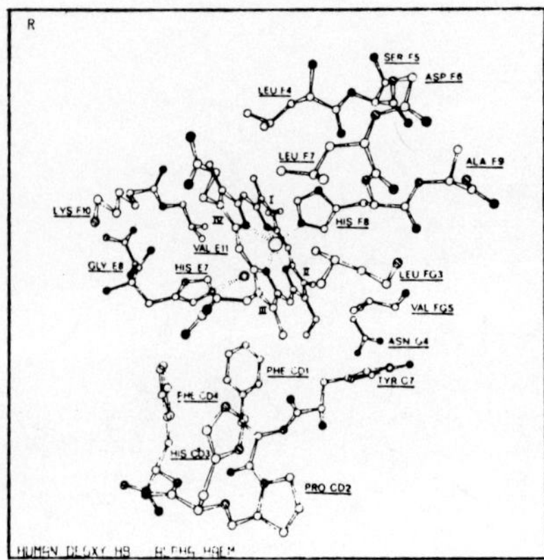

FIGURE 18. Stereo-pair drawing of the heme environment in the α subunit of human deoxyhemoglobin. ''Lys F10'' should read ''Lys E10''. There is a solvent molecule present in the heme pocket of the α-subunit, but not in that of the β-subunit. (From Fermi, G., *J. Mol. Biol.*, 97, 237, 1975. Copyright by Academic Press, London. With permission.)

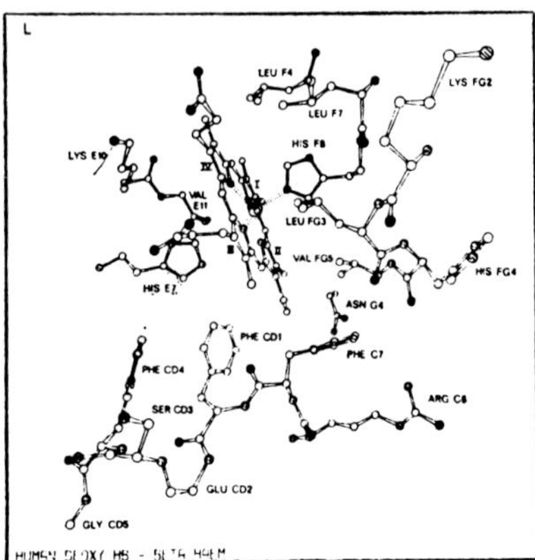

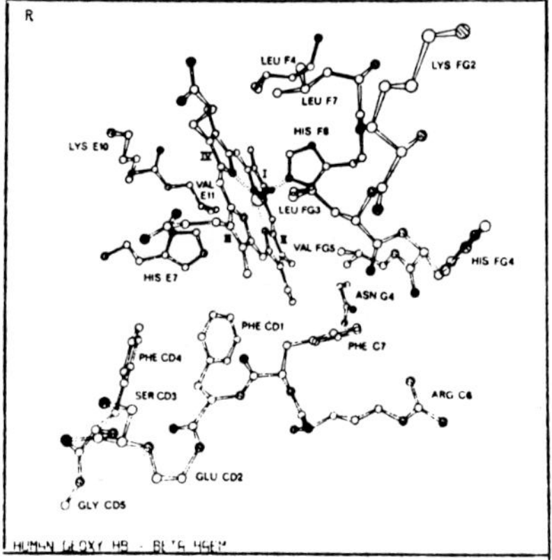

FIGURE 19. Stereo-pair drawing of the heme environment in the β-subunit of human deoxyhemoglobin. The position of Val E11 is closer to the iron atom in the β-subunit than in the α-subunit. (From Fermi, G., *J. Mol. Biol.*, 97, 237, 1975. Copyright by Academic Press, London. With permission.)

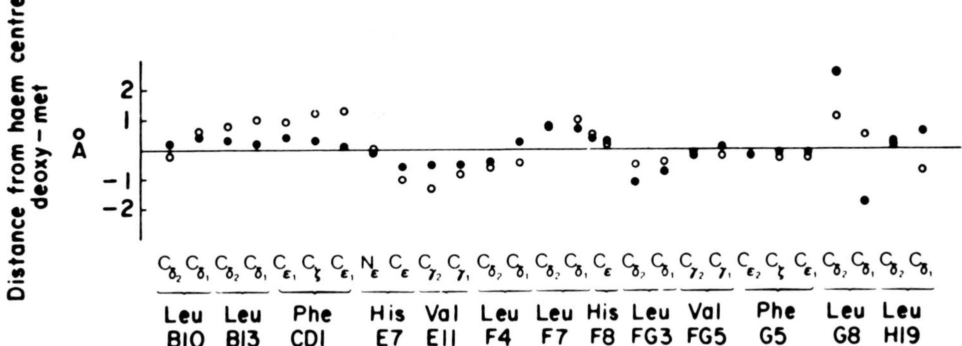

FIGURE 20. Movements of the heme environment relative to the heme center due to the transition from met- to deoxyhemoglobin; (●) α-chain, (○) β-chain. (From Ladner, R. C., Heidner, E. J., and Perutz, M. F., *J. Mol. Biol.*, 114, 385, 1977. Copyright by Academic Press, London. With permission.)

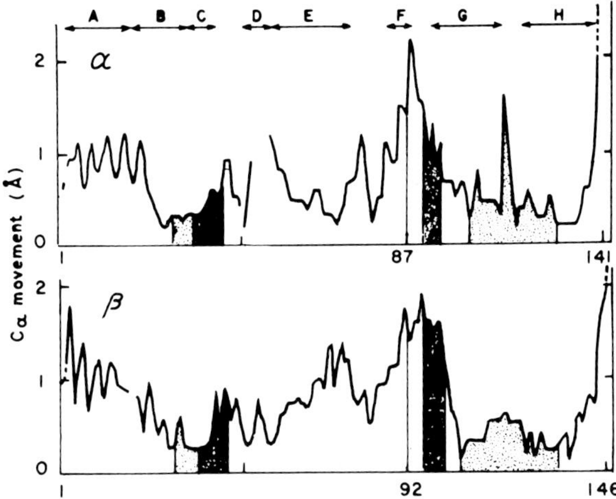

FIGURE 21. Tertiary structure changes during oxygenation. The distance between equivalent α-carbon atoms in deoxy- and met-hemoglobin is plotted against residue number. This diagram shows that the movements of the two types of chains are quite similar. The proximal His F8 is residue 87α and 92β. The $\alpha_1\beta_2$ contact residues are lightly shaded; the $\alpha_1\beta_2$ residues are more strongly shaded. The positions of the amino- and carboxy-terminal residues are shown with dashed lines, because they are not clearly defined in methemoglobin. Random errors in the structures are expected to give distances of 0.4 Å in this diagram. (Courtesy of Chothia, C., Wodak, S., and Janin, J., *Proc. Natl. Acad. Sci. U.S.A.*, 73, 3793, 1976.)

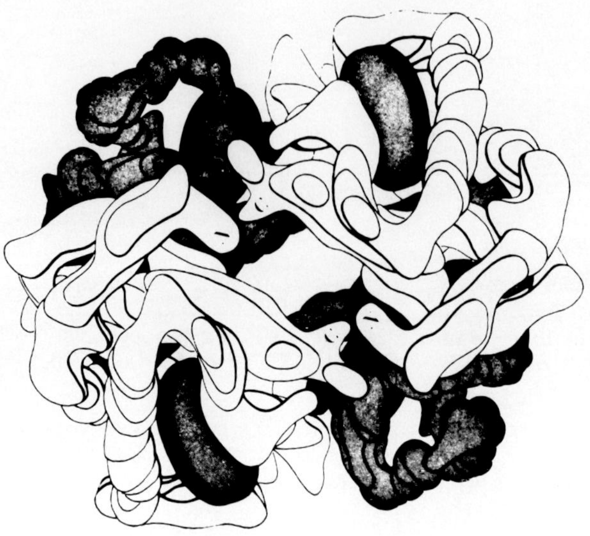

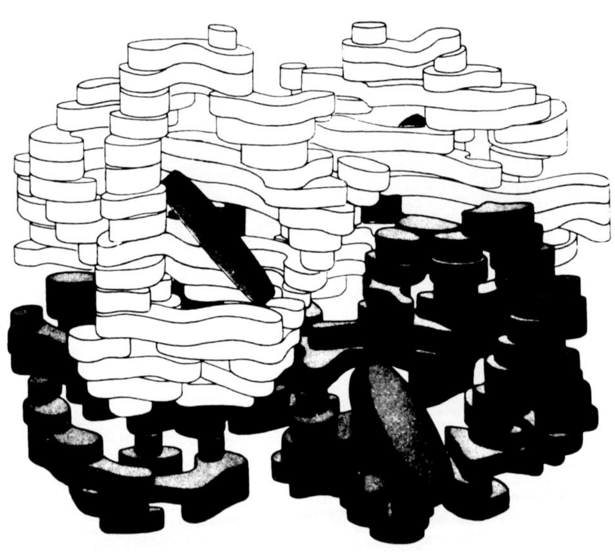

FIGURE 22. Quaternary structure of hemoglobin. The irregular block represents the electron-density pattern of the molecule. The α-chains are the light blocks; the β-chains are the dark blocks. The disks are the four heme groups. In the top view, the letter "N" denotes the amino termini of the α-chains; the letter "C" denotes the carboxyl termini. (From Perutz, M. F., The Hemoglobin Molecule, *Sci. Am.*, 211, 64, 1964. Copyright 1964 by Scientific American, Inc. All rights reserved.)

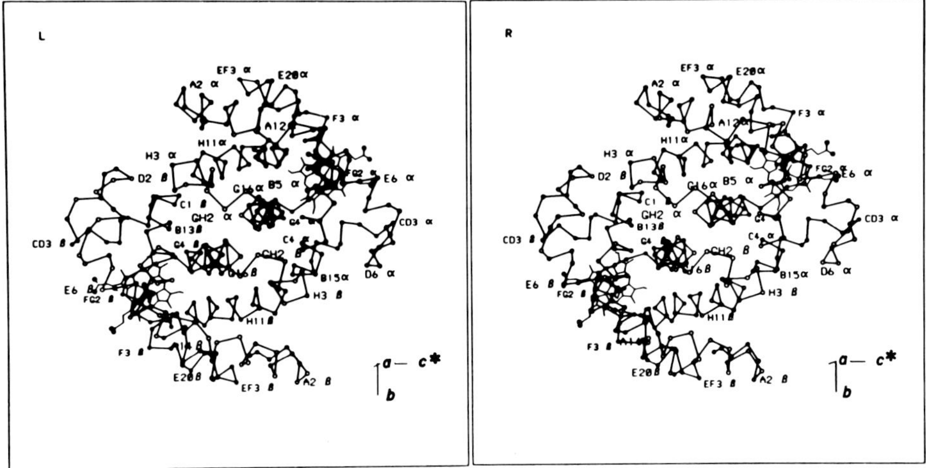

FIGURE 23. Stereo-pair drawing of the $\alpha_1\beta_1$ dimer in horse methemoglobin viewed along the pseudodyad symmetry axis between the two G helices. (From Ladner, R. C., Heidner, E. J., and Perutz, M. F., *J. Mol. Biol.*, 114, 385, 1977. Copyright by Academic Press, London. With permission.)

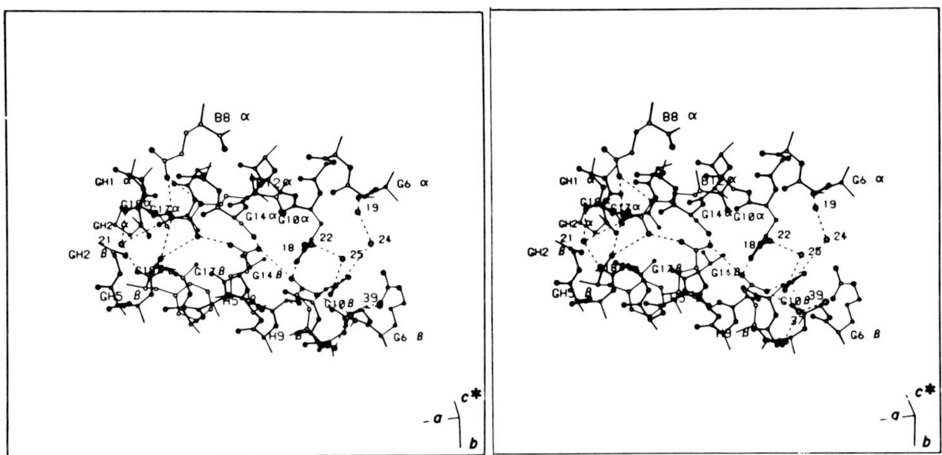

FIGURE 24. Stereo-pair drawing of the hydrogen bonding between the G helices in the $\alpha_1\beta_1$ contact of horse methemoglobin. (From Ladner, R. C., Heidner, E. J., and Perutz, M. F., *J. Mol. Biol.*, 114, 385, 1977. Copyright by Academic Press, London. With permission.)

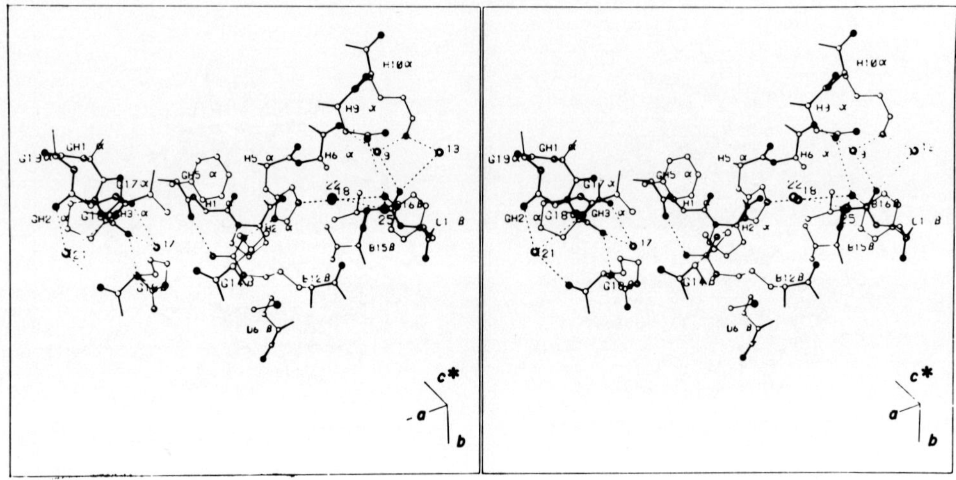

FIGURE 25. Stereo-pair drawing of the hydrogen bonding in the $\alpha_1\beta_1$ contact near the molecular center of horse methemoglobin. Water molecules 18, 22, and 25 are also seen in Figure 24. (From Ladner, R. C., Heidner, E. J., and Perutz, M. F., *J. Mol. Biol.*, 114, 385, 1977. Copyright by Academic Press, London. With permission.)

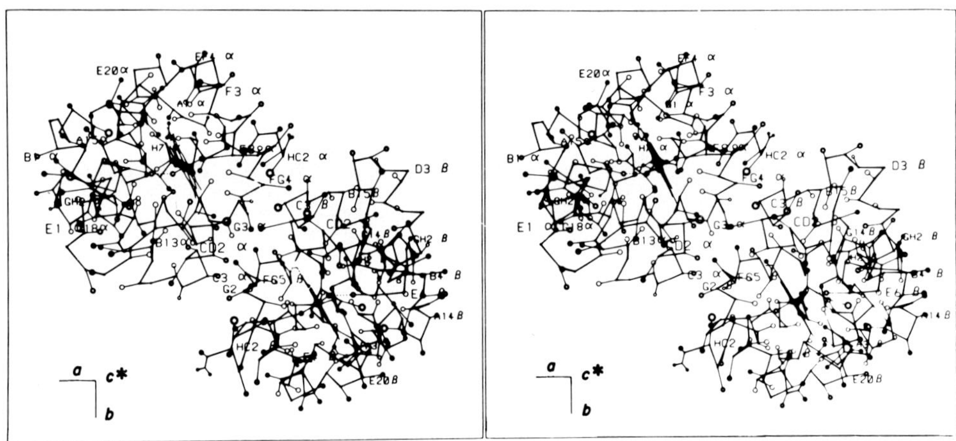

FIGURE 26. Stereo-pair drawing of the $\alpha_1\beta_2$ dimer in horse methemoglobin viewed along the pseudodyad that relates the subunits. The α-carbons and an atom at the center of mass of each side chain are shown. Open circles indicate hydrophobic side chains; cross-hatched circles, acidic ones; striped circles, basic ones; small double circles, neutral hydrophilic ones; large double circles, Tyr and Trp. (From Ladner, R. C., Heidner, E. J., and Perutz, M. F., *J. Mol. Biol.*, 114, 385, 1977. Copyright by Academic Press, London. With permission.)

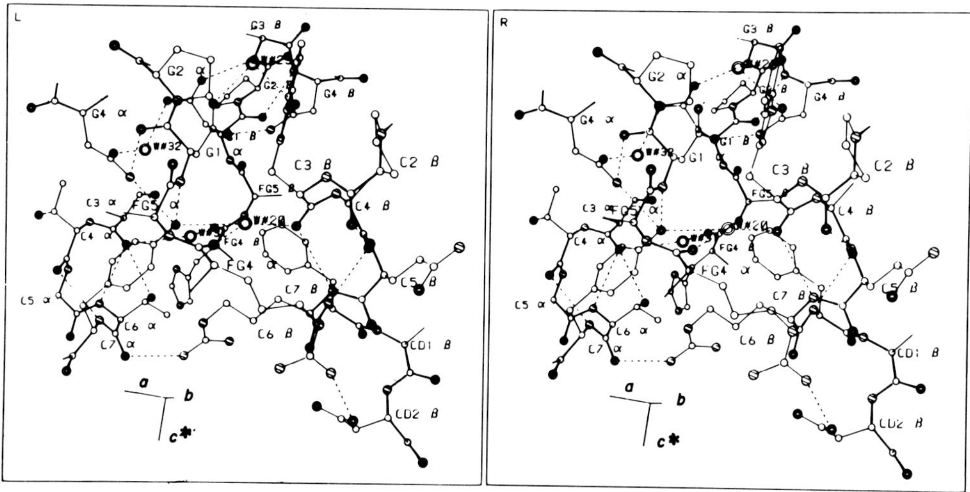

FIGURE 27. Stereo-pair drawing of the $\alpha_1\beta_2$ contact in horse methemoglobin showing the dove-tailing of helix Cβ with FGα at the top and of helix Cα with FGβ underneath. The double circles indicate hydrogen-bonded water molecules. (From Ladner, R. C., Heidner, E. J., and Perutz, M. F., *J. Mol. Biol.*, 114, 385, 1977. Copyright by Academic Press, London. With permission.)

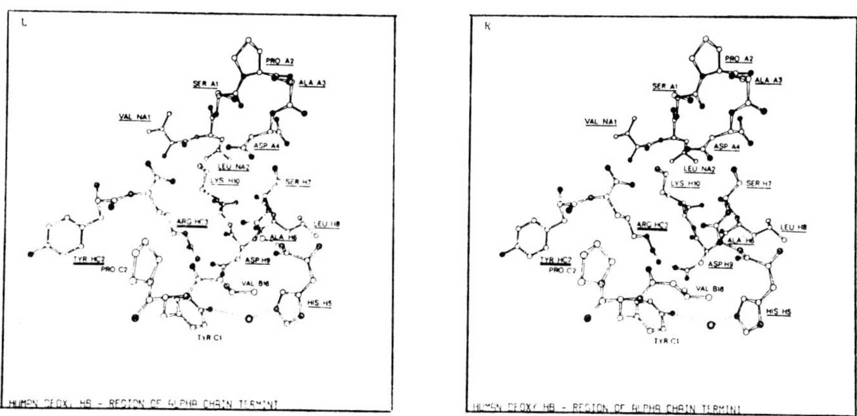

FIGURE 28. Stereo-pair drawing showing parts of segments NA, A, and H of the α_2-chain, segments B and C of the β_2-chains, and segment HC of the α_1-chain in human deoxyhemoglobin. Residue labels of the α_2-chain are underlined once. Those of the α_1-chain are underlined twice. (From Fermi, G., *J. Mol. Biol.*, 97, 237, 1975. Copyright by Academic Press, London. With permission.)

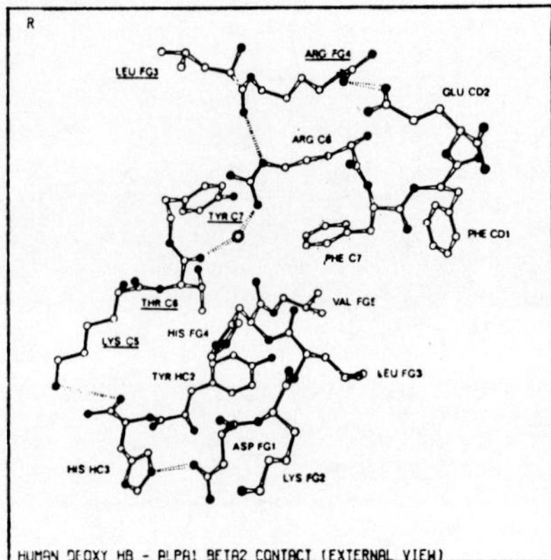

FIGURE 29. Stereo-pair drawing of the external residues of the $\alpha_1\beta_2$ contacts in human deoxy-hemoglobin. The salt bridges involving His HC3(146)β are shown. There is a water molecule linking the side chain of Arg C6(40)β and the carbonyl group of Thr C6(41)α. The hydrogen bond involving the γ-carboxyl group of Glu CD2(43)β is questionable, since this group is poorly resolved in the electron density map. (From Fermi, G., *J. Mol. Biol.*, 97, 237, 1975. Copyright by Academic Press, London. With permission.)

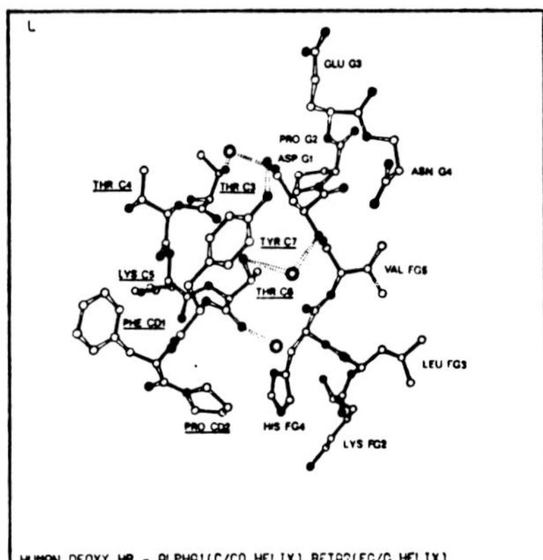

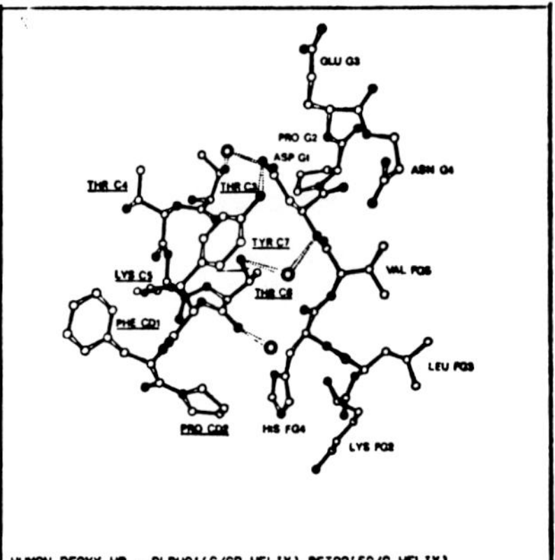

FIGURE 30. Stereo-pair drawing of the dovetailing in the $\alpha_1\beta_2$ contact of human deoxyhemoglobin. Underlined residues are in the α subunit. The side chain of Thr C6(41)α fits into the groove at the α-carbon of Val FG5(98)β. (From Fermi, G., *J. Mol. Biol.*, 97, 237, 1975. Copyright by Academic Press, London. With permission.)

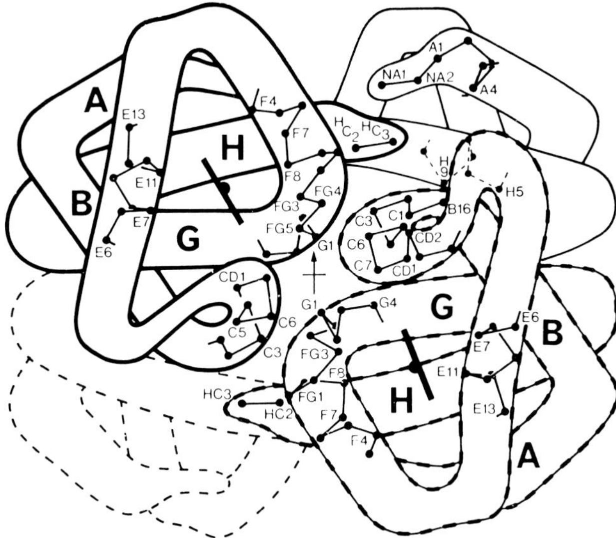

FIGURE 31. The deoxyhemoglobin tetramer. The α-subunits are drawn in the solid line; the β-subunits, in the broken line. The $\alpha_1\beta_2$ dimer is drawn closer to the reader than the $\alpha_2\beta_1$ dimer. The figure is viewed along one of the pseudo-dyads. The molecular twofold axis is the vertical arrow in the plane of the figure. (From Fermi, G., *J. Mol. Biol.*, 97, 237, 1975. Copyright by Academic Press, London. With permission.)

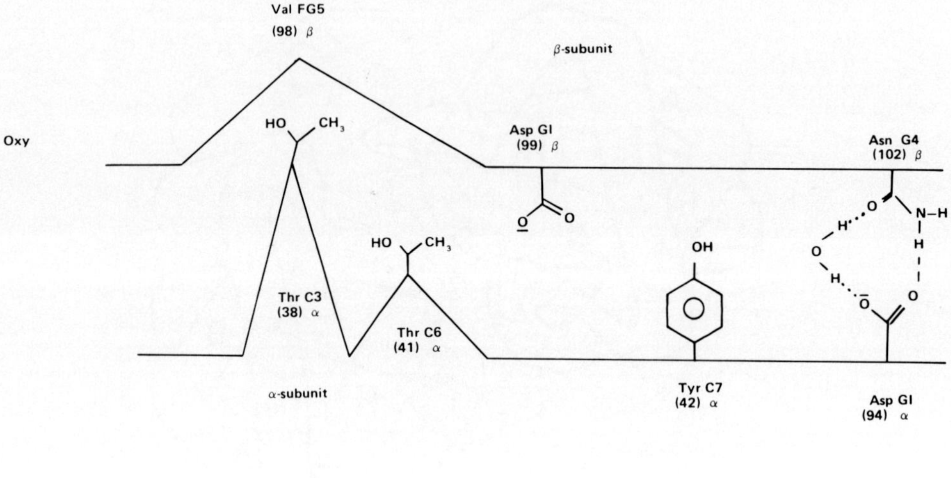

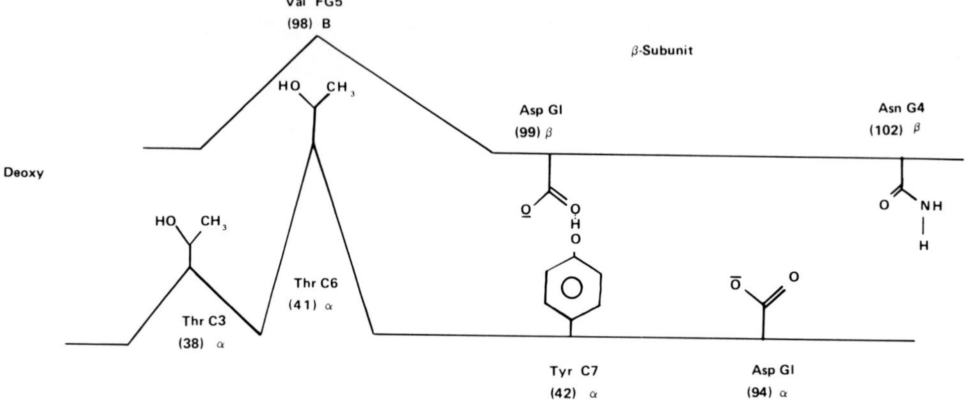

FIGURE 32. Schematic drawing of the changes in the $\alpha_1\beta_2$ contact during oxygenation, showing the two possible interactions between the C helix of the α-chain and Val FG5(98)β.

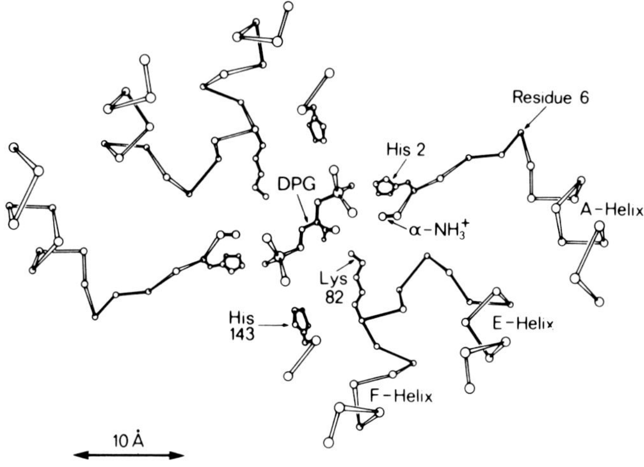

FIGURE 33. Drawing of the binding of diphosphoglycerate to human deoxyhemoglobin. (From Arnone, A., *Nature (London)*, 237, 146, 1972. With permission.)

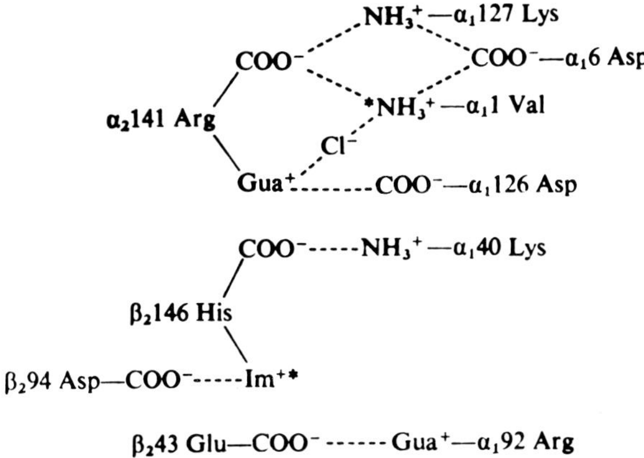

FIGURE 34. Schematic drawing of the salt bridges in deoxyhemoglobin that are not present in oxyhemoglobin. (From Baldwin, J. D., *Br. Med. Bull.*, 32, 213, 1976. Reproduced by permission of the Medical Department, The British Council.)

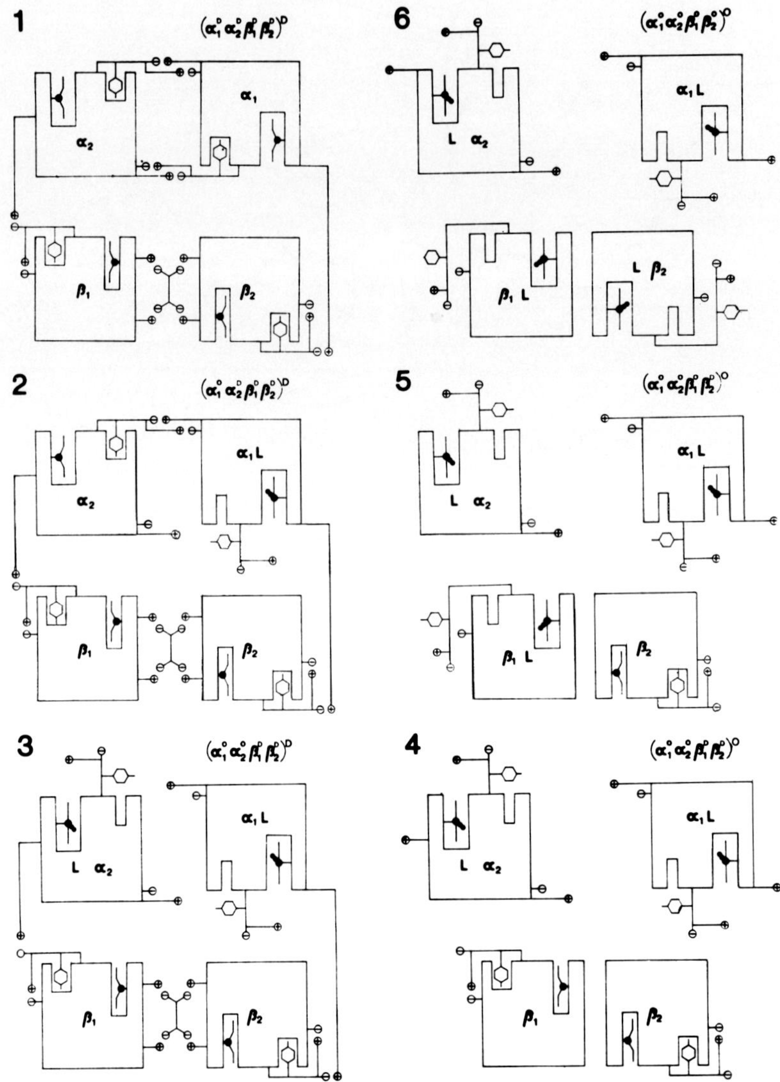

FIGURE 35. Schematic drawing of the proposed sequence of conformational changes that occur during oxygenation. One molecule of DPG is bound between the β-subunits in the deoxy quaternary structure. Panel 1 shows deoxyhemoglobin. The α-chains are oxygenated between panels 1 and 2 and between panels 2 and 3; while the β-chains are oxygenated between panels 4 and 5 and between panels 5 and 6. The quaternary structure changes from deoxy to oxy between panels 3 and 4, accompanied by the expulsion of DPG and the breaking of the salt bridges between subunits α_1 and β_2 and between α_2 and β_1. This change of quaternary structure could occur at any stage of the reaction. More recent work by Perutz and colleagues has confirmed that the rupture of salt bridges in the quaternary deoxy structure is linked to oxygen uptake, but has shown no evidence that the rupture of any particular salt bridge is linked to uptake of oxygen by any particular heme. Their work has confirmed that the penultimate tyrosines are firmly bonded in their pockets in the quaternary deoxy structure, and that they are loose in the quaternary oxy structure, but it has failed to show evidence of the release of tyrosines from their pockets being directly linked to oxygen uptake — it may be linked to the change in quaternary structure instead. (From Perutz, M. F., *Nature (London)*, 228, 726, 1970. With permission.)

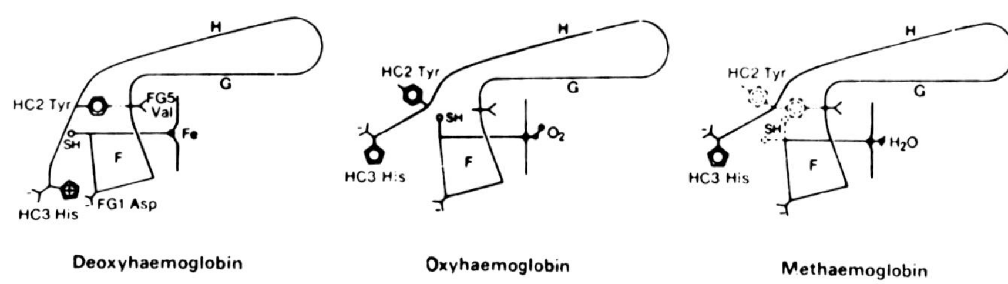

FIGURE 36. Schematic drawing of the conformational changes involving Tyr HC2 and Cys F9 during oxygenation. The Tyr side chain is forced out of its pocket during oxygenation. The Cys side chain faces outward in deoxyhemoglobin, but it is screened from solution by His HC3. In liganded hemoglobin, this screening effect is absent, and there is an equilibrium: Cys in, Tyr out $\rightleftharpoons$ Cys out, Tyr in. Low spin ligands, such as oxygen, strongly favor the Cys in, Tyr out position. On the other hand, high spin ligands, as in methemoglobin, shift the equilibrium toward the Cys out, Tyr in position. (From Perutz, M. F., *Br. Med. Biol.*, 32, 195, 1976. Reproduced by permission of the Medical Department, The British Council.)

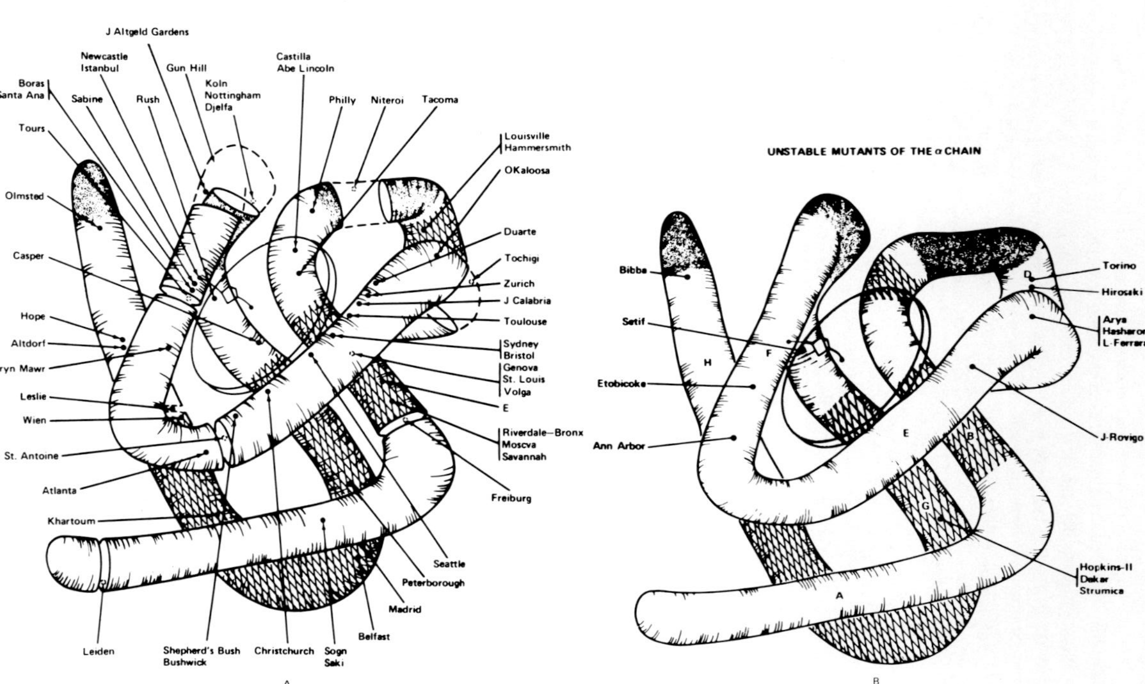

FIGURE 37. Locations of amino acid substitutions in the α (B) and β (A) chains of unstable hemoglobins. The $\alpha_1\beta_1$ contact regions are indicated by the dotted areas. The $\alpha_1\beta_2$ contact regions are indicated by the cross-hatched areas. Deletions, which have been found only in the β-chain, are also known. (From Winslow, R. M. and Anderson, W. F., in *The Metabolic Basis of Inherited Disease*, 4th ed., Stanbury, J. B., Wyngaarden, J. B., and Fredrickson, D. S., Eds., McGraw-Hill, 1978, 1465. With permission.)

Table 1
X-RAY STRUCTURE DETERMINATIONS OF MONOMERIC GLOBINS

Species	Derivative	Resolution (Å)	Ref.
Sperm-whale myoglobin	Aquomet-	2.0	11, 12
	Deoxy-	2.0	13
	Azidomet	2.8	14
	Cyanmet	2.8	15
	CO-	1.8	16
	CO[a]	1.8	152
	Oxy-	1.6	153
	Imidazole	2.5	154
Seal myoglobin	Aquomet-	2.5	17, 170
Tuna myoglobin	Aquomet-	6.0	18
Aplysia myoglobin	Imidazole	3.6	154
Chironomus erythrocruorin	Aquomet-	1.4	19, 169
	CO-	1.4	20, 169
	Deoxy-	1.4	20, 169
	Oxy-	1.4	167
	Cyanmet-	1.4	169
Glycera hemoglobin	Cyanmet-	5.5	21, 22
Lamprey hemoglobin	Cyanmet-	2.0	23, 168
Leghemoglobin	Aquomet-	5.0	24

[a] Neutron diffraction study.

Modified from Perutz, M. F., *Br. Med. Bull.*, 32, 195, 1976.
Reproduced by permission of the Medical Department, the British Council.

Table 2
X-RAY STRUCTURE DETERMINATIONS OF TETRAMERIC HEMOGLOBINS

Species	Derivative	Resolution (Å)	Ref.
Human Hb A	Deoxy	2.5	25, 26
	Deoxy Co(II)	2.5	155
	CO	2.7	27, 156
	Deoxy, α-carbamylated	3.5	157
	Deoxy, Arg-14α hydrazide	3.5	158
	Deoxy, Zn(II) bound	3.5	159
	Deoxy, cross-linked	4.4	160, 161
	Fluoromet	3.5	62
Human Hb F	Deoxy	3.5	28
Horse	Aquomet	2.0	29
	Deoxy	2.8	30
	CO	2.8	31
	Azidomet	2.8	32, 162
	Cyanmet	2.8	33
	Fluoromet	2.8	34
	Deuteromet	2.8	35
	Metmangano	2.8	36
	NO met	2.8	163
	Isothiocyanate met	2.8	164
	Imidazole met	2.7	165
	Mesomet	2.8	166

Modified from Perutz, M. F., *Br. Med. Bull.*, 32,195, 1976.
Reproduced by permission of the Medical Department, The British Council.

Table 3
AMINO ACID SEQUENCES AND POSITIONS OF HUMAN HEMOGLOBINS AND MYOGLOBIN

Structural position		α-Chain		β-, γ-, and δ-Chains				Myoglobin	
		Number	Sequence	Number	β-Sequence	γ-Sequence	δ-Sequence	Number	Sequence
NA	1			1	Val	Gly	Val		
	2	1	Val	2	His	His	His	1	Gly
	3	2	Leu	3	Leu	Phe	Leu	2	Leu
A	1	3	Ser	4	Thr	Thr	Thr	3	Ser
	2	4	Pro	5	Pro	Glu	Pro	4	Asp
	3	5	Ala	6	Glu	Glu	Glu	5	Gly
	4	6	Asp	7	Glu	Asp	Glu	6	Glu
	5	7	Lys	8	Lys	Lys	Lys	7	Trp
	6	8	Thr	9	Ser	Ala	Thr	8	Gln
	7	9	Asn	10	Ala	Thr	Ala	9	Leu
	8	10	Val	11	Val	Ile	Val	10	Val
	9	11	Lys	12	Thr	Thr	Asn	11	Leu
	10	12	Ala	13	Ala	Ser	Ala	12	Asn
	11	13	Ala	14	Leu	Leu	Leu	13	Val
	12	14	Trp	15	Trp	Trp	Trp	14	Trp
	13	15	Gly	16	Gly	Gly	Gly	15	Gly
	14	16	Lys	17	Lys	Lys	Lys	16	Lys
	15	17	Val	18	Val	Val	Val	17	Val
	16	18	Gly	—	—	—	—	18	Glu
AB	1	19	Ala	—	—	—	—	19	Ala
B	1	20	His	19	Asn	Asn	Asn	20	Asp
	2	21	Ala	20	Val	Val	Val	21	Ile
	3	22	Gly	21	Asp	Glu	Asp	22	Pro
	4	23	Glu	22	Glu	Asp	Ala	23	Gly
	5	24	Try	23	Val	Ala	Val	24	His
	6	25	Gly	24	Gly	Gly	Gly	25	Gly
	7	26	Ala	25	Gly	Gly	Gly	26	Gln
	8	27	Glu	26	Glu	Glu	Glu	27	Glu
	9	28	Ala	27	Ala	Thr	Ala	28	Val

	10	29	Leu	28	Leu	Leu	Leu	29	Leu
	11	30	Glu	29	Gly	Gly	Gly	30	Ile
	12	31	Arg	30	Arg	Arg	Arg	31	Arg
	13	32	Met	31	Leu	Leu	Leu	32	Leu
	14	33	Phe	32	Leu	Leu	Leu	33	Phe
	15	34	Leu	33	Val	Val	Val	34	Lys
	16	35	Ser	34	Val	Val	Val	35	Gly
C	1	36	Phe	35	Tyr	Tyr	Tyr	36	His
	2	37	Pro	36	Pro	Pro	Pro	37	Pro
	3	38	Thr	37	Trp	Trp	Trp	38	Glu
	4	39	Thr	38	Thr	Thr	Thr	39	Thr
	5	40	Lys	39	Gln	Gln	Gln	40	Leu
	6	41	Thr	40	Arg	Arg	Arg	41	Glu
	7	42	Tyr	41	Phe	Phe	Phe	42	Lys
CD	1	43	Phe	42	Phe	Phe	Phe	43	Phe
	2	44	Pro	43	Glu	Asp	Glu	44	Asp
	3	45	His	44	Ser	Ser	Ser	45	Lys
	4	46	Phe	45	Phe	Phe	Phe	46	Phe
	5	—	—	46	Gly	Gly	Gly	47	Lys
	6	47	Asp	47	Asp	Asn	Asp	48	His
	7	48	Leu	48	Leu	Leu	Leu	49	Leu
	8	49	Ser	49	Ser	Ser	Ser	50	Lys
D	1	—	—	50	Thr	Ser	Ser	51	Ser
	2	—	—	51	Pro	Ala	Pro	52	Glu
	3	—	—	52	Asp	Ser	Asp	53	Asp
	4	—	—	53	Ala	Ala	Ala	54	Glu
	5	—	—	54	Val	Ile	Val	55	Met
	6	50	His	55	Met	Met	Met	56	Lys
	7	51	Gly	56	Gly	Gly	Gly	57	Ala
E	1	52	Ser	57	Asn	Asn	Asn	58	Ser
	2	53	Ala	58	Pro	Pro	Pro	59	Glu
	3	54	Gln	59	Lys	Lys	Lys	60	Asp
	4	55	Val	60	Val	Val	Val	61	Leu
	5	56	Lys	61	Lys	Lys	Lys	62	Lys
	6	57	Gly	62	Ala	Ala	Ala	63	Lys
	7	58	His	63	His	His	His	64	His
	8	59	Gly	64	Gly	Gly	Gly	65	Gly

Table 3 (continued)
AMINO ACID SEQUENCES AND POSITIONS OF HUMAN HEMOGLOBINS AND MYOGLOBIN

Structural position	α-Chain		β-, γ-, and δ-Chains				Myoglobin	
	Number	Sequence	Number	β-Sequence	γ-Sequence	δ-Sequence	Number	Sequence
9	60	Lys	65	Lys	Lys	Lys	66	Ala
10	61	Lys	66	Lys	Lys	Lys	67	Thr
11	62	Val	67	Val	Val	Val	68	Val
12	63	Ala	68	Leu	Leu	Leu	69	Leu
13	64	Asp	69	Gly	Thr	Gly	70	Thr
14	65	Ala	70	Ala	Ser	Ala	71	Ala
15	66	Leu	71	Phe	Leu	Phe	72	Leu
16	67	Thr	72	Ser	Gly	Ser	73	Gly
17	68	Asn	73	Asp	Asp	Asp	74	Gly
18	69	Ala	74	Gly	Ala	Gly	75	Ile
19	70	Val	75	Leu	Ile	Leu	76	Leu
20	71	Ala	76	Ala	Lys	Ala	77	Lys
EF 1	72	His	77	His	His	His	78	Lys
2	73	Val	78	Leu	Leu	Leu	79	Lys
3	74	Asp	79	Asp	Asp	Asp	80	Gly
4	75	Asp	80	Asn	Asp	Asn	81	His
5	76	Met	81	Leu	Leu	Leu	82	His
6	77	Pro	82	Lys	Lys	Lys	83	Glu
7	78	Asn	83	Gly	Gly	Gly	84	Ala
8	79	Ala	84	Thr	Thr	Thr	85	Glu
F 1	80	Leu	85	Phe	Phe	Phe	86	Ile
2	81	Ser	86	Ala	Ala	Ser	87	Lys
3	82	Ala	87	Thr	Gln	Gln	88	Pro
4	83	Leu	88	Leu	Leu	Leu	89	Leu
5	84	Ser	89	Ser	Ser	Ser	90	Ala
6	85	Asp	90	Glu	Glu	Glu	91	Gln
7	86	Leu	91	Leu	Leu	Leu	92	Ser
8	87	His	92	His	His	His	93	His
9	88	Ala	93	Cys	Cys	Cys	94	Ala

FG	1	89	His	94	Asp	Asp	Asp	95	Thr
	2	90	Lys	95	Lys	Lys	Lys	96	Lys
	3	91	Leu	96	Leu	Leu	Leu	97	His
	4	92	Arg	97	His	His	His	98	Lys
	5	93	Val	98	Val	Val	Val	99	Ile
G	1	94	Asp	99	Asp	Asp	Asp	100	Pro
	2	95	Pro	100	Pro	Pro	Pro	101	Val
	3	96	Val	101	Glu	Glu	Glu	102	Lys
	4	97	Asn	102	Asn	Asn	Asn	103	Tyr
	5	98	Phe	103	Phe	Phe	Phe	104	Leu
	6	99	Lys	104	Arg	Lys	Arg	105	Glu
	7	100	Leu	105	Leu	Leu	Leu	106	Phe
	8	101	Leu	106	Leu	Leu	Leu	107	Ile
	9	102	Ser	107	Gly	Gly	Gly	108	Ser
	10	103	His	108	Asn	Asn	Asn	109	Glu
	11	104	Cys	109	Val	Val	Val	110	Cys
	12	105	Leu	110	Leu	Leu	Leu	111	Ile
	13	106	Leu	111	Val	Val	Val	112	Ile
	14	107	Val	112	Cys	Thr	Cys	113	Gln
	15	108	Thr	113	Val	Val	Val	114	Val
	16	109	Leu	114	Leu	Leu	Leu	115	Leu
	17	110	Ala	115	Ala	Ala	Ala	116	Gln
	18	111	Ala	116	His	Ile	Arg	117	Ser
	19	112	His	117	His	His	Asn	118	Lys
GH	1	113	Leu	118	Phe	Phe	Phe	119	His
	2	114	Pro	119	Gly	Gly	Gly	120	Pro
	3	115	Ala	120	Lys	Lys	Lys	121	Gly
	4	116	Glu	121	Glu	Glu	Glu	122	Asp
	5	117	Phe	122	Phe	Phe	Phe	123	Phe
H	1	118	Thr	123	Thr	Thr	Thr	124	Gly
	2	119	Pro	124	Pro	Pro	Pro	125	Ala
	3	120	Ala	125	Pro	Glu	Gln	126	Asp
	4	121	Val	126	Val	Val	Met	127	Ala
	5	122	His	127	Gln	Gln	Gln	128	Gln
	6	123	Ala	128	Ala	Ala	Ala	129	Gly
	7	124	Ser	129	Ala	Ser	Ala	130	Ala
	8	125	Leu	130	Tyr	Trp	Tyr	131	Met

Table 3 (continued)
AMINO ACID SEQUENCES AND POSITIONS OF HUMAN HEMOGLOBINS AND MYOGLOBIN

Structural position		α-Chain		β-, γ-, and δ-Chains				Myoglobin	
		Number	Sequence	Number	β-Sequence	γ-Sequence	δ-Sequence	Number	Sequence
	9	126	Asp	131	Gln	Gln	Gln	132	Asn
	10	127	Lys	132	Lys	Lys	Lys	133	Lys
	11	128	Phe	133	Val	Met	Val	134	Ala
	12	129	Leu	134	Val	Val	Val	135	Leu
	13	130	Ala	135	Ala	Thr	Ala	136	Glu
	14	131	Ser	136	Gly	Gly	Gly	137	Leu
	15	132	Val	137	Val	Val	Val	138	Phe
	16	133	Ser	138	Ala	Ala	Ala	139	Arg
	17	134	Thr	139	Asn	Ser	Asn	140	Lys
	18	135	Val	140	Ala	Ala	Ala	141	Asp
	19	136	Leu	141	Leu	Leu	Leu	142	Met
	20	137	Thr	142	Ala	Ser	Ala	143	Ala
	21	138	Ser	143	His	Ser	His	144	Ser
HC	1	139	Lys	144	Lys	Arg	Lys	145	Asn
	2	140	Tyr	145	Tyr	Tyr	Tyr	146	Tyr

Table 4
DIFFERENCES BETWEEN THE α- AND β-CHAINS AND MYOGLOBIN (M)

	α	β	M
Number of residues	141	146	153
Segment			
NA	= M	Contains 3 residues	Contains 2 residues
A	= M	= M	—
AB	2 Amides A16-B1 differ	−2 Residues	—
B	= M	= M	—
BC	= M	= M	—
C	$3 \cdot 0_{10}$ Helix	$3 \cdot 0_{10}$ Helix	α-Helix
CD	All different	2 Amides CD5—7 differ	—
D	Absent	= M	—
E	Irregular	E18—20 Irregular	1 Kink
EF	3 Amides EF2 − 5 differ, but α = β	—	—
F	= M	= M	—
FG	= M	= M	—
G	—	G1—3 in $3 \cdot 0_{10}$ helix differ	—
GH	= M	Amide GH1—2	—
H	Contains 21 residues	Contains 21 residues	Contains 26 residues
HC	Contains 3 residues	Contains 3 residues	Contains 4 residues

From Perutz, M. F., *Proc. Roy. Soc. Ser. B,* 173, 113, 1969. With permission.

Table 5
CONFORMATIONAL PARAMETERS OF HELICES

Type	Residues/turn	Atoms/turn	ϕ^a	ψ^b	h (Å)[c]	Ref.
3_{10}	3	10	130.7	154.3	2.00	44, 46
α	3.615	13	133.0	122.8	1.495	43, 46
π	4.4	16	122.9	110.3	1.15	45, 46

[a] Dihedral angle between the plane of the peptide bond containing the amino group of a residue, and the plane containing amino nitrogen atom, the α-carbon atom, and the carbonyl carbon atom of the same residue. See Reference 46 for a detailed explanation.

[b] Dihedral angle between the plane of the peptide bond containing the carbonyl group of a residue, and the plane containing the amino nitrogen atom, the α-carbon atom of the same residue. See Reference 46 for a detailed explanation.

[c] Height of one residue along the axis of the helix.

Table 6
REPLACEMENTS AMONG THE 33 INTERNAL SITES[a]

Residue	Observed
A8	Val, Ile
11	Ala, Thr, Ile, Leu, Cys, Ser, Phe, Val, Met
12	Trp, Phe, Val
15	Val, Ile, Ala, Asn
B6	Gly, Ala
9	Ala, Tyr, Gly, Val, Ile
10	Leu, Val
13	Met, Thr, Leu
14	Phe, Leu
C4	Thr
CD1	Phe
4	Phe, Met, Trp, Lys, Ile, Leu
D5	Val, Ile, Met
E4	Val, Ile, Leu, Met
8	Gly
11	Val, Ile
12	Ala, Ile, Ser, Met, Leu
15	Leu, Ile, Val, Phe
18	Ala, Gly, Ile
19	Val, Gly, Ala, Ile, Leu, Met
F1	Leu, Phe, Tyr, Ile, Val
FG5	Val, Ile
G5	Phe, Leu
8	Leu, Ile
11	Cys, Ser, Gly, Asn, His, Val, Ile, Met, Ala
12	Leu, Phe, Ile
16	Leu, Ile, Met, Phe
H8	Leu, Val, Met, Tyr, Phe, Trp, His
11	Phe, Val, Leu, Met, His, Ala
12	Leu, Phe, Val
15	Val, Leu, Phe
19	Leu, Ile, Met, Ala
HC2	Tyr

[a] The internal sites are the ones listed by Perutz et al[49] The sequences used include 20 α-chains, 22 β-type chains, and 17 myoglobin chains listed in alignments 33, 34, and 35 of Reference 37.

Table 7
REPLACEMENTS AMONG NONPOLAR SURFACE RESIDUES[a]

Residue	Observed
NA2	Val, Ser, Met, His, Gln, Gly
3	Leu, Phe, Trp
A3	Ala, Glu, Asp, Lys, Pro, Ser, Gly, Gln
5	Lys, Arg, Ser, Trp
7	Asn, Glu, His, Arg, Ala, Asp, Leu, Gln, Ser, Thr
9	Lys, Thr, Arg, Ser, Leu, Asn, Ala, Ile
13	Gly, Glu, Asp, Ala, Thr, Ser
AB1	Gly, Ala, Ser, Pro, Glu, Thr
B2	Ala, Gly, Pro, Glu, Val, Ile, Glu, Leu
3	Gly, Glu, Ala, Asp, Pro, Asn, His, Val
4	Glu, Asp, Ala, Gly, Gln, Lys, Ser
11	Glu, Gly, Gln, Thr, Phe, Asp, Ala, Ile, Met
C2	Pro, Thr
5	Lys, Arg, Gln, Ser, Leu, Met
CD7	Leu, Val, Phe
D3	Asp, Ser, Lys, Asn, Gly, Thr, Glu
7	Gly, Asn, Ser, Asp, Ala, His
E9	Lys, Ala, Glu, Ser, Asn, Val, Thr, Asp, Ile
14	Ala, Gly, Ser
6	Thr, Gly, Ala, Asp, Ser, Cys
17	Asn, Lys, Thr, Asp, Leu, Asn, Glu, Gly, Ala
EF3	Asp, Asn, Glu, Gly
7	Gly, Ser, Asn, Ala, Val, Ala
E3	Ala, Lys, Asp, Thr, Ser, Glu, Gln, Pro, His
4	Leu
5	Ser, Ala
9	Ala, Cys, Ser
G1	Asp, Pro, Ser, Ala
2	Pro, Ile, Val
4	Asn, Tyr, Phe
7	Leu, Ile, Phe, Lys, Arg
13	Leu, Val, Thr, Ile, Ala
15	Thr, Val, Gly, Cys
GH2	Pro, Gly, Asn, Lys, Ser, Gln
3	Ala, Ser, Gly, Thr, Asn, Asp, Glu, Pro, Lys, His
5	Phe, Leu
H1	Thr, Pro, Gly, Ala, Asx, Ser
2	Pro, Tyr, Ile, Ala, Thr
4	Val, Ala, Met, Leu, Thr, Cys
6	Ala, Cys, Met, Val, Ser, His, Gly
7	Ser, Ala, Glu, Asx, Ala, Asp
14	Ser, Asn, Ala, Arg, Asp, Val, Gly, Leu
20	Thr, Glu, Asx, Ser, Gly, Ala
21	Ser, Ala, Glu, Gln, His, Arg, Lys, Thr

[a] The nonpolar surface residues are the ones listed by Perutz et al.[49] The sequences used are the same as for Table 6.

Table 8
CONSERVATION OF RESIDUES IN THE GLOBIN FOLD

Conservation of Polar and Nonpolar Residues in Internal and Surface Positions[a]

Structural position	Residue type	Number of residues	Position (%)	Total (%)
Internal	—	33	—	22
	Polar	1	3	1
	Nonpolar	24	73	16
	Either	8	24	5
Surface	—	115	—	78
	Polar	14	12	9
	Nonpolar	6	5	4
	Either	95	83	64

Completely Conserved Positions

Position	Residue	Roll
C4	Thr	Unknown
E7	His	Distal histidine
E8	Gly	Unknown
F4	Leu	Heme contact
F8	His	Proximal histidine
HC2	Tyr	Hydrogen bond holds H and F helices together

[a] The positions used to obtain these data are the ones listed by Perutz et al.[49] The sequences used are the same as for Table 6.

Table 9
SOME DERIVATIVES OF HEMOGLOBINS AND THEIR SPINS

	Ligand in sixth position	Spin
Ferrous derivatives		
Oxyhemoglobin (HbO_2)	O_2	0
Carboxyhemoglobin (HbCO)	CO	0
Deoxyhemoglobin (Hb)	None	2
NO-hemoglobin (HbNO)	NO	0
Ferric derivatives		
Acid methemoglobin (HbH_2O) (methemoglobin, ferrihemoglobin)	H_2O	5/2
Alkaline methemoglobin (HbOH) (ferrihemoglobin hydroxide)	OH^-	1/2, 5/2
Ferrihemoglobin fluoride (HbF)	F^-	5/2
Ferrihemoglobin azide (HbN_3)	N_3^-	1/2
Ferrihemoglobin cyanide (HbCN) (cyanomethemoglobin)	CN^-	1/2

Note: Each molecule of hemoglobin binds four ligands; thus, for example, HbO_2 is an abbreviated version of $Hb(O_2)_4$. The same nomenclature applies to the other derivatives.

From Weissbluth, M., *Hemoglobin: Cooperativity and Electronic Properties*, Springer-Verlag, New York, 1974, 3. With permission.

Table 10
HEME STEREOCHEMISTRY

Distances (Å)	Myoglobin		Hemoglobin				2-Methylimidazole iron(II)[52] TPP[a]	Picket-fence oxygen adduct[53]
			α-Chain		β-Chain			
	Aquomet	Deoxy	Aquomet	Deoxy	Aquomet	Deoxy		
Fe to porphyrin plane	0.40	0.55	0.07	0.60	0.21	0.63	0.55	0
His N_ϵ to porphyrin plane	2.5	2.6	2.2	2.6	2.4	2.8	2.68	2.07
Fe to N_ϵ	2.1	2.1	2.1	2.0	2.2	2.2	2.16	2.07
Fe to $N_{pyrrole}$ (average)	2.04	2.06	2.0[b]	2.1	2.0[b]	2.1	—	—
Imidazole angle[c]	19°	19°	21°	20°	15°	25°	—	—

[a] Abbreviation: TPP, tetraphenylporphyrin.
[b] Constrained to be equidistant.
[c] Angle between plane of imidazole projected on to heme plane and line joining heme center to the nitrogens of pyrroles I and III, as defined in Figures 2 and 3 of Fermi (1975).[25]

From Perutz, M. F., *Br. Med. Bull.*, 32, 195, 1976. Reproduced by permission of the Medical Department, The British Council.

Table 11
INTERATOMIC CONTACTS OF THE HEME GROUPS AND THEIR SURROUNDING RESIDUES, AND NUMBERS OF ATOMS INVOLVED IN HEME-GLOBIN CONTACTS

Myoglobin			α-Heme			β-Heme		
	Number of atoms			Number of atoms			Number of atoms	
Residue	Globin	Heme	Residue	Globin	Heme	Residue	Globin	Heme
CDI Phe	4	6	C7 Tyr	2	2	C7 Phe	1	1
CD3 Arg	2	4	CD1 Phe	3	5	CD1 Phe	2	2
E7 His	2	7	CD3 His	1	1	E7 His	3	10
E10 Thr	1	3	CD4 Phe	2	1	E10 Lys	1	1
E11 Val	2	5	E7 His	2	7	E11 Val	4	10
E14 Ala	1	2	E10 Lys	1	1	E14 Ala	1	3
E15 Leu	1	1	E11 Val	1	1	F1 Phe	1	1
F7 Ser	2	2	F4 Leu	3	2	F4 Leu	3	6
F8 His	3	12	F7 Leu	1	2	F7 Leu	1	2
FG2 His	3	7	F8 His	3	7	F8 His	2	6
FG4 Ile	2	2	FG3 Leu	2	5	FG3 Leu	1	3
G4 Tyr	2	1	FG5 Val	3	6	FG5 Val	1	1
G5 Leu	1	1	G4 Asn	3	1	G4 Asn	5	2
G8 Ile	1	1	G5 Phe	4	4	G5 Phe	2	3
			G8 Leu	1	3	G8 Leu	1	1
			H19 Leu	1	4	H19 Leu	1	4
Total	27	54		33	52		30	56

Note: All interatomic distances of 4 Å or less were counted. In metmyoglobin the distal water molecule was taken as part of the heme.

From Perutz, M. F., *Br. Med. Bull.*, 32, 195, 1976. Reproduced by permission of the Medical Department, The British Council.

Table 12
DISTANCES (Å) FROM HEME TO SURROUNDING AMINO ACID SIDE CHAINS IN HORSE MET- AND HUMAN DEOXYHEMOGLOBIN

Group	Residue	Atom	1 Distance to porphyrin plane[a]		2 Distance to heme axis		3 Distance to porphyrin center		4 Distance to Fe		5 Distance to heme-linked water	
					α							
B10	Leu 29	Cδ2	6.3	6.5	2.4	2.5	6.8	7.0	6.9	7.5	5.0	—
		Cδ1	7.7	8.1	0.5	0.6	7.7	8.1	7.8	8.7	5.8	—
B13	Met 32	Cε	5.1	5.2	6.2	6.5	8.0	8.3	8.1	8.7	6.9	—
		Sδ	4.6	4.6	7.3	7.5	8.6	8.8	8.7	9.1	7.7	—
CD1	Phe 43	Cε2	3.7	3.9	4.7	5.1	6.0	6.4	6.0	6.8	4.9	—
		Cζ	3.4	3.4	4.4	4.6	5.5	5.8	5.6	6.1	4.6	—
		Cε1	3.5	3.3	5.5	5.7	6.5	6.6	6.6	6.9	5.6	—
E7	His 58	Nε	3.6	3.8	2.3	1.7	4.3	4.2	4.4	4.7	2.8	—
		Cε	3.3	3.1	3.4	2.4	4.7	4.0	4.8	4.5	3.7	—
E11	Val 62	Cγ2	4.3	3.8	2.8	2.5	5.1	4.6	5.2	5.1	3.8	—
		Cγ1	4.7	4.4	4.8	4.3	6.7	6.2	6.8	6.7	5.7	—
F4	Leu 83	Cδ2	−3.3	−2.8	7.1	6.9	7.8	7.4	7.8	7.3	8.9	—
		Cδ1	−3.5	−3.8	5.6	5.7	6.6	6.9	6.6	6.6	7.9	—
F7	Leu 86	Cδ2	−3.8	−4.3	4.8	5.4	6.1	6.9	6.0	6.6	7.4	—
		Cδ1	−5.3	−6.1	5.7	5.9	7.8	8.5	7.8	8.1	9.2	—
F8	His 87	H_2O	1.9	—	0.1	—	1.9	—	2.0[b]	—	—	—
		Fe	−0.1	−0.6	0[b]	0[b]	0.1	0.6	—	—	2.0[b]	—
		Nε	−2.2	−2.6	0.2	0.3	2.2	2.6	2.1	2.0	4.1	—
		Cε	−2.8	−3.1	1.2	1.5	3.1	3.4	3.0	2.9	4.9	—
FG3	Leu 91	Cδ2	−3.9	−3.7	7.0	5.8	8.0	6.9	7.9	6.6	9.0	—
		Cδ1	−3.3	−3.5	4.6	3.3	5.6	4.9	5.6	4.5	6.9	—
FG5	Val 93	Cγ2	−3.8	−3.0	4.9	5.4	6.3	6.2	6.2	5.9	7.5	—
		Cγ1	−3.3	−2.8	6.3	6.4	7.1	7.0	7.0	6.7	8.0	—

Table 12 (continued)

DISTANCES (Å) FROM HEME TO SURROUNDING AMINO ACID SIDE CHAINS IN HORSE MET- AND HUMAN DEOXYHEMOGLOBIN

Group	Residue	Atom	1 Distance to porphyrin plane[a]		2 Distance to heme axis		3 Distance to porphyrin center		4 Distance to Fe		5 Distance to heme-linked water	
G5	Phe 98	Cε2	−4.3	−4.4	5.8	5.4	7.2	7.0	7.1	6.6	8.4	—
		Cζ	−4.0	−4.0	4.7	4.4	6.1	6.0	6.1	5.5	7.5	—
		Cε1	−3.2	−3.2	5.0	4.9	5.9	5.8	5.9	5.5	7.1	—
G8	Leu 101	Cδ2	3.0	5.3	4.9	6.6	5.8	8.4	5.8	8.8	5.1	—
		Cδ1	5.1	3.2	6.2	5.3	8.0	6.2	8.1	6.5	7.0	—
H19	Leu 136	Cδ2	−5.5	−5.1	4.8	5.3	7.3	7.4	7.2	7.0	8.9	—
		Cδ1	−3.5	−3.4	4.5	5.5	5.7	6.4	5.6	6.2	7.1	—
					β							
B10	Leu 28	Cδ2	6.8	6.8	3.2	2.7	7.5	7.3	7.7	7.8	5.9	—
		Cδ1	7.6	5.5	1.7	4.6	7.8	7.2	8.0	7.7	6.1	—
B13	Leu 31	Cδ2	4.6	3.7	6.3	7.8	7.8	8.6	7.9	8.9	6.8	—
		Cδ1	4.7	3.4	8.4	10.2	9.7	10.7	9.8	10.9	8.8	—
CD1	Phe 42	Cε2	3.6	3.2	4.5	7.2	5.8	7.9	5.9	8.1	4.8	—
		Cζ	3.3	3.0	4.4	6.0	5.5	6.7	5.6	7.0	4.5	—
		Cε1	3.6	3.3	5.5	6.0	6.6	6.8	6.7	7.1	5.7	—
E7	His 63	Nε	3.3	3.2	2.4	2.4	4.0	4.0	4.2	4.5	2.8	—
		Cε	3.0	2.9	3.5	2.2	4.6	3.6	4.7	4.1	3.8	—
E11	Val 67	Cγ2	3.9	3.0	2.3	1.4	4.6	3.3	4.8	3.9	3.3	—
		Cγ1	4.2	3.6	4.2	3.7	5.9	5.2	6.0	5.7	4.8	—
F4	Leu 88	Cδ2	−3.6	−3.2	5.7	5.3	6.8	6.2	6.6	5.9	7.9	—
		Cδ1	−3.9	−2.5	6.6	6.3	7.2	6.8	7.1	6.6	8.2	—
F7	Leu 91	Cδ2	−4.2	−4.7	4.8	5.4	6.4	7.2	6.3	6.8	7.7	—
		Cδ1	−5.8	−6.4	5.9	6.8	8.3	9.3	8.1	8.9	9.7	—

F8	His 92	H_2O	1.8	—	0.1	—	1.8	—	2.0[b]	—	—	—
		Fe	−0.2	−0.6	0[b]	0[b]	0.2	0.6	—	—	2.0[b]	—
		Nϵ	−2.4	−2.9	0.2	0.3	2.4	2.9	2.2	2.2	4.2	—
		Cϵ	−3.0	−3.4	1.2	1.5	3.3	3.7	3.1	3.1	5.0	—
FG3	Leu 96	Cδ2	−4.2	−4.1	6.6	6.1	7.8	7.3	7.7	7.0	8.8	—
		Cδ1	−3.5	−3.6	4.2	3.6	5.5	5.1	5.3	4.7	6.7	—
FG5	Val 98	Cγ2	−3.6	−4.3	5.4	4.7	6.6	6.4	6.4	6.0	7.6	—
		Cγ1	−3.4	−3.9	6.1	5.5	7.0	6.8	6.9	6.4	7.9	—
G5	Phe 103	Cϵ2	−5.7	−5.8	5.3	5.0	7.8	7.6	7.7	7.1	9.1	—
		Cζ	−5.0	−4.9	4.4	4.0	6.7	6.4	6.5	5.2	8.1	—
		Cϵ1	−3.7	−3.6	4.6	4.3	5.9	5.6	5.8	5.9	7.1	—
G8	Leu 106	Cδ2	3.1	2.8	4.9	6.4	5.8	6.9	5.9	7.2	5.0	—
		Cδ1	5.1	4.6	6.3	7.3	8.1	8.6	8.3	9.0	7.1	—
H19	Leu 141	Cδ2	−4.8	−4.9	4.8	5.2	6.8	7.1	6.6	6.7	8.2	—
		Cδ1	−3.1	−3.4	5.9	4.9	6.7	6.0	6.6	5.7	7.7	—

Note: In each column met is first and deoxy second. Plus on distal, minus on proximal side; the probable errors of these distances are 0.20 Å for met and 0.32 Å for deoxy. Angle between plane of imidazole F8 projected onto heme plane and line joining heme center to nitrogens of pyrroles I and III, as defined in Figures 2 and 3 of Fermi (1975):[25] α, met 21°, deoxy 20°; β, met 15°, deoxy 25°. The probable errors are based on the assumption that the positions of side chains surrounding the hemes are as well-defined as those of the hemes, so that the probable error in their positions is 0.57 × the overall error, which is 0.25 Å for this structure and 0.40 for human deoxyhemoglobin. ($0.57 \times 0.25 \times \sqrt{2} = 0.20$; $0.57 \times 0.40 \times \sqrt{2} = 0.32$).

[a] The porphyrin plane is defined as the mean plane of the ring nitrogens and carbons and the first carbons of all the side chains.

[b] Constrained.

From Ladner, R. C., Heidner, E. J., and Perutz, M. F., *J. Mol. Biol.*, 114, 385, 1977.

Table 13
COMPARISON OF THE MODEL ATOMIC COORDINATES OF HUMAN AND HORSE DEOXYHEMOGLOBIN BEFORE AND AFTER RIGID-BODY FITTING

	r.m.s. Difference (Å)		Rigid-body motion		
Portion fitted	**Before fitting**	**After fitting**	**r.m.s. Shift (Å)[a]**	**Translation (Å)**	**Rotation (degree)[b]**
Overall	1.18	—	—	—	—
α-Subunit					
Globin chain	1.06	1.03	0.28	0.24	0.7
A helix	1.10	0.97	0.52	0.50	1.3
B helix	1.10	0.97	0.52	0.38	4.1
C helix	1.42	1.32	0.53	0.35	6.2
E helix	1.13	1.08	0.36	0.33	1.5
F helix	0.74	0.63	0.39	0.35	2.2
G helix	0.97	0.89	0.38	0.23	3.7
H helix	0.68	0.65	0.18	0.16	1.1
Heme	0.53	0.38	0.37	0.31	2.6
β-Subunit					
Globin chain	1.30	1.19	0.52	0.38	1.7
A helix	1.85	1.06	1.51	1.28	12.4
B helix	1.27	1.15	0.55	0.49	3.4
C helix	0.76	0.73	0.21	0.16	1.4
D helix	0.96	0.74	0.62	0.58	4.5
E helix	1.38	1.09	0.85	0.58	4.0
F helix	0.62	0.49	0.38	0.28	3.5
G helix	0.80	0.59	0.54	0.30	3.7
H helix	0.89	0.81	0.37	0.33	1.9
Heme	0.70	0.56	0.41	0.28	4.2

[a] Calculated as $\sqrt{(\Delta_{X_b})^2 - (\Delta_{X_a})^2}$, where Δ_{X_b} and Δ_{X_a} are the r.m.s. difference in the coordinates of the two structures before and after fitting. This assumes that the mean inner product between the vector shift due to rotation (about the center mass) and the residual vectors is zero, an assumption that could either overestimate or underestimate the shift during rigid-body motion.

[b] About center of mass.

From Fermi, G., *J. Mol. Biol.*, 97, 237, 1975. With permission.

Table 14
SURFACE AREA BURIED IN CONTACTS

	Human deoxyhemoglobin		**Horse methemoglobin**	
	Surface area (Å²)	**Polar fraction (%)[b]**	**Surface area (Å²)**	**Polar fraction (%)**
Accessible surface area of subunit[a]				
α	7100	37	6900	37
β	7500	41	7200	40
Surface area buried in contact				
$\alpha_1\beta_1$ or $\alpha_2\beta_2$	1650	37	1750	32
$\alpha_1\beta_2$ or $\alpha_2\beta_1$	1300	40	950	38
$\alpha_1\alpha_2$	500	65	<200[c]	—
$\beta_1\beta_2$	0	—	<200[c]	—
Total buried surface area[d]	6400	40	~5800	35

[a] The accessible surface area of isolated subunits is calculated in the conformation observed in the tetrameric molecules. Values near 7200 Å² are expected on the basis of the molecular weights. After differences due to amino acid substitutions are subtracted, the values obtained for α-chains in the deoxy- and in methemoglobin are the same to within 3%, and to within 2% for the β-chains. This yields an estimate of the precision in determining accessible (or buried) surface areas from two independent crystallographic structure determinations.

[b] Fraction of surface area contributed by nitrogen, oxygen, and, marginally, sulfur atoms.

[c] The calculations based on atomic coordinates provided by Ladner give significant values for the surface buried between the subunits in methemoglobin. However, most of this comes from the amino and carboxyl terminal residues for which little density is seen in the electron density map, and which are probably free to move in solution.

[d] Contacts between α- and β-chains occur twice; contacts between like chains, once.

From Chothia, C., Wodak, S., and Janin, J., *Proc. Natl. Acad. Sci. U.S.A.*, 73, 3793, 1976. With permission.

Table 15
SUBUNIT CONTACTS IN HORSE METHEMOGLOBIN

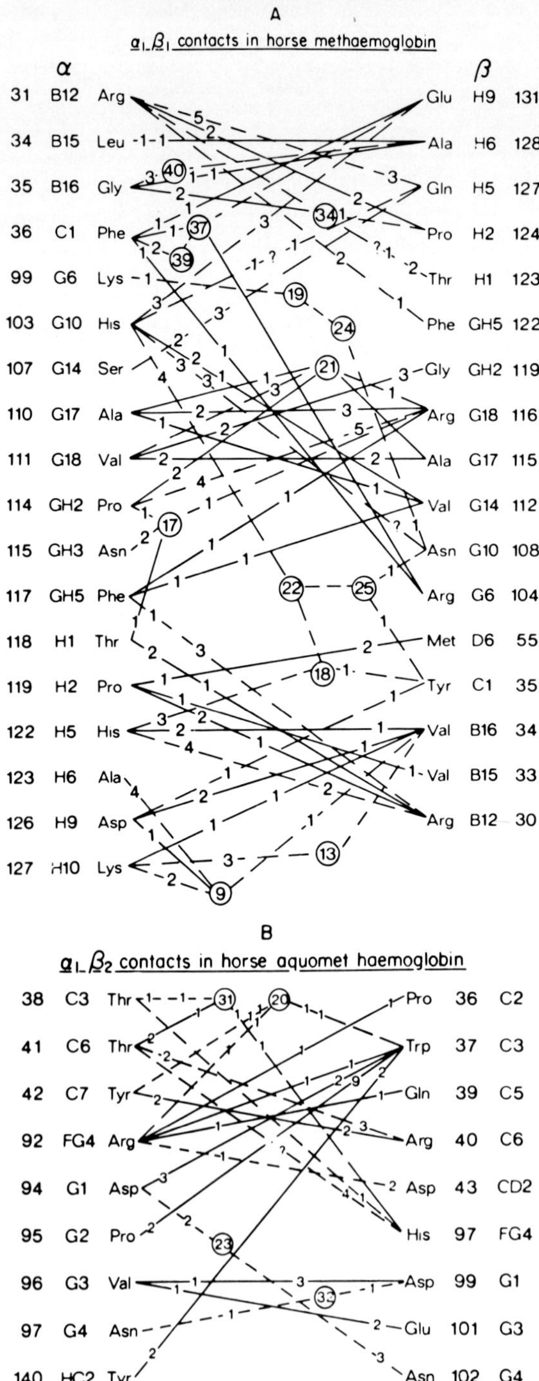

Table 16
SUBUNIT CONTACTS IN HUMAN DEOXYHEMOGLOBIN

Interatomic contacts between residues in unlike chains†

(a) *The contact* $\alpha_1\beta_1$

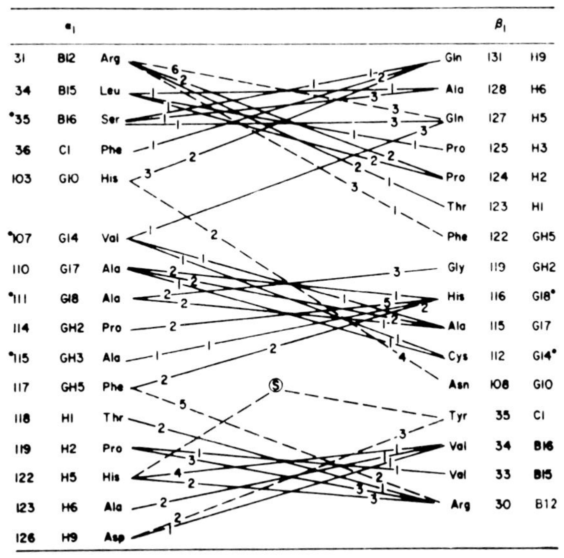

(b) *The contact* $\alpha_1\beta_2$

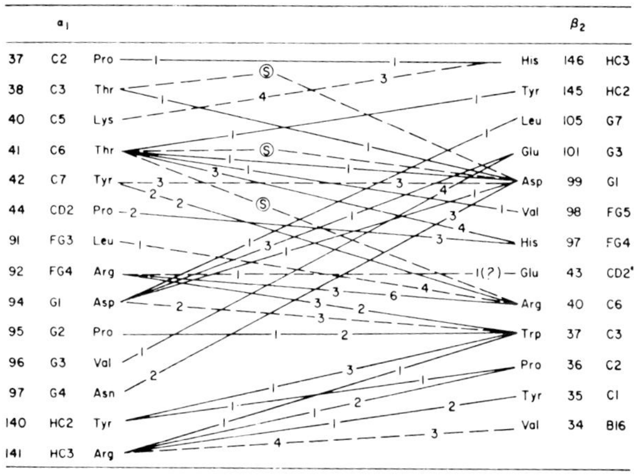

27 residues including about 107 atoms in contact.

Note: All interatomic distances of 4.0 Å or less were counted as contacts. Plain lines indicate van der Waals' contacts; broken ones indicate that the contact includes a hydrogen bond. The symbol S represents a solvent molecule (identified as a positive peak in a difference map of observed minus calculated structure-factor amplitudes). Numbers on the lines give the number of atoms, contributed to the contact by the residues on each side. For future reference in studies of the differences between oxy- and deoxyhemoglobin, it is noted that the distance between the imidazole of His H5(122)α_1 and the guanidinium of Arg B12(30)β_1 is 3.2 Å. Residues marked with an asterisk differ in horse and human hemoglobin.

From Fermi, G., *J. Mol. Biol.*, 97, 237, 1975. With permission.

Table 17
RESIDUES IN CONTACT WITH HEME GROUPS

Designation	Residue		Replacement		Variability[a]	Clinical symptoms	Abnormal properties	Structural effects of replacement	Ref.
	No.	Position	From	To					
α-Chain variants									
Torino	43	CDI	Phe	Val	I	Hemolytic anemia[b]	Unstable	Substitution removes the contact of the heme group with Cδ and Cζ of Phe, leaving the gap at the surface of the heme pocket; Cγ2 of Val makes a short contact with Cβ of the Phe CD4(46) which would disturb the conformation of the CD segment	75
M-Boston	58	E7	His	Tyr	I	Cyanosis[c]	Difficult to reduce; α-chains do not combine with O_2	Phenol group of tyrosine probably forms ionic links with Fe(III), thus stabilizing it in the ferric state	76
M-Iwate	87	F8	His	Tyr	I	Methemoglobinemia		In addition to the effects described for Hb Boston, the heme group must be displaced towards helix E; X-ray studies show that Hb M-Iwate has a conformation similar to normal deoxyhemoglobin in both the reduced and oxidized states; a small conformational change occurs, but does not alter the crystal lattice	77, 129
Bibba	136	H19	Leu	Pro	I	Hemolytic anemia	Unstable; separable by electrophoresis at pH 8.6	Substitution removes contact of $C\delta_2$ with the heme group and leads to unfolding of residues 136 to 138 of helix H; should inhibit normal function of the α-chains	78
β-Chain variants									

Hammersmith	42	CD_1	Phe	Ser	I	Hemolytic anemia: cyanosis	Unstable, easily oxidized, then loses heme; low oxygen affinity	Substitution removes the contact of the heme group with the $C\epsilon$ and $C\zeta$ of Phe, leaving a gap at the surface of the heme pocket; the presence of the hydrophilic OH opens the pocket to water	79, 80
M-Saskatoon	63	E7	His	Tyr	I	Cyanosis; methemoglobinemia			
Zürich	63	E7	His	Arg	I	Hemolytic anemia on treatment with sulfonamides	Combines reversibly with O_2 but is more easily oxidized and precipitated	The arginine side chain cannot be accommodated in the heme pocket, but must protrude at the surface leaving a large cavity at the ligand site of the iron atom; γ-COO^- of Glu forms a salt bridge with Fe(III) and pushes the side chain of His E7 out of the heme pocket	81, 82
M-Milwaukee	67	E11	Val	Glu	I	Cyanosis; methemoglobinemia			76
Sydney	67	E11	Val	Ala	I	Hemolytic anemia; inclusion bodies formed on incubation of blood at 37°C	Unstable; easily oxidized; loss of heme on heating	Breaks contact of the heme group with both $C\gamma$'s of Val; loosens heme group	83
Santa Ana	88	F4	Leu	Pro	I	Hemolytic anemia; inclusion bodies in erythrocytes after splenectomy	No heme in β-chain	Proline occurs at the amino end of helix F and may not cause any change in the conformation of the main chain, but the replacement removes the contact of the heme group with $C\gamma$ and $C\delta$ of Leu; this opens a crevice on the proximal side into which water could enter	84, 129
M-Hyde Park	92	F8	His	Tyr	I	Cyanosis; methemoglobinemia	Difficult to reduce; β-chains do combine with O_2; unstable	See Hb M-Iwate	89

Table 17 (continued)
RESIDUES IN CONTACT WITH HEME GROUPS

	Residue		Replacement						
Designation	No.	Position	From	To	Variability[a]	Clinical symptoms	Abnormal properties	Structural effects of replacement	Ref.
Köln	98	FG5	Val	Met	I	Hemolytic anemia; inclusion bodies in erythrocytes after splenectomy	Slightly increased + charge at pK 8.6, suggesting a rise in the pK of a histidine; high oxygen affinity	There are two possibilities: (1) the side chain of Met could go into an internal position by the heme group; this would displace the heme towards the distal histidine or cause a change in conformation of the FG corner; (2) the side chain of Met could be external, which could happen only at the expense of a change in conformation of the FG corner	86, 87
Kansas	102	G4	Asn	Thr	I	Cyanosis	Unstable; decreased oxygen affinity; decreased Hill's constant;[d] large Bohr effect;[e] high rate of autoxidation; oxyhemoglobin dissociates into $\alpha\beta$ dimers	$C\gamma$ of Thr probably makes short contact with vinyl and methyl of pyrrol II; this would displace either the heme or helix G. Also Asn G4 of chain β normally forms a hydrogen bond with Asp G1 of chain α. This would be broken by the replacement, which should favor dissociation into $\alpha\beta$ dimers	88

[a] Variability refers to whether the amino acid position that is substituted is variable (V) or invariable (I) among mammalian hemoglobins, and if variable, whether the variability is restricted to either polar (Vp) or nonpolar (Vn) amino acid residues.
[b] Inclusion body anemia: precipitated hemoglobin forms inclusion bodies in the red cell and shortens its lifespan.
[c] Cyanosis: blue color of skin due to deoxyhemoglobin in the capillaries; can be due to the oxygen affinity of hemoglobin being too low.
[d] Hill's constant: a measure of the interaction between the four heme groups causing the sigmoid shape of the oxygen dissociation curve.
[e] Bohr effect: dependence of the oxygen affinity on pH.

Modified from Perutz, M. F. and Lehmann, H., *Nature (London)*, 219, 902, 1968. With permission.

Table 18
RESIDUES AT CONTACTS BETWEEN SUBUNITS

Designation	Residue		Replacement		Variability	Clinical symptoms	Abnormal properties	Structural effects of replacement in oxyhemoglobin	Contact affected	Ref.
	No.	Position	From	To						
α-Chain variants										
G-Chinese	30	B11	Glu	Gln	I	None	None	Glu B11α_1 makes contact with Pro H2β_1, but replacement of OH by NH_2 should not matter	$\alpha_1\beta_1$	89
J-Capetown	92	FG4	Arg	Gln	I	Mild polycythemia in homozygote	High oxygen affinity; diminished heme-heme interaction	Arg GF4α_1 is Van der Waals contact with Arg C6β_2; in addition its guanidinium group may make a hydrogen bond with a recipient group in β_2; replacement may interfere with structural transition between oxy and deoxy forms	$\alpha_1\beta_2$	90, 91
Chesapeake	92	FG4	Arg	Leu	I	Polycythemia[a]	High oxygen affinity; diminished heme-heme interaction; normal Bohr effect	See Hb J-Capetown.	$\alpha_1\beta_2$	92, 93
Chiapas	114	GH2	Pro	Arg	I	None	None	Would be expected to weaken GH corner and make α-chain and $\alpha_1\beta_1$ contact less stable	$\alpha_1\beta_1$	94
β-Chain variants										
E	26	B8	Glu	Lys	I	Microcytosis	Diminished affinity of normal α-chains for these abnormal β-chains; unstable in vitro	Replacement of the Glu B8β_1, removes one of the residues designed to neutralize Arg B12, introducing instead an extra + charge; this would disturb the hydrogen bonding between the arginine and the α_1-chain	$\alpha_1\beta_1$	95, 96

Table 18 (continued)
RESIDUES AT CONTACTS BETWEEN SUBUNITS

	Residue		Replacement							
Designation	No.	Position	From	To	Variability	Clinical symptoms	Abnormal properties	Structural effects of replacement in oxyhemoglobin	Contact affected	Ref.
Tacoma	30	B12	Arg	Ser	I	None reported	Increased oxygen affinity; unstable in vitro	Removes the hydrogen bond between Arg B12β_1 and Phe GH5α_1, thus weakening bonds between α_1 and β_1	$\alpha_1\beta_1$	97, 130
Philly	35	C1	Tyr	Phe	I	Mild hemolytic anemia	All six cysteines react with PMB; unstable in vitro	Removes the hydrogen bond between Tyr C1β_1 and Asp H9α_1, thus weakening bonds between α_1 and β_1	$\alpha_1\beta_1$	98, 131
β-Chain variants										
Yakima	99	G1	Asp	His	I	Polycythemia	Increased oxygen affinity; diminished heme-heme interaction; normal Bohr effect	The carboxyl group of Asp G1β_2 normally forms a hydrogen bond with NH of Glu G3β_2; it also touches Cγ of Val G3α_1; the imidazole ring of histidine could still make the same hydrogen bond, though it would be weaker, and touch Val G3α_1; in addition it would make a new contact with Leu G7α_1	$\alpha_1\beta_2$	99, 100
Kempsey	99	G1	Asp	Asn	I	Polycythemia	Increased oxygen affinity; diminished heme-heme interaction; Bohr effect present	Replacement of OH by NH_2 would weaken internal hydrogen bond and alter contact with Val G3α_1	$\alpha_1\beta_2$	101
Kansas	102	G4	Asn	Thr	I	See Table 17			$\alpha_1\beta_2$	88

New York	113	G15	Val	Glu	I	None reported	No increased electrophoretic mobility at pH 8.6, despite extra − charge	Introduces a − charge deep in a surface crevice; might cause rearrangement of Arg B12, Glu B8, and His G19; unchanged electrophoretic mobility might be due to a rise in pK of His G19	$\alpha_1\beta_1$	102
K-Woolwich	132	H10	Lys	Glu	I	None	None	Lys H10β is in a position to form a hydrogen bond with the α-carboxyl group of histidine H24 of the opposite β-chain in oxy, but not in deoxyhemoglobin; in deoxyhemoglobin it may bind diphosphoglycerate; its replacement by glutamic acid may affect the oxygen dissociation curve	$\beta_1\beta_2$	103

[a] Polycythemia: excess of red blood cells. Can be caused by stimulation of red cell production by shortage of oxygen in the tissues; for example, if the oxygen affinity of hemoglobin is too high.

Modified from Perutz, M. F. and Lehmann, H., *Nature (London),* 219, 902, 1968. With permission.

Table 19
RESIDUES IN GENERAL POSITIONS

Designation	Residue		Replacement		Variability	Clinical symptoms	Abnormal properties	Structural effects of replacement	Ref.
	No.	Position	From	To					
α-Chain variants									
Etobicoke	84	F5	Ser	Arg	I	None reported	Unstable	In Hb A the OH of serine F5 probably forms a hydrogen bond with CO of Leu H19. Substitution of Arg would force a conformational change, either within helix F (short contact between Cy (Arg) and OH (Ser F2)), or by prying helices F and G apart	104
Manitoba	102	G9	Ser	Arg	I	None; present only in small proportion	Difficult to separate from HB A by electrophoresis at pH 8.6	In central cavity. May introduce instability through excess of + charges in central cavity	105, 132
β-Chain variants									
Tokuchi	2	NA2	His	Tyr	V	None	Little evidence	The imidazole ring of His 2 is probably external; the phenyl ring of tyrosine is more hydrophobic and is rarely found in external positions; the replacement is likely to lead to a conformational change in the NA segment	106
Sogn	14	All	Leu	Arg	Vn	None	Unstable; appearance of free α-chains	Removes contact of $C\delta_1$ of Leu All with Cδ and Cϵ of Phe GH5 and of $C\delta_2$ with Cϵ of Phe GH1; also of Cδ of Leu All with $C\delta_1$ and $C\delta_2$ of Leu H4. Could form salt bridge with Asp GH4	107

Freiburg	23	B5	Val	—	Vn	Cyanosis[a]	High oxygen affinity	Deletion would draw the carboxyl group of Glu 22 (B4) into a crevice about 4 Å below the protein surface; it would also remove the last turn of the B helix and disturb the conformation of the AB corner	108
Genova	28	B10	Leu	Pro	I	Hemolytic anemia	Unstable	Introduction of proline disrupts helix B	
Gun Hill	Deletion of 5 residues between 91 and 97					Hemolytic anemia	No heme in β-chain	Removes section of polypeptide chain which forms essential heme contacts and contacts with α-subunits	
Wien	130	H8	Tyr	Asp	Vn	Hemolytic anemia	Unstable; no increased electrophoretic mobility at pH 8.6 despite extra − charge	In Hb A the phenyl ring of tyrosine is internal; its hydroxyl emerges in a surface crevice near helix A, probably forming a hydrogen bond with CO of Val A8(11)β Its replacement by Asp creates an internal − charge which would be unstable and draw a + charge near it; the absence of an increased electrophoretic mobility at pH 8.6 suggests that a new + charge is created by a rise in pK of a previously uncharged group; this could be the imidazole of His NA2 or the α-amino group of Val NA1; either of these could be drawn in to neutralize Asp H8 at the expense of a displacement of helix A	111, 133

Table 19 (continued)
RESIDUES IN GENERAL POSITIONS

Designation	Residue		Replacement		Variability	Clinical symptoms	Abnormal properties	Structural effects of replacement	Ref.
	No.	Position	From	To					
Hope	136	H14	Gly	Asp	I	None	Difficult to separate from Hb A by electrophoresis at pH 8.6; unstable in vitro	Could form salt bridge with α-amino group of Val NA1 and by raising its pK produce a compensating charge	112
Rainier	145	HC2	Tyr	His	I	Polycythemia[b]	Increased oxygen affinity; unusual resistance to alkali	Hb A the phenolic OH forms a hydrogen bond with CO of Val FG5, and the phenyl ring acts as a spacer between helix H and the FG segment; the imidazole ring is too short to make this bond but could instead form a hydrogen bond with CO of Leu H19; while the former hydrogen bond would be broken by alkali, the latter might not	113

[a] Cyanosis: blue color of skin due to deoxyhemoglobin in the capillaries; can be due to the oxygen affinity of hemoglobin being too low.
[b] Polycythemia: excess of red blood cells. Can be caused by stimulation of red cell production by tissue hypoxia; for example, if the oxygen affinity of hemoglobin is too high to permit efficient delivery of O_2 to tissues.

Modified from Perutz, M. F. and Lehmann, H., *Nature (London)*, 219, 902, 1968. With permission.

Table 20
RESULTS OF CRYSTALLOGRAPHIC STUDIES OF ABNORMAL HEMOGLOBINS

Name	Mutation	Hill constant (n)	O_2 affinity	Bohr effect	Comments	Resolution (Å)	Structural changes	Ref.
Barcelona	Asp FG1(94)β →His	—	High	Low	Asp FG(94)β forms a salt bridge to His HC3(146)β in HbA	3.2	The new imidazole is rotated so that it is farther away from the C terminal His than the carboxylate was in Hb A; His HC3(146)β has also moved away His FG(194)β in Hb Barcelona, but the salt bridge between the C-terminus and Lys C5(40)α has been maintained	137
Bart's	γ4	—	High	Absent	Hb Bart's is found in neonates who have α-thalassemia trait; it is noncooperative	—	Only a preliminary study has been done; trigonal space group is unique for hemoglobins	134
M-Boston	His E7(58)α →Tyr (distal His)	1.2	Low	Absent	Hb M-Boston is more stable to heat denaturation than Hb A; carriers show cyanosis	3.5	The iron atom is on the distal side of the α-heme and bonded to the phenolate side chain; thus the changes in the α-chain stabilized the deoxy quaternary structure, causing abnormal properties; heat stability is due to strong bond between ferric iron and the phenolate	114

Table 20 (continued)
RESULTS OF CRYSTALLOGRAPHIC STUDIES OF ABNORMAL HEMOGLOBINS

Name	Mutation	Hill constant (n)	O_2 affinity	Bohr effect	Comments	Resolution (Å)	Structural changes	Ref.
C	Glu A3(6)β →Lys	—	—	—	Deoxy Hb C crystallizes inside the red blood cell; it is the second most common abnormal hemoglobin in the U.S.	5	Several crystal forms were studied; energetically favorable intermolecular interactions involving the β6 Lys occur in both Hb C crystal forms and could explain the tendency to crystallize in vivo	135
J-Capetown	Arg FG4(92)α →Gln	2.2	Slightly high	—	See Hb Chesapeake	5.5	Deoxy Hb J-Capetown showed no significant distortions compared to Hb A; the oxy structure has not been determined	115
Chesapeake	Arg FG4(92)α →Leu	1.3	High	—	See Hb J-Capetown	5.5	Deoxy Hb Chesapeake showed no significant distortions, but oxy structure did; helices C, B, D, and G of the β-chain, which lies across the $\alpha_1\beta_2$ interface, move away from the FG4α position and toward the $\alpha_1\beta_2$ interface	115
Cochin-Port Royal	His HC3(146) β →Arg	3.0	Normal	Low (73%)	See Hb Hiroshima	3.5	Only the intrasubunit salt bridge between His HC3(146)β and Asp FG1(94)β is lost; no other structural changes were detected; deoxy-form studied	116

Cranston	Elongation mutation; 11 additional residues and changes at positions 145 and 146 of the β-chain	1.1	High	Markedly reduced	Elongation is the result of a frameshift mutation; inositol hexophosphate decreases oxygen affinity and increases cooperativity and the Bohr effect	3.5	Crystals contain an equal molar mixture of Hb A and Hb Cranston in asymmetric hybrid molecules with the hydrophobic tail of Hb Cranston accommodated in the central cavity between the two β-chains	136
Creteil	Ser FS(89)β →Asn	1.2	High	Reduced	DPG has no effect on oxygen affinity	3.5	The hydrogen bonds normally associated with Ser 89β are lost and the additional side chain atoms of Asn 89β sterically hinder the tight packing between helices F and H; thus, 143β—146β are disordered similar to Hb Nancy (see below)	138
H	β4	—	Very high	—	Although Hb H is found in patients with α-thalassemia trait, the sample used in the crystallographic studies was prepared from isolated β-chains; Hb H binds DPG with an affinity similar to that of Hb A	2.5	Examination of the $\alpha_1\beta_2$ interface shows that CO-β is more like liganded Hb A (the R state) than deoxy-Hb A; in CO-β_4, residues His 143β_1 and His 143β_2 move apart by about 3 Å, which creates inorganic anion binding sites spaced 6.5 Å from each other, explaining the ability to bind DPG	146
Hiroshima	His HC3(146)β →Asp	2.4	Low	Low (approx. 50% of normal)	See Hb Cochin-Port-Royal	3.5	Only the intrasubunit salt bridge between His HC3(146)β and Asp FG1(94)β is lost; other structural changes are small; deoxy form studied	117

Table 20 (continued)
RESULTS OF CRYSTALLOGRAPHIC STUDIES OF ABNORMAL HEMOGLOBINS

Name	Mutation	Hill constant (n)	O_2 affinity	Bohr effect	Comments	Resolution (Å)	Structural changes	Ref.
M-Hyde Park	His F8(92)β →Tyr (proximal His)	1.3	Normal	Normal	See Hb M-Iwate	3.5	Approximately 25% of the β-chains have lost their hemes; the resulting distortions are restricted to the heme pocket and are not significant in the rest of the molecule	118
M-Iwate	His F8(87)β →Tyr	1.1	Low	Very low	See Hb M-Hyde Park	5.5	Two crystal forms were observed; α-chains were in the met state in both but the β-chains are deoxy in one and met in the other; in both forms the α-hemes are bound to both the distal His E7(58)α and the proximal Tyr F8(87)α; both forms are in the deoxy quaternary structure, although the β-chain does undergo some conformational changes when it is liganded	

Kansas	Asn G4(102)β →Thr	1.3	Low	Large	Dissociates to dimers more easily than Hb A; inositol hexaphosphate keeps it in the deoxy quaternary structure, even when it is liganded	3.5, 5.5	In deoxy Hb Kansas, Asp (99)β moves towards the hole caused by a smaller residue at residue G4, provoking a series of small movements across the $\alpha_1\beta_2$ interface, and in the α-subunit; in carboxy Hb Kansas, there are marked changes in the tertiary structure similar to oxidation of Hb A, but the salt bridges are not broken and the penultimate tyrosines HC2(140)α and (145)β are not displaced	119, 120, 139
M-Milwaukee	Val E11(67)β →Glu	1.4	Low	Large	—	3.5	The introduction of Glu into the heme pocket of the β-chains leads to a link between the α-carboxyl group and the ferric iron; in the crystal structures, the quaternary conformation is controlled by the state of ligation of the ferrous α-subunits; if the abnormal β-chain favors the deoxy tertiary and quaternary structures in solution, the abnormal properties can be explained	121
Nancy	Tyr HC2(145)β →Asp	1.1	Very high	Low (50%)	Inositol hexaphosphate increase the Hill constant to 2, but this effect is less than with Hb A	3.5	The C-terminal tetrapeptide is severely disordered, resulting in the rupture of the salt bridges; the decreased inositol hexaphosphate is due to the movement of His HC3(143)β, which forms part of its binding site	116

Table 20 (continued)
RESULTS OF CRYSTALLOGRAPHIC STUDIES OF ABNORMAL HEMOGLOBINS

Name	Mutation	Hill constant (n)	O_2 affinity	Bohr effect	Comments	Resolution (Å)	Structural changes	Ref.
Rainier	Tyr HC2(145)β →Cys	1.5	High	Low (68%)	—	3.5	Structure of deoxy Hb Rainier shows that a disulfide bridge is formed between the new Cys and Cys F9(93)β, the resulting distortions of the C-terminus break the salt bridges associated with His HC3(146)β, as well as the hydrogen bond between Tyr HC(145)β and Val FG5(98)β, thereby inhibiting the Bohr effect and cooperativity	122
Richmond	Asn G4(102)β →Lys	2.5	Normal	Normal	Dissociates into dimers more easily than Hb A, but not as easily as Hb Kansas	4.0	The deoxy structure shows small changes surrounding the mutated residue, but the heme group is not perturbed, except for a small rotation of a vinyl group	120

S	Glu A3(6)β →Val	—	—	—	Deoxy Hb S is much less soluble than Hb A and forms rods inside erythrocytes and in cell-free solution	5.0	There are no large conformational differences between Hb S and Hb A; in the crystal, the molecules form double strands running parallel to one of the crystallographic axes; Val A3(6)β is involved in side-to-side contacts between adjacent strands, these contacts must stabilize the strands, which are likely to be very similar to the fibers seen in electron micrographs of sickle cells	125, 140, 141
St. Louis	Leu B10(28)β →Gln	2.2	High	Normal	Hb St. Louis is a valency hybrid, $\alpha_2\beta_2^{+}$; diphosphoglycerate effect is decreased	3.5	Gln B10(28)β and the distal His E7(63)β swing towards each other and stabilize a water molecule between them with hydrogen bonds; the introduction of this water into the normally hydrophobic heme pocket causes the oxidation of the β-hemes to the *met*-state; since these two *met*-state chains would closely resemble oxygenated subunits, the molecule always appears to be at least half saturated, which accounts for the low cooperativity and high oxygen affinity; in the deoxy structure reported, there are no additional changes other than a small increase in the tilt of the heme	126

Table 20 (continued)
RESULTS OF CRYSTALLOGRAPHIC STUDIES OF ABNORMAL HEMOGLOBINS

Name	Mutation	Hill constant (n)	O_2 affinity	Bohr effect	Comments	Resolution (Å)	Structural changes	Ref.
San Diego	Val G11(109)β →Met	2.1	High	Normal	—	3.5	The side chain at G11β acts as a spacer between the β-G helix and the β-G and α-H helices; this substitution allows β-G to move closer, while α-H is pushed away; the movements in the $\alpha_1\beta_1$ contact weaken the hydrogen bond between Tyr C1(35)β and Asp H9(126)α, and allow the formation of an intrachain hydrogen bond between Asp H9(126)α and His H5(122)α; these changes destabilize the deoxy form and, thus, increase oxygen affinity	123
Seattle	Ala E14(70)β →Asp	—	Low	Normal	Hb Seattle shows an increased rate of methemoglobin formation in vitro and an increased heat lability	3.5	This mutation introduces a negatively charged carboxy group into the heme binding pocket, which may lower the oxygen affinity by polarizing the β-hemes; in addition, the tilt of the heme has changed	124
Suresnes	Arg HC3(141)α →His	1.43	High	Reduced	Arg 141α plays a major role in both cooperativity and the alkaline Bohr effect in Hb A; Hb Suresnes has increased subunit dissociation	3.5	Deoxy Hb Suresnes has lost the normal intersubunit salt bridge to Lys 127α and has a decreased occupancy of α-chain anion binding site	142

Sydney	Val E11(67)β →Ala	—	See comment	—	Hb Sydney has an abnormally high oxygen affinity at low and abnormally low affinity at high partial pressures of oxygen	2.73	A water molecule is bound to the distal histidine in deoxy-Hb Sydney, replacing the steric hindrance of Val E11 in Hb A; this leads to more autoxidation; the gap in the heme pocket must also be responsible for the instability of Hb Sydney which results in hemolytic anemia	143, 144
Tacoma	Arg B12(30)β →Ser	Low	Low	Low	In spite of the loss of two arginines per tetramer, Hb Tacoma has only slightly more anodic mobility than Hb A in alkaline media	3.5	The carboxylate of Glu B8(26)β, which forms a salt bridge with the guanidinium group of Arg B12(30)β in Hb A, swings around its α–β carbon bond towards the imidazoles of His G18(116) and G19(117)β in Hb Tacoma; this interaction raises the pK values of the histidines, and their increased positive charge may compensate for the loss of the arginine on the electrophoretic mobility; the loss of the hydrogen bonds across the $\alpha_1\beta_1$ interface made by Arg B12(30)β would loosen the deoxy structure, explaining the decreases in the allosterism and stability, but not in the Bohr effect	127

Table 20 (continued)
RESULTS OF CRYSTALLOGRAPHIC STUDIES OF ABNORMAL HEMOGLOBINS

Name	Mutation	Hill constant (n)	O_2 affinity	Bohr effect	Comments	Resolution (Å)	Structural changes	Ref.
Yakima	Asp G1(99)β →His	Low	High	Normal		3.5	The His G1(99)β_2 does not form a hydrogen bond to Tyr C7(42)α_1; since His is bulkier than Asp, it makes additional contacts with Pro G2(100)β_2, Glu G3(101)β_2, Thr C3(38)α_1, which causes rearrangements in the contact; the subunits slide past each other so that deoxy Hb Yakima is partially in the oxy conformation, which lowers the cooperativity and raises the oxygen affinity; since the salt bridges are not broken, the Bohr effect is normal	128
Zürich	His E7(63)β→Arg	—	High	—	Both CO-(143,144) and deoxy-(145) Hb Zürich structures have been determined	2.8	In CO-Hb-Zürich the side chain of the distal Arg attaches itself to the propionate of the heme, leaving the heme pocket wide open; in the deoxy form this side chain has rotated toward the CD corner; the propionate, which is still hydrogen bonding to the Arg, is rotated and the CD corner is slightly rearranged	143, 144, 145

Table 21
MUTATIONS THAT INCREASE THE SOLUBILITY OF HEMOGLOBIN S HYBRIDS

Hemoglobin	Mutation	Ref.
Ananthara	Lys A9(11)α→Glu	203
I	Lys A14(16)α→Glu	203, 205
Mugino	Asp CD6(47)α→Gly	203
Sealy	Asp CD6(47)α→His	203, 205
Montgomery	Leu CD7(48)α→Arg	203
J-Mexico	Gln E3(54)α→Glu	203
Shimonoseki	Gln E3(54)α→Arg	203
G-Philadelphia	Asn E17(68)α→Lys	203
Ube II	Asn E17(68)α→Asp	203
O-Indonesia	Glu GH4(116)α→Lys	203
J-Baltimore	Gly A13(16)β→Asp	204
J-Amiens	Lys A14(17)β→Gln	204
D-Ouled Rabah	Asn B1(19)β→Lys	204
Pyrgos	Gly EF7(83)β→Asp	204
Detroit	Lys FG2(95)β→Asn	204
N-Baltimore	Lys FG2(95)β→Glu	204

REFERENCES

1. **Perutz, M. F.,** Structure and mechanism of haemoglobin, *Br. Med. Bull.*, 32, 195, 1976.
2. **Baldwin, J. M.,** Structure and function of haemoglobin, *Prog. Biophys. Mol. Biol.*, 29, 225, 1975.
3. **Weissbluth, M.,** *Hemoglobin: Cooperativity and Electronic Properties*, Springer-Verlag, New York, 1974, 1.
4. **Perutz, M. F.,** The haemoglobin molecule, *Proc. R. Soc. London Ser. B*, 173, 113, 1969.
5. **Perutz, M. F.,** The hemoglobin molecule, *Sci. Am.*, 211, 64, 1964.
6. **Stryer, L.,** *Biochemistry*, W. H. Freeman, San Francisco, 1975, 46.
7. **Lehninger, A.,** *Biochemistry: The Molecular Basis of Cell Structure and Function*, 2nd ed., Worth, New York, 1975, 145.
8. **Metzler, D. E.,** *Biochemistry: The Chemical Reactions of Living Cells*, Academic Press, New York, 1977, 226.
9. **Orten, J. M. and Neuhaus, O. W.,** *Human Biochemistry*, 9th ed., C. V. Mosby, St. Louis, 1975, 776.
10. **White, A., Handler, P., and Smith, E. L.,** *Principles of Biochemistry*, 5th ed., McGraw-Hill, New York, 1973, 1971.
11. **Kendrew, J. C., Dickerson, R. E., Strandberg, B. E., Hart, R. G., Davies, D. R., Phillips, D. C., and Shore, V. C.,** Structure of myoglobin, *Nature (London)*, 185, 422, 1960.
12. **Takano, T.,** Structure of myoglobin refined at 2.0 Å resolution. I. Crystallographic refinement of metmyoglobin from sperm whale, *J. Mol. Biol.*, 110, 537, 1976.
13. **Takano, T.,** Structure of myoglobin refined at 2.0 Å resolution. II. Structure of deoxymyoglobin from sperm whale, *J. Mol. Biol.*, 110, 569, 1976.
14. **Stryer, L., Kendrew, J. C., and Watson, H. C.,** The mode of attachment of the azide ion to sperm whale metmyoglobin, *J. Mol. Biol.*, 8, 96, 1964.
15. **Bretscher, P. A.,** The X-ray Analysis of Cyanide and Carboxymethylated Metmyoglobin, Ph.D. thesis, University of Cambridge, Cambridge, England, 1968, 1.
16. **Norvell, J. C., Nunes, A. C., and Schoenborn, B. P.,** Neutron diffraction analysis of myoglobin: structure of the carbon monoxide derivative, *Science*, 190, 568, 1975.
17. **Scouloudi, H.,** X-ray crystallographic studies of seal myoglobin: the molecule at 6 Å and 5 Å resolution, *J. Mol. Biol.*, 40, 353, 1969.
18. **Lattman, E. E., Nockolds, C. E., Kretsinger, R. H., and Love, W. E.,** Structure of yellow fin tuna metmyoglobin at 6 Å resolution, *J. Mol. Biol.*, 60, 271, 1971.
19. **Huber, R., Epp, O., Steigemenn, W., and Formanek, G.,** The atomic structure of erythrocruorin in the light of the chemical sequence and its comparison with myoglobin, *Eur. J. Biochem.*, 19, 42, 1971.

20. **Huber, R., Epp, O., and Formanek, H.,** Structures of deoxy- and carbomonoxy-erythrocruorin, *J. Mol. Biol.,* 52, 349, 1970.
21. **Padlan, E. A. and Love, W. E.,** Structure of the haemoglobin of the marine annelid worm, *Glycera dibranchiata,* at 5.5 Å resolution, *Nature (London),* 220, 376, 1968.
22. **Padlan, E. A. and Love, W. E.,** Three-dimensional structure of hemoglobin from the polychaete annelid, *Glycera dibranchiata,* at 2.5 Å resolution, *J. Biol. Chem.,* 249, 4067, 1974.
23. **Hendrickson, W. A. and Love, W. E.,** Structure of lamprey haemoglobin, *Nature (London) New Biol.,* 232, 197, 1971.
24. **Vainshtein, B. K., Harutyunyan, E. H., Kuranova, I. P., Borisov, V. V., Sosfenov, N. I., Pavlovsky, A. G., Grebenko, A. I., and Konareva, N. V.,** Structure of leghaemoglobin from lupin root nodules at 5 Å resolution, *Nature (London),* 254, 163, 1975.
25. **Fermi, G.,** Three-dimensional Fourier synthesis of human deoxyhaemoglobin at 2.5 Å resolution: refinement of the atomic model, *J. Mol. Biol.,* 97, 237, 1975.
26. **Ten Eyck, L. F. and Arnone, A.,** Three-dimensional Fourier synthesis of human deoxyhemoglobin at 2.5 Å resolution. I. X-ray analysis, *J. Mol. Biol.,* 100, 3, 1976.
27. **Baldwin, J. M.,** in preparation.
28. **Frier, J. A. and Perutz, M. F.,** Structure of human foetal deoxyhaemoglobin, *J. Mol. Biol.,* 112, 97, 1977.
29. **Ladner, R. C., Heidner, E. J., and Perutz, M. F.,** The structure of horse methaemoglobin at 2.0 Å resolution, *J. Mol. Biol.,* 114, 385, 1977.
30. **Bolton, W. and Perutz, M. F.,** Three-dimensional Fourier synthesis of horse deoxyhaemoglobin at 2.8 Å resolution, *Nature (London),* 228, 551, 1970.
31. **Heidner, E. J., Ladner, R. C., and Perutz, M. F.,** Structure of horse carbonmonoxyhaemoglobin, *J. Mol. Biol.,* 104, 707, 1976.
32. **Perutz, M. F. and Mathews, F. S.,** An X-ray study of azide methaemoglobin, *J. Mol. Biol.,* 21, 199, 1966.
33. **Deatherage, J. F., Loe, R. S., Anderson, C. M., and Moffat, K.,** Structure of cyanide methemoglobin, *J. Mol. Biol.,* 104, 687, 1976.
34. **Deatherage, J. F., Loe, R. S., and Moffat, K.,** Structure of fluoride methemoglobin, *J. Mol. Biol.,* 104, 723, 1976.
35. **Seybert, D. W. and Moffat, K.,** The structure of hemoglobin reconstituted with deuteroheme, *J. Mol. Biol.,* 106, 895, 1976.
36. **Moffat, K., Loe, R. S., and Hoffman, B. M.,** The structure of metamanganoglobin, *J. Mol. Biol.,* 104, 669, 1976.
37. **Dayhoff, M. O.,** Atlas of protein sequence and structure, *Natl. Biomed. Res. Found,* 5 (Suppl. 2), 191, 1976.
38. **Hill, R. L., Harris, C. M., Naylor, J. T., and Sams, W. M.,** The partial amino acid sequence of human myoglobin, *J. Biol. Chem.,* 244, 2182, 1969.
39. **Hill, R. J. and Konigsberg, W.,** The structure of human hemoglobin, *J. Biol. Chem.,* 237, 3151, 1962.
40. **Braunitzer, G., Gehring-Muller, R., Hilschmann, N., Helse, K., Halom, G., Rudloff, V., and Wittmann-Liebold, B.,** Die Konstitution des normalen adulten Humanhämoglobins, *Hoppe-Seyler's Z. Physiol. Chem.,* 325, 283, 1961.
41. **Schroeder, W. A., Shelton, J. R., Shelton, J. B., Cormick, J., and Jones, R. T.,** The amino acid sequence of the γ chain of human fetal hemoglobin, *Biochemistry,* 2, 992, 1963.
42. **Jones, R. T.,** Structural studies of aminoethylated hemoglobins by automatic peptide chromatography, *Cold Spring Harbor Symp. Quant. Biol.,* 29, 297, 1964.
43. **Pauling, L., Corey, R. B., and Branson, H. R.,** The structure of proteins: two hydrogen bonded helical configurations of the polypeptide chain, *Proc. Natl. Acad. Sci. U.S.A.,* 37, 205, 1951.
44. **Donohue, J.,** Hydrogen bonded helical configurations of the polypeptide chain, *Proc. Natl. Acad. Sci. U.S.A.,* 39, 470, 1953.
45. **Low, B. W. and Grenville-Wells, H. J.,** Generalized mathematical relationships for polypeptide chain helices. The coordinates of the II helix, *Proc. Natl. Acad. Sci. U.S.A.,* 39, 785, 1953.
46. **Ramachandran, G. N. and Sasisekharan, V.,** Conformation of polypeptides and proteins, *Adv. Prot. Chem.,* 23, 283, 1968.
47. **Kauzmann, W.,** Some factors in the interpretation of protein denaturation, *Adv. Prot. Chem.,* 14, 1, 1959.
48. **Tanford, C.,** Contribution of hydrophobic interactions to the stability of the globular conformation of proteins, *J. Am. Chem. Soc.,* 84, 4240, 1962.
49. **Perutz, M. F., Kendrew, J. C., and Watson, H. C.,** Structure and function of haemoglobin. II. Some relations between polypeptide chain configuration and amino acid sequence, *J. Mol. Biol.,* 13, 669, 1965.
50. **Olsen, K. W.,** Relationship of Sequence and Three-Dimensional Structure in Proteins, 10th International Congress of Biochemistry, Hamburg, 1976.

51. **Perutz, M. F. and Lehmann, H.,** Molecular pathology of human haemoglobin, *Nature (London),* 219, 902, 1968.
52. **Hoard, J. L. and Scheidt, W. R.,** Stereochemical trigger for initiating cooperative interaction of the subunits during the oxygenation of cobalthemoglobin, *Proc. Natl. Acad. Sci. U.S.A.,* 70, 3919, 1973.
53. **Collman, J. P., Gagne, R. R., Reed, C. A., Robinson, W. F., and Rodley, G. A.,** Structure of an iron (II) dioxygen complex; a model for oxygen carrying hemeproteins, *Proc. Natl. Acad. Sci. U.S.A.,* 71, 1326, 1974.
54. **Chothia, C., Wodak, S., and Janin, J.,** Role of subunit interfaces in the allosteric mechanism of hemoglobin, *Proc. Natl. Acad. Sci. U.S.A.,* 73, 3793, 1976.
55. **Perutz, M. F.,** Stereochemistry of cooperative effects of haemoglobin, *Nature (London),* 228, 726, 1970.
56. **Perutz, M. F. and Ten Eyck, L. F.,** Stereochemistry of cooperative effects of hemoglobin, *Cold Spring Harbor Symp. Quant. Biol.,* 36, 295, 1971.
57. **Perutz, M. F., Muirhead, H., Cox, J. M., Goaman, L. C. G., Mathews, F. S., McGandy, E. L., and Webb, L. E.,** Three-dimensional Fourier synthesis of horse oxyhaemoglobin at 2.8 Å resolution: (1) X-ray analysis, *Nature (London),* 219, 29, 1968.
58. **Perutz, M. F., Muirhead, H., Cox, J. M., and Goaman, L. C. G.,** Three-dimensional Fourier synthesis of horse oxyhaemoglobin at 2.8 Å resolution: the atomic model, *Nature (London),* 219, 131, 1968.
59. **Muirhead, H., Cox, J. M., Mazzarella, L., and Perutz, M. F.,** Structure and function of haemoglobin, III. A three-dimensional Fourier synthesis of human deoxyhaemoglobin at 5.5 Å resolution, *J. Mol. Biol.,* 28, 117, 1967.
60. **Arnone, A.,** X-ray diffraction study of binding of 2,3-diphosphoglycerate to human deoxyhaemoglobin, *Nature (London),* 237, 146, 1972.
61. **Arnone, A. and Perutz, M. F.,** Structure of inositol hexaphosphate-human deoxyhaemoglobin complex, *Nature (London),* 249, 34, 1974.
62. **Fermi, G. and Perutz, M. F.,** Structure of human fluoromethaemoglobin with inositol hexaphosphate, *J. Mol. Biol.,* 114, 421, 1977.
63. **Kilmartin, J. V. and Rossi-Bernardi, L.,** Inhibition of CO_2 combination and reduction of the Bohr effect in haemoglobin chemically modified at its α-amino group, *Nature (London),* 222, 1243, 1969.
64. **Arnone, A., O'Donnell, S., and Schuster, T.,** X-ray diffraction studies of carbamylated human deoxyhemoglobin, *Fed. Proc.,* 35, 1604, 1976.
65. **Garner, M. H., Bogardt, R. A., Jr., and Gurd, F. R. N.,** Determination of the pK values for the α amino groups of human hemoglobin, *J. Biol. Chem.,* 250, 4398, 1975.
66. **Kibmartin, J. V.,** Interaction of haemoglobin with protons, CO_2 and 2,3-diphosphoglycerate, *Br. Med. Bull.,* 32, 209, 1976.
67. **Roughton, F. J. W.,** Some recent work on the interactions of oxygen, carbon dioxide, and haemoglobin. The Seventh Hopkins Memorial Lecture, *Biochem. J.,* 117, 801, 1970.
68. **Arnone, A.,** X-ray studies of the interaction of CO_2 with human deoxyhaemoglobin, *Nature (London),* 247, 143, 1974.
69. **Monod, J., Wyman, J., and Changeux, J.-B.,** On the nature of allosteric transitions: a plausible model, *J. Mol. Biol.,* 12, 88, 1965.
70. **Koshland, D. E., Jr., Nemethy, G., and Filmer, D.,** Comparison of experimental binding data and theoretical models in proteins containing subunits, *Biochemistry,* 5, 365, 1966.
71. **Perutz, M. F.,** Nature of haem-haem interaction, *Nature (London),* 237, 495, 1972.
72. **Lindstrom, T. R. and Ho, C.,** Functional nonequivalence of α and β hemes in human adult hemoglobin, *Proc. Natl. Acad. Sci. U.S.A.,* 69, 1707, 1972.
73. **Winslow, R. M. and Anderson, W. F.,** The hemoglobinopathies, in *Metabolic Basis of Inherited Disease,* 4th ed., Stanbury, J. B., Wyngaarden, J. B., and Fredrickson, D. S., Eds., McGraw-Hill, New York, 1978, 1465.
74. **Morimoto, H., Lehmann, H., and Perutz, M. F.,** Molecular pathology of human haemoglobin: stereochemical interpretation of abnormal oxygen affinities, *Nature (London),* 232, 408, 1971.
75. **Beretta, A., Prato, V., Gallo, E., and Lehmann, H.,** Haemoglobin Torino-α43 (CDI) phenylalanine $\rightarrow$ valine, *Nature (London),* 217, 1016, 1968.
76. **Gerald, P. S. and Efron, M. L.,** Chemical studies of several varieties of HbM, *Proc. Natl. Acad. Sci. U.S.A.,* 47, 1758, 1958.
77. **Miyaji, T., Iuchi, I., Shibata, S., Takeda, I., and Tamura, A.,** Possible amino acid substitution in the alpha chain (alpha-87tyr) of HbM-lwate, *Acta Haematol. Jpn.,* 26, 538, 1963.
78. **Kleihauer, E. F., Reynolds, C. A., Dozy, A. M., Wilson, J. B., Moores, R. R., Berenson, M. P., Wright, C. S., and Huisman, T. H. J.,** Hemoglobin$_{Bibba}$ or $\alpha_2{}^{136}$ Pro β_2, an unstable α chain abnormal hemoglobin, *Biochim. Biophys. Acta,* 154, 220, 1968.
79. **Dacie, J. V., Shinton, N. K., Gaffney, P. J., Jr., Carrell, R. W., and Lehmann, H.,** Haemoglobin Hammersmith (β42(CD1)Phe $\rightarrow$ Ser), *Nature (London),* 216, 663, 1967.

80. **Jacob, H. S., Brain, M. C., Dacie, J. V., Carrell, R. W., and Lehmann, H.,** Abnormal haem binding and globin SH group blockade in unstable haemoglobins, *Nature (London),* 218, 1214, 1968.
81. **Muller, C. J. and Kingma, A.,** Haemoglobin Zurich: $\alpha_2{}^A\beta_{2\,63Arg}$. *Biochim. Biophys. Acta,* 50, 595, 1961.
82. **Hitzig, W. H., Frick, P. G., Betke, K., and Huisman, T. H. J.,** Hemoglobin Zurich: a new hemoglobin anomaly with sulfonamide-induced inclusion body anemia, *Helv. Paediatr. Acta,* 15, 499, 1960.
83. **Carrell, R. W., Lehmann, H., Lorkin, P. A., Raik, E., and Hunter, E.,** Haemoglobin Sydney: β67(E11) Valine → Alanine: an emerging pattern of unstable haemoglobins, *Nature (London),* 215, 626, 1967.
84. **Opfell, R. W., Lorkin, P. A., and Lehmann, H.,** Hereditary non-spherocytic haemolytic anaemia with post-splenectomy inclusion bodies and pigmenturia caused by an unstable haemoglobin Santa Ana β88 (F4) Leucine → Proline, *J. Med. Genet.,* 5, 292, 1968.
85. **Heller, P., Coleman, R. D., and Yakulis, J.,** Structural Studies of Hemoglobin M Hyde Park, *Proc. Eleventh Cong. Int. Soc. Haematol.,* 1966, 427.
86. **Carrell, R. W., Lehmann, H., and Hutchison, H. E.,** Haemoglobin Koln (β-98 valine → methionine); an unstable protein causing inclusion-body anaemia, *Nature (London),* 210, 915, 1966.
87. **Vaughan-Jones, R., Grimes, A. J., Carrell, R. W., and Lehmann, H.,** Koln haemoglobinopathy, further data and a comparison with other hereditary Heinz body anaemias, *Br. J. Haematol.,* 13, 394, 1976.
88. **Bonaventura, J. and Riggs, A.,** Hemoglobin Kansas, a human hemoglobin with a neutral amino acid substitution and an abnormal oxygen equilibrium, *J. Biol. Chem.,* 243, 980, 1968.
89. **Swenson, R. T., Hill, R. L., Lehmann, H., and Jim, R. T. S.,** A chemical abnormality in hemoglobin G from Chinese individuals, *J. Biol. Chem.,* 237, 1517, 1962.
90. **Botha, M. C., Beale, D., Isaacs, W. A., and Lehmann, H.,** Haemoglobin J-Cape Town — α_2 92 Arginine → Glutamine, *Nature (London),* 212, 792, 1966.
91. **Lines, J. G. and McIntosh, R.,** Oxygen binding by haemoglobin J-Cape Town (α_2 92 Arg → Gln), *Nature (London),* 215, 297, 1967.
92. **Clegg, J. B., Naughton, M. A., and Weatherall, D. J.,** Abnormal human haemoglobins separation and characterization of the α and β chains by chromatography, and the determination of two new variants, Hb Chesapeake and HbJ (Bangkok), *J. Mol. Biol.,* 19, 91, 1966.
93. **Nagel, R. L., Gibson, Q. H., and Charache, S.,** Relation between structure and function in hemoglobin Chesapeake, *Biochemistry,* 6, 2395, 1967.
94. **Jones, R. T., Brimhall, B., and Lisker, R.,** Chemical characterization of Haemoglobin Mexico and Haemoglobin Chiapas, *Biochim. Biophys. Acta,* 154, 488, 1968.
95. **Hunt, J. A. and Ingram, V. M.,** Abnormal human haemoglobins: human haemoglobin E: the chemical effect of gene mutation, *Nature (London),* 184, 870, 1959.
96. **Bellingham, A. J. and Huehns, E. R.,** Compensation in haemolytic anaemias caused by abnormal haemoglobins, *Nature (London),* 218, 924, 1968.
97. **Baur, E. W. and Motulsky, A. G.,** Hemoglobin Tacoma — a β chain variant associated with increased HbA_2, *Humangenetik,* 1, 621, 1965.
98. **Rieder, R. F., Oski, F. A., and Clegg, J. B.,** Hemoglobin Philly (β35 tyrosine → phenylalanine): studies in the molecular pathology of hemoglobin, *J. Clin. Invest.,* 48, 1627, 1969.
99. **Jones, R. T., Osgood, E. E., Brimhall, B., and Koler, R. D.,** Hemoglobin Yakima. I. Clinical and biochemical studies, *J. Clin. Invest.,* 46, 1840, 1967.
100. **Miles, J. N., Miles, J. E., and Metcalfe, J.,** Hemoglobin Yakima. II. High blood oxygen affinity associated with compensatory erythrocytosis and normal hemodynamics, *J. Clin. Invest.,* 46, 1848, 1967.
101. **Reed, C. S., Hanpson, R., Gordon, S., Jones, R. T., Navy, M. J., Brimhall, B., Edwards, M. J., and Koler, R. D.,** Erythrocytosis secondary to increased oxygen affinity of a mutant hemoglobin, hemoglobin Kempsey, *Blood,* 31, 623, 1968.
102. **Ranney, H. M., Jacobs, A. S., and Nagel, L. L.,** Haemoglobin New York, *Nature (London),* 213, 876, 1976.
103. **Allan, N., Beale, D., Irvine, D., and Lehmann, H.,** Three haemoglobins K: Woolwich, an abnormal Cameroon and Ibadan, two unusual variants of human haemoglobin A, *Nature (London),* 208, 658, 1965.
104. **Crookston, J. H., Farquarson, H. A., Beale, D., and Lehmann, H.,** Hemoglobin Etobicoke: alpha-84(F5) serine replaced by arginine, *Can. J. Biochem.,* 47, 143, 1969.
105. **Crookston, J. H., Goldstein, J., Lehmann, H., and Beale, D.,** unpublished results.
106. **Shibata, S., Iuchi, I., Miyaji, T., and Takeda, I.,** Spectrophotometric determination of Hb M-Iwate in the hemolysate of hereditary Nigremia, *Bull. Yamaguchi Med. School,* 10, 31, 1963.
107. **Monn, E., Gaffney, P. J., and Lehmann, H.,** Haemoglobin Sogn (beta 14 arginine) a new haemoglobin variant, *Scand. J. Haematol.,* 5, 353, 1968.
108. **Jones, R. T., Brimhall, B., Huisman, J. H. J., Kleihaver, E. F., and Betke, K.,** Hemoglobin Freiburg: abnormal hemoglobin due to deletion of a single amino acid residue, *Science,* 154, 1024, 1976.

109. **Sansone, G., Carrell, R. W., and Lehmann, H.,** Haemoglobin Genova: β28 (B10) leucine → proline, *Nature (London),* 214, 877, 1967.
110. **Bradley, T. B., Wohl, R. C., and Rieder, R. F.,** Hemoglobin Gunn Hill: deletion of five amino acid residues and impaired heme-globin binding, *Science,* 157, 1581, 1967.
111. **Lorkin, P. A., Pietschmann, H., Braunsteiner, H., and Lehmann, H.,** Structure of Haemoglobin Wien β130(H8) tyrosine → aspartic acid: an unstable haemoglobin variant, *Acta Haematol.,* 51, 351, 1974.
112. **Minnich, V., Hill, R. L., Khuri, P. D., and Anderson, M. E.,** Hemoglobin hope: a beta chain variant, *Blood,* 25, 830, 1965.
113. **Stanmatoyannopoulos, G., Adamson, J., Yoshida, A., and Heinenberg, S.,** Hemoglobin Rainier: an adult alkali resistant hemoglobin associated with erythrocytosis, *Blood,* 30, 879, 1967.
114. **Pulsinelli, P. D., Perutz, M. F., and Nagel, R. L.,** Structure of hemoglobin M Boston, a variant with a five-coordinated ferric heme, *Proc. Natl. Acad. Sci. U.S.A.,* 70, 3870, 1973.
115. **Greer, J.,** Three-dimensional structure of abnormal haemoglobins Chesapeake and J. Capetown, *J. Mol. Biol.,* 62, 241, 1971.
116. **Arnone, A., Gacon, G., and Wajcman, H.,** X-ray and functional studies of hemoglobins Nancy and Cochin-Port-Royal, *J. Biol. Chem.,* 251, 5875, 1976.
117. **Perutz, M. F., Pulsinelli, P. D., Ten Eyck, L., Kilmartin, J. V., Shibata, S., Iuchi, I., Miyaji, T., and Hamilton, H. B.,** Haemoglobin Hiroshima and the mechanism of the alkaline Bohr effect, *Nature (London) New Biol.,* 232, 147, 1971.
118. **Greer, J.,** Three-dimensional structure of abnormal human haemoglobins M Hyde Park and M Iwate, *J. Mol. Biol.,* 59, 107, 1971.
119. **Anderson, L.,** Structures of deoxy and carbonmonoxy haemoglobin Kansas in the deoxy quaternary conformation, *J. Mol. Biol.,* 94, 33, 1975.
120. **Greer, J.,** Three-dimensional structure of abnormal human haemoglobin Kansas and Richmond, *J. Mol. Biol.,* 59, 99, 1971.
121. **Perutz, M. F., Pulsinelli, P. D., and Ranney, A. M.,** Structure and subunit interaction of haemoglobin M Milwaukee, *Nature (London) New Biol.,* 237, 259, 1972.
122. **Greer, J. and Perutz, M. F.,** Three-dimensional structure of haemoglobin Rainier, *Nature (London) New Biol.,* 230, 261, 1971.
123. **Anderson, N. L.,** Hemoglobin San Diego, (β109 (G 11) Val → Met) crystal structure of the deoxy form, *J. Clin. Invest.,* 53, 329, 1974.
124. **Anderson, N. L., Perutz, M. F., and Stamatoyannopoulos, G.,** Site of the amino acid substitution in haemoglobin Seattle (α_2^A β_2^{oAsp}), *Nature (London) New Biol.,* 243, 274, 1973.
125. **Wishner, B. C., Ward, K. B., Lattman, E. E., and Love, W. E.,** Crystal structure of sickle-cell deoxyhemoglobin at 5 Å resolution, *J. Mol. Biol.,* 98, 179, 1975.
126. **Anderson, N. L.,** Hemoglobin St. Louis β28(B10 Leu → Gln) crystal structure of the fully reduced (deoxy) form, *J. Clin. Invest.,* 58, 1107, 1976.
127. **Tucker, P. W. and Perutz, M. F.,** Mechanism of charge compensation and impairment of cooperative functions in haemoglobin Tacoma (Arg B12(30β) → Ser), *J. Mol. Biol.,* 114, 415, 1977.
128. **Pulsinelli, P. D.,** Structure of deoxyhaemoglobin Yakima: a high-affinity mutant form exhibiting oxylike $\alpha_1\beta_2$ subunit interactions, *J. Mol. Biol.,* 74, 57, 1973.
129. **Green, J.,** personal communication.
130. **Jones, R. T.,** personal communications.
131. **Rieder, R. F., Oski, F. A., and Clegg, J. B.,** personal communication.
132. **Crookston, J. H., Goldstein, J., Lehmann, H., and Beale, O.,** unpublished results.
133. **Pietschmann, H., Lorkin, P. A., Lehman, H., and Braunsteiner, H.,** unpublished results.
134. **Czerwinski, E. W., Risk, M., and Matustik, M. C.,** Crystallization and preliminary X-ray diffraction studies of methemoglobin Bart's, *J. Biol. Chem.,* 256, 13128, 1981.
135. **Fitzgerald, P. M. D. and Love, W. E.,** Structure of deoxy hemoglobin C (beta six Glu → Lys) in two crystal forms, *J. Mol. Biol.,* 132, 603, 1979.
136. **McDonald, M. J., Lund, D. P., Bleichman, M., Bunn, H. T., De Young, A., Noble, R. W., Foster, B., and Arnone, A.,** Equilibrium, kinetic and structural properties of hemoglobin Cranston, an elongated β chain variant, *J. Mol. Biol.,* 140, 357, 1980.
137. **Phillips, S. E. V., Perutz, M. F., Poyart, C., and Wajcman, H.,** Structure and function of Haemoglobin Barcelona Asp FG1(94)β→ His, *J. Mol. Biol.,* 164, 477, 1983.
138. **Arnone, A., Thillet, J., and Rosa, J.,** Structure of hemoglobin Creteil (β89Ser → Asn) is similar to that of abnormal human hemoglobins having sequence changes at Tyr145β, *J. Biol. Chem.,* 256, 8545, 1981.
139. **Kilmartin, J. V., Anderson, N. L., and Ogawa, S.,** Response of the Bohr group salt bridges to ligation of the T state of haemoglobin Kansas, *J. Mol. Biol.,* 123, 71, 1978.
140. **Rosen, L. S. and Magdoff-Fairchild, B.,** Molecular packing in a second monoclinic crystal of deoxygenated sickle hemoglobin, *J. Mol. Biol.,* 157, 181, 1982.

141. **Magdoff-Fairchild, B., Rosen, L. S., and Chiu, C. C.,** Triclinic crystal associated with fibers of deoxygenated sickle hemoglobin, *EMBO J.*, 1, 121, 1982.
142. **Poyart, C., Bursaux, E., Arnone, A., Bonaventura, J., and Bonaventura, C.,** Structural and functional studies of hemoglobin Suresnes (Arg141$\alpha_2 \rightarrow$ HisB_2), Consequences of disrupting an oxygen-linked anion-binding site, *J. Biol. Chem.*, 255, 9465, 1980.
143. **Tucker, P. W., Phillips, S. E. V., Perutz, M. F., Houtchens, R., and Caughey, W. S.,** Structure of hemoglobins Zürich [His E7(63)$\beta \rightarrow$ Arg] and Sydney [Val E11(67)$\beta \rightarrow$ Ala] and role of the distal residues in ligand binding, *Proc. Acad. Natl. Sci. U.S.A.*, 75, 1076, 1978.
144. **Tucker, P. W., Phillips, S. E. V., Perutz, M. F., Houtchens, R., and Caughey, W. S.,** Structure of haemoglobins Zürich (His E7(63)$\beta \rightarrow$ Arg) and Sydney (Val E11(67)$\beta \rightarrow$ Ala) and the role of the distal residues in ligand binding, in *The Red Blood Cell*, Brewer, G. J., Ed., Alan R. Liss, New York, 1978, 3.
145. **Phillips, S. E. V., Hall, D., and Perutz, M. F.,** Structure of deoxyhaemoglobin Zürich (His E7(63β) $\rightarrow$ Arg), *J. Mol. Biol.*, 150, 137, 1981.
146. **Arnone, A., Briley, P. D., Rogers, P. H., and Hendrickson, W. A.,** Structure-function relationships in carbonmonoxy β_4 hemoglobin, in *Hemoglobin and Oxygen Binding*, Ho, C., Ed., Elsevier Biomedical, New York, 1982, 127.
147. **Dickerson, R. E. and Geis, I.,** *Hemoglobin: Structure, Function, Evolution, and Pathology*, Benjamin Cummings, Menlo Park, Calif., 1983.
148. **Ho, C.,** *Hemoglobin and Oxygen Binding*, Elsevier Biomedical, New York, 1982.
149. **Perutz, M. F.,** Regulation of oxygen affinity of hemoglobin: influence of structure of the globin on the heme iron, *Ann. Rev. Biochem.*, 48, 327, 1979.
150. **Perutz, M. F.,** Stereochemical mechanism of oxygen transport by haemoglobin, *Proc. R. Soc. London*, B208, 135, 1980.
151. **Perutz, M. F.,** Hemoglobin structure and respiratory transport, *Sci. Am.*, 239, 92, 1978.
152. **Hanson, J. C. and Schoenborn, B. P.,** Real space refinement of neutron diffraction data from sperm whale carbonmonoxy myoglobin, *J. Mol. Biol.*, 153, 117, 1981.
153. **Phillips, S. E. V.,** Structure and refinement of oxymyoglobin at 1.6 Å resolution, *J. Mol. Biol.*, 142, 531, 1980.
154. **Bolognesi, M., Cannillo, E., Ascenzi, Giacometti, G. M., Merli, A., and Brunori, M.,** Reactivity of ferric *Aplysia* and sperm whale myoglobins towards imidazole, X-ray and binding study, *J. Mol. Biol.*, 158, 305, 1982.
155. **Fermi, G., Perutz, M. F., Dickinson, L. C., and Chien, J. C. W.,** Structure of human deoxy cobalt haemoglobin, *J. Mol. Biol.*, 155, 495, 1982.
156. **Baldwin, J. M.,** Structure of human carbonmonoxy haemoglobin at 2.7 Å resolution, *J. Mol. Biol.*, 136, 103, 1980.
157. **O'Donnell, S., Mandaro, R., Schuster, T. M., and Arnone, A.,** X-ray diffraction and solution studies of specifically carbamylated human hemoglobin A. Evidence for the location of a proton- and oxygen-linked chloride binding site at valine 1α, *J. Biol. Chem.*, 254, 12204, 1979.
158. **Kilmartin, J. V., Arnone, A., and Fogg, J.,** Specific modification of the α chain C-terminal carboxyl group of hemoglobin by trypsin-catalyzed hydrazinolysis, *Biochemistry*, 16, 5393, 1977.
159. **Arnone, A. and Williams, D.,** Binding of zinc to human deoxyhemoglobin and its possible relevance to the anti-sickling effect of zinc, in *Zinc Metabolism: Current Aspects in Health and Disease*, Brewer, G. J. and Prasad, A. S., Ed., Alan R. Liss, New York, 1977, 317.
160. **Walder, J. A., Walder, R. Y., and Arnone, A.,** Development of antisickling compounds that chemically modify hemoglobin S specificity within the 2,3-diphosphoglycerate binding site, *J. Mol. Biol.*, 141, 195, 1980.
161. **Chatterjee, R., Walder, R. Y., Arnone, A., and Walder, J. A.,** Mechanism for the increase in solubility of deoxyhemoglobin S due to crosslinking the β chains between lysine-82β_1 and lysine-82β_2, *Biochemistry*, 21, 5901, 1982.
162. **Deatherage, J. F., Obendorf, S. K., and Moffat, K.,** Structure of azide methemoglobin, *J. Mol. Biol.*, 134, 419, 1979.
163. **Deatherage, J. F. and Moffat, K.,** Structure of nitric oxide hemoglobin, *J. Mol. Biol.*, 134, 401, 1979.
164. **Korszun, Z. R. and Moffat, K.,** Structure of isothiocyanate methemoglobin, J. *Mol. Biol.*, 145, 815, 1981.
165. **Bell, J. A., Korszun, Z. R., and Moffat, K.,** Structure of imidazole methemoglobin, *J. Mol. Biol.*, 147, 325, 1981.
166. **Seybert, D. W. and Moffat, K.,** Structure of hemoglobin reconstituted with mesoheme, *J. Mol. Biol.*, 113, 419, 1977.
167. **Weber, E., Steigemann, W., Jones, T. A., and Huber, R.,** Structure of oxy-erythrocruorin at 1.4 Å resolution, *J. Mol. Biol.*, 120, 327, 1978.

168. **Hendrickson, W. A., Love, W. E., and Karle, J.,** Crystal structure analysis of sea lamprey hemoglobin at 2 Å resolution, *J. Mol. Biol.*, 74, 331, 1973.
169. **Steigemann, W. and Weber, E.,** Structure of erythrocruorin in different ligand states refined at 1.4 Å resolution, *J. Mol. Biol.*, 127, 309, 1979.
170. **Scouloudi, H. and Baker, E. N.,** X-ray crystallographic studies of seal myoglobin; the molecule at 2.5 Å resolution, *J. Mol. Biol.*, 126, 637, 1978.
171. **Scouloudi, H.,** A preliminary comparison of metmyoglobin molecules from seal and sperm whale, *J. Mol. Biol.*, 126, 661, 1978.
172. **Friend, S. H. and Gurd, F. R. N.,** Electrostatic stabilization in myoglobin. pH dependence of summed electrostatic contributions, *Biochemistry*, 18, 4612, 1979.
173. **Friend, S. H. and Gurd, F. R. N.,** Electrostatic stabilization in myoglobin. Interactive free energies between individual sites, *Biochemistry*, 18, 4620, 1979.
174. **Friend, S. H., Matthew, J. B., and Gurd, F. R. N.,** Protein-protein interactions: Nature of the electrostatic stabilization of deoxyhemoglobin tetramer formation, *Biochemistry*, 20, 580, 1981.
175. **Flanagan, M. A., Ackers, G. K., Matthew, J. B., Hanania, G. I. H., and Gurd, F. R. N.,** Electrostatic contributions to the energetics of dimer-tetramer assembly in human hemoglobin: pH dependence and effect of specifically bound chloride ions, *Biochemistry*, 20, 7439, 1981.
176. **Hol, G. J. W., Halie, L. M., and Sander, C.,** Dipoles of the α-helix and β-sheet: their role in protein folding, *Nature (London)*, 294, 532, 1981.
177. **Russu, I. M., Ho, N. T., and Ho, C.,** A proton nuclear magnetic resonance investigation of histidyl residues in human normal adult hemoglobin, *Biochemistry*, 21, 5031, 1982.
178. **Kilmartin, J. V., Fogg, J. H., and Perutz, M. F.,** Role of C-terminal histidine in the alkaline Bohr effect of human hemoglobin, *Biochemistry*, 19, 3189, 1980.
179. **Kwiatkowski, L. D. and Noble, R. W.,** The contribution of histidine (HC3) (146β) to the R state Bohr effect of human hemoglobin, *J. Biol. Chem.*, 257, 8891, 1982.
180. **Matthew, J. B., Hanania, G. I. H., and Gurd, F. R. N.,** Electrostatic effects in hemoglobin: Bohr effect and ionic strength dependence of individual groups, *Biochemistry*, 18, 1928, 1979.
181. **Perutz, M. F., Kilmartin, J. V., Nishikura, K., Fogg, J. H., Butler, P. J. G., and Rollema, H. S.,** Identification of residues contributing to the Bohr effect of human haemoglobin, *J. Mol. Biol.*, 138, 649, 1980.
182. **Kilmartin, J. V., Imai, K., Jones, R. T., Faruqui, A. R., Fogg, J., and Baldwin, J. M.,** Role of Bohr group salt bridges in cooperativity in hemoglobin, *Biochim. Biophys. Acta*, 534, 15, 1978.
183. **Kilmartin, J. V.,** The Bohr effect of human hemoglobin, *Trends Biochem. Sci.*, 2, 247, 1977.
184. **Nasuda-Kouyama, A., Tachibana, H., and Wada, A.,** Preference of oxygenation between α and β subunits of haemoglobin; results of multidimensional spectroscopic observation, *J. Mol. Biol.*, 164, 451, 1983.
185. **Phillips, S. E. V. and Schoenborn, B. P.,** Neutron diffraction reveals oxygen-histidine hydrogen bond in oxymyoglobin, *Nature (London)*, 292, 81, 1981.
186. **Perutz, M. F. and Imai, K.,** Regulation of oxygen affinity of mammalian haemoglobins, *J. Mol. Biol.*, 136, 183, 1980.
187. **Matthew, J. B., Friend, S. H., and Gurd, F. R. N.,** Electrostatic effects in hemoglobin: electrostatic energy associated with allosteric transition and effector binding, *Biochemistry*, 20, 571, 1981.
188. **Baldwin, J. and Chothia, C.,** Haemoglobin: the structural changes related to ligand binding and its allosteric mechanism, *J. Mol. Biol.*, 129, 175, 1979.
189. **Perutz, M. F., Sanders, J. K. M., Chenery, D. H., Noble, R. W., Penelly, R. R., Fung, L. W.-M., Ho, C., Giannini, I., Prosohke, D., and Winkler, H.,** Interaction between the quaternary structure of the globin and the spin state of the heme in ferric mixed spin derivatives of hemoglobin, *Biochemistry*, 17, 3640, 1978.
190. **Messana, C., Cerdonio, M., Shenkin, P., Noble, R. W., Fermi, G., Perutz, K. N., and Perutz, M. F.,** Influence of quarternary structure of the globin on thermal spin equilibria in different methemoglobin derivatives, *Biochemistry*, 17, 3652, 1978.
191. **Weber, G.,** Asymmetric ligand binding by haemoglobin, *Nature (London)*, 300, 603, 1982.
192. **Johnson, M. L. and Ackers, G. A.,** Thermodynamic analysis of human hemoglobins in terms of the Perutz mechanism: extension of the Szabo-Karplus model to include subunit assembly, *Biochemistry*, 21, 201, 1982.
193. **Moffat, K., Deatherage, J. F., and Seybert, D. W.,** A structural model for the kinetic behavior of hemoglobin, *Science*, 206, 1035, 1979.
194. **Dykes, G., Crepeau, R. H., and Edelstein, S. J.,** Three-dimensional reconstruction of the fibres of sickle cell hemoglobin, *Nature (London)*, 272, 506, 1978.
195. **Crepeau, R. H., Dykes, G., Garrell, R., and Edelstein, S. J.,** Diameter of haemoglobin S fibres in sickled cells, *Nature (London)*, 274, 616, 1978.

196. **Dykes, G. W., Crepeau, R. H., and Edelstein, S. J.,** Three-dimensional reconstruction of the 14-filament fibers of hemoglobin S, *J. Mol. Biol.,* 130, 451, 1979.
197. **Garrell, R. L., Crepeau, R. H., and Edelstein, S. J.,** Cross-sectional views of hemoglobin S fibers by electron microscopy and computer modeling, *Proc. Natl. Acad. Sci. U.S.A.,* 76, 1140, 1979.
198. **Edelstein, S. J.,** Patterns in the quinary structures of proteins, Plasticity and inequivalence of individual molecules in helical arrays of sickle cell hemoglobin and tubulin, *Biophys. J.,* 32, 347, 1980.
199. **Wellems, T. E. and Josephs, R.,** Helical crystals of sickle cell hemoglobin, *J. Mol. Biol.,* 137, 443, 1980.
200. **Wellems, T. E., Vassar, R. J., and Josephs, R.,** Polymorphic assemblies of double strands of sickle cell hemoglobin, Manifold pathways of deoxyhemoglobin S crystallization, *J. Mol. Biol.,* 153, 1011, 1981.
201. **Vassar, R. J., Potel, M. J., and Josephs, R.,** Studies of the fiber to crystal transition of sickle cell hemoglobin in acidic polyetheylene glycol, *J. Mol. Biol.,* 157, 395, 1982.
202. **Magdoff-Fairchild, B. and Chiu, C. C.,** X-ray diffraction studies of fibers and crystals of deoxygenated sickle cell hemoglobin, *Proc. Natl. Acad. Sci. U.S.A.,* 76, 223, 1979.
203. **Benesch, R. E., Kwong, S., Benesch, R., and Edalji, R.,** Location and bond type of intermolecular contacts in the polymerization of haemoglobin S., *Nature (London),* 269, 772, 1977.
204. **Nagel, R. L., Johnson, J., Bookchin, R. M., Garel, M. C., Rosa, J., Schiliro, G., Wajcman, H., Labie, D., Moo-Penn, W., and Castro, O.,** β-Chain contact sites in the haemoglobin S polymer, *Nature (London),* 283, 832, 1980.
205. **Benesch, R. E., Kwong, S., and Benesch, R.,** The effects of α chain mutations *cis* and *trans* to the β6 mutation on the polymerization of sickle cell haemoglobin, *Nature (London),* 299, 231, 1982.
206. **Arnone, A., Chatterjee, R., Rogers, P., Musso, G. F., Kaiser, E. T., Steck, T. L., and Walder, J.,** Hemoglobin's binding site for the NH_2-terminal peptide of the erythrocyte band 3 protein, *Fed. Proc.,* 42, 2196, 1983.

ELECTROPHORETIC MOBILITIES OF MUTANT HEMOGLOBINS AND MUTANT GLOBIN CHAINS

Rose G. Schneider and Ronald C. Barwick

Electrophoresis in alkaline buffers (most conveniently on cellulose acetate) and on citrate agar are two especially useful complementary procedures for identifying abnormal hemoglobins. The rationale of these methods differs substantially; in the former, mobility is largely a function of the net charge of the hemoglobin, whereas on citrate agar, mobilities are related to many additional factors, particularly the molecular location of the substituted residue.[1,2] Because these analyses reveal different aspects of molecular structure, the combined data often provide presumptive, or in some cases, highly specific identifications of mutant hemoglobins. When the data are supplemented by those of globin chain electrophoresis at acidic and alkaline pH, the scope of the identification is greatly enlarged.

In globin electrophoresis, urea and mercaptoethanol promote removal of heme, unfolding of the helices, and separation of globin chains. Charge differences are thereby unmasked and sharpened. However, molecular unfolding may be incomplete in 6 *M* urea and some conformational effects may persist. Their electrophoretic manifestations may vary with pH, perhaps explaining some pH-related differences in mobility, such as the characteristic proximity of $\beta^{\text{D-Los Angeles}}$ to β^{A} in acidic compared to alkaline buffers.

Performing the globin electrophoresis at both alkaline and acidic pH (values 8.9 and 6.0) also permits the detection of mutant globin chains whose alterations involve histidine. For example, the β-chain of Hb P Galveston (β117 His→Arg) separates from β^{A} at pH 8.9, in which histidine is neutral and arginine is basic, but not at pH 6.0, in which histidine and arginine are both basic. Conversely, a mutant β-chain with a His→Leu (or Gln) substitution, such as Hb $\beta^{\text{Cowtown }(\beta 146\text{ His}\rightarrow\text{Leu})}$, does not separate from β^{A} in alkaline buffers, in which histidine and leucine are both neutral, but it does separate in acidic buffers, in which leucine is neutral but histidine is basic.

Previous evaluations of mobilities have usually depended on direct visual comparison of the hemoglobin being tested with reference samples analyzed simultaneously. Mobilities are often recorded by lines representing comparative distances. In an attempt to make the comparisons more uniform and objective, we have instituted a system of calculating relative mobilities.[3] For cellulose acetate electrophoresis the method is as follows:

1. The mobility of Hb A is designated as zero (0).
2. The distance between the mutant and Hb A is measured from the middle of each electrophoretically separated fraction (or the corresponding densitometric peak), divided by the distance between Hb A and Hb C, and then arbitrarily multiplied by 10. This procedure is expressed in the equation:

$$N = \frac{D(\text{A to X})}{D(\text{A to C})} \times 10$$

   where N = ratio, X = mutant being analyzed, and D = distance between electrophoretically separated fractions.
3. Mobilities of hemoglobins anodic to HbA are marked plus (+); those cathodic to HbA are marked minus (−).

Hb C was chosen as the reference because it moves farther from Hb A than any other readily available mutant, both in cellulose acetate and citrate agar electrophoresis. In the latter method, anodic and cathodic mobilities may vary independently according to electrophoretic conditions; we therefore measured anodic and cathodic mobilities in relation to separate controls, the anodic control being Hb C (the equation applied is the same as above) and the cathodic control, Hb F. For cathodic mobilities, the distance between Hb A and the mutant was divided by the distance between Hb A and Hb F, and the quotient was multiplied by 4.4, a value that generally reflects the relationship of the mobility of the Hb F control to the 10 value of the Hb C control. The equation for cathodic mobilities on citrate agar electrophoresis is

$$N = -4.4 \times \frac{D(A \text{ to } X)}{D(A \text{ to } F)}$$

In areas where Hb C is not available, Hb E or Hb A_2 may be substituted in electrophoresis on cellulose acetate. Citrate agar electrophoresis is apt to be less useful in areas where Hb S and Hb C are not found.

In globin electrophoresis, the migrations of mutant chains in alkaline (pH 8.9) and acidic (pH 6.0) urea buffers are related to those of α^A- and β^A-globin chains analyzed simultaneously, often in the same sample. For purposes of calculating ratios, the α^A- and β^A-globins are assigned values of 10 and 20, respectively. The following equation is applied:

$$N = \left[\frac{D(\alpha^A \text{ to } X)}{D(\alpha^A \text{ to } \beta^A)} \times 10\right] + 10$$

where $D(\alpha^A$ to $X)$ is the distance from α^A to the mutant globin chain, entered as positive if the mutant chain is anodic to α^A, and as negative if it is cathodic to α^A; $D(\alpha^A$ to $\beta^A)$ is the distance from α^A to β^A. The arbitrary addition of 10 to the expression conveniently partitions the mobilities into three regions: (1) those cathodic to α^A, for which N is less than 10; (2) those between α^A and β^A, for which N lies between 10 and 20; (3) those anodic to β^A, for which N is greater than 20. Figure 1 shows the visual relationship for selected hemoglobins of electrophoretic mobility to the value of N in each of the four methods. The following examples illustrate the quantitation:

1. $\alpha^{G\ Philadelphia}$ moves cathodically to α^A; the α^A to β^A distance, $D(\alpha^A$ to $\beta^A)$, is 4.53 cm (on a densitometric tracing); the α^A to X distance, $D(\alpha^A$ to $X)$, is 0.95 cm. The calculations are as follows:

$$\begin{aligned} N &= 10 \times (-0.95/4.53) + 10; \quad D(\alpha^A \text{ to } X) \text{ is entered as negative because the mutant chain is cathodic to } \alpha^A \\ &= (-0.21 \times 10) + 10 \\ &= -2.1 + 10 \\ &= 7.9 \end{aligned}$$

2. $\beta^{J\ Baltimore}$ moves anodically to β^A; $D(\alpha^A$ to $\beta^A)$ = 4.62 cm; $D(\alpha^A$ to $X)$ = 5.96 cm. The calculation are as follows:

$$\begin{aligned} N &= 10 \times (5.96/4.62) + 10 \\ &= (1.29 \times 10) + 10 \\ &= 1.29 + 10 = 22.9 \end{aligned}$$

Globin electrophoresis usually indicates whether it is the α- or non-α-chain that is altered because the mutant globin chain usually moves closer to its parent chain than to the other

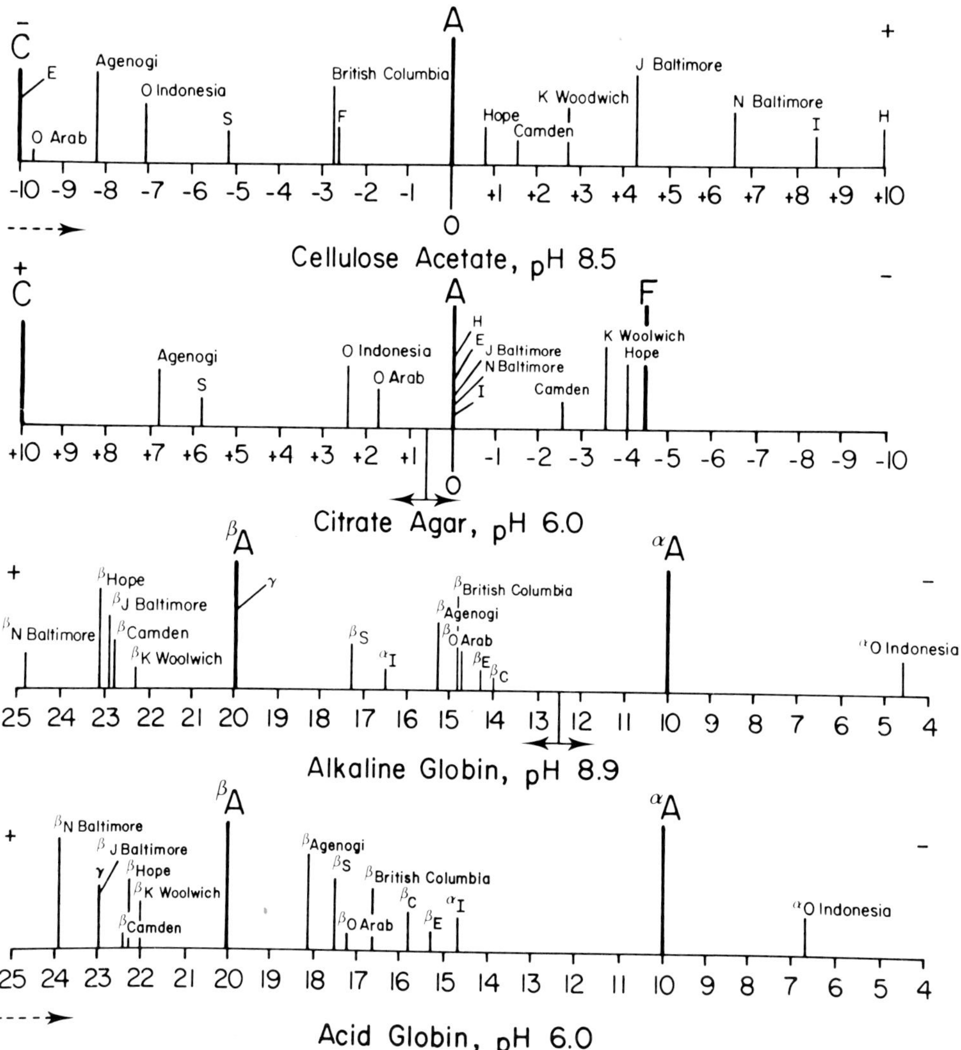

FIGURE 1. The relationship of visual electrophoretic mobility of selected hemoglobins to N values in the four methods. Electrophoretic mobilities are shown above the line for each method; N values (see text) are shown below the line. Controls which define the numerical scale are depicted with heavy lines. Arrows indicate the electrophoretic point of origin in each method. (From Schneider, R. G. and Barwick, R. C., *Hemoglobin*, 2(5), 417—435, 1978. With permission.)

chain. β^S, for example, moves closer to β^A than to α^A (N = 17.3). However, some mutants with Lys→Glu or Glu→Lys substitutions do not follow this rule. A globin chain that moves halfway between α^A and β^A (i.e., N = 15), could be a negatively charged α-chain mutant or a positively charged β-chain mutant. In these cases its mobility relative to Hb A in cellulose acetate electrophoresis would indicate the charge, and allow it to be identified as an α- or β-chain mutant. For example, the mutant chain of a hemoglobin that moves anodically to Hb A in cellulose acetate electrophoresis moves anodically to its parent chain in globin electrophoresis. Also, in most cases, α-chain mutants are usually easily recognized by the presence of an "extra Hb A_2" in cellulose acetate electrophoresis.

When an unknown mutant chain does not separate from its parent chain in either alkaline or acidic globin electrophoresis, N for these methods is given as "10/20", because the mutant chain migrates with either the α- or β-chain, but which of the two cannot be determined from the electrophoresis. However, if the mutant chain separates at only one pH value, N for the other pH can be specified either as "10" (normal α) or "20" (normal β), since the altered chain is now known (see, for example, Hb Hasharon, α47 Asp→His).

The ratios provide a more objective measure of comparative mobilities than visual comparisons. They also make it possible to compare hemoglobins analyzed at different times and to computerize the data.

QUALIFICATIONS

Relative electrophoretic mobilities on citrate agar vary considerably according to technique. Mobilities on cellulose acetate and in globin electrophoresis may also vary, especially according to: (1) type of buffer and its ionic strength, (2) electrical conditions, (3) duration of electrophoresis, (4) temperature, (5) method of preparation of hemolysate, and (6) kind and amount of accompanying hemoglobin. These conditions should be kept as constant as possible.

The mobilities of the hemoglobins examined in this laboratory are marked with an asterisk. At least ten separate analyses were made for each of the more frequent ones, but some rare mutants were only examined once or twice. Standard deviations were calculated where possible for relative mobilities (N) in all four methods. In general, these were as follows: 0.23 for cellulose acetate electrophoresis; 0.47 for citrate agar electrophoresis; 0.18 for alkaline globin electrophoresis; 0.31 for acidic globin electrophoresis. Mobilities of hemoglobins not examined here were obtained either from the data compiled by Lehmann and Kynoch[4] or from the original description of the mutant. These figures are approximations and are so marked; however, when the mobility was described as being like that of Hb S (or Hb C), it was given the numerical designation of Hb S (or Hb C). A dash (—) indicates that the data were not available.

Data derived from the literature represent a variety of methods (including filter paper or, in a few cases, starch gel). Moreover, descriptions were often scanty, with some hemoglobins characterized merely as "slow" or "fast". Data from different laboratories may not therefore be strictly comparable.

METHODS

Cellulose Acetate Electrophoresis[1]

Apparatus — Details of technique may vary slightly with the type of apparatus, which generally consists of: Mylar®-backed cellulose acetate plates, a zone electrophoresis chamber, applicators, and a power supply with variable voltage control.

Reagents — All procedures use deionized water.

1. Tris, EDTA, borate buffer (TEB): 10.2 g tris, 0.6 g EDTA, and 3.2 boric acid per liter
2. Ponceau S stain; 0.3 g Ponceau S in 100 mℓ of 3% trichloracetic acid
3. Glacial acetic acid (3%)
4. Tolidine reagent: 1.0 g *o*-Tolidine dihydrochloride in 25 mℓ glacial acetic acid made up to 100 mℓ with H_2O
5. Tolidine stain: 20 mℓ tolidine reagent, 10 mℓ 3 to 5% acetic acid, and 2 mℓ 3% H_2O_2

Procedures — Hemolysates (containing 5 to 10 g Hb per 100 mℓ) may be prepared by any of the standard methods.

1. Pour TEB buffer into chambers; soak and position wicks.

2. Soak cellulose acetate plates in TEB buffer for at least 20 min before use.
3. Blot plate between two pieces of absorbent paper quickly and evenly to absorb excess buffer.
4. Apply samples with an applicator to the cellulose acetate at about 2.5 cm from the cathodic end.
5. Put plate on wicks in chamber with glass slide (3″ × 2″) on top to assure even contact. Three plates may be analyzed simultaneously.
6. Apply 450 V for 20 min at room temperature.
7. Remove plates from chamber and stain immediately 1 to 3 min in Ponceau S stain.
8. Remove plate from stain and place in three consecutive 3-min washes in 3% acetic acid or until background is clear.
9. Optional: counterstain in freshly made tolidine stain about 1 to 2 min. Rinse in distilled water for at least 20 min.
10. If desired, clear plate by soaking it for 2 min in absolute methanol, then for 10 min in 25% glacial acetic acid in absolute methanol. Allow plate to dry.

Citrate Agar Electrophoresis[5]

Many methods are available. The following is the method used in this study.

Apparatus — The apparatus is the same as for cellulose acetate.

Reagents — The reagents used include:

1. Sodium citrate buffer — 0.5 *M*, stock solution: 147 g sodium citrate ($Na_3C_6H_5O_7 \cdot 2H_2O$) per liter; adjust to pH 6 with citric acid (300 g/ℓ).
2. Working buffer — 0.05 *M*, dilute stock buffer tenfold with water and adjust to pH 6 with citric acid solution (300 g/ℓ). All solutions should be stored at 4°C.
3. Dilute hemolysate to 1 g/100 mℓ for adult samples and 3 g/100 mℓ for umbilical cord blood samples.
4. Tolidine stain — same as for cellulose acetate; make fresh just before use.

Procedures —Preparation of citrate agar plates is as follows:

1. Soak Mylar®-backed cellulose acetate plates (Helena or Gelman) in working buffer for at least 30 min. A rack to hold the plates is convenient.
2. Add 1.0 g Bacto Agar® (Difco® certified) to 100 mℓ working buffer; add 2 drops 5% KCN as preservative. Heat in boiling water bath until agar is completely dissolved.
3. Cool agar to 60 to 70°C.
4. Remove rack of cellulose acetate plates from buffer and drain for about 30 sec. Place rack into agar solution for 30 min; maintain the temperature between 60 and 70°C.
5. Remove plates. Place individually (or two, back to back) in plastic bag with 1 to 2 mℓ of working buffer added.
6. Store in tightly closed box in refrigerator. They may be stored for several weeks.

Electrophoretic procedure is as follows:

1. Add working buffer to each side of electrophoresis chamber. Volume depends on type of chamber. Position wicks.
2. Remove citrate agar plate from package and blot to remove excess buffer and agar.
3. Apply sample lightly with applicator approximately 3 cm from anodic end of plate.
4. Immediately invert plate on wicks in electrophoresis chamber and apply 80 V for 30 min. Cover plate with a glass slide (3″ × 2″) to assure proper contact with the wicks. Several plates may be analyzed simultaneously.

5. Stain in freshly made tolidine stain until bands become distinct, about 1 to 2 min.
6. Rinse in distilled water for at least 20 min.

Alkaline Globin Electrophoresis[6]

Reagents — The reagents for this procedure are as follows:

1. TEB buffer: Tris, 10.2 g; EDTA, 0.6 g; boric acid, 3.2 g; deionized water, to 1 ℓ
2. Urea-TEB buffer: dissolve 108 g urea in about 210 mℓ TEB buffer and add TEB buffer to 300 mℓ
3. Ponceau S stain: Ponceau S, 0.3 g; trichloroacetic acid 5 g; water to 100 mℓ
4. Acetic acid (3%)

Procedure — The procedure is as follows:

1. To 200 mℓ TEB-urea buffer, add 1.6 mℓ mercaptoethanol. Soak Gelman Super Sepraphore plates overnight in 100 mℓ and divide the other 100 mℓ evenly (i.e., 50 mℓ each) between the sides of the electrophoresis chamber. Soak and position double thickness wicks.
2. Just before electrophoresis, add 20 μℓ hemolysate to 20 μℓ TEB-urea buffer and 20 μℓ mercaptoethanol.
3. Blot plates carefully and apply samples to the center of the plate. Application should be even but without using any more pressure than absolutely necessary.
4. Trim plate and position on wicks. Cover with glass slides.
5. Apply 200 V for 1 hr.
6. Stain plates for about 30 sec with Ponceau S stain and decolorize with 3% acetic acid until background is clear. Air-dry.

Acidic Globin Electrophoresis[7]

Reagents — The reagents for this procedure are as follows:

1. TEB buffer: Tris, 10.2 g; EDTA, 0.6 g; boric acid, 3.2 g; deionized water up to 1 ℓ
2. 2-Mercaptoethanol
3. Citric acid (30%)
4. Ponceau S stain: Ponceau S, 0.3 g; trichloroacetic acid, 5 g; deionized water up to 100 mℓ
5. Acetic acid (3%)
6. Chamber buffer: dissolve 72 g urea in 100 to 130 mℓ of TEB buffer; adjust pH to 6.0 with 30% citric acid; add TEB buffer to 200 mℓ; add 0.8 mℓ mercaptoethanol to 100 mℓ of this buffer and divide evenly (i.e., 50 mℓ each) between sides of electrophoresis chamber. Use the other 100 mℓ for diluting the hemolysate (see step 3 of electrophoretic procedure, below).
7. Soak buffer: add 50 mℓ water to 50 mℓ TEB buffer; in about 60 to 70 mℓ of this 1:1 buffer dissolve 36 g urea; adjust pH to 6.0 with 30% citric acid and adjust volume to 100 mℓ with 1:1 buffer. Keep no longer than 2 days.

Procedure — The procedure is as follows:

1. Soak Gelman Sepraphore™ X plates overnight in soak buffer.
2. Soak and apply double thickness wicks to electrophoresis chamber.
3. To 20 μℓ hemolysate add 10 μℓ chamber buffer (w/o mercaptoethanol) and 20 μℓ mercaptoethanol.

4. Apply above hemolysate to plates 2 cm from anodal end of plate.
5. Place on wicks and cover with glass slides.
6. Perform electrophoresis at 200 V for 75 min.
7. Stain with Ponceau S stain for about 30 sec and rinse with 3% acetic acid until background is clear. Air-dry.

Table 1
RELATIVE ELECTROPHORETIC MOBILITIES OF MUTANT HEMOGLOBINS

α-Chains

Name	Residue	Substitution	Cellulose acetate	Citrate agar	Alkaline globin	Acidic globin
J Toronto*	α5	Ala-Asp	+4.5	0	12.5	12.8
Sawara*	α6	Asp-Ala	−2.8	+1.25	7.5	8.2
Dunn*	α6	Asp-Asn	−3.2	2.4	7.4	8.7
Ferndown	α6	Asp-Val	~−5	—	—	—
Anantharaj*	α11	Lys-Glu	+5.8	0	12.5	11.9
J-Wenchang-Wuming	α11	Lys-Gln	~+4.5	—	—	—
J Paris*	α12	Ala-Asp	+4.7	0	11.8	11.8
J Oxford*	α15	Gly-Asp	+4.6	0	12.5	12.3
Ottawa	α15	Gly-Arg	~+4	0	—	—
I*	α16	Lys-Glu	+8.5	0	15.9	14.6
Handsworth	α18	Gly-Arg	—	—	~8.0	—
J Kurosh	α19	Ala-Asp	~+4	—	~12.0	—
Necker Enfants-Malades	α20	His-Tyr	0	—	—	—
J Nyanza	α21	Ala-Asp	~+4	—	—	—
J Medellin	α22	Gly-Asp	~+4	0	—	—
Memphis	α23	Glu-Gln	−5.2	~+6.25	—	—
Chad	α23	Glu-Lys	−10	—	—	—
G Audhali	α23	Glu-Val	~−5	—	—	—
Fort Worth*	α27	Glu-Gly	−2.7	0	7.3	8.6
Spanish Town	α27	Glu-Val	~−2.8	0	—	—
Shuangfeng	α27	Glu-Lys	~−9.0	—	—	—
O Padova*	α30	Glu-Lys	−8.2	+7.9	5.7	6.6
G Honolulu	α30	Glu-Gln	−5.0	0	—	—
Prato	α31	Arg-Ser	—	—	—	—
Queens	α34	Leu-Arg	—	—	—	—
Torino	α43	Phe-Val	0	—	—	—
Hirosaki	α43	Phe-Leu	0	0	20	20
Milledgeville	α44	Pro-Leu	—	—	—	—
Kawachi	α44	Pro-Arg	0	—	—	—
Fort de France*	α45	His-Arg	−5.6	0	7.4	10
Bari	α45	His-Gln	~+0.5	0	10	~12.5
Kokura*	α47	Asp-Gly	−5.8	+2.0	7.9	10
Hasharon*	α47	Asp-His	−5.5	+6.25	7.9	10
Arya*	α47	Asp-Asn	−5.2	0	8.4	10
Montgomery*	α48	Leu-Arg	−4.6	+2.5	7.9	8.4
Savaria	α49	Ser-Arg	~−5	—	—	—
J Sardegna	α50	His-Asp	~+4	0	—	—
J Abidjan	α51	Gly-Asp	~+2	0	~12.5	—
Russ*	α51	Gly-Arg	−5.2	0	7.6	10
J Rovigo*	α53	Ala-Asp	+4.5	0	12.5	11.2
Shimonoseki*	α54	Gln-Arg	+5.6	+0.5	7.8	10
J Mexico*	α54	Gln-Glu	+4.6	0	12.5	10
Thailand	α56	Lys-Thr	~+2	—	—	—
Shaare Zedek	α56	Lys-Glu	~+8	—	—	—
L Persian Gulf	α57	Gly-Arg	~−5	0	~7.5	—

Table 1 (continued)
RELATIVE ELECTROPHORETIC MOBILITIES OF MUTANT HEMOGLOBINS

Name	Residue	Substitution	Cellulose acetate	Citrate agar	Alkaline globin	Acidic globin
J Norfolk*	α57	Gly-Asp	+4.6	0	12.4	11.0
M Boston	α58	His-Tyr	0	—	—	—
Tottori	α59	Gly-Val	0	—	—	—
Zambia	α60	Lys-Asn	∼+4	—	—	—
Dagestan	α60	Lys-Glu	∼+8	—	—	—
J Buda	α61	Lys-Asn	∼+4	—	∼12.5	—
Pontoise*	α63	Ala-Asp	+5.2	0	13	10
Aida*	α64	Asp-Asn	−5.1	0	8	8.8
Q India*	α64	Asp-His	−4.8	+3.4	8.1	8.25
Persepolis	α64	Asp-Tyr	∼−4.5	∼+2.0	∼8.0	—
Ube-2*	α68	Asn-Asp	+4.3	0	12.5	12.3
G Philadelphia*	α68	Asn-Lys	−5.2	0	7.9	8.6
J Habana	α71	Ala-Glu	∼+4	—	—	—
Daneskgah-Tehran*	α72	Asp-His	−4.9	0	7.8	10
Mahidol*	α74	Asp-His	−4.3	−2.25	7.5	6.6
G Pest	α74	Asp- Asn	∼−5	—	—	—
Chapel Hill	α74	Asp-Gly	—	—	—	—
Lille	α74	Asp-Ala	∼−5	—	—	—
Q Iran*	α75	Asp-His	−4.8	+1	7.7	7.8
Duan	α75	Asp-Ala	∼−5?	—	—	—
Winnipeg*	α75	Asp-Tyr	−4.6	0	8.0	8.2
Matsue-Oki*	α75	Asp-Asn	−5.1	+1.5	7.9	8.1
Mizushi*	α75	Asp-Gly	−4.7	+1.9	7.9	8.6
Noko	α76	Met-Lys	—	—	—	—
Stanleyville-II*	α78	Asn-Lys	−5.1	0	7.3	8.7
Ann Arbor	α80	Leu-Arg	∼−6	—	—	—
Nigeria	α81	Ser-Cys	0	—	—	—
Garden State	α82	Ala-Asp	—	— —	—	
Etobicoke	α84	Ser-Arg	0	0	—	—
G Norfolk*	α85	Asp-Asn	−4.9	0	7.9	8.6
Atago*	α85	Asp-Tyr	−4.2	0	8.1	9.0
Inkster*	α85	Asp-Val	−5.0	0	7.9	9.0
Moabit	α86	Leu-Arg	∼−4.5	—	—	—
M Iwate*	α87	His-Tyr	−1.9	0	10	10
M Iwata	α87	His-Arg	∼−5	—	—	—
J Broussais*	α90	Lys-Asn	4.1	0	12.2	10.3
J Rajappen	α90	Lys-Thr	∼+4.0	—	∼12.0	—
Handa	α90	Lys-Met	—	—	—	—
Port Phillip	α91	Leu-Pro	∼−a2.5	—	—	—
J Capetown*	α92	Arg-Gln	+3.3	0	12.6	10
Chesapeake*	α92	Arg-Leu	+3.1	+0.75	12.2	10.9
Setif*	α94	Asp-Tyr	−5.6	+6.5	7.9	10
Titusville*	α94	Asp-Asn	−5.4	+6.0	8.2	10
Sunshine Seth	α94	Asp-His	−6.5	—	—	—
G Georgia*	α95	Pro-Leu	−5.3	−1.5	10	10
Rampa*	α95	Pro-Ser	−5.5	−1.5	10	10
Denmark Hill	α95	Pro-Ala	∼−1	—	10	10
St. Lukes	α95	Pro-Arg	∼−1	—	—	—
Dallas*	α97	Asn-Lys	−1.5	+5.0	8.0	8.8
Manitoba*	α102	Ser-Arg	−3.6	−5.6	7.6	8.4
Suan-Dok	α109	Leu-Arg	∼−3.0	—	—	—
Petah-Tikva	α110	Ala-Asp	0	—	—	—
Hopkins-II*	α112	His-Asp	+4.1	0	12.7	14.2
Strumica	α112	His-Arg	∼−3.0	—	∼8.0	10
Chiapas	α114	Pro-Arg	∼−5	—	—	—
J Tongariki	α115	Ala-Asp	∼+4.0	—	∼12.0	—

Table 1 (continued) RELATIVE ELECTROPHORETIC MOBILITIES OF MUTANT HEMOGLOBINS

Name	Residue	Substitution	Cellulose acetate	Citrate agar	Alkaline globin	Acidic globin
O Indonesia*	α116	Glu-Lys	−7.1	+2.5	4.6	6.7
Ube-4	α116	Glu-Ala	∼−4.0	—	—	—
Oleander*	α116	Glu-Gln	−4.5	0	7.3	7.4
J Birmingham	α120	Ala-Glu	∼+4.0	—	∼12.0	—
Westmead	α122	His-Gln	0	—	—	—
Quong Sze	α125	Leu-Pro	0	—	—	—
Tarrant*	α126	Asp-Asn	−2.3	+5.4	7.9	7.6
St. Claude*	α127	Lys-Thr	+2.6	0	12.7	12.75
Jackson*	α127	Lys-Asn	+3.3	0	12.5	12.6
Bibba	α136	Leu-Pro	∼−5	—	—	—
Singapore	α141	Arg-Pro	∼−2	—	—	—
Suresnes	α141	Arg-His	—	—	—	—
J Cubujuqui*	α141	Arg-Ser	+3.8	0	12.9	13.3
Legnano	α141	Arg-Leu	∼+5.0	—	—	—
J Camagüey	α141	Arg-Gly	∼+4.0	—	—	—
		β-Chains				
Raleigh*	β1	Val-Ac-Ala	0	−4.2	20	22
Deer Lodge*	β2	His-Arg	−2.6	0	17.2	20
S*	β6	Glu-Val	−5.2	+5.8	17.3	17.5
C*	β6	Glu-Lys	10.0	+10.0	14.0	15.8
G Makassar	β6	Glu-Ala	∼+1.0	—	∼22.0	—
G San José*	β7	Glu-Gly	−3.6	+7.5	17.3	17.2
Siriraj	β7	Glu-Lys	∼−4	+10.0	—	—
Porto Alegre	β9	Ser-Cys	∼+0.4	+10.0	—	—
Ankara	β10	Ala-Asp	∼+4	—	—	—
J Lens	β13	Ala-Asp	∼+4.5	—	∼23.0	—
Sogn	β14	Leu-Arg	−5.2	—	—	—
Saki*	β14	Leu-Pro	−5.2	0	17.0	16.9
Belfast*	β15	Trp-Arg	−5.5	0	16.9	17.9
J Baltimore*	β16	Gly-Asp	+4.3	0	22.9	23.0
D Bushman	β16	Gly-Arg	−5.2	—	—	—
Nagasaki	β17	Lys-Glu	∼+5	—	—	—
D Ouled Rabah	β19	Asn-Lys	−5.2	—	—	—
Alamo	β19	Asn-Asp	∼+1.0	0	—	—
Olympia	β20	Val-Met	0	0	20	20
Strasbourg*	β20	Val-Asp	+0.5	0	22.7	22.3
Yusa*	β21	Asp-Tyr	−5.0	0	17.6	17.3
Connecticut*	β21	Asp-Gly	−5.3	0	17.3	17.2
Cocody	β21	Asp-Asn	∼−5.0	—	—	—
E Saskatoon	β22	Glu-Lys	−10	0	∼16.0	—
G Taipei	β22	Glu-Gly	∼−5	—	—	—
G Coushatta*	β22	Glu-Ala	−4.8	0	17.5	17.6
D Iran*	β22	Glu-Gln	−5.2	0	17.4	16.9
Miyashiro	β23	Val-Gly	0	—	—	—
Riverdale-Bronx	β24	Gly-Arg	∼−5	0	—	—
Savannah	β24	Gly-Val	∼−3	—	∼18.0	—
Moscva	β24	Gly-Asp	∼+2	0	—	—
G Taiwan Ami	β25	Gly-Arg	∼−5	—	—	—
E*	β26	Glu-Lys	−10	0	14.1	15.3
Henri Mondor*	β26	Glu-Val	−5.2	0	17.4	16.6
Volga	β27	Ala-Asp	0	0	∼22.0	—
St. Louis*	β28	Leu-Gln	−3.1	0	20	20
Genova	β28	Leu-Pro	0	—	—	—

Table 1 (continued)
RELATIVE ELECTROPHORETIC MOBILITIES OF MUTANT HEMOGLOBINS

Name	Residue	Substitution	Cellulose acetate	Citrate agar	Alkaline globin	Acidic globin
Lufkin*	β29	Gly-Asp	+3.2	0	22.6	23.1
Tacoma*	β30	Arg-Ser	+0.9	0	22.6	23.7
Yokohama	β31	Leu-Pro	0	—	—	—
Perth	β32	Leu-Pro	0	0	—	—
Castilla*	β32	Leu-Arg	−5.0	0	17.3	18.0
Pitie-Salpetriere	β34	Val-Phe	0	—	—	—
Philly	β35	Tyr-Phe	0	—	20	20
Hirose	β37	Trp-Ser	∼−5	0	—	—
Rothschild	β37	Trp-Arg	—	—	—	—
Alabama*	β39	Gln-Lys	−4.9	0	18.1	18.2
Vaasa	β39	Gln-Glu	—	—	—	—
Waco*	β40	Arg-Lys	−0.4	−2.0	20	22
Austin*	β40	Arg-Ser	+2.5	−2.1	22.8	22.4
Mequon	β41	Phe-Tyr	—	—	—	—
Hammersmith*	β42	Phe-Ser	0	0	20	20
Bucuresti	β42	Phe-Leu	0	—	—	—
G Galveston*	β43	Glu-Ala	−4.8	0	17.3	17.9
Hoshida	β43	Glu-Gln	—	—	—	—
Cheverly	β45	Phe-Ser	0	—	—	—
K Ibadan	β46	Gly-Glu	∼+0.5	—	—	—
G Copenhagen	β47	Asp-Asn	∼−5	—	—	—
Gavello	β47	Asp-Gly	−5.2	—	—	—
Avicenna	β47	Asp-Ala	∼−5.0	0	—	—
Okaloosa*	β48	Leu-Arg	−4.7	0	16.7	17.5
Edmonton	β50	Thr-Lys	−5.2	0	—	—
Willamette*	β51	Pro-Arg	−5.1	0	16.5	17.3
Osu-Christianborg*	β52	Asp-Asn	−5.2	0	16.9	18.1
Ocho Rios	β52	Asp-Ala	−5.2	0	∼18.0	—
Summer Hill	β52	Asp-His	∼−5.0	—	—	—
J Bangkok*	β56	Gly-Asp	+4.2	0	22.5	22.1
Hamadan*	β56	Gly-Arg	−5.1	+0.25	17.8	18.8
G Ferrara*	β57	Asn-Lys	−5.2	0	18.2	20
Dhofar	β58	Pro-Arg	∼−5	—	—	—
I High Wycombe	β59	Lys-Glu	∼+7.0	—	—	—
J Honolulu*	β59	Lys-Thr	+4.9	0	22	20.4
J Lome	β59	Lys-Asn	∼+4.0	—	—	—
Yatsushiro	β60	Val-Leu	∼−3?	—	—	—
N Seattle*	β61	Lys-Glu	+7.4	0	24.7	22
Hikari	β61	Lys-Asn	∼+6	0	∼22.0	—
Bologna	β61	Lys-Met	∼+3.5	0	∼23.0	—
Duarte	β62	Ala-Pro	0	—	—	—
Zürich*	β63	His-Arg	−5.2	0	18.5	20
M Saskatoon*	β63	His-Tyr	−1.9	0	20	20
Bicetre	β63	His-Pro	—	—	—	—
J Calabria*	β64	Gly-Asp	+3.6	0	22.0	20
J Sicilia	β65	Lys-Asn	—	—	—	—
J Cairo*	β65	Lys-Gln	+4.7	0	21.7	20
I Toulouse	β66	Lys-Glu	∼+5.0	—	∼23.0	—
Bristol	β67	Val-Asp	0	—	—	—
M Milwaukee-I	β67	Val-Glu	0	—	—	—
Sydney	β67	Val-Ala	−5.2	—	20	20
Mizuho	β68	Leu-Pro	0	—	—	—
Brisbane	β68	Leu-His	0	0	20	—
J Cambridge	β69	Gly-Asp	∼+4.0	—	—	—
Seattle	β70	Ala-Asp	∼+4.0	—	—	—

Table 1 (continued)
RELATIVE ELECTROPHORETIC MOBILITIES OF MUTANT HEMOGLOBINS

Name	Residue	Substitution	Cellulose acetate	Citrate agar	Alkaline globin	Acidic globin
Christchurch	β71	Phe-Ser	0	—	20	20
Vancouver*	β73	Asp-Tyr	−4.9	+0.5	17.7	18.2
Korle Bu*	β73	Asp-Asn	−4.9	+0.5	17.5	18.2
Mobile*	β73	Asp-Val	−4.9	+0.55	17.65	18.2
Bushwick	β74	Gly-Val	~−8	—	20	20
Shepherds Bush	β74	Gly-Asp	~+0.5	0	~22.0	—
Atlanta	β75	Leu-Pro	0	—	—	—
Pasadena	β75	Leu-Arg	−3.5	0	—	—
J Chicago	β76	Ala-Asp	~+4.0	0	—	—
J Iran	β77	His-Asp	~+4.0	—	~22.0	—
G Hsi-Tsou	β79	Asp-Gly	~−5	—	~17.5	—
Tampa*	β79	Asp-Tyr	−3.8	+6.5	17.6	19.1
G Szuhu*	β80	Asn-Lys	−3.0	+6.25	17.7	18.4
Baylor*	β81	Leu-Arg	−4.4	+2.75	17.0	17.8
Providence*	β82	Lys-Asn-Asp	+1.6	−3.0		
			+2.2	−4.2	25.2	24.75
Rahere	β82	Lys-Thr	0	~−4.4	~22.0	—
Helsinki	β82	Lys-Met	0	—	~22.0	—
Ta-Li	β83	Gly-Cys	0	—	—	—
Pyrgos*	β83	Gly-Asp	+3.2	−2.75	22.7	21.4
Byrn Mawr	β85	Phe-Ser	~−0.4	—	—	—
D Ibadan*	β87	Thr-Lys	−4.8	+1.1	17.55	18.3
Borås	β88	Leu-Arg	~−2.5	—	—	—
Santa Ana	β88	Leu-Pro	~−2.5	—	—	—
Creteil*	β89	Ser-Asn	+0.2	0	20	20
Vanderbilt*	β89	Ser-Arg	−2.7	+3.7	17.6	18.2
Agenogi*	β90	Glu-Lys	−8.2	+6.8	15.3	18.0
Sabine*	β91	Leu-Pro	−5.9			
			−8.6	0	20	20
Caribbean	β91	Leu-Arg	−5.2	0	—	—
M Hyde Park	β92	His-Tyr	~+0.3	—	—	—
St. Etienne*	β92	His-Gln	−8.9	0	20	20
J Altegeld						
Gardens	β92	His-Asp	~+5.0	—	—	—
Newcastle	β92	His-Pro	~−2.6	—	20	~22.0
Mozhaisk	β92	His-Arg	—	—	—	—
Barcelona	β94	Asp-His	—	—	—	—
N Baltimore*	β95	Lys-Glu	+6.6	0	24.8	23.9
Detroit*	β95	Lys-Asn	+3.7	0	22.6	21.6
Malmö*	β97	His-Gln	+0.5	−1.1	20	21.3
Wood*	β97	His-Leu	0	−2.2	20	21.3
Köln*	β98	Val-Met	−7.5	−2.2	20	20
Nottingham*	β98	Val-Gly	−8.4			
			−9.1	0	20	20
Djelfa*	β98	Val-Ala	0	0	20	20
Kempsey*	β99	Asp-Asn	−2.5	+2.2	17.5	17.9
Yakima*	β99	Asp-His	−1.0			
			−2.3	+6.5	17.4	17.9
Radcliffe	β99	Asp-Ala	~−3	—	—	—
Ypsilanti	β99	Asp-Tyr	~−3.4			
			~−2.2	—	—	—
Hotel-Dieu	β99	Asp-Gly	~−5.0	—	—	—
Brigham	β100	Pro-Leu	0	—	—	—
British Columbia*	β101	Gly-Lys	−2.7	+10.7	14.8	16.6
Rush*	β101	Glu-Gln	−2.7	+7.3	17.6	18.0

Table 1 (continued)
RELATIVE ELECTROPHORETIC MOBILITIES OF MUTANT HEMOGLOBINS

Name	Residue	Substitution	Cellulose acetate	Citrate agar	Alkaline globin	Acidic globin
Alberta*	β101	Glu-Gly	−2.7	+7.4	17.7	18.1
Potomac*	β101	Glu-Asp	0	0	20	20
Richmond*	β102	Asn-Lys	−0.5			
			−2.7	+5.75	17.8	18.2
Kansas	β102	Asn-Thr	—	—	20	20
Beth Israel	β102	Asn-Ser	~+0.3	—	20	—
St. Mandé	β102	Asn-Tyr	~−2.5	—	—	—
Heathrow	β103	Phe-Leu	0	0	20	—
Camperdown	β104	Asp-Ser	0	—	~17.5	—
Sherwood Forest	β104	Arg-Thr	—	—	—	—
Southampton	β106	Leu-Pro	0	—	—	—
Tübingen	β106	Leu-Gln	~−3.1	—	20	20
Burke*	β107	Gly-Arg	−2.2	+5.75	17.3	18.3
Yoshizuka	β108	Asn-Asp	—	—	—	—
Presbyterian*	β108	Asn-Lys	−1.7	+8.0	17.5	18.3
San Diego	β109	Val-Met	0	—	20	—
Peterborough	β111	Val-Phe	0	~−5	—	—
Indianapolis	β112	Cys-Arg	0	0	—	—
New York*	β113	Val-Glu	+1.5	0	22.7	21.9
Madrid	β115	Ala-Pro	0	0	20	—
P Galveston*	β117	His-Arg	−5.2	0	17.6	20
Fannin-Lubbock*	β119	Gly-Asp	+2.6	0	22.7	21.6
Bougardirey-Mali	β119	Gly-Val	0	—	—	—
Hijiyama*	β120	Lys-Glu	+6.6	0	25.0	24.7
Riyadh*	β120	Lys-Asn	+3.3	0	22.9	22.2
Takamatsu*	β120	Lys-Gln	+3.8	−1	22.7	21.6
D Los Angeles*	β121	Glu-Gln	−5.2	0	17.4	18.6
O Arab*	β121	Glu-Lys	−9.7	+1.8	14.7	17.2
Beograd	β121	Glu-Val	—	—	—	—
Khartoum	β124	Pro-Arg	—	—	—	—
Ty Gard	β124	Pro-Gln	0	—	—	—
Hofu*	β126	Val-Glu	+4.5	0	21.7	22.9
Hacettepe	β127	Gln-Glu	~+4.0	—	—	—
J Guantanamo	β128	Ala-Asp	~+4	—	—	—
J Taichung	β129	Ala-Asp	~+4.0	—	—	—
K Cameroon	β129	Ala-Glu-Asp	—	—	—	—
Crete	β129	Ala-Pro	—	—	—	—
Wien	β130	Tyr-Asp	0	—	~22.0	—
Camden*	β131	Gln-Glu	+1.6	−2.5	22.8	22.4
K Woolwich*	β132	Lys-Gln	+2.7	−3.5	22.3	22.1
North Shore	β134	Val-Glu	—	—	—	—
Altdorf	β135	Ala-Pro	0	—	—	—
Hope*	β136	Gly-Asp	+0.8	−4.0	23.1	22.3
Brockton*	β138	Ala-Pro	0	0	20	20
Olmsted	β141	Leu-Arg	0	—	~17.5	—
Ohio*	β142	Ala-Asp	−2.7	−3.7	23.1	22.2
Toyoake	β142	Ala-Pro	~−5.0	—	—	—
Abruzzo*	β143	His-Arg	−2.9	+3.0	17.1	20
Little Rock*	β143	His-Gln	—	—	—	—
Syracuse	β143	His-Pro	0	—	—	—
Andrew-Minneapolis*	β144	Lys-Asn	+2.9	−3.8	22.9	21.8
Bethesda*	β145	Tyr-His	0	+2.75	20	20
Rainer*	β145	Tyr-Cys	0	+2.5	20	20
Fort Gordon*	β145	Tyr-Asp	+2.1	−2.0	22.5	21.6
McKees Rocks*	β145	Tyr-Term	+2.6	−3.5	20	20

Table 1 (continued)
RELATIVE ELECTROPHORETIC MOBILITIES OF MUTANT HEMOGLOBINS

Name	Residue	Substitution	Cellulose acetate	Citrate agar	Alkaline globin	Acidic globin
Hiroshima*	β146	His-Asp	+2.4	−4.4	23.2	24.8
York	β146	His-Pro	0	∼−2	—	—
Cochin-Port Royal*	β146	His-Arg	−2.7	+0.25	17.1	20
Cowtown*	β146	His-Leu	0	−3.5	20	21.8
		δ-Chains				
A_2 Sphakia	δ2	His-Arg	—	—	—	—
A_2 NYU	δ12	Asn-Lys	∼−10.8	—	—	—
A_2I*	δ16	Gly-Arg	−11.1	0	—	—
A_2 Roosevelt	δ20	Val-Glu	—	—	—	—
A_2 Flatbush*	δ22	Ala-Glu	−4.5	0	—	—
A_2 Melbourne	δ43	Glu-Lys	∼−11.7	—	—	—
A_2 Adria	δ51	Pro-Arg	—	—	—	—
A_2 Indonesia	δ69	Gly-Arg	—	—	—	—
A_2 Coburg	δ116	Arg-His	∼−3.4	—	—	—
A_2 Babinga*	δ136	Gly-Asp	−9.2	−4.0	—	—
		γ-Chains				
F Malaysia	γ1	Gly-Cys	—	—	—	—
F Texas I*	γ5	Glu-Lys	−10.6	−3.5	—	—
F Meinohama	γ5	Glu-Gly	∼−4.0	—	—	—
F Texas II	γ6	Glu-Lys	∼−10.5	—	—	—
F Kotobuke	γ6	Glu-Gly	∼−6.5	—	—	—
F Auckland	γ7	Asp-Asn	—	—	—	—
F Alexandra	γ12	Thr-Lys	∼−9.2	—	—	—
F Melbourne	γ16	Gly-Arg	—	—	—	—
F Kuala Lumpur	γ22	Asp-Gly	∼−10.9	0	—	—
F Jamaica	γ61	Lys-Glu	—	—	—	—
F M-Osaka	γ63	His-Tyr	∼−3.5	—	—	—
F Iwata	γ72	Gly-Arg	∼−5.0	—	—	—
F Sardinia	γ75	Ile-Thr	−2.6	—	—	—
F Victoria Jubilee	γ80	Asp-Tyr	∼−5.4	—	—	—
F Yamaguchi	γ80	Asp-Asn	∼−5.0	—	—	—
F Dickinson*	γ97	His-Arg	−5.45	−4.4	—	—
F Ube	γ108	Asn-Lys	—	—	—	—
F Malta-I	γ117	His-Arg	∼−7.5	—	—	—
F Hull	γ121	Glu-Lys(A)	∼−10.1	—	—	—
F Carlton	γ121	Glu-Lys(G)	—	—	—	—
F Port Royal	γ125	Glu-Ala	—	−4.4	—	—
F Poole	γ130	Trp-Gly	—	—	—	—
		Fusion Mutants				
Lepore-Hollandia	δβ		∼−5	0	—	—
Lepore-Baltimore	δβ		∼−5	0	—	—
Lepore-Washington-Boston*	δβ		−4.6	3.6?	17.3	16.6
Parchman	δββδ		—	—	—	—
Miyada	βδ		—	—	—	—
P Congo	βδ		∼−5	0	—	—
P Nilotic*	βδ		−4.3	0	17.65	20
Lincoln Park	βδ		—	—	—	—
Kenya*	γβ		−6.9	0	17.8	20

Table 1 (continued)
RELATIVE ELECTROPHORETIC MOBILITIES OF MUTANT HEMOGLOBINS

Name	Residue	Substitution	Cellulose acetate	Citrate agar	Alkaline globin	Acidic globin
		Added Residues				
Constant Spring*	31add,α		−11.9	0	6.3	8.5
Icaria	31add,α		—	—	—	—
Koya Dora	16add,α		—	—	—	—
Tak	11add,β		∼−3	∼+5	—	—
Wayne	Frameshift		—	—	—	—
Cranston	Frameshift		−5.2	0	—	—
Grady*	3 inserted α		+3.0	0	—	—
		Deleted Residues				
Leiden	β6 or 7 del		∼−5	0	∼7.5?	—
Lyon	β17-18 del		∼3.3	—	—	—
Freiburg	β23 del		∼−3	—	—	—
Niteroi	β43-45 del		∼−0.5	—	—	—
Tochigi	β56-59 del		—	—	—	—
St. Antoine	β74-75 del		0	—	—	—
Vicksburg	β75 del		0	0	—	—
Tours	β87 del		—	—	—	—
Gun Hill*	β91-95 del		−6.0, −9.4	3.0	—	—
Deaconess*	β131 del		−2.1	8.4	20	17.5
Coventry	β141 del		0	—	—	—
Boyle Heights	α6 del		∼−3.5	0	—	—
		More Than One Substitution				
C Harlem*	β6	Glu-Val				
	β73	Asp-Asn	−10.0	+5.8	14.4	15.2
Arlington Park	β6	Glu-Lys				
	β95	Lys-Glu	0	0	—	—
J Singapore	α78	Asn-Asp				
	α79	Ala-Gly	—	—	—	—
C Ziguinchor*	β6	Glu-Val				
	β58	Pro-Arg	−10.3	+5.8	—	—
S Travis*	β6	Glu-Val				
	β142	Ala-Val	−4.3	+4.0	17.2	17.0

REFERENCES

1. **Schneider, R. G. and Hightower, B. J.,** Structure in relation to behavior of mutant hemoglobins in citrate agar electrophoresis, *Hemoglobin,* 1, 427, 1977.
2. **Barwick, R. C. and Schneider, R. G.,** Correlation of mobilities of mutant hemoglobins in citrate agar electrophoresis with specific molecular locations of affected residues, *Biochim. Biophys. Acta,* 668, 485, 1981.
3. **Schneider, R. G. and Barwick, R. C.,** Measuring electrophoretic mobilities of mutant hemoglobins and globin chains, *Hemoglobin,* 2(5), 417—435, 1978.
4. **Lehmann, H. and Kynoch, P. A. M.,** *Human Haemoglobin Variants and Their Characteristics,* Elsevier/North-Holland, Amsterdam, 1976.

5. **Schneider, R. G., Hosty, T. S., Tomlin, G., and Atkins, R.,** Identification of hemoglobins and hemoglobinopathies by electrophoresis on cellulose acetate plates impregnated with citrate agar, *Clin. Chem.*, 20, 74, 1974.
6. **Ueda, S. and Schneider, R. G.,** Rapid differentiation of polypeptide chains of hemoglobin by cellulose acetate electrophoresis of hemolysates, *Blood*, 34, 230—235, 1969.
7. **Schneider, R. G.,** Differentiation of electrophoretically similar hemoglobins such as S, D, G and P, or A_2, C, E, and O by electrophoresis of the globin chains, *Clin. Chem.*, 20, 1111—1115, 1974.

THE CHROMATOGRAPHY OF HEMOGLOBIN

William P. Winter

INTRODUCTION

Of the methods available to the investigator for separating hemoglobin either from nonhemoglobin proteins or from other hemoglobin types, some form of ion exchange chromatography is most often the method of choice. Preparative electrophoresis is capable of yielding high-purity hemoglobin preparations, but the amount of material which can be accommodated per run is small and the dilution factor is large, necessitating a concentration step after the run. Isoelectric focusing affords very high purity and can be adapted to preparative runs, as can polyacrylamide gel electrophoresis (PAGE). However, in most cases chromatography remains the quickest, simplest, and most economical method to obtain large quantities of specific hemoglobins.

Ion exchange chromatography refers to any liquid chromatography system in which the molecules being separated are partitioned between a soluble and an insoluble ion of the opposite charge to that of the molecule whose purification is desired. Generally, all molecular species in the sample — hemoglobins in this discussion — start out bound to the column, i.e., to the insoluble ion. When the conditions are adjusted, usually either pH or ionic strength, the equilibrium is shifted so that the hemoglobin dissociates from the stationary ion and associates with the soluble or mobile ion. The value of the equilibrium constant for this reaction for any hemoglobin type is a function of the hemoglobin net surface charge or pK, and hence, a separation occurs. The actual value of the equilibrium constant or the pK, is of little practical consequence in the purification.

Three other types of chromatography are in widespread use although their applications in hemoglobin purification are somewhat limited. These are gel filtration, affinity chromatography, and paper chromatography. Paper chromatography has no current applications in hemoglobin purification. It is used in fingerprinting tryptic peptides of hemoglobin in the course of structural studies, but that goes beyond the scope of this chapter. For a discussion, see Winter and Rucknagel.[1]

Since gel filtration entails a separation based on molecule size,[2] this technique has relatively little application in hemoglobin work. The variant Hb Porto Alegro, (β9 Ser→Cys) forms dimers of tetramers (octomers) which separate well from Hb A on gel filtration with Sephadex G-100.[3] Sephadex G-75 has also been used to separate free hemoglobin subunits, primarily α-subunits, from hemoglobin tetramers.[4]

Affinity chromatography[5] similarly has relatively few applications in hemoglobin chromatography. Affinity chromatography of heme-proteins has been reported,[6] but the technique was designed for separating heme-proteins from nonheme-proteins and requires the conversion of heme-proteins to their apo form. A novel method based on affinity chromatography has been devised for the purification of high oxygen affinity variants.[7] With this method, the exposure of SH groups in high-affinity hemoglobin variants, which results from their being stabilized in the R conformational state, is used as the basis of their separation from Hb A.

In recent years, high pressure (or high performance) liquid chromatography (HPLC) has come into prominence as a major separation method. Its principal advantages are speed and resolution. Its principal drawback is initial cost of the equipment. A feature which may be either an advantage or a drawback is that sample size is quite small compared with traditional liquid chromatography. If the amount of sample is limited and the object of the chromatography is quantitation or preparation of small quantities, as for high-sensitivity sequencing procedures, this feature is a boon. On the other hand, if traditional peptide mapping, function studies, or similar procedures are planned, HPLC has serious limitations.

HPLC embodies a variety of separation modalities including ion exchange, gel permentation, and reverse-phase chromatography.

HPLC methods have been described for a wide variety of applications. Hanash and Shapiro[8] and Gardiner et al.[9] have developed methods for hemoglobin quantitation by HPLC. Methods have been published for the determination of Hb A_2,[10] Hb Ab_{1c}, and other gycosylated hemoglobins,[11-13] and the G_γ and A_γ forms of Hb F.[14,15] Shelton et al.[16] and Petrides[17] have devised chain separation methodologies and Shelton et al.[18] have reported the use of HPLC in the characterization of several human variants has been described.[92,22] (See also related chapters by Jones and by Schroeder in this volume.)

While HPLC has much to recommend it, it is a somewhat specialized technique and will not be dealt with in detail in this chapter. The reader should consult the above references for details.

CHOICE OF ION EXCHANGER

There are two primary considerations in choosing an ion exchange medium: the exchange properties (anionic vs. cationic) and the properties of the polymer or resin. The term "resin" as applied to cellulose or dextrans is technically inappropriate since it is borrowed from the synthetic polymer field and does not apply to natural carbohydrate polymers. However, the term is in wide use in this context and will be used in this discussion to denote polymeric materials, natural or synthetic, which form the insoluble matrix for ion exchange chromatography.

There are few firm rules to guide the user in choosing between anionic and cationic exchangers. Some investigators prefer to have the hemoglobin of interest elute first from the column. This would dictate an anion exchanger such as DEAE for hemoglobins, S, C, E, D, G, O, and other slow* types but a cation exchanger such as CM for hemoglobins J, I, H, and other fast* variants. However, the quality of the separation is of paramount importance and should be the first consideration in selecting and ion exchange media. In general, DEAE probably is the best, and it is the most widely used. However, for the separation of Hb A_2 from slow-moving variants such as Hb C, C-Harlem, O-Arab, O-Indonesia, and Agenogi, CM is the medium of choice.

There are three basic types of resin to choose from: cellulose, dextran, and polystyrene. As a rule, polystyrene-based resins (Dowex®, Amberlite®, Aminex®, and Duolite®) do not work well for chromatography of proteins. An important exception to this is Amberlite® IRC-50 (BioRex®-70), which gives superb separation of some hemoglobins. In most polystyrene resins, however, the cross-linked beads have pores which are extremely small and are not well penetrated by macromolecules. Thus most of the exchange groups are inaccessible to the proteins. Moreover, there is some evidence that proteins become denatured on the surface of the beads and the resin is extremely slow in coming to equilibrium with the starting buffer. For this reason, Amberlite® is most often used in conjunction with equilibrium elution where there is no change in the buffer pH or ionic strength during the course of elution.

The cyclic dextrans (Sephadex®) are natural carbohydrate polymers produced by bacteria of the genus *Leuconostoc* and are available as ion exchange resins, both anion (A) and cation (C) exchangers, in two porosity grades, 50 and 25. For protein chromatography, the A-50 or C-50 (anion and cation exchangers, respectively) are the desired grades. DEAE and CM Sephadex yield very good, high-resolution separations. The principal drawbacks to Seph-

* "Slow" and "fast" in this context refer to the rate of migration relative to Hb A on electrophoresis at alkaline pH.

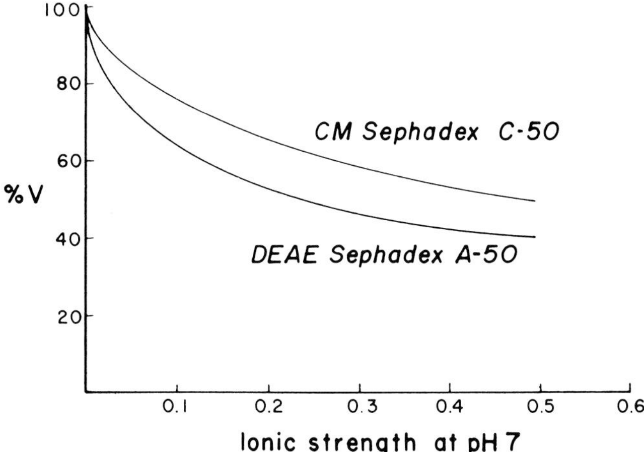

FIGURE 1. Effect of ionic strength on the column volume of ion exchange Sephadexes at pH 7. The volume at ionic strength 0.01 has arbitrarily been taken as 100%. (Redrawn from manufacturer's data.)

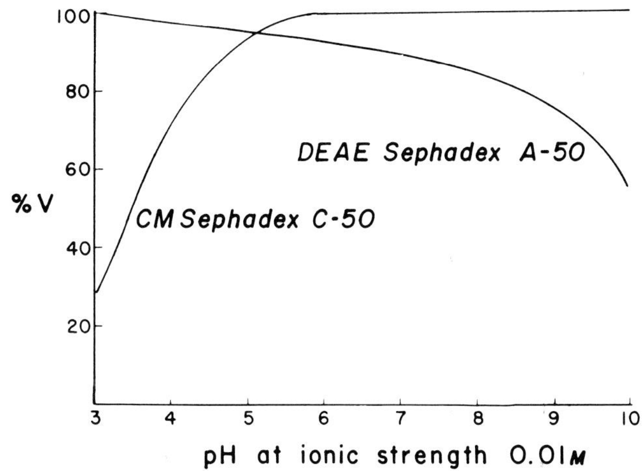

FIGURE 2. Effect of pH on the column volume of ion exchange Sephadexes at ionic strength 0.01. The volume of DEAE Sephadex was taken to be 100% at pH 3 while that of CM Sephadex was taken as 100% at pH 10. (Redrawn from manufacturer's data.)

adex® in comparison to cellulose are the initial swelling time, the annoying tendency of the swollen Sephadex® to stick to glassware, sinks, pH electrodes, etc., and the striking volume changes it undergoes as the result of pH or ionic strength changes (Figures 1 and 2). Both DEAE Sephadex® and CM Sephadex® shrink to about half their original volume in going from 0.01 to 0.5 *M* ionic strength. DEAE Sephadex® shrinks with increasing pH, while CM Sephadex® expands under the same conditions. Volume changes in turn lower the flow rate by increasing the resistance to flow; if the column is being pumped, this often results in the buildup of excessive back pressure, compression of the resin bed, and ultimately the complete cessation of flow with concomitant ''blow-out'' of the supply lines on the high-pressure side.

Cellulose ion exchangers are available in several grades according to the uniformity of the particle dimensions. The best grade — microgranular — has high uniformity and an expanded fibril structure which maximizes the exposure of the charged groups to the solvent.

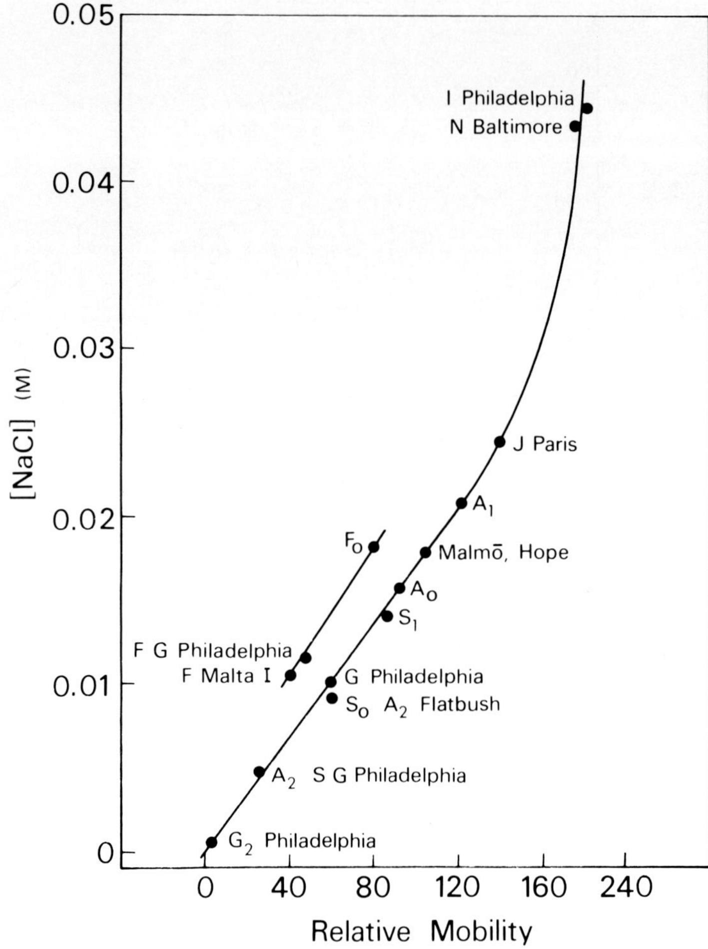

FIGURE 3. Chromatographic properties of selected hemoglobin variants of DE-52 in glycine-NaCl buffers. The abcissa is relative electrophoretic mobility on cellulose acetate at alkaline pH. The mobility of Hb A is taken arbitrarily as 100. Ordinate gives NaCl concentration in milliosmolarity. (Modified from Abraham, E. C., Reese, A., Stallings, M., and Huisman, T. H. J., *Hemoglobin*, 1, 27, 1976.)

Cellulose requires no significant swelling time to rehydrate and does not exhibit any swelling or shrinking during the run. The Whatman Company produces a grade called CM 52 or DE 52 which has never been dried and hence, needs no rehydrating at all. It is considered by many to be the grade of choice for high-resolution separations although it is somewhat more costly than the dry grades CM 32 or DE 32 (Figures 3 and 4).

An ion exchanger with properties similar to both cellulose and Sephadex® is DEAE-Sephacel (Pharmacia). This material is a beaded cellulose gel matrix which, according to the manufacturer, possesses flow properties superior to either Sephadex® or cellulose.

It has been found in the laboratory of the author and others to effect excellent, high-capacity, high-resolution chromatography of hemoglobin. A detailed method for its use is included below.

CHOICE OF BUFFER

In theory, a buffer system capable of maintaining the pH should be usable in ion exchange chromatography. However, the rule of thumb is that best results can be obtained by using

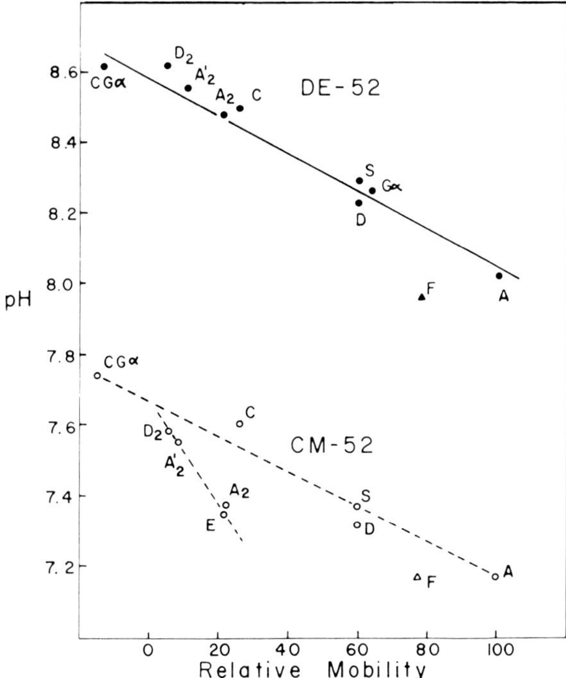

FIGURE 4. Relationship between chromatographic behavior and electrophoretic mobility of selected hemoglobins variants. Electrophoresis is indicated on the abcissa as relative mobility on cellulose acetate at alkaline pH. Hb A = 100. Chromatography was carried out on preswollen microgranular celluloses DE-52 and CM-52 in tris and phosphate buffers, respectively. (Modified from Huisman, T. H. J., *Standardization of Laboratory Reagents and Methods for Detection of Hemoglobinopathies,* Schmidt, R. M., Huisman, T. H. J., and Lehmann, M., Eds., CRC Press, Boca Raton, Fla., 1974, 73.)

cationic buffers (Tris-HCl, etc.) with anion exchanger and anionic buffers (phosphate, acetate, etc.) with cation exchangers. As previously explained, the reason for this is that elution from an ion exchange column is the result of the competition between the stationary ion and a mobile ion of the same charge for association with the protein. Thus, in a DEAE column, Tris is a better cation to compete with DEAE than is, for example, sodium, which would be the cation if sodium phosphate or acetate were used. However, this is not a "hard" rule and there are some examples in the literature in which phosphate buffers have been used with great success in DEAE columns.

In a recent article a novel buffer system was reported to have widespread applicability with DEAE cellulose in the purification of hemoglobins.[23] High-resolution and compact symmetrical zones have been described. The buffer is 0.2 *M* glycine, 0.01% KCN, pH 7.7 to 7.9. Varying amounts of NaCl [0.005 *M* (0.293 g/ℓ) to 0.2 *M* (11.7 g/ℓ)] are added to eluting buffers. From the standpoint of convenience, the buffers are attractive since the zwitterion glycine is a natural buffer and requires no pH adjustment.

This system has been used to great advantage in the author's laboratory. In the original method, the authors expressed the salt concentration in terms of milliosmolality. Since this is an unfamiliar unit for many laboratories, a conversion to sodium chloride concentration in moles per liter is given in Figure 3.

An important — in fact essential — consideration in choosing a buffer is that its pH must be below the pK of the resin of anion exchangers or above it for cation exchangers. If DEAE

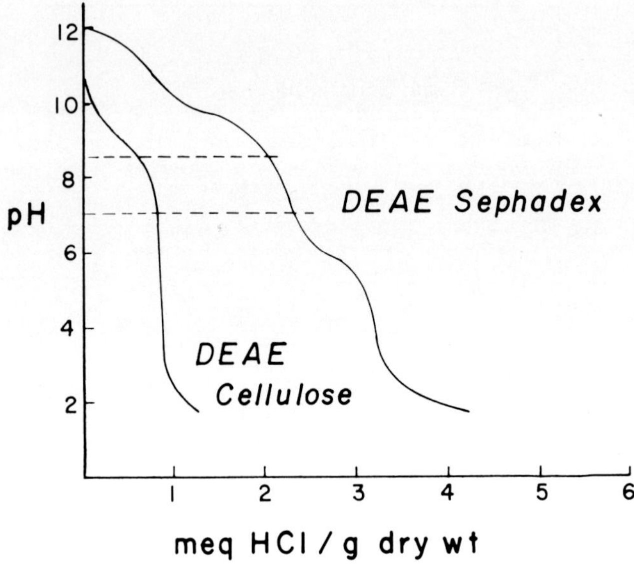

FIGURE 5. Titration curves of diethylaminoethyl ion exchangers. The broken lines indicate the pH range over which the exchangers are normally used. The apparently greater binding capacity of the Sephadex is offset by the much greater water regain of that resin. (Redrawn from manufacturer's data.)

cellulose is used at pH 10, for example, the ion exchange groups will be almost totally uncharged and binding capacity of the resin will be greatly reduced. Titration curves of typical anion and cation exchangers are shown in Figures 5 to 7.

GRADIENTS

In theory, the number of column volumes of starting buffer required to elute a protein is equal to the equilibrium constant for the association of the protein to the immobile phase. If this value is on the order of 1000 or greater, as is often the case, the volume of starting buffer required to effect an elution would be prohibitively large. Therefore, it is convenient to bring about the elution of the protein by gradually changing the properties of the buffer to lower the equilibrium constant to a value approaching 1. Under these conditions, the elution of the protein becomes rapid and quantitative.

Numerous types of gradients have been used successfully in hemoglobin chromatography. One of the simplest gradients to construct and use is a two-chamber gradient (Figure 8). If the vessels are of equal size and identical shape, the gradient will be linear in concentration from the buffer in chamber 1 (the mixing chamber) to that in chamber 2 (the reservoir). If the volumes or shapes are not identical, the instantaneous concentration can be calculated from Equation 1:

$$C_{(t)} = C_2 - (C_2 - C_1)(1 - V)\ A_2/A_1 \quad (1)$$

where $C_{(t)}$ = concentration at time t, C_2 = reservoir concentration, C_1 = initial concentration in mixing vessel, V = volume fraction used at time t, and A_2/A_1 = ratio of cross-sectional area of reservoir (A_2) and mixer (A_1).

The most commonly employed gradients are pH gradients. While in most cases a linear pH change is desired, a simple two-chamber gradient between two pH values is often

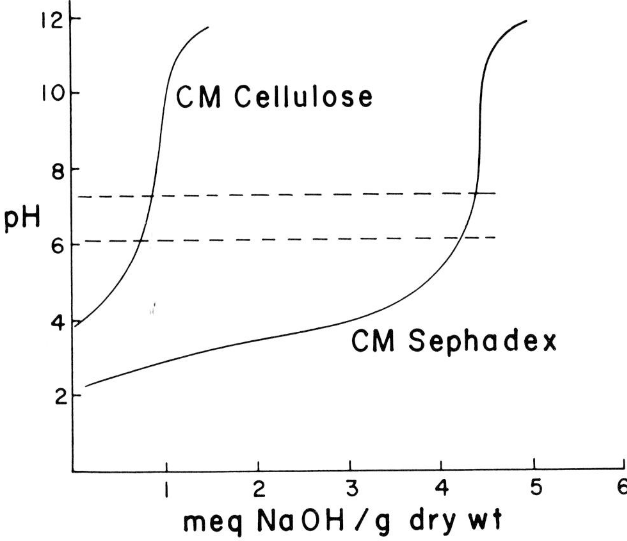

FIGURE 6. Titration curves of carboxymethyl ion exchangers. The broken lines indicate the pH range over which the exchangers are normally used. The apparently greater binding capacity of the Sephadex is offset by the much greater water regain of that resin. (Redrawn from manufacturer's data.)

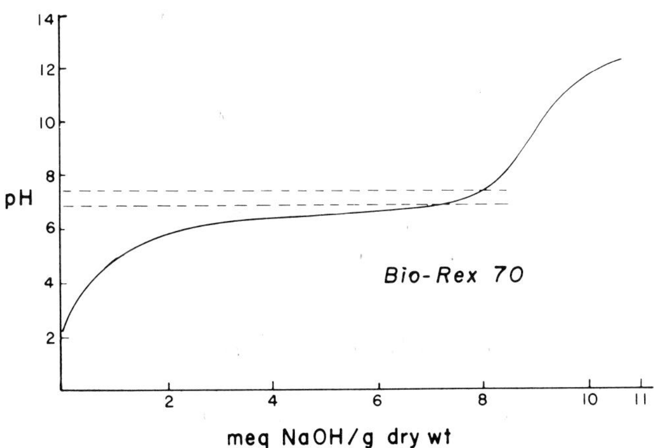

FIGURE 7. Titration curve of carboxymethylated polystyrene resin. A similar curve would be obtained from other resins of this group such as Amberlite® IRC-50 and CG-50. (Redrawn from manufacturer's data.)

unsatisfactory because the capacities of the two buffers may differ. The result is a gradient which tends to maintain the pH of the buffer at higher capacity. Therefore, an approach to linearity is employed either by a multichamber gradient or by a series of convex gradients using different limit buffers which are changed at specified times. For a multichamber gradient a Varigrad or its equivalent is employed.[24] The chambers are filled with buffers approximately 0.2 pH units apart. A typical multichamber gradient for DEAE column involves buffers at pH 8.3, 8.1, 7.9, 7.7, 7.5, 7.3, 7.1, 6.9, and 6.7. Equal volumes of each are generally used.

In the multiple convex gradient, a closed mixing chamber is constructed as shown in

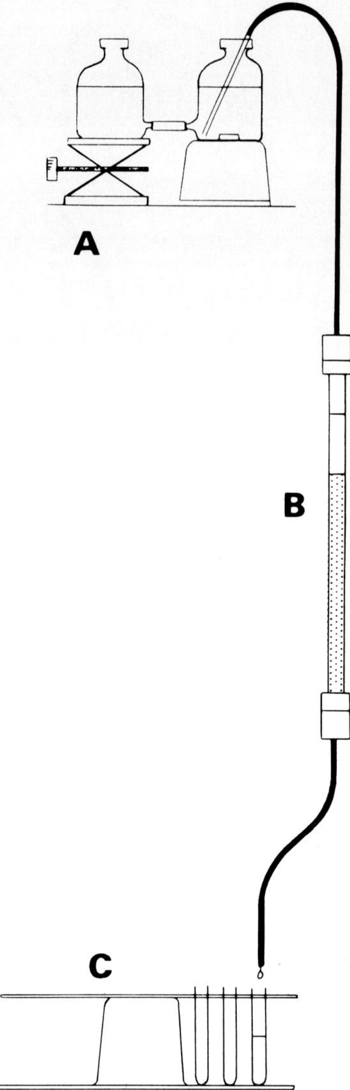

FIGURE 8. Typical equipment assembly for gravity flow chromatography: (A) linear gradient mixer, (B) column, and (C) fraction collector.

Figure 9. The chamber is filled with starting buffer, and the reservoir vessel is filled with a second buffer. The column is started, and after a specified volume has passed through the column (most readily measured as a time interval at constant flow rate), the buffer in the reservoir is replaced by a third buffer. A typical schedule of reservoir buffers and changeover times is shown in Table 1. For use with anion exchangers (DEAE), decreasing pH gradients are used; for use with cation exchangers (CM), rising pH gradients are used. Salt gradients are always rising gradients whether they are used with anion or cation exchangers.

SAMPLE PREPARATION

The sample should be in solution in a buffer that has pH and ionic strength close to or

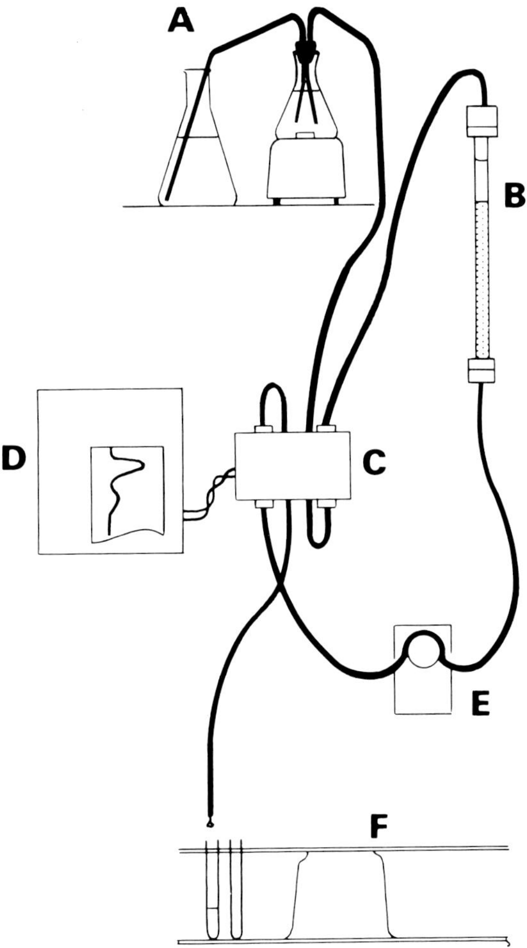

FIGURE 9. Typical equipment assembly for pumped chromatography: (A) constant volume gradient mixer, (B) column, (C) monitor, (D) recorder, (E) pump, and (F) fraction collector. Note that in this assembly, the pump is *below* the column generating a *negative* pressure on the bottom of the column.

Table 1
SCHEDULE OF BUFFER CHANGES FOR CONSTANT VOLUME MIXING CHAMBER GRADIENT

	Column diameter and flow rate		
V_i	**0.9 cm @ 15 mℓ/hr**	**1.5 cm @ 25 mℓ/hr**	**Change buffer reservoir to**
After	55[a] mℓ (3.6 hr)[a]	110[a] mℓ (4.6 hr)	pH 7.7
After	130 mℓ (8.6 hr)	260 mℓ (10.6 hr)	pH 7.4
After	425 mℓ (28.3 hr)	850 mℓ (34 hr)	pH 7.0
After	550 mℓ (36.6 hr)	1100 mℓ (44 hr)	pH 6.5[b]

Note: In constant volume mixing chamber (for details of gradient assembly, see Figure 9). V_i pH 8.3 buffer. (All buffers are 0.05 *M* Tris HCl containing 10^{-4} *M* EDTA and 0.01% KCN.) In reservoir: pH 8.0 buffer.

[a] Times and volumes are cumulative rather than interval.

[b] Continue with the final buffer until the column is fully developed.

Table 2
SOME FREQUENTLY SPECIFIED COLUMN DIMENSIONS, THEIR TYPICAL APPLICATIONS, APPROXIMATE SAMPLE SIZE OF HEMOGLOBIN ACCOMMODATED ON SUCH COLUMNS, AND APPROXIMATE FLOW RATE

Column size				
Diameter (cm)	Length (cm)	Application	Sample size (mg)	Approximate flow rate (cm^3/hr)
0.5	6—8	Microanalytical	2—5	25
0.9—1.0	30—50	Analytical or small-scale prep	50—100	15—25
1.8—2.0	35	Preparative	100—200	75—90
5.0	35	Large-scale preparative	300—500	500—600

identical with those of the column. In order to promote good binding to the top of the bed, the sample pH may be slightly higher (for anion exchangers) or lower (for cation exchangers) than that of the column. For example, DEAE columns are often equilibrated at pH 8.3 with the sample prepared at pH 8.5.

The best general method for sample preparation is dialysis. This ensures that, within differences due to Donnan equilibrium, the pH and ionic strength will be those which are desired. However, if time does not permit lengthy dialysis, the sample may be diluted in the starting buffer to approximate the correct values. There is no advantage to highly concentrated samples in ion exchange chromatography; in fact, a more dilute sample may have better flow properties and may be easier to apply.

COLUMN SIZE

In ion exchange chromatography, the column dimensions are much less critical than in gel filtration, where a pure equilibrium process is taking place. Length to diameter ratios of 10:1 to 20:1 are generally satisfactory, and highly satisfactory results can often be obtained with even shorter columns. However, to achieve desired resolution, still higher length to diameter ratios such as 50:1 or 60:1 are frequently specified. Table 2 gives some frequently specified column dimensions together with typical applications of columns of such sizes and the approximate sample size for hemoglobin accommodated on each.

In general, in modifying an existing column to achieve desired results, or in designing a column system for a particular application, the following rules apply to choice of dimensions:[25]

1. The sample capacity is proportional to the square of the column diameter. It is largely unaffected by length.
2. The flow rate is proportional to the square of the column diameter for any constant bed height.
3. The resolution (relative separation between peaks) is proportional to the square root of the length of the resin column.
4. The pressure required is also proportional to the length of the resin column.

Thus, if one wished to double the sample load with little or no loss of resolution, he should increase the column diameter by the $\sqrt{2}$, keep the length of the column constant, and allow for a doubling of the flow rate at the same back pressure. The total volume of buffer would also be approximately doubled.

COLUMN PREPARATION

In order to produce satisfactory and reproducible columns, careful attention must be given to the preparation of the columns. Generally, manufacturer's directions for the preparation and the equilibrium of the resin of choice should be followed. It is important to realize that equilibrium has been achieved only when the pH and ionic strength of the buffer flowing into a column are exactly equal to the pH and ionic strength of the buffer leaving the column. The use of high concentrations of acid or base to adjust the pH in equilibrating ion exchange resins must be avoided. If an exchanger is being equilibrated at pH 8.5 in 0.05 *M* tris HCl buffer, for example, and it becomes necessary to raise the pH, this may be done simply by adding 0.05 *M* tris alone. Adjustment with 1 *M* tris or, worse yet, with NaOH, will change the ionic strength of the buffer and may adversely affect the performance of the column.

In packing a column, best results will be achieved when the bed is uniform both from top to bottom and side to side. Channeling, hard spots, cracks, air bubbles, and other irregularities are to be assiduously avoided. The problem of irregularities is relatively minor in small columns (1.5 cm diameter or smaller) but is greatly magnified in large columns. The best slurry from which to pour the column is a 1:1 or 50% slurry in which after a reasonable time (30 min) the settled resin volume (depth) approximately equals the supernatant volume (depth).

In order to avoid air entrapment, it is advisable to place a few centimeters of buffer in the column and open the bottom briefly so as to fill the dead space with liquid. The slurry is then poured. If an extension tube can be arranged, the whole bed may be poured at once. Otherwise, at intervals before the bed has settled, clear supernatant is aspirated and more slurry is added. When the packing is complete, the column is run at the flow rate or pressure that is to be used in the separation until the bed is stabilized. The effluent pH should be checked and compared with that of the initial buffer.

FLOW RATE PUMPING

A typical flow rate for an ion exchange column is 30 mℓ/cm^2/hr. Approximate flow rates for various standard size columns are shown in Table 2. While these flow rates need not be regarded as optimal, they do provide some clue as to the quality of a particular column.

Low flow rates of one tenth or less of the suggested flow rate will often lead to unnecessary delays in completing the experiment, loss of sample due to denaturation, or loss of resolution due to diffusion of bands. Excessively high flow rates, which are usually due to channeling, may lead to distorted zones or poor resolution due to incomplete equilibrium of the sample bands with the columns.

The use of a pump to maintain the desired flow rate is generally desirable. Pumping generally minimizes the total run time, improves resolution by reducing time-dependent diffusion, and prevents changes in flow rate with time. The latter consequence permits precise calculation of buffer change schedules and fraction collector schedules, and, if a monitor is being used, makes quantitation by peak area calculation possible. Most columns can be used at flow rates higher than those obtained by gravity flow at reasonable pressure. However, caution should be exercised in attempting to achieve greatly increased flow rates by pumping, since bed packing may occur that leads to the development of pressures greater than the joints in the system can withstand. A typical pressure-flow rate curve is shown in Figure 10.

For cellulose and Sephadex® columns, a peristaltic pump should be used, whereas either a peristaltic or a piston pump may be used with polystyrene-type resins. This is because the piston pump tends to deliver high-pressure "spikes" which pack the column. Since the expansion of the bed is generally slow in relation to the pump stroke rate, a progressive

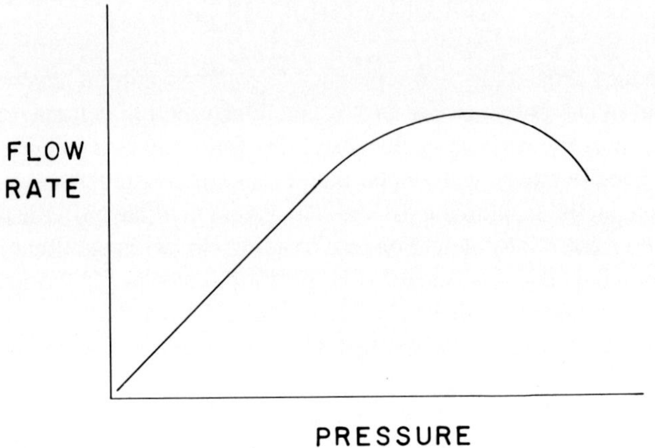

FIGURE 10. The effect of pressure on flow rate in a chromatographic column. The deviation from linearity is the result of "drag" of the solvent on the particles of the column bed. The effect is accentuated as the viscosity of the solvent increases.

packing with concomitant pressure increase will occur. Polystyrene resins have less tendency to compress and are much less susceptible to this effect. On the other hand, Sephadex® is highly subject to compression and should be pumped with caution if it is to be pumped at all.

The pump may be placed either at the inlet or outlet of the column. Typical arrangements are shown in Figure 10. Note that the pump is connected directly to the column in either case. Flow cells or other monitoring devices should be placed on the atmospheric pressure side of the pump. The principal advantage of placing the pump on the outlet side of the column is that in the event of an increase in column packing, high backpressure does not develop, and fittings are not "blown". A disadvantage is that the amount of dead volume below the column is increased and this may lead to loss of resolution.

MONITORING AND FRACTION COLLECTING

Hemoglobin has the extremely helpful property of absorbing light in the visible spectrum and thus can be monitored with the human eye. When gross separations are required, this is probably as satisfactory a method as any for determining what volume to collect and save. However, when separations are marginal, when minor components are the object of the chromatography, or when quantitation is desired, an absorbance monitor can be a useful device. However, it is rarely essential and is best regarded as a time- and labor-saving device.

A fraction collector, on the other hand, is almost essential unless the chromatography is to be of a very short duration or in the event that the preparative method described below is to be used. Most fraction collectors measure fractions by one or more of three criteria: volume, drop counts, or time. If the flow rate is reasonably constant, then all three will yield the same final result. If the flow rate changes during the run, a volume or drop counter will yield more satisfactory results. However, volume and drop counter heads are usually more expensive than timers and are less reliable mechanically. Since fraction collectors are governed by Murphy's Law,* the more dependable timer is to be highly recommended, glowing claims from instrument manufacturers notwithstanding.

* If something can go wrong, it will.

Table 3
PROBLEMS OF COLUMN CHROMATOGRAPHY OF HEMOGLOBIN AND POSSIBLE SOLUTIONS

Problem	Causes	Solutions
Flow rate too slow	Excessive fines	Define and pour again
Before addition of sample	Bottom screen or sinter clogged (check flow rate of empty column);	Clean or replace clogged piece
	Incomplete swollen resin (Sephadex)	Complete swelling, repack
After addition of sample	Sample precipitated on column	Check column pH, ionic strength for compatibility with sample
	Particulate matter in sample	Centrifuge sample (this can sometimes be corrected *in situ* by stirring up the top of the bed)
	Sample-induced swelling (Sephadex)	Stir up as far down as sample goes, dilute sample
During run	Packing due to high pressure	Reduce pressure (pumping rate); in extreme cases, abort run
	Too rapid change in pH, ionic strength	Change gradient
Flow rate too rapid	Channeling through bed, resin too coarse	Repour column; choose finer mesh resin
Sample does not bind to top of bed	pH of sample too low (DEAE) or high (CM); resin pore size grade too small (Sephadex)	Check pH, ionic strength; make sure Sephadex A or C 25 was not used
Sample binds irregularly	Channeling; non-flat bed top, trapped air	Repack top of column; smooth bed top, use top screen
Poor resolution irregular zones, good zones — poorly separated	Bad column packing, gradient too steep, or volume too small	Repack column, use narrower range of buffers, increase volume
	Poor choice of resin	Try another exchanger or better grade resin
All bands run at beginning (end) of column	Poor choice of starting (ending) conditions	Make appropriate adjustments in buffers

If no fraction collector is available, preparative hemoglobin chromatography can still be done.

A column of CM cellulose is prepared and the chromatography is begun. When the bands are well separated, the development is stopped and the cellulose with the hemoglobin bound is collected by digging it out of the column. It is suspended in starting buffer and repacked in another column. The hemoglobin is then eluted with 2% KCN in water, and the purified, concentrated sample is collected. If fractions have been collected, this method is also useful for the pooled fractions. The pool must be diluted roughly 1:1 with water and its pH adjusted to 6 to 6.5. The CM cellulose, equilibrated with 0.05 *M* Tris-maleate containing 10^{-3} *M* EDTA and adjusted to pH 6.5, is poured to yield a short column. The diluted hemoglobin, when passed through the column, should concentrate in the top several millimeters of the columns. It can then be eluted in concentrated form with 2% KCN.

TROUBLESHOOTING

It is impossible, of course, to anticipate every troublesome situation which might arise in the course of column chromatography of hemoglobin. It would be presumptuous of the author to suppose that he had the answer for every such problem. However, in this section some troublesome problems and possible remedies will be tabulated (Table 3).

In addition, several general techniques that are useful in trouble shooting are listed below.

Backwashing — If a column goes dry and develops cracks or pulls away from the tube walls, the run can sometimes be rescued by attaching the output of a pump to the bottom of the column and slowly pumping starting buffer up the column. Addition of buffer to the top of a dry, cracked column bed usually leads to trapped air and serious channeling.

Bottom screen replacement — If a flow adapter is available, remove the buffer from the top of the bed and install the adapter. Clamp the exit tube from the adapter and invert the column. The bottom of the column may now be removed and the screen inspected or replaced.

Stripping — CM cellulose and CM Sephadex® columns may be rapidly and quantitatively stripped with unbuffered 2% KCN. The column may be re-equilibrated by washing it with 4 to 5 column volumes of buffer. DEAE cellulose may be similarly stripped with 5% NaCl.

Recycling — While some manufacturers do not recommend recycling cellulose or Sephadex® resins, it may be done, with some loss of exchange capacity, by the following procedure. Suspend anion exchange resins (DEAE) in 1 *M* NaOH. Cation exchangers (CM) are suspended in 1 *M* HCl. EDTA (10^{-3} *M*) may be added to scavenge heavy metals. The suspension is gently stirred for 30 to 60 min and filtered. The cake is washed to within 2 pH units of neutrality and then suspended in 1 *M* HCl or 1 *M* NaOH, respectively. The resin is again stirred gently and washed. The resins may be stored in this form without drying and equilibrated with the desired buffer for use. Sodium azide may be added as a preservative.

SYSTEMS FOR GENERAL USE

Hemoglobin Chain Separation

Clegg et al.[26,27] introduced the first practical chromatographic method for globin chain purification and this method, presented in detail below, is still in wide use under the appellation "Clegg column". This procedure yields heme-free protein or globin. Investigators wishing to purify subunits are referred to the method of Bucci and Fronticelli[28] and related methods.[29] The Clegg column is particularly useful in structural studies of new hemoglobin variants and in thalassemia studies for the determination of the α/non-α biosynthesis ratio.[30]

Materials:

- CM-32 (Whatman) Dry carboxymethyl cellulose
- $Na_2HPO_4 \cdot 7H_2O$
- H_3PO_4 25% aqueous solution
- Urea
- Mixed bed ion exchange resin
- Acetone
- HCl
- 2-Mercaptoethanol
- Lo-temp cooler
- Conductivity meter
- Peristaltic pump
- UV monitor
- Fraction collector
- Gradient maker
- 0.9 × 20 cm column

Preparation of urea — An 8-*M* urea stock solution should be made in advance. A convenient way to do this is to mark on a 5-lb bottle of urea the height which corresponds

Table 4
BUFFER COMPOSITION FOR CHAIN SEPARATION CHROMATOGRAPHY

Phosphate concentration (M)	0.005	0.040	0.045	0.050
		Limit buffer for		
Use	Start	Fast β, γ	Slow β, Fast α	Slow α
$Na_2HPO_4 \cdot 7H_2O$	0.68 g	1.08 g	1.21 g	1.35
8 M Urea	500 mℓ	100 mℓ	100 mℓ	100 mℓ
pH adj with 25% H_3PO_4	6.7	6.7	6.7	6.7
2-Mercaptoethanol	2.2 mℓ	0.63 mℓ	0.63 mℓ	0.63 mℓ

to 4.7 ℓ. Add water to this mark and stir with a stirring paddle and drive motor. Urea may be warmed gently to speed dissolution but strong heating is to be avoided since it hastens decomposition of the urea. Decomposition products accumulate with time in the stock solution and must be removed by deionization. For a single run involving up to 100 mg of hemoglobin, about 700 mℓ of urea must be deionized. Add several common tablespoons of mixed bed ion exchange resin to the urea solution and stir with a magnetic spin bar. From time to time check the conductivity. It should be 20 mmho/cm or lower. Filter the urea through a pad of Pyrex wool in a large funnel. The urea should be crystal clear; further filtration may be necessary if turbidity is observed.

Preparation of buffers — The composition of the buffer is given in Table 4. If a pH electrode containing 4 M KCl, saturated AgCl is used the pH should be adjusted before adding the 2-mercaptoethanol to avoid formation of silver mercaptide in the electrode. The pH must be exactly 6.7 and cannot be back-titrated if the pH drops below that value.

Preparation of resin — Weigh 3.5 g of CM-32. Add 100 mℓ of 0.005 M pH 6.7 urea buffer (start buffer) and stir magnetically for 5 to 10 min. Adjust pH back to 6.7 with 25% H_3PO_4 (about 1 drop). Pour the suspension into a 100-mℓ graduated cylinder and allow the resin to settle for 30 min. Aspirate the top 80 mℓ. Add 80 mℓ of start buffer, mix, allow to settle, and aspirate as above. Do this once more. After the final settling leave sufficient buffer to yield a 50% suspension (i.e., if settled volume is 11 mℓ, leave a total of 22 mℓ in the cylinder).

Preparation of sample — Prepare 50 mℓ of 1% HCl in acetone at −10°C. Arrange this in a beaker with a magnetic stirring unit. Take the desired volume of 10 g/dℓ hemolysate and dilute 1:1 with water. Add the hemoglobin solution slowly dropwise to the rapidly stirred, chilled HCl-acetone. If dark red lumps form, dilute the hemoglobin further. When all the hemoglobin has been added, allow to stir for 15 min or more and filter through Whatman #1 paper. Wash the precipitate with acetone at −10°C at least three times. Air-dry the precipitate at room temperature, breaking up the cake with the tip of a spatula. When nearly dry, add sample to 1 mℓ of start buffer. Dissolving the slightly moist precipitate greatly speeds the redissolution of the "de-hemed" globin. In the author's experience, dialyzing, which is sometimes recommended, is not necessary at this step.

Column preparation and running — A column setup similar to that in Figure 9 is used. A column is poured to a packed depth of 11 cm. It is then pumped with start buffer at 40 mℓ/hr to check for leaks and establish the bed height and recorder baseline. The column is then opened, the liquid supernatant removed, and the sample placed on the top of the bed. It is allowed to flow on under gravity, the column refilled with start buffer and pumping started again. After a few minutes a "breakthrough" peak will be detected. When the pen has returned to baseline, the gradient may be started. Fractions are then collected every 7 min (5 mℓ per fraction).

Table 5
BUFFER COMPOSITION FOR DEAE SEPHACEL CHROMATOGRAPHY

	Buffer designation			
	A	**A × 10**	**A′**	**B**
Tris 1 *M* (mℓ)	200	500	40	200
HCl 1 *M* (mℓ)	88	300	17.5	170
EDTA 0.2 *M* (mℓ)	2.0	5	0.4	2.0
Dilute to (mℓ)	4000	1000	4000	4000
Final Tris conc.	0.05 *M*	0.5 *M*	0.01	0.05
pH	8.2	8.2	8.2	7.3
Final EDTA	10^{-4} *M*	10^{-3} *M*	2×10^{-5}	10^{-4}

Gradient — A two-chamber gradient consisting of 100 mℓ of start buffer is satisfactory. However, better resolution toward the beginning of the column can be obtained with a three-chamber gradient in which the first two chambers are start buffer and the last is limit buffer. If a slow α-chain variant is suspected (e.g., G-Philadelphia or O-Indonesia) a 0.050 *M* limit buffer or two 0.045 *M* limit buffer chambers should be used. Following the run, all lines should be cleaned before the urea can crystallize in them. Since urea decomposes to cyanate, which will react with amino groups, the globin should be freed from the urea as soon as possible. If dialysis is used, be sure to use 6000 to 8000 mol wt cutoff dialysis tubing to minimize losses. Counting of radioactivity may be done directly using 1 mℓ of each fraction and 10 mℓ of RIA Fluor® (New England Nuclear). Most other scintillation cocktails will not support the urea in solution and may cause errors in the radioactivity determination.

Hemoglobin Purification Using DEAE Sephacel

The following method has been used with success in the laboratory of the author and others. It is based on the method of Huisman and Dozy[31] for DEAE cellulose and adapted for large-scale preparation. The author is indebted to John A. Kark for details of the procedure. The required materials are listed below.

DEAE Sephacel (2 ℓ)
Tris (1 *M*)
HCl (1 *N*)
EDTA (0.2 *M*)
Column (5 cm × 50 cm)

Preparation of buffers — The preparation of buffers is given in Table 5.

Preparation of sample —Wash and hemolyze blood. Dialyze the hemolysate using two changes of 2 ℓ of buffer A′ in the cold over a 24-hr period. The sample volume should be about 100 mℓ with a hemoglobin concentration of 15 g/dℓ.

Preparation of resin — Use a volume of DEAE Sephacel suspension sufficient to yield about 800 mℓ packed volume. Decant the supernatant liquid and suspend the Sephacel in excess of buffer A × 10 and allow to stand overnight. Wash two times with buffer A′, suspend in buffer A, and pour the column. Equilibrate overnight with 2 ℓ of buffer A. Final column dimensions should be about 5 × 45 cm.

Application of sample — Remove excess buffer from the top of the column. Add the dialyzed hemolysate carefully so as not to disturb the bed. Use a volume of hemolysate equivalent to 5 to 20 g of hemoglobin. Allow the sample to flow onto the column. Add about 100 mℓ of buffer A to the top of the column and start elution.

Table 6
CHROMATOGRAPHY OF HEMOGLOBIN C-LIKE VARIANTS

Variant	Substitution	Ref.	Chromatography system	Ref.
Chad	α23 glu→lys	32	DEAE Sephadex A-50	a
O Padova	α30 glu→lys	33	DEAE Sephadex A-50	l
O Indonesia	α116 glu→lys	34	CM Cellulose	u
E	β26 glu→lys	35	CM Cellulose,	i
			DEAE Sephadex A-50	a
C Ziguinchor	β6 glu→val,	36	DEAE Cellulose	h
	β58 pro→arg			
Agenogi	β90 glu→lys	37	CM Cellulose	u
St. Etienne	β92 his→glu	38,39	DEAE Sephadex A-50	a,b
Gunn Hill	β91—95 Deleted,	40	CM Cellulose	i
	β92—96, or β93—97			
O Arab	β121 glu→lys	34	CM Cellulose	u

Table 7
CHROMATOGRAPHY OF HEMOGLOBIN S-LIKE VARIANTS

Variant	Substitution	Ref.	Chromatography system	Ref.
Ottawa	α15 gly→arg	41	DEAE Sephadex A-50	a
Arya	α47 asp→asn	42	DEAE Sephadex A-50	a
Hasharon	α47 asp→his	43	DEAE Sephadex A-50	a
			IRC-50	f
Shimonoseki	α54 glu→arg	44	CG-50	d
L Persian Gulf	α57 gly→lys	45	IRC-50	f
Daneshgan Tehran	α72 his→arg	46	DEAE Cellulose	a
G Taichung	α74 asp→his	47	DEAE Sephadex A-50	a
Q Iran	α75 asp→his	47	DEAE Sephadex A-50	a
Stanleyville II	α78 asn→lys	48	IRC-50	m
G Norfolk	α85 asp→asn	49	DEAE Sephadex A-50	a
G Georgia	α95 pro→leu	50	DEAE Cellulose	v
Chiapas	α114 pro→arg	51	IRC-50	e
Bibba	α136 leu→pro	52	DEAE Sephadex A-50	a,b
S	β6 glu→val		DEAE Cellulose	v
D Iran	β22 glu→gln	53	DEAE Cellulose	a
Alabama	β39 gln→lys	54	DEAE Sephadex A-50	a
D Ibadan	β87 thr→lys	55	IRC-50	f
Tours	β87 thr→0	56	Biorex-70	k
D Punjab	β121 glu→gln	57	DEAE Cellulose	a
Richmond	β102 asn→lys	58	DEAE Sephadex A-50	a,b

Elution — A 4-ℓ gradient consisting of 2 ℓ of buffer A and 2 ℓ of buffer B is used as shown in Figure 8. Gravity flow is sufficient. This system has provided excellent resolution.

Systems for Selected Variants

Tables 6 to 12 are presented as an aid in planning the chromatographic separation of variant hemoglobins. Not all variants have been successfully chromatographed, either because they do not separate well from Hb A by ion exchange methods or, as is more often the case, because the variant chain was purified directly by the method of Clegg et al. In many cases, one or more of a relatively small number of published methods was referred to by the authors of those papers in which hemoglobins were purified by these methods. Therefore, in these tables an internal referencing system is used in which a key reference to the original description of the variant is given as well as the reference within that key

Table 8
CHROMATOGRAPHY OF HEMOGLOBIN A-LIKE VARIANTS

Variant	Substitution	Ref.	Chromatography system	Ref.
Aida	α64 asp→asn	59	DEAE Sephadex A-50	—
Rampa	α95 pro→ser	60	DEAE Cellulose	s
Denmark Hill	α95 pro→ala	61	CM Sephadex C-50	r
St. Lukes	α95 pro→arg	62	DEAE Sephadex A-50	a
Athens-Georgia	β40 arg→lys	63	DEAE Cellulose	v
M Saskatoon	β63 his→tyr	65	Biorex-70, CG-50	g
M Milwaukee	β67 his→tyr	66	CG-50, Biorex-70	g
M Hyde Park	β92 his→tyr	67	CG-50	—
Malmö	β97 his→gln	68	DEAE Cellulose	v
Kansas	β102 asn→thr	69	CM Cellulose	t
San Diego	β109 val→met	70	CM Sephadex C-50	a
Hope	β136 gly→asp	71	IRC-50, DEAE Cellulose	f,v
Little Rock	β143 his→gln	72	CM Cellulose	n
Syracuse	β143 his→pro	73	CM Cellulose	o

Table 9
CHROMATOGRAPHY OF HEMOGLOBIN J-LIKE VARIANTS

Variant	Substitution	Ref.	Chromatography system	Ref.
J Paris	α12 ala→asp	74	DEAE Cellulose	v
J Kurosh	α19 ala→asp	75	DEAE Sephadex A-50	a
J Nyanza	α21 ala→asp	76	DEAE Sephadex A-50	a
Norfolk	α57 gly→asp	77	CM Cellulose	c
Lyon	β17,18 lys,val→0	78	Biorex-70	q
J Sicilia	β65 lys→asn	79	DEAE Sephadex A-50	a
J Cairo	β65 lys→gln	80	DEAE Sephadex A-50	—
J Chicago	β76 ala→asp	81	DEAE Sephadex A-50	b
J Habana	β71 ala→glu	82	DEAE Sephadex A-50	a
J Meerut	β120 ala→glu	83	DEAE Sephadex A-50	a

Table 10
CHROMATOGRAPHY OF HEMOGLOBIN I-LIKE VARIANTS

Variant	Substitution	Ref.	Chromatography system	Ref.
I	α16 lys→glu	84	CM Cellulose, DEAE Cellulose	p,v
Nagasaki	β17 lys→glu	85	CM Cellulose	p,q
Hikari	β61 lys→asn	86	IRC-50	f
N Baltimore	β95 lys→glu	27	DEAE Cellulose	v

citation which gives the chromatographic methods. It is hoped that in this way, investigators can more quickly gain access to the literature in this field.

Chromatographic Systems Diagrams

Figures 8 and 9 are presented as an aid to those who may be unfamiliar with the laboratory methods of column chromatography. Each of these systems is intended as an example of one possible way — not as the only way or even the best way — in which the equipment could be arranged. The investigator should use these drawings as a guide and adapt whatever equipment he has to the job.

Table 11
CHROMATOGRAPHY OF MINOR HEMOGLOBIN TYPES

Hemoglobin	Chain notation	Ref.	Chromatography system	Ref.
Portland	$\zeta_2\gamma_2$	87,88	DEAE Sephadex A-50	a
A_2	$\alpha_2\delta_2$	—	DEAE Cellulose	a,v
F	$\alpha_2\gamma_2$	—	CM Sephadex, DEAE Cellulose	b,r,u,v
Kenya	$\alpha_2\gamma\beta_2$	89	DEAE Sephadex A-50	b
Lepore	$\alpha_2\delta\beta_2$	—	DEAE Cellulose, DEAE Sephadex A-50	a
Constant Spring	α Extension	90	IRC-50	d
Icaria	α Extension	91	IRC-50	d
F Port Royal	G_γ 125 glu→ala		CM Sephadex C-50	r

Table 12
COMPOSITION AND PROPERTIES OF THE SCHROEDER DEVELOPERS (d,q)

Number	pH @ 25°C	Na^+ (*M*)	KCN (*M*)	$NaH_2PO_4H_2O$[a] (g/4 ℓ)	Na_2HPO_4[a] (g/4 ℓ)	KCN (g/4 ℓ)
1	7.22 ± 0.02	0.075	0.01	13.80	14.20	2.6
2	7.18 ± 0.02	0.0625	0.01	13.80	10.65	2.6
3	7.02 ± 0.02	0.050	0.01	13.80	7.10	2.6
4	6.91 ± 0.02	0.050	0.01	16.56	5.68	2.6
5	6.85 ± 0.05	0.055	0.01	16.56	7.10	2.6
6	6.70 ± 0.02	0.055	0.01	18.37	4.74	2.6

[a] It is recommended by Dr. Schroeder that for best results the hydrates specified be used.

REFERENCES FOR TABLES 6 TO 12

a. **Huisman, T. H. J. and Dozy, A. M. M.,** *Chromatography,* 19, 160, 1965.
b. **Dozy, A. M. J., Kleihauer, T., and Huisman, T. H. J.,** *J. Chromatogr.,* 32, 723, 1968.
c. **Huisman, T. H. J. and Meyring, C. A.,** *Clin. Chem. Acta,* 5, 103, 1960.
d. **Allen, D. W., Schroeder, W. A., and Balog, J.,** *J. Am. Chem. Soc.,* 80, 1628, 1958.
e. **Jones, R. T. and Schroeder, W. A. J.,** *Chromatography,* 10, 421, 1963.
f. **Huisman, T. H. J. and Prins, H. K.,** *J. Lab. Clin. Med.,* 46, 255, 1955.
g. **Ranney, H. M., Nagel, R., Heller, P., and Udem, L.,** *Biochim. Biophys. Acta,* 160, 112, 1968.
h. **Efremov, G. D., Huisman, T. H. J., Bowman, K., and Wrightstone, R. N.,** *J. Lab. Clin. Med.,* 83, 657, 1974.
i. **Chernoff, A. I., Pettit, N., and Northrop, O.,** *J. Blood,* 25, 646, 1965.
j. **Charache, S., Weatherall, D. J., and Clegg, J. B.,** *J. Clin. Invest.,* 45, 813, 1966.
k. **Hayashi, A., Suzuki, T., Schimizu, T., and Yamamura, Y.,** *Biochim. Biophys. Acta,* 160, 252, 1968.
l. **Vettore, L., DeSandre, G., Dilorio, E. E., Winterhalter, K. H., Lan, A., and Lehman, K.,** *Blood,* 44, 869, 1974.
m. **Van Ros, G., Beale, D., and Lehmann, H.,** *Br. Med. J.,* 4, 92, 1968.
n. **Bromberg, P. A., Alben, J. O., Bare, G. H., Balcerzak, S. P., Jones, R. T., Brimhall, B., and Padilla, F.,** *Nature (New Biol.),* 243, 177, 1973.
o. **Jensen, M., Oski, F. A., Nathan, D. G., and Bunn, H. F.,** *J. Clin. Invest.,* 55, 469, 1975.
p. **Huisman, T. H. J., Martis, E. A., and Dozy, A. M.,** *J. Lab. Clin. Med.,* 52, 312, 1958.
q. **Clegg, M. D. and Schroeder, W. A.,** *J. Am. Chem. Soc.,* 81, 6065, 1959.
r. **Dozy, A. M. and Huisman, T. H. J.,** *J. Chromatogr.,* 40, 62, 1969.
s. **Bernini, L. F.,** *Biochem. Genet.,* 2, 305, 1969.
t. **Bonaventura, J. and Riggs, A.,** *J. Biol. Chem.,* 243, 980, 1968.
u. **Huisman, T. H. J.,** *Standardization of Laboratory Reagents and Methods for Detection of Hemoglobinopathies,* Schmidt, R. M., Huisman, T. H. J., and Lehmann, H., Eds., CRC Press, Boca Raton, Fla., 1974, 73.
v. **Abraham, E. C., Reese, A., Stallings, M., and Huisman, T. H. J.,** *Hemoglobin,* 1, 27, 1976.
w. **Ahern, E., Holder, W., Ahern, V., Serjeant, G. R., Serjeant, B. E., Forbes, M., Brimhall, B., and Jones, R. T.,** *Biochim. Biophys. Acta,* 393, 188, 1975.

REFERENCES

1. **Winter, W. P. and Rucknagel, D. L.,** Peptide mapping, in *Standardization of Laboratory Reagents and Methods for the Detection of Hemoglobinopathies,* Schmidt, R. M., Huisman, T. H. J., and Lehmann, H., Eds., CRC Press, Boca Raton, Fla., 1974, 81.
2. **Porath, J. and Flodin, P.,** Gel filtration, in *Protides of the Biological Fluids,* Vol. 10, Elsevier, Amsterdam, 1963, 290.
3. **Seid-Akhavan, M., Ayres, M., Salzano, F. M., Winter, W. P., and Rucknagel, D. L.,** Two more examples of Hb Porto Alegre, $\alpha_2\beta_2\ 9^{Ser \rightarrow Cys}$, in Belem, Brazil, *Hum. Hered.,* 23, 175, 1973.
4. **Gill, F. M. and Schwartz, E.,** Free α-globin pool in human bone marrow, *J. Clin. Invest.,* 52, 3057, 1973.
5. **Killander, J.,** Separation of human heme- and hemoglobin-binding plasma proteins, ceruloplasmin and albumin by gel filtration, *Biochim. Biophys. Acta,* 93, 1, 1964.
6. **Olsen, K. W.,** Affinity chromatography of heme binding proteins, *Fed. Proc. Abstr.,* 36, 2550, 1977.
7. **Brenne, S. O., Winterbourn, C. C., and Carrell, R. W.,** Isolation of high oxygen affinity hemoglobins, *Hemoglobin,* 1, 479, 1977.
8. **Hanash, S. M. and Shapiro, D. N.,** Separation of human hemoglobin by ion exchange high pressure liquid chromatography, *Hemoglobin,* 5, 165, 1981.
9. **Gardiner, M. B., Carver, J., Abraham, B. L., Wilson, J. B., and Huisman, T. H. J.,** Further studies on the quantitation of the hemoglobinopathies using high pressure liquid chromatography, *Hemoglobin,* 6, 1, 1982.
10. **Gooding, K. M., Lu, K.-C., and Regnier, F. E.,** High performance liquid chromatography of hemoglobin. I. Determination of Hb A_2, *J. Chromatogr.,* 164, 506, 1979.
11. **Cole, R. A., Soeldner, J. S., Dunn, P. J., and Bunn, H. F.,** An automated method for the determination of hemoglobin A_{1c} and total fast hemoglobins using high pressure liquid chromatography, *Chromatogr. Sci.,* 10, 659, 1979.
12. **Davis, J. E., McDonald, J. M., and Jarett, M.,** A high performance liquid chromatography method for hemoglobin A_{1c}, *Diabetes,* 27, 102, 1978.
13. **Dunn, P. J., Cole, R. A., and Soeldner, J. S.,** Further development and automation of a high pressure liquid chromatography method for the determination of glycosylated hemoglobins, *Metabolism,* 28, 777, 1979.
14. **Shimizu, K., Wilson, J. B., and Huisman, T. H. J.,** Determination of the percentages of $^G\gamma$ and $^A\gamma$ chains in human fetal hemoglobin by HPLC, *Hemoglobin,* 4, 487, 1980.
15. **Congote, L. F., Bennett, H. P. J., and Solomon, S.,** Rapid separation of the α, β, $^G\gamma$ and $^A\gamma$ human globin chains by reversed-phase high pressure liquid chromatography, *Biochem. Biophys. Res. Commun.,* 89, 851, 1979.
16. **Shelton, J. B., Shelton, J. R., and Schroeder, W. A.,** Preliminary experiments in the separation of globin chains by high performance liquid chromatography, *Hemoglobin,* 3, 353, 1979.
17. **Petrides, P. E., Jones, R. T., and Bohlen, P.,** Reverse-phase high performance liquid chromatography of proteins: the separation of hemoglobin chain variants, *Anal. Biochem.,* 105, 383, 1980.
18. **Shelton, J. B., Shelton, J. R., Schroeder, W. A., and DeSimone, J.,** Detection of Hb Papio B, a silent mutation of the baboon β chain by high performance liquid chromatography. Improved procedures for the separation of globin chains by HPLC, *Hemoglobin,* 6, 451, 1982.
19. **Schroeder, W. A., Shelton, J. B., Shelton, J. R., and Powars, D.,** Separation of peptides by high pressure liquid chromatography for the identification of a human variant, *J. Chromatogr.,* 174, 385, 1979.
20. **Wilson, J. B., Lam, H., Pravatmuang, P., and Huisman, T. H. J.,** Separation of tryptic peptides of normal and abnormal alpha, beta, gamma and delta hemoglobin chains by high pressure liquid chromatography, *J. Chromatogr.,* 179, 271, 1979.
21. **Stoming, T. A., Garver, F. A., Gangorosa, M. A., Harrison, J. M., and Huisman, T. H. J.,** Separation of the $^A\gamma$ and $^G\gamma$ cyanogen bromide peptides of human fetal hemoglobin by high pressure liquid chromatography, *Anal. Biochem.,* 96, 113, 1979.
22. **Nakatsuji, T., Headlee, M., Lam, H., Wilson, J. B., and Huisman, T. H. J.,** Hb F-Bonaire, Ga. or $\alpha_2{}^A\gamma_2 39(C5)gln \rightarrow arg$ characterized by high pressure liquid chromatographic and microsequencing procedures, *Hemoglobin,* 6, 599, 1982.
23. **Abraham, E. C., Reese, A., Stallings, M., and Huisman, T. H. J.,** Separation of human hemoglobin by DEAE cellulose chromatography using glycine-KCN-NaCl developers, *Hemoglobin,* 1, 27, 1976.
24. **Peterson, E. A. and Sober, H. A.,** A variable gradient device for chromatography, *Anal. Chem.,* 31, 857, 1959.
25. **Kirkland, J. J.,** *Modern Practice of Liquid Chromatography,* Wiley-Interscience, New York, 1971.
26. **Clegg, J. B., Naughton, M. A., and Weatherall, D. J.,** Abnormal human haemoglobins. Separation and characterization of the α and β chains by chromatography and the determination of two new variants, Hb Chesapeake and Hb J (Bangkok), *J. Mol. Biol.,* 19, 91, 1966.

27. **Clegg, J. B., Naughton, M. A., and Weatherall, D. J.,** An improved method for the characterization of human hemoglobin mutants: identification $\alpha_2\beta_2^{95glu}$, Hb N Baltimore, *Nature (London),* 207, 945, 1965.
28. **Bucci, E. and Fronticelli, C.,** A new method for the preparation of α and β subunits of human hemoglobin, *J. Biol. Chem.,* 240, 551, 1965.
29. **DeRenzo, E. C., Toppolo, C., Aniconi, G., Antonini, E., and Wyman, T.,** Properties of α and β chains of hemoglobin prepared from their mercuribenzoate derivatives by treatment with 1-dodecanethiol, *J. Biol. Chem.,* 242, 4850, 1967.
30. **Huisman, T. H. J. and Jonxis, J. H. P.,** *The Hemoglobinopathies. Techniques of Identification,* Marcell Dekker, New York, 1977, 192.
31. **Huisman, T. H. J. and Dozy, A. M.,** Studies on the heterogeneity of hemoglobin IX. The use of Trishydroxymethylaminomethane buffer in the anion exchange chromatography of hemoglobins, *J. Chromatogr.,* 19, 160, 1965.
32. **Vettore, L., DeSandre, G., Dilorio, E. E., Boyer, S. H., Crosby, E. F., Fuller, G. F., Ulenurm, L., and Buck, A. A.,** A survey of hemoglobin in the republic of Chad and characterization of Hb Chad: $\alpha_2^{23glu\rightarrow lyz}\beta_2$, *Am. J. Hum. Genet.,* 20, 570, 1969.
33. **Vettore, L., DeSandre, G., Dilorio, E. E., Winterhalter, K. H., Lang, A., and Lehmann, H.,** A new abnormal hemoglobin O Padova α30 (B11) glu→lys and a dyserythropoietic anemia with erythroblastic multinuclearity coexisting in the same patient, *Blood,* 44, 869, 1974.
34. **Baglioni, C. and Lehmann, H.,** Chemical heterogeneity of Haemoglobin O, *Nature (London),* 196, 229, 1962.
35. **Bunn, H. F., Meriwether, W. D., Balcerzak, S. P., and Rucknagel, D. L.,** Oxygen equilibria of hemoglobin, E, *J. Clin. Invest.,* 51, 2984, 1972.
36. **Gossens, M., Garel, M. C., Aurinet, J., Basset, P., Gomes, P., and Rosa, J.,** Hemoglobin C Ziguinchor $\alpha_2{}^A\beta_2$ 6(A3)$^{glu\rightarrow val}$K 58(E2) pro→arg. The second sickling variant with amino acid substitutions in 2 residues of the polypeptide chain, *FEBS Lett.,* 58, 149, 1975.
37. **Miyaji, T., Suzuki, H., Ohba, Y., and Shibata, S.,** Hemoglobin Agenogi ($\alpha_2\beta_2^{90lys}$), a slow moving hemoglobin of a Japanese family resembling Hb E, *Clin. Chim. Acta,* 14, 624, 1966.
38. **Beuzard, Y., Courvalin, J. C., Cohen-Solal, M., Garel, M. C., Rosa, J., Brizand, C. P., and Giband, A.,** Structural studies of hemoglobin St. Etienne β92(F8) his→gln: a new abnormal hemoglobin with loss of proximal histidine and absence of heme in the chains, *FEBS Lett.,* 27, 76, 1972.
39. **Aksoy, M., Erdem, S., Efremov, G. D., Wilson, J. B., Huisman, T. H. J., Schroeder, W. F., Shelton, J. R., Shelton, J. B., Ulitin, O. N., and Muftuoglu, A.,** Hemoglobin Istanbul: substitution of glutamine for histidine in a proximal histidine (F8(92)β), *J. Clin. Invest.,* 51, 2380, 1977.
40. **Bradley, T. B., Jr., Wohl, R. C., and Reider, R. F.,** Hemoglobin Gunn Hill: deletion of five amino acid residues and impaired heme-globin binding, *Science,* 157, 1581, 1967.
41. **Vella, F., Casey, R., Lehmann, H., Labossiere, A., and Jones, T. G.,** Hb Ottawa, α_2 15 (A13)gly→arg β_2, *Biochim. Biophys. Acta,* 336, 25, 1974.
42. **Rahbar, S., Mahdavi, N., Nowzari, R., and Mustafaus, I.,** Hemoglobin Arya: α_2 47 (CD 5) asp→asn, *Biochim. Biophys. Acta,* 386, 525, 1975.
43. **Halbrecht, I., Issacs, W. A., Lehmann, H., and Ben-Porat, F.,** Hemoglobin Hasharon (α47 asp→his), *Isr. J. Med. Sci.,* 3, 827, 1967; **Schneider, R. G., Veda, S., Alperin, J. B., Brimhall, B., and Jones, R. T.,** Hemoglobin Sealey ($\alpha_2^{47\ his}\beta_2$): a new variant in a Jewish family, *Am. J. Hum. Genet.,* 20, 151, 1968.
44. **Hanada, M. and Rucknagel, D. L.,** The abnormality in the primary structure of Hb Shimonoseki, *Biochem. Biophys. Res. Commun.,* 11, 229, 1963.
45. **Rahbar, S., Kinderlehrer, J. L., and Lehmann, H.,** Hemoglobin L Persian Gulf, α57 (E6) gly→arg, *Acta Haematol.,* 42, 169, 1969.
46. **Rahbar, S., Nowzari, G., and Daneshmand, P.,** Hb Daneshgah-Tehran α_2 72 (EFI) his→arg $\beta_2{}^A$, *Nature (New Biol.),* 245, 268, 1973.
47. **Lorkin, P. A., Charlesworth, D., Lehmann, H., Rahbar, S., Tuchinda, S., and Lie Injo Luan Eng.,** Two haemoglobins Q, α74 (EF3) and α75 (EF4) asp→his, *Br. J. Haematol.,* 19, 117, 1970.
48. **Van Ros, G., Beale, D., and Lehmann, H.,** Haemoglobin Stanleyville II (α78 asn→lys), *Br. Med. J.,* 4, 92, 1968.
49. **Lorkin, P. A., Huntsman, R. G., Ager, J. A. M., Lehman, H., Vella, F., and Darbre, P. D.,** Haemoglobin G. Norfolk α85 (F6) asp→asn, *Biochim. Biophys. Acta,* 379, 22, 1975.
50. **Huisman, T. H. J., Adams, H. R., Wilson, J. B., Efremov, G. D., Reynolds, C. A., and Wrightstone, R. N.,** Hemoglobin G Georgia or $\alpha_2^{95leu(G2)}\beta_2$, *Biochim. Biophys. Acta,* 200, 578, 1970.
51. **Jones, R. T., Brimhall, B., and Lisker, R.,** Chemical characterization of Hb Mexico and Hb Chiapas, *Biochim. Biophys. Acta,* 154, 488, 1968.
52. **Smith, L. L., Barton, B. P., and Huisman, T. H. J.,** Subunit dissociation of the unstable hemoglobin Bibba (α_2 136 pro (H19)β_2), *J. Biol. Chem.,* 245, 2185, 1970.

53. **Rahbar, S.,** Haemoglobin D Iran: β_2 22 glutamic acid→glutamine (β4), *Br. J. Haematol.,* 24, 31, 1973.
54. **Brimhall, B., Jones, R. T., Schneider, R. G., Hosty, J. S., Tomlin, G., and Atkins, R.,** Hemoglobin Alabama (β39(C5) glyn→lys) and Hb Montgomery (α48(CD6)leu→arg), *Biochim. Biophys. Acta,* 379, 28, 1975.
55. **Watson-Williams, E. J., Beale, D., Irvine, D., and Lehmann, H.,** A new hemoglobin D Ibadan, (β87 thr→lys) producing no sickle cell-Hb D disease with Hb S, *Nature (London),* 205, 1273, 1965.
56. **Wajcman, H., Labie, D., and Schapira, G.,** Hemoglobin tours: Thr β87 (F3) deleted and hemoglobin St. Antoine, Gly→leu β74-75 (E18-19) deleted. Consequences for oxygen affinity and protein stability, *Biochim. Biophys. Acta,* 295, 495, 1973.
57. **Schneider, R. G., Veda, S., Alperin, J. B., Levin, W. C., Jones, R. T., and Brimhall, B.,** Hemoglobin D Los Angeles in two Caucasian families. Hemoglobin SD disease and Hemoglobin D Thalassemia, *Blood,* 32, 250, 1968.
58. **Efremov, G. D., Huisman, T. H. J., Smith, L. L., Wilson, J. B., Kitchens, J. L., Wrightstone, R. N., and Adams, H. R.,** Hemoglobin Richmond, a human hemoglobin which forms asymmetric hybrids with other hemoglobins, *J. Biol. Chem.,* 244, 6105, 1969.
59. **Blackwell, R. Q., Jim, R. T. S., Tan, I. G. H., Weng, M.-I., Liu, C.-S., and Wang, C.-L.,** Hemoglobin G Waimanalo α 64 asp→asn, *Biochim. Biophys. Acta,* 322, 27, 1973.
60. **DeJong, W. W. W., Bernini, L. F., and Khan, P. M.,** Hemoglobin Rampa: α95 pro→ser, *Biochim. Biophys. Acta,* 236, 197, 1971.
61. **Wiltshire, B. G., Clark, K. G. A., Lorkin, P. A., and Lehmann, H.,** Haemoglobin Denmark Hill α95 (G2) pro→ala; a variant with unusual electrophoretic and oxygen binding properties, *Biochim. Biophys. Acta,* 278, 459, 1972.
62. **Bannister, W. H., Grech, J. L., Plese, C. F., Smith, L. L., Barton, B. P., Wilson, J. B., Reynolds, C. A., and Huisman, T. H. J.,** Hemoglobin St. Luke's or $\alpha_2^{95\ Arg(G2)}\ \beta_2$, *Eur. J. Biochem.,* 29, 301, 1972.
63. **Brown, W. J., Niazi, G. A., Jayakalshmi, M., Abraham, E. C., and Huisman, T. H. J.,** Hemoglobin Athens-Georgia or $\alpha_2\beta_2$ 40 (C6) arg→lys. A hemoglobin variant with an increased oxygen affinity. To be published; cited in Lehmann, H. and Kynoch, P. A. M., *Human Hemoglobin Variants and their Characteristics,* North-Holland, Amsterdam, 1976.
64. **Byckova, V., Wajcman, H., Labie, D., and Travers, F.,** Hemoglobin M Saskatoon: further data on biophysics and oxygen equilibrium, *Biochim. Biophys. Acta,* 243, 117, 1971.
65. **Gerald, P. S. and Efron, M. L.,** Chemical studies of several varieties of Hb M, *Proc. Natl. Acad. Sci. U.S.A.,* 47, 1758, 1961.
66. **Udem, L., Ranney, H. M., Bunn, H. F., and Pisciotta, A.,** Some observations on the properties of hemoglobin M Milwaukee I, *J. Mol. Biol.,* 48, 489, 1970.
67. **Heller, P., Coleman, R. D., and Yakulis, V.,** Hemoglobin M Hyde Park: a new variant of abnormal methemoglobin, *J. Clin. Invest.,* 45, 1021, 1966.
68. **Lorkin, P. A., Lehmann, H., Fairbanks, V. F., Berglund, G., and Leonhardt, T.,** Two new pathological haemoglobins: Olmsted, β141 (H19) Leu→arg and Malmö, β97 (FG4) his→gln, *Biochem. J.,* 119, 68P, 1970.
69. **Bonaventura, J. and Riggs, A.,** Hemoglobin Kansas, a human hemoglobin with a neutral amino acid substitution and an abnormal oxygen equilibrium, *J. Biol. Chem.,* 243, 980, 1968.
70. **Nute, P. E., Stamatoyannopoules, G., Hermodson, M. A., Roth, D., and Hornung, S.,** Hemoglobinopathic erythrocytosis due to a new electrophoretically silent variant hemoglobin San Diego (β109 (G11) val→met), *J. Clin. Invest.,* 53, 320, 1974.
71. **Minnich, V., Hill, R. J., Khuri, P. D., and Anderson, M. D.,** Hemoglobin Hope: a beta chain variant, *Blood,* 25, 830, 1965.
72. **Bromberg, P. A., Alben, J. O., Bare, G. H., Balcerzak, S. P., Jones, R. T., Brimhall, B., and Padilla, F.,** High oxygen affinity variant of haemoglobin Little Rock with unique properties, *Nature (London) New Biol.,* 243, 177, 1973.
73. **Jensen, M., Oski, F. A., Nathan, D. G., and Bunn, H. F.,** Hemoglobin Syracuse ($\alpha_2\beta_2$ 143 (H21) his→pro) a new high affinity variant detected by special electrophoretic methods, *J. Clin. Invest.,* 55, 469, 1975.
74. **Rosa, J., Maleknia, N., Vergoz, D., and Dumet, R.,** Une nouvelle hemoglobine abnormale: l'hemoglobine $J\alpha_{Paris}$ 12 ala→asp, *Nouv. Rev. Fr. Hematol.,* 6, 423, 1966.
75. **Rahbar, S., Ala, F., Akhavan, E., Nowzari, G., Shoai, I., and Zamanianpoor, M. H.,** Two new haemoglobins: haemoglobin Persopolis (α64(E13) asp→tyr) and haemoglobin J Kurosh (α19(AB1) ala→asp), *Biochim. Biophys. Acta,* 119, 1976.
76. **Kendall, A. G., Barr, R. D., Lang, A., and Lehmann, H.,** Haemoglobin J Nyanza:α21(B2) ala→asp, *Biochim. Biophys. Acta,* 310, 357, 1973.
77. **Baglioni, C. A.,** Chemical study of Hemoglobin Norfolk, *J. Biol. Chem.,* 237, 69, 1962.

78. **Rosa, J.,** Haemoglobin Lyon (β17-18(A14-15) lys val→0). Determination by sequenator analysis, *Biochim. Biophys. Acta,* 351, 306, 1974.
79. **Ricco, G., Pich, P. G., Mazza, U., Rossi, G., Ajmar, F., Arese, P., and Gallo, E.,** Hb J Sicilia: β65(E9)lys→asn, a beta chain homologue of Hb Zambia, *FEBS Lett.,* 39, 200, 1974.
80. **Garel, M. C., Hassan, W., Coquelet, M. T., Gossens, M., Rosa, J., and Arous, N.,** Hemoglobin J Cairo: β65 (E9) lys→gln, a new hemoglobin variant discovered in an Egyptian family, *Biochim. Biophys. Acta,* 420, 97, 1976.
81. **Romain, P. L., Schwartz, A. D., Shamsuddin, M., Adams, J. G., Mason, R. G., Vidda, L. N., and Honing, G. R.,** Hemoglobin J Chicago (β76 (E20) ala→asp): a new variant resulting from substitution of an external residue, *Blood,* 45, 387, 1975.
82. **Colombo, B., Vidal, H., Kamuzora, H., and Lehmann, H.,** A new Haemoglobin J Habana α71 (E20) alanine→glutamic acid, *Biochim. Biophys. Acta,* 351, 1, 1974.
83. **Blackwell, R. Q., Wong, H. B., Wang, C.-L., Weng, M.-I., and Liu, C.-S.,** Hemoglobin J Meerut: α120 ala→glu, *Biochim. Biophys. Acta,* 351, 7, 1974.
84. **Schneider, R. G., Alperin, J. B., Beale, D., and Lehmann, H.,** Hemoglobin I in an American Negro family: structural and hematological studies, *J. Lab. Clin. Med.,* 68, 940, 1966.
85. **Maekawa, M., Maekawa, T., Fujiwara, N., Tabara, K., and Matsuda, G.,** Hemoglobin Nagasaki: ($\alpha_2{}^A\beta_2{}^{17\ glu}$). A new abnormal hemoglobin found in one family in Nagasaki, *Int. J. Prot. Res.,* 2, 147, 1970.
86. **Shibata, S., Miyaji, T., Iuchi, I., Veda, S., and Takeda, I.,** Hemoglobin Hikari: ($\alpha_2{}^A\beta_2{}^{61asn}$) a fast moving hemoglobin found in two unrelated Japanese families, *Clin. Chem. Acta,* 10, 101, 1964.
87. **Capp, G. L., Rigas, D. A., and Jones, R. T.,** Hemoglobin Portland I: a new human haemoglobin in structure, *Nature (London),* 228, 278, 1970.
88. **Kamuzora, H. and Lehmann, H.,** Human embryonic haemoglobins including a comparison by homology of the human ζ and α chains, *Nature (London),* 256, 511, 1975.
89. **Smith, D. H., Clegg, J. B., Weatherall, D. J., and Giles, H. M.,** Hereditary persistence of foetal haemoglobin associated with a $\gamma\beta$ fusion variant Haemoglobin Kenya, *Nature (London) New Biol.,* 246, 184, 1973.
90. **Clegg, J. B., Weatherall, D. J., and Milner, P. F.,** Haemoglobin Constant Spring, a chain termination mutant?, *Nature (London),* 234, 337, 1971.
91. **Clegg, J. B., Weatherall, D. J., Contopolou, I., Caroutsos, K., Poungouras, P., and Tsevrenis, H.,** Haemoglobin Icaria, a new chain termination mutant which causes thalassemia, *Nature (London),* 251, 245, 1974.
92. **Ibarra, B., Franco-Gambog, E., Ramirez, M. L., Contu, J. M., Wilson, J. B., Lam, H., and Huisman, T. H. J.,** Hb Chiapas, $\alpha_2{}^{114\ pro\rightarrow arg}\beta_2$. Identification by high pressure liquid chromatography, *Hemoglobin,* 5, 605, 1981.

STRUCTURAL CHARACTERIZATION OF HEMOGLOBINS BY HIGH PERFORMANCE LIQUID CHROMATOGRAPHY

Richard T. Jones

INTRODUCTION

The structural characterization of hemoglobins depends, in large part, on determining the primary structure or the sequence of amino acid residues in each of the globin chains of the hemoglobin. Because of the size of the globin chains (either 141 or 146 residues in length), it is convenient to determine their primary structure by examining fragments of the polypeptide chains produced by chemical or enzymatic cleavage of specific peptide bonds. The resultant fragments, such as the tryptic peptides formed by enzymatic hydrolysis of a globin chain with trypsin, must be separated and subjected to further primary structure analysis. In this way the amino acid sequence of each region of the original chain represented by its peptide fragment can be deduced. In the case of a globin chain for which the primary structure is unknown, the sequence of all of its fragments must be determined. In the case of most abnormal human hemoglobins, only the peptide fragments which are different from the fragments of the corresponding normal chain need to be sequenced. However, in both cases, the isolation of single, pure peptide fragments represents an essential step in structural characterization.

To date, three different procedures have been used to separate peptide fragments. The first method used for determining the structure of abnormal hemoglobins was the "finger printing" procedure of Ingram[1] which utilized a combination of paper electrophoresis and chromatography to separate tryptic and chymotryptic peptides. This method, and modifications of it, are still used by many laboratories for the structural characterization of abnormal hemoglobins. A second approach to the separation of peptide fragments of hemoglobins or globin chains was by conventional or low-pressure column chromatography. Schroeder and co-workers[2] applied both cation and anion exchange procedures with volatile organic developers to the structural studies of hemoglobin. The cation procedure was automated by this author and used to separate the tryptic peptides of aminoethylated globin chains.[3,4] The third and newest method for separating peptide fragments of hemoglobin is by reverse-phase high-performance liquid chromatography (HPLC). Although the initial investment in the HPLC equipment and columns needed for this third procedure may be greater than for the other two methods, it has the advantages of being much more rapid, reproducible, dependable, and very sensitive. Results published since 1979 amply demonstrate that the HPLC separation of peptide fragments of hemoglobin is a very powerful technique for the structural analysis of abnormal hemoglobins and as yet unsequenced globin chains of humans and other animals. It is the HPLC method of separating peptide fragments of hemoglobin chains that is the subject of this chapter.

HISTORY OF HPLC APPLIED TO THE SEPARATION OF HEMOGLOBIN PEPTIDE FRAGMENTS

Soon after Congote et al.[5] described the first HPLC separation of the globin chains of normal Hb A and Hb F in 1979, Schroeder and associates[6-11] and Huisman and coworkers[12-14] demonstrated the application of HPLC to the separation and isolation of peptide fragments of hemoglobin. Schroeder et al.[6] used a Waters μBondapak® C_{18} reverse-phase column (3.9 × 300 mm, 10 μm) and the ammonium acetate and acetonitrile developer solutions to detect the differences between the tryptic digests of Hb A, Hb C, and Hb E.

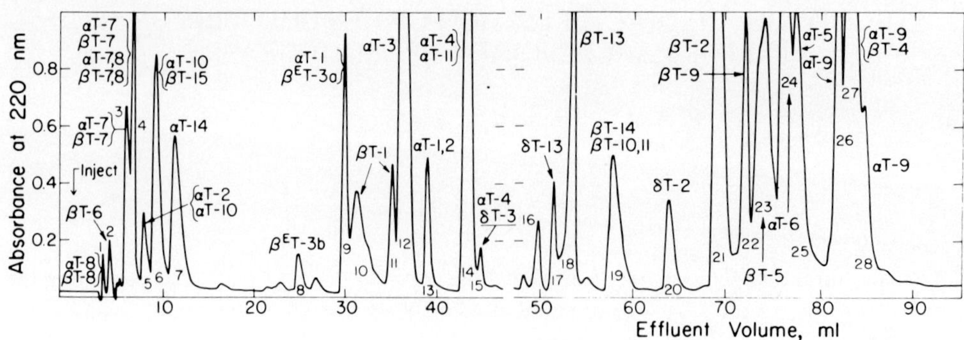

FIGURE 1. HPLC separation of the tryptic peptides of the α- and β-chains of Hb E on a 3.9 × 300 mm Waters μBondapak C_{18} column using a 0.01 *M* ammonium acetate (pH 6.07) and acetonitrile gradient starting with 0% acetonitrile and ending with 40% acetonitrile after 100 mℓ (66.7 min at 1.5 mℓ/min flow rate). (From Schroeder, W. A. et al., *J. Chromatogr.*, 174, 385, 1979. With permission.)

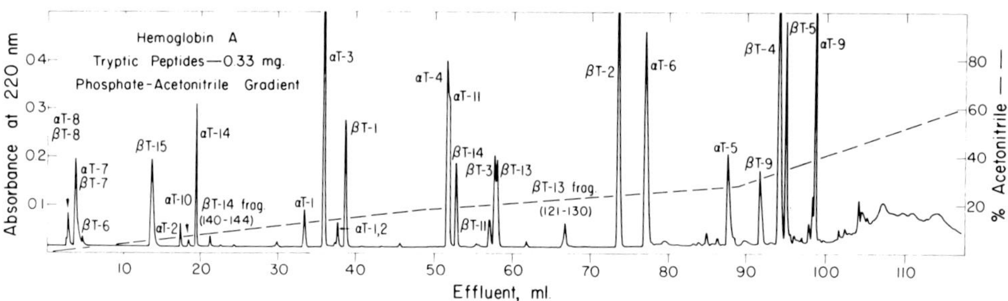

FIGURE 2. HPLC separation of tryptic peptides of 0.33 mg normal adult globin (from Hb A) on a 4.6 × 250 mm Altex Ultrasphere ODS column using a gradient of potassium phosphate (pH 2.95) and acetonitrile at 1 mℓ/min (0 to 18% acetonitrile in 48 mℓ, to 28% in 40 mℓ, to 40% in 10 mℓ, and to 62% in 20 mℓ). (From Schroeder, W. A., et al., *Clin. Biol. Res.*, 60, 1, 1981. With permission.)

Their chromatogram for the tryptic peptides of Hb E is shown in Figure 1. Sufficient amounts of pure peptides were obtained from about 5 mg of hemoglobin to determine the amino acid composition of the peptides by automatic amino acid analysis. At essentially the same time, Efremov et al.[12] reported using a similar procedure to isolate the 9th and 15th tryptic peptides of the T_γ, I_γ, G_γ, and A_γ chains of different human fetal hemoglobins. They found that 1 to 2 mg of tryptic digests was sufficient for satisfactory amino acid analyses. In the same year, Stroming et al.[13] reported the separation of the cyanogen bromide peptide fragments of G_γ and A_γ chains by HPLC and applied this to the determination of the ratio of these two types of chains in Hb F samples without the need for amino acid analysis of glycine and alanine. The first new abnormal hemoglobin to be structurally characterized by HPLC was Hb Sunshine-Seth [α94 (G1) Asp → His].[7] Although Schroeder et al. used the ammonium acetate-acetonitrile developer system for the characterization of this hemoglobin, these investigators introduced the low pH (2.86 to 2.95), potassium phosphate-acetonitrile developer system for the characterization of their next new variant, Hb Pasadena [α75 (E19) Leu → Arg].[8] Schroeder and co-workers[9] have carefully compared HPLC procedures including different types of columns, developer solvents, and gradients, as well as sample preparations and load amounts required to produce satisfactory separations of tryptic peptides. Figure 2 was obtained by Schroeder et al.[10] for a tryptic hydrolysate of 0.33 mg of Hb A separated on a 4.6 × 250 mm column of Altex Ultrasphere ODS using their phosphate-acetonitrile gradient. These investigators prefer the phosphate-acetonitrile developer system over the ammonium acetate-acetonitrile system because the former produces sharper peaks, better

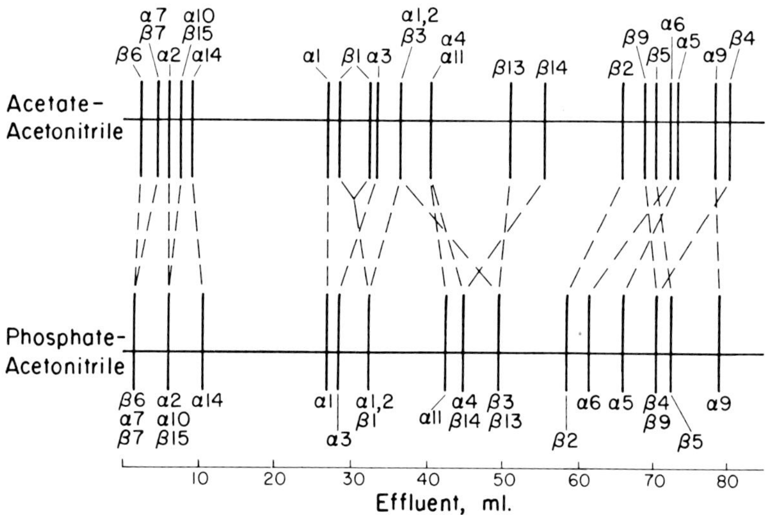

FIGURE 3. Comparison of the elution volumes of the tryptic peptides of Hb A using ammonium acetate-acetonitrile above and potassium phosphate-acetonitrile below. A 3.9 × 300 mm Waters μBondapack C_{18} column was used with a linear gradient from 0 to 40% acetonitrile in a total of 100 mℓ at 1 mℓ/min for both developer systems. (From Schroeder, W. A. et al., *Hemoglobin*, 4, 551, 1980. With permission.)

resolution of most tryptic peptides, and cleaner removal of material from the column with only one serious limitation, namely the involatility of the potassium phosphate. Because many of the tryptic peptides of hemoglobin behave rather differently with these two developer systems, as shown in Figure 3 from a comparison done by Schroeder et al.,[9] it is possible to use the phosphate developers for the initial separation and then rechromatograph any zone with the ammonium acetate developers, using the same column, if desalting or further purification is necessary.

As described in a paper by Wilson et al.,[14] Huisman and co-workers continued to use only the ammonium acetate-acetonitrile developer system with the Waters μBondapak C_{18} column to separate and isolate the tryptic peptides of normal and abnormal α-chain, aminoethylated β-, γ-, and δ-chains, and the chymotryptic peptides of the oxidized core of α-chains. As will be discussed later, they demonstrated the application of this HPLC method to the identification of abnormal peptides from 25 previously characterized hemoglobin variants.[14] These investigators have continued to apply this HPLC procedure, with only minor modification, to the study of other abnormal hemoglobins, including Hb Chiapas [α114 (GH2) Pro → Arg],[15] Hb Wuming [α11 (A9) Glu → Lys],[16] and Hb Olympia [β20 (B2) Val→ Met] and Hb San Diego [β109 (G11) Val → Met].[17] Although the laboratories headed by Schroeder and Huisman have led the development and application of HPLC to the isolation of hemoglobin peptide fragments for structural characterization, other investigators have begun to publish their results using HPLC for studies of human hemoglobins. These are listed in Table 1.

EQUIPMENT

Except for the specific column to be used, the choice of HPLC equipment is of little importance, provided the system can generate a gradient change between the developer solutions and meet other general requirements of HPLC.

A simple HPLC system is diagrammed in Figure 4 and consists of a two-chamber linear gradient device with open reservoir and mixing cylinders of equal diameters, a valve for

Table 1
ABNORMAL HEMOGLOBIN DETERMINED BY HPLC

A. α-Chain Variants

Name	Residue position	Substitution	Abnormal tryptic peptide #	Developer system	Ref.
Boyle Heights	6	Asp→o	1	PO_4	28
Wuming	11	Lys→Gln	2,3	NH_4Ac	16
Albany-GA	11	Lys→Asn	2,3	NH_4Ac	29
I-Interlaken	15	Gly→Asp	3	NH_4Ac	14
I	16	Lys→Glu	3,4	NH_4Ac	14
I	16	Lys→Glu	3,4	PO_4	11
Handsworth	18	Gly→Arg	4	PO_4	11
G-Montgomery	48	Leu→Arg	6	NH_4Ac	14
J-Sardegna	50	His→Asp	6	NH_4Ac	14
Russ	51	Gly→Arg	6	NH_4Ac	14
Shimonoseki	54	Gln→Arg	6	NH_4Ac	14
G-Philadelphia	68	Asn→Lys	9	PO_4	11
Winnipeg	75	Asp→Tyr	9	NH_4Ac	30
Etobicoke	85	Ser→Arg	9	NH_4Ac	31
Sunshine Seth	94	Asp→His	11	NH_4Ac	7
Rampa	95	Pro→Ser	11	PO_4	11
Chiapas	114	Pro→Arg	12	PO_4	15
Oleander	116	Glu→Gln	12	NH_4Ac	27
Tarrant	126	Asp→Asn	12	PO_4	11
Suresnes	141	Arg→His	14	NH_4Ac	14

B. β-Chain Variants

Name	Residue position	Substitution	Abnormal tryptic peptide #	Developer system	Ref.
S	6	Glu→Val	1	NH_4Ac, PO_4	14, 11
C	6	Glu→Lys	1	NH_4Ac, PO_4	6, 11
G-San Jose	7	Glu→Gly	1	NH_4Ac	14
Rio Grande	8	Lys→Thr	1, 2	NaAc	32
Saki	14	Leu→Pro	2	NH_4Ac	14
J-Georgia	16	Gly → Asp	2, 3	NH_4Ac	14
Alamo	19	Asn→Asp	3	NH_4Ac	14
Olympia	20	Val→Met	3	NH_4Ac	17
Connecticut	21	Asp→Gly	3	NH_4Ac	14
Cocody	21	Asp→Asn	3	NH_4Ac	33
Palmerston North	23	Val→Phe	3	PO_4	34
E	26	Glu→Lys	3	NH_4Ac, PO_4	6, 14, 11
Tacoma	30	Arg→Ser	3, 4	NH_4Ac	14
Austin	40	Arg→Ser	4, 5	NH_4Ac	14
Hammersmith	42	Phe→Ser	5	PO_4	11
Cheverly	45	Phe→Ser	5	NH_4Ac	35
Avicenna	47	Asp→Ala	5	NH_4Ac	33
Osu-Christianborg	52	Asp→Asn	5	PO_4	11
J-Bangkok	56	Gly→Asp	5	PO_4	36
J-Daloa	57	Asn→Asp	5	NH_4Ac	37
N-Seattle	61	Lys→Glu	6, 7	PO_4	11
Korle Bu	73	Asp→Asn	9	NH_4Ac, PO_4	33, 38
Pasadena	75	Leu→Arg	9	PO_4	8
Sabine	91	Leu→Pro	10	NH_4Ac	39
Malmö	97	His→Gln	11	NH_4Ac	14
Köln	98	Val→Met	11	PO_4	11
San Diego	109	Val→Met	12A	NH_4Ac	17
P-Galveston	117	His→Arg	12B	NH_4Ac	14
Fannin-Lubbock	119	Gly→Asp	12	PO_4	11
Riyadh	120	Lys→Asn	12B, 13	NH_4Ac	14

Table 1 (continued)
ABNORMAL HEMOGLOBIN DETERMINED BY HPLC

A. α-Chain Variants

Name	Residue position	Substitution	Abnormal tryptic peptide #	Developer system	Ref.
O-Arab	121	Glu→Lys	13	PO_4	11
Hacettepe	127	Gln→Glu	13	NH_4Ac	14
Andrew-Minneapolis	144	Lys→Asn	13, 14	PO_4	11
C. γ-Chain Variants					
F-Meinohama	5	Glu→Gly	1	NH_4Ac	40
F-Pordenone	6	Glu→Gln	1	NH_4Ac	41
F-Bonaire-Ga	39	Gln→Arg	5	NH_4Ac	42
F-Kennestone	77	His→Arg	10	NH_4Ac	43
F-Marietta	80	Asp→Asn	10	NH_4Ac	44
F-Columbus-Ga	94	Asp→Asn	11	NH_4Ac	45
F-Malta I	117	His→Arg	13	NH_4Ac	14
F-Caltech	120	Lys→Gln	13, 14	TFA	46
D. δ-Chain Variants					
A'_2	16	Gly→Arg	2	NH_4Ac	14
A_2 Flatbush	22	Ala→Glu	3	NH_4Ac	14

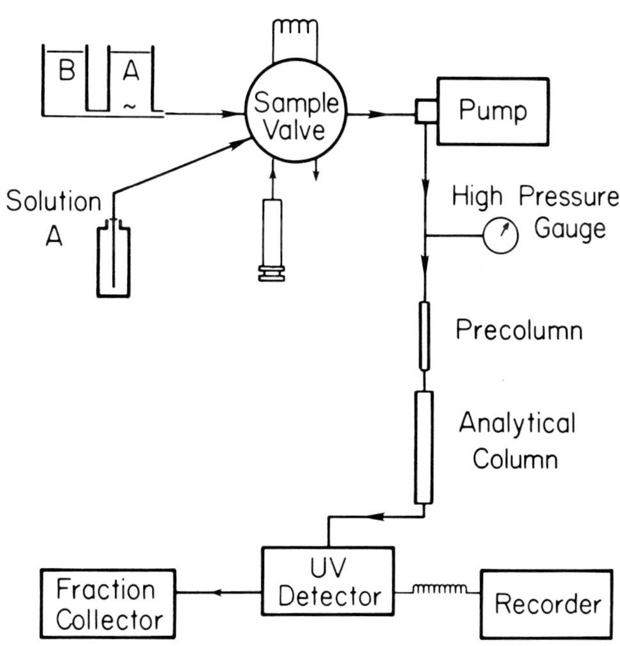

FIGURE 4. A diagram of a simple HPLC system which can be assembled from parts and used for separating peptide fragments of hemoglobins.

sample injection and alternate solvent reservoirs, a high-pressure pump and pressure gauge, a pre- or guard column, the analytical column, a flow-through photometer with UV detection at 220 nm, a chart recorder, and a fraction collector. Schroeder et al.[6] have used such a system for the separation of tryptic peptides of hemoglobins and Congote et al.[18] have described it in more detail for separation of globin chains of hemoglobin. Such a simple

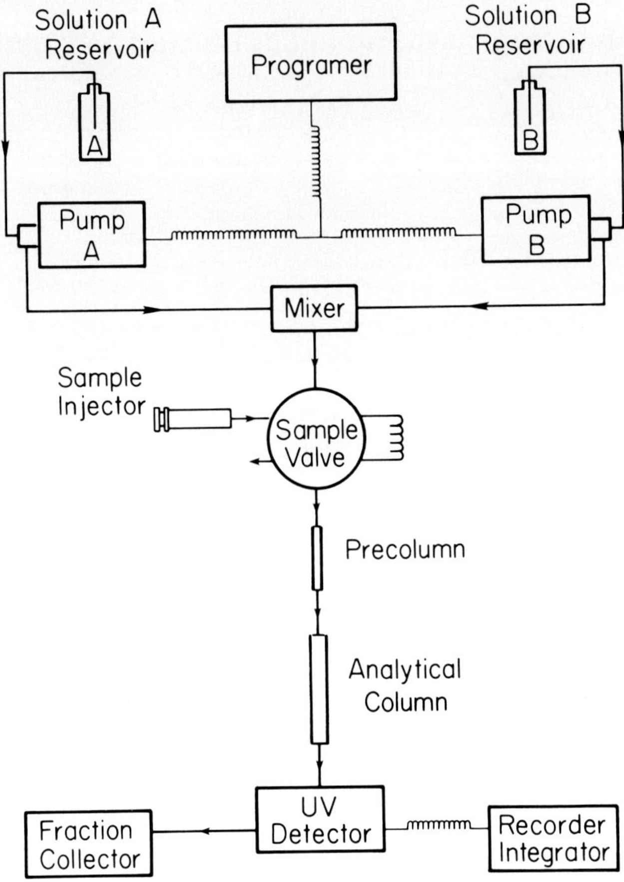

FIGURE 5. Diagram of a complete, programmable two-pump HPLC system used for automatic separation of peptide fragments of hemoglobin.

system can be assembled using spare components from peptide analyzers[4] or amino acid analyzers and other laboratory equipment with minimal expense.

A more contemporary and versatile two-pump, programmable HPLC system is diagrammed in Figure 5. It consists of a microprocessor programming unit, two HPLC pumps, a mixing chamber, a sample injection valve, a guard column, an analytical column, a UV detector, a recorder-integrator, and a fraction collector. Although several different complete systems are commercially available and in use (see References 10 and 14 for examples), the author has successfully employed a Beckman-Altex Model 332 HPLC system which is comprised of a Model 420 microprocessor controller unit, two Model 110A single-piston, reciprocating pumps, a gradient mixing chamber, a Model 210 syringe-loading sample injection valve with a 250-$\mu\ell$ sample loop; a Waters μBondapak C_{18}/Corasil guard column, a 10 × 250 mm Altex Ultrasphere-ODS C_{18} reverse-phase column, a model 100-30 Altex/Hitachi UV-Vis variable-wavelength detector modified with an 8-$\mu\ell$ analytical flow cell, and the printer-plotter of a Hewlett Packard HP 5830A gas chromatograph system. A simple strip chart recorder (Brinkman Model 2541) has been substituted for the Hewlett Packard printer-plotter from time to time when the latter is unavailable for use with the HPLC system. A Gilson Model FC-80K microfraction collector with either 10 × 75 mm borosilicate glass culture tubes or a Gilson Model 26107 disposable plastic collecting plate is used to collect effluent from tubing connected to the spectrophotometer flow cell.

Three different analytical columns and one preparative column have been evaluated in the author's laboratory for separation of tryptic peptides of aminoethylated and nonaminoethylated globin chains. These are the 4.6 × 250 mm Altex Lichrosorb C18 5 μm column, the 3.9 × 300 mm Waters μBondapak C_{18} column, the 4.6 × 250 mm Altex Ultrasphere ODS C18 5 μm analytical column, and the 10 × 250 mm Altex Ultrasphere ODS C18 5 μm preparative column. Although all of these columns give good separations of tryptic peptides, we are currently using the 10 × 250 mm Altex Ultrasphere ODS C_{18} preparative column for structural characterizations of abnormal hemoglobins. Schroeder et al.[9,10] have compared a variety of HPLC columns and prefer the separations obtained with the 4.6 × 250 mm Altex Ultrasphere ODS column.[10,11] Huisman and co-workers[14,17] continue to use the 3.9 × 300 mm Waters μBondapak C_{18} column. Although Schroeder et al.[10] point out that a guard column is not necessary, a precolumn packed with μBondapak C_{18}/Corasil is used with the author's system in the hope that it will prolong the useful lifetime of the main column.

PROCEDURES FOR SEPARATION OF TRYPTIC PEPTIDES OF HEMOGLOBIN BY HPLC

HPLC can be applied to the separation of peptides from the tryptic hydrolysis of hemoglobin,[10] globin,[10] unmodified globin chains,[14] aminoethylated globin chains,[14] and aminoethylated-glycinamidated globin chains.[10,19] The reader should consult appropriate references for the procedures used in isolating pure hemoglobin components,[20] preparing globin,[21] separating globin chains,[22] chemically modifying to form the aminoethylated[3,22] and/or glycinamidated[23] chains, oxidizing chains,[24,25] and further enzymatic hydrolysis of tryptic cores.[26] The procedures and formulations used in the author's laboratory for tryptic hydrolysis, sample preparation and application, developer solutions, gradient and other HPLC conditions, and rechromatography are described below.

Tryptic Hydrolysis and Sample Preparation

Between 10 and 20 mg of globin chain is dissolved in 1 mℓ of distilled or deionized water. To this are added 0.1 mℓ of 0.8 *M* ammonium bicarbonate and 100 μℓ TPCK-treated trypsin (2 mg/mℓ, Worthington). The pH is checked with narrow-range pH paper, and more 0.8 *M* ammonium bicarbonate is added if the pH is below 8.0. The hydrolysis is carried out at 37°C for 2 hr in the case of aminoethylated or glycinamidated globin chains, and 4 hr in the case of chemically unmodified globin chains. The mixture is then adjusted to a pH between 2 and 3 with 2 *M* acetic acid, and dried by lyophylization. The dried peptide mixture is redissolved with 0.625 mℓ of the starting or A developer solution per 10 mg of original protein, and any solid material is removed first by centrifugation for 10 min at 3000 rpm, and then by filtering the supernatant through a 0.45-μm Millipore filter; 250 μℓ containing the tryptic peptides of 4 mg of original material is then loaded into the sample application loop.

Developer Conditions

Two different pairs of developer solutions have been in general use for separating tryptic peptides of hemoglobin. Both are used with several different linear gradient conditions. The composition of developer solutions and gradient conditions used in the author's laboratory are given below.

The ammonium acetate-acetonitrile developer system, originally described by Stoming et al.[13] and adapted by Schroeder et al.[6] for peptide separation, has the following composition: Solution A is 0.01 *M* ammonium acetate (0.77 g/ℓ) adjusted to pH 6.07 with about 4 drops of 5 *M* acetic acid. If a system with a two-chamber gradient device and one HPLC pump is used, then solution B should be prepared to contain 40% acetonitrile by volume and 60% of Solution A (0.01 ammonium acetate, pH 6.07). If a two-pump, programmable HPLC system is to be used, Solution B can be 100% acetonitrile. Reagent grade ammonium acetate and glacial acetic acid, such as "Baker Analyzed Reagents", and deionized water which has passed a 0.22-μm filter in the water line are used in the author's laboratory for preparing Solution A. After the pH of Solution A has been adjusted to 6.07, it is filtered through a 0.45-μm HA aqueous filter (Millipore Corporation) and used fresh or stored at 0°C for up to 2 weeks before using. Because of impurities present in some sources of acetonitrile which absorb strongly at and above 220 nm, this reagent must either be purified further, or a special reagent grade suitable for spectrophotometry and liquid chromatography must be obtained. Many laboratories, including the author's, have found the Burdick and Jackson Laboratories Inc. "Distilled in Glass" spectrophotometric grade to be satisfactory. It can be used directly without further purification or filtration. Another commercial source of acetonitrile reported to be satisfactory is Aldrich gold label 99+% spectrophotometric grade.[6] Probably any prefiltered, HPLC grade acetonitrile would be satisfactory.[10]

The phosphate-acetonitrile developer system originally described by Johnson et al.[8] has the following composition: Solution A is 0.049 *M* KH_2PO_4 (6.66 g/ℓ Baker Analyzed Reagents) and 0.0054 *M* H_3PO_4 (0.37 mℓ 86.3% H_3PO_4 per liter, Baker Analyzed Reagent). The pH of this solution has been reported to be 2.86[8] and 2.95.[10] In the author's laboratory, no adjustment of pH is made as long as it is in the range of 2.9 to 3.0 and the molarities of the constituents are correct. This is also prepared from deionized water and the solution is passed through a 0.45-μm HA aqueous filter (Millipore Corporation). It is used fresh or stored at room temperature for up to 1 month. If a two-chamber gradient device is used, Solution B is prepared to contain 40% acetonitrile by volume and 60% Solution A. A third Solution C is also prepared to contain 55% acetonitrile and 45% Solution A. For the two pump-programmable HPLC system, the second or B Solution can be 100% acetonitrile. The need for a "spectrophotometer" grade of acetonitrile noted above also applies to this phosphate-acetonitrile developer system.

The conditions for pre-equilibration of the column, application of sample development of the chromatogram, and re-equilibration of the column using either the ammonium acetate-acetonitrile or the phosphate-acetonitrile developer systems for routine purposes are the same and as follows: the column is pre-equilibrated by pumping Solution A at 1 mℓ/min for the 3.9 × 300 mm Waters μBondapak C_{18} column or 1.5 mℓ/min for the 10 × 250 mm Altex Ultrasphere ODS C_{18} column for 20 min or longer. At the time the development program is started, 250 μℓ of a sample containing 4 mg of tryptic hydrolysate dissolved in Solution A is injected into the HPLC system. Development of the chromatogram is begun at the time the sample is injected. A simple development can be obtained by pumping 100% Solution A for 5 min followed by a gradient beginning at 100% of Solution A and 0% Solution B and going to 60% Solution A and 40% Solution B by the end of 85 min. The developer condition is then changed back to 100% Solution A in 5 min and pumped for another 5 min before stopping. Under these conditions the column is ready for another sample without requiring further equilibration. As suggested by Schroeder et al.,[6,7] the column can be cleaned while the developer ratio is 60% Solution A and 40% Solution B by injecting a series of 2-mℓ quantities of 100% acetonitrile followed by 60:40 ratio of Solution A to Solution B.

Different gradients that are more or less steep and either interrupted or not can be used. A prolonged ammonium acetate-acetonitrile gradient program which takes 210 min has been described by Nakatsuji et al.[17] and gives excellent separations of most tryptic peptides, but at the expense of time and reagents. Schroeder et al.[10,11] have demonstrated very good separations of tryptic peptides of globin containing both α- and β-chains using a phosphate-acetonitrile gradient program with four different steps. The developer conditions for the chromatogram illustrated in this chapter are given in the legends of the figures.

Detection and Recovery of Peptides

The peptides are detected in the column effluent by the absorption of the carbonyl bond

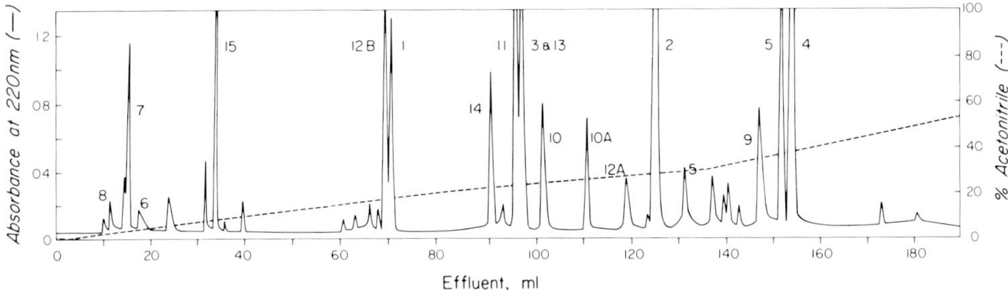

FIGURE 6. HPLC separation of the tryptic peptides of 4 mg of aminoethylated β-chain from normal Hb A, using a 10 × 250 mm Altex Ultrasphere ODS C_{18} column and a gradient of potassium phosphate and acetonitrile developers at 1.5 mℓ/min (0% acetonitrile for 3 mℓ, to 18% in 72 mℓ, to 28% in 60 mℓ, to 62% in 68 mℓ, and back to 0% in 15 mℓ).

which can be measured at 220 nm, a wavelength at which the developers have relatively low and constant absorption. An appropriate combination of sensitivity settings of the spectrophotometer and recorder is made to give 0.5 to 1.5 absorbance units for full scale recorder sensitivity (AUFS). The effluent is collected in small fraction volumes of 0.5 to 2 mℓ per tube. The effluent containing a single peptide peak is dried by rotary evaporation or lyophylization and either hydrolyzed with 6 *M* HCl for amino acid analysis or dissolved in the starting developer solution for rechromatography with a different developer system, gradient, or HPLC column.

EXAMPLES OF SEPARATION OF PEPTIDES FROM ABNORMAL HEMOGLOBINS AND GLOBIN CHAINS

Many examples of HPLC separations of tryptic peptides of hemoglobins and their separated chains can be found in the References given for this chapter. In addition to those shown in Figures 1 to 3, a few other examples may be helpful. The actual chromatographic patterns obtained will vary mostly with the type of developer solutions and gradient used and less with different columns of the same basic structure.

Figure 6 shows the separation of the tryptic peptides of about 4 mg of aminoethylated β-chains of normal hemoglobin A (Hb A). This was obtained using a 10 × 250 mm Altex Ultrasphere ODS C_{18} column and the 49 m*M* KH_2PO_4 and 5.4 m*M* H_3PO_4 developer as Solution A and 100% acetonitrile as Solution B. A flow rate of 1.5 mℓ/min was used with developer ratios as given in the figure legend. Although many of the β-chain tryptic peptides can be isolated in pure form from this single chromatographic step, some peptides like βT-3, βT-11, and βT-13 elute close together under the conditions used. These peptides, which elute between 94 and 98 mℓ with the potassium phosphate-acetonitrile developer, can be separated more completely by rechromatography using the same column but with a gradient of ammonium acetate-acetonitrile, as shown in Figure 7. The gradient conditions are given in the figure legend. Rechromatography of the peptides which elute near the front of chromatograms developed with the potassium phosphate-acetonitrile buffers generally results in good separations when done with an initial isocratic step with only the ammonium acetate Solution A, followed by a slowly changing gradient with acetonitrile.

Figure 8 shows the separation of the tryptic peptides of the aminoethylated α-chains of Hb Oleander [$\alpha_2$116 (GH4) Glu → Glnβ_2][27] using the potassium phosphate-acetonitrile developer gradient and the 10 × 250 mm Altex Ultrasphere ODS C_{18} column. The location of each peptide is given. The position of the abnormal αT-12B peptide is indicated by the arrow. Rechromatography of the region of this chromatogram containing this abnormal tryptic peptide and the normal αT-9 is illustrated in Figure 9. In this case, the same gradient and

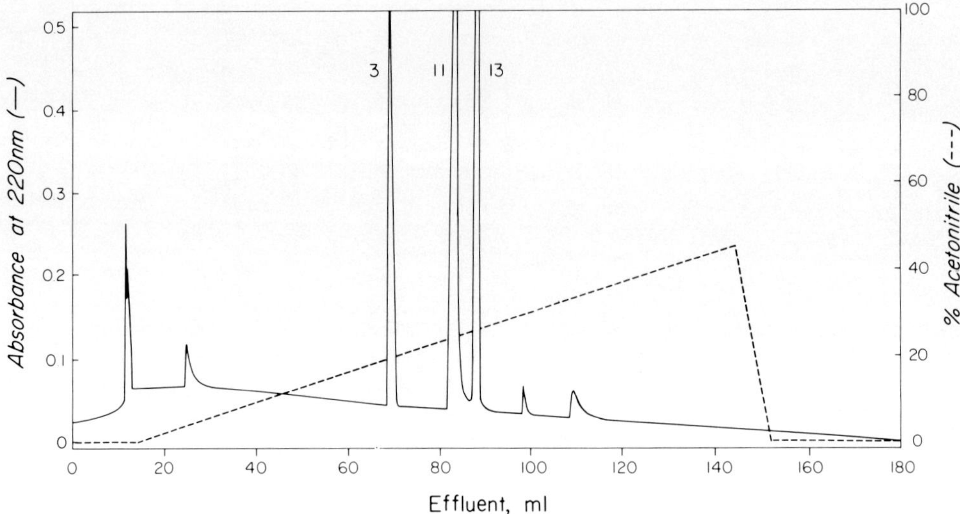

FIGURE 7. Rechromatography of the region of the chromatogram shown in Figure 6, containing βT-11, βT-3, and βT-13 (94 and 98 mℓ of effluent). The same column as for Figure 6 was used for this rechromatography; however, the development was made with an ammonium acetate-acetonitrile gradient at 1.5 mℓ/min (0% acetonitrile for 15 mℓ and then to 45% acetonitrile in 135 mℓ).

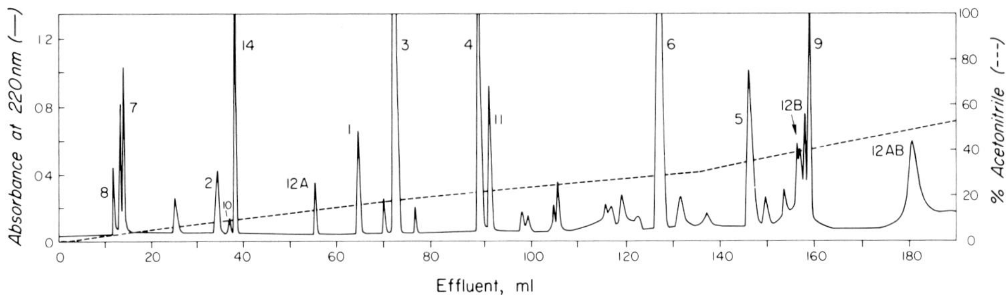

FIGURE 8. HPLC separation of the tryptic peptides of the abnormal aminoethylated α-chain of Hb Oleander [α_2 116 (GH4) Glu→Gln β_2] on a 10 × 250 mm Altex Ultrasphere ODS C_{18} column using a gradient of potassium phosphate and acetonitrile at 1.5 mℓ/min (0% acetonitrile for 3 mℓ, to 18% to 72 mℓ, to 28% in 60 mℓ, to 62% in 68 mℓ, and to 0% in 15 mℓ). Approximately 4 mg of tryptic hydrolysate was loaded. The abnormal αT-12B peptide is identified by an arrow. This was not shifted appreciably from the position of the normal αT-12B peptide under these conditions.

column were used with the ammonium acetate-acetonitrile developer system. For comparison, the rechromatography of the same region from the separation of a tryptic hydrolysate of normal aminoethylated α-chain is shown in Figure 10.

For the determination of the abnormal structure of Hb Oleander, Schneider et al.[27] isolated the chymotryptic peptides of the aminoethylated abnormal αT-12B tryptic peptide by HPLC. This separation is illustrated in Figure 11. The amino acid compositions of the peptides in the five main peaks provided sufficient information to deduce the location of the substituted residue in this abnormal hemoglobin.

Figure 12 shows the location of aberrant tryptic peptides of 11 different mutant hemoglobins studied by Schroeder et al.[11] This illustrates the utility of the potassium phosphate-acetonitrile HPLC developer system to separate the tryptic peptides of samples of whole hemoglobin. Schroeder and co-workers have demonstrated that many variants can be identified in this way without separating chains or even removing the heme before tryptic

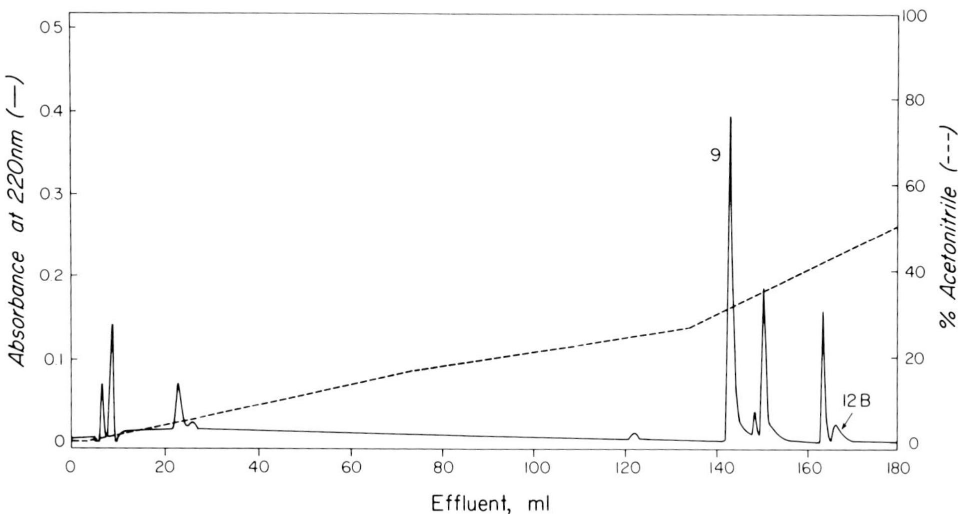

FIGURE 9. Rechromatography of the region of the chromatogram shown in Figure 6 which contained the abnormal αT-12B and the normal αT-9 tryptic peptides of Hb Oleander (154 to 160 mℓ effluent volumes). The same column as for Figure 8 was used for the rechromatography; however, the development was made with an ammonium acetate-acetonitrile gradient at 1.5 mℓ/min (changes in percent acetonitrile same as for Figure 8).

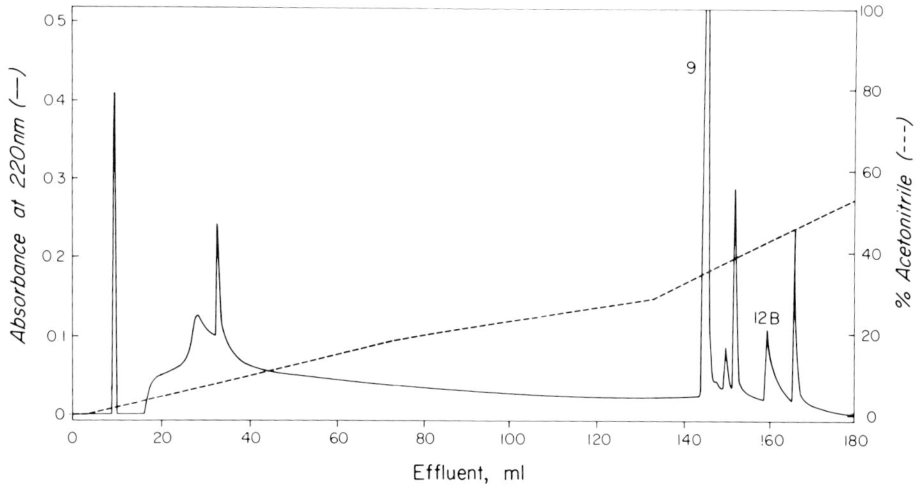

FIGURE 10. Rechromatography of the same region as used for Figure 9, but from an initial chromatogram prepared from the aminoethylated α-chain of normal Hb A. Otherwise, all of the conditions were the same as given in Figures 8 and 9.

hydrolysis. As can be seen from this figure, all of these variants can be differentiated from normal Hb A by a change in position of one or more tryptic peptides. Wilson et al.[14] have demonstrated the utility of the ammonium acetate-acetonitrile HPLC developer system for identification of 25 different hemoglobin variants by separating the tryptic peptides of the soluble tryptic peptides of the α-chain and aminoethylated (AE) β-, γ-, and δ-chains; 23 of these are illustrated in Figure 13, which is a composite of three figures from the paper by Wilson et al.[14] The location of the normal and aberrant tryptic peptides is shown for each chain. Although these authors examined the insoluble or core region of the α-chain by separating the chymotryptic peptides of the oxidized α-chain core, it is possible to isolate

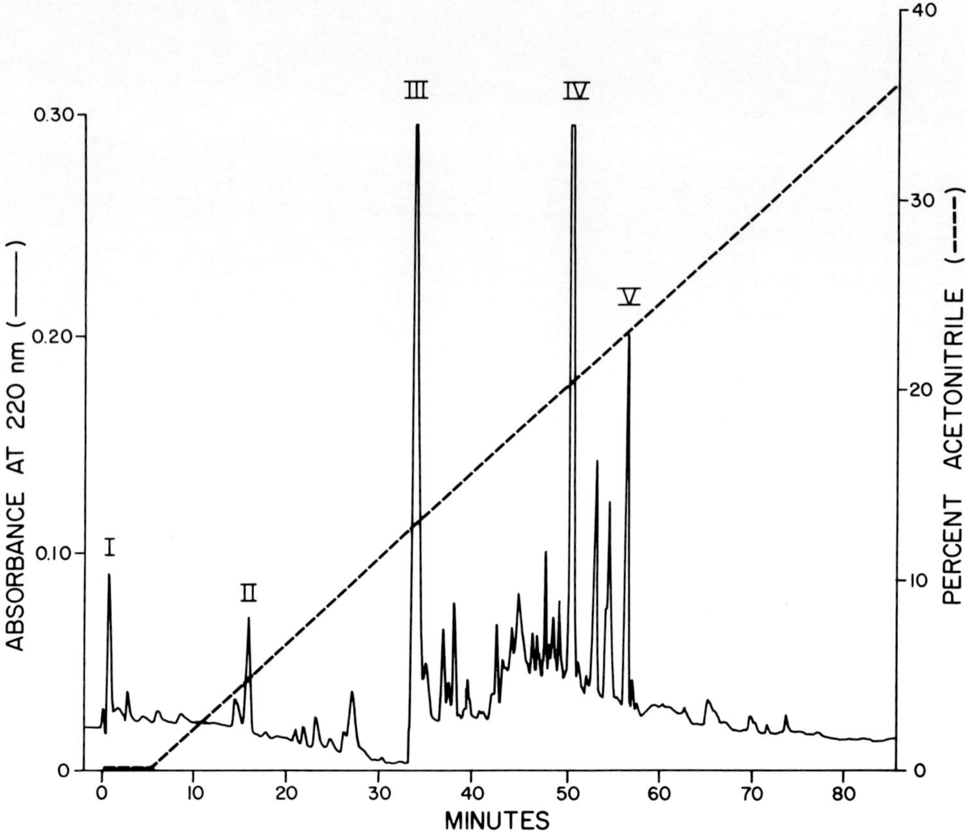

FIGURE 11. Separation of the chymotryptic peptides of glycinamidated αT-12B from Hb Oleander. A 4.6 × 250 mm Altex Ultrasphere ODS C_{18} column was used with a gradient of ammonium acetate-acetonitrile developer at 1 mℓ/min (0% acetonitrile for 5 mℓ and then 0 to 40% acetonitrile in 95 mℓ). (From Schneider, R. G. et al., *Hemoglobin,* 6, 465, 1982. With permission.)

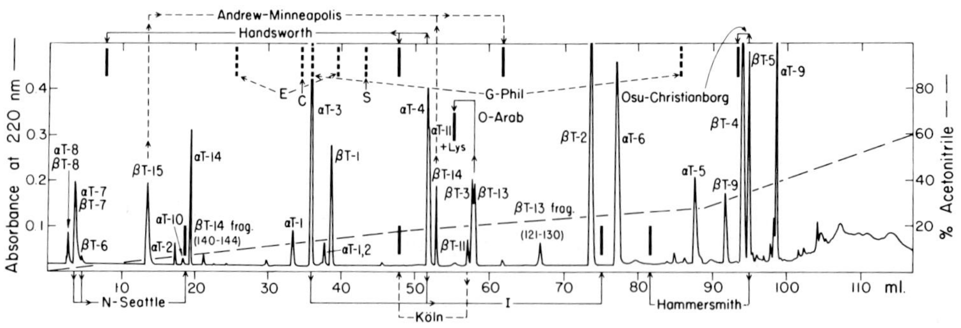

FIGURE 12. HPLC separation of the tryptic peptides of Hb A as shown in Figure 2 with the positions of aberrant peptides of 12 different mutant human hemoglobins. The positions of the abnormal peptides of the more common variants are shown by dashed bars. The solid bars are for the positions of the peptides of less common mutants. The chromatographic conditions are those given in Figure 2. (From Schroeder, W. A. et al., *Biochem. Genet.,* 20, 133, 1982. With permission.)

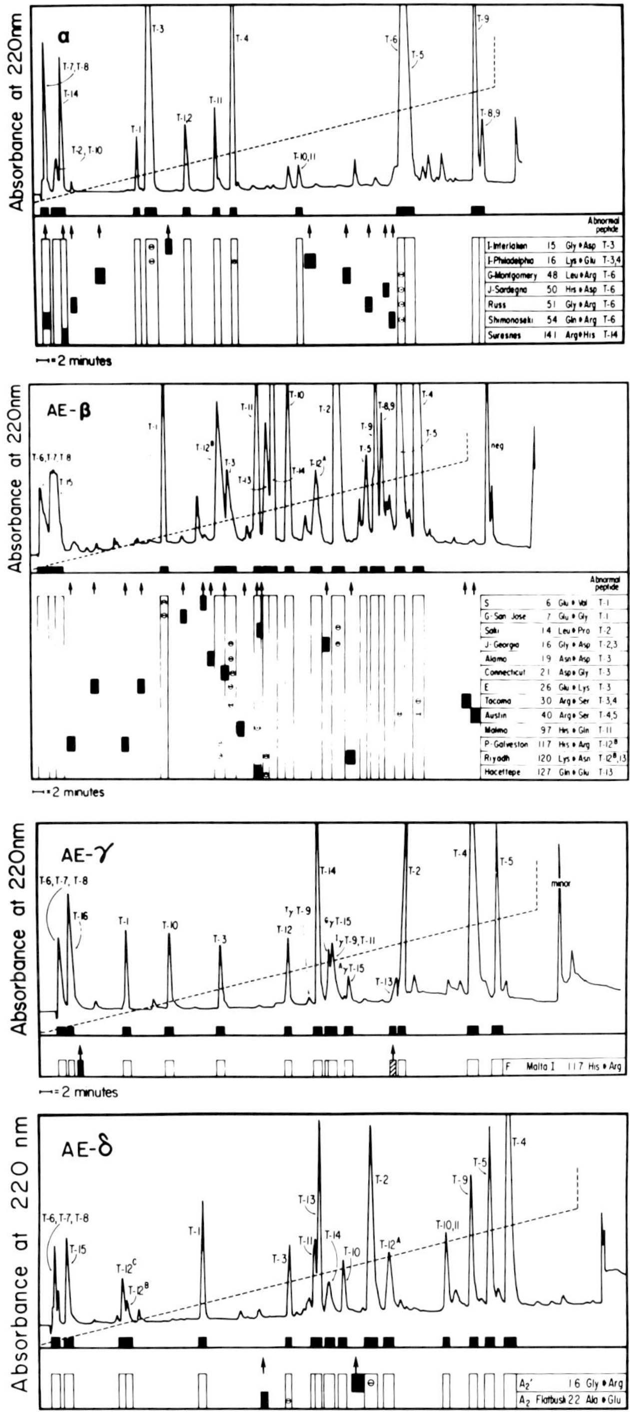

FIGURE 13. The HPLC separations of the tryptic peptides, from top to bottom, are native α-; aminoethylated β-; aminoethylated γ-; aminoethylated δ-chains. The positions of aberrant peptides of 23 different human hemoglobin variants are also shown. In each case, about 2 to 3 mg of tryptic digests were separated on a 3.9 × 300 mm Waters μBondapak C_{18} column using a linear gradient of ammonium acetate-acetonitrile developers at 1.5 mℓ/min beginning at 0% acetonitrile and going to 30% acetonitrile in 120 min or 180 mℓ effluent volume. The θ denotes the absence of a normally occurring peptide from the chromatogram of the variant and the replacement by one or two others indicated by ■ and ↑ .[14] (From Wilson, J. B., et al., *J. Chromatogr.*, 179, 271, 1979. With permission.)

αT-12A and αT-12B from tryptic digests of aminoethylated α-chain as illustrated in Figure 8.

Table 1 lists the publications of abnormal hemoglobins which have been examined to date by HPLC and includes the chain, residue, amino acid substitution, abnormal tryptic peptide, developer system used, and reference for each.

SUMMARY

As reported in the literature and illustrated above, reverse-phase HPLC has been applied with considerable success to the chemical characterization of abnormal human hemoglobins. Although various combinations of samples, columns, developers, and HPLC equipment have been reported, all of these variations have in common high sensitivity, rapid and reproducible separations, and nondestructive recovery of pure or partially purified peptides. This method of separating tryptic peptides of abnormal hemoglobins appears to be superior to the paper "finger printing" and conventional ion exchange column chromatography. Its potential for application to studies of chemical modification of hemoglobins, biosynthesis, and sequence studies of other animal hemoglobin appears to be as great as the ingenuity of the experimenter who chooses to employ this approach. One limitation which requires further work and improvement is the variable yield or recovery of some peptides.[9] This limits the application of HPLC separation of peptides in cases where yields approaching 100% recovery are required.

ACKNOWLEDGMENT

Technical assistance from Mrs. Charlotte Head is gratefully acknowledged. Appreciation is expressed to the authors and publishers who hold the copyrights, for permission to reproduce their illustrations in Figures 1, 2, 3, 11, 12, and 13 and for which specific references are cited. Dr. W. A. Schroeder and Dr. T. H. J. Huisman considerately supplied photographs of their original drawings. Some of the work described in this chapter was supported by USPHS Research Grant AM17850.

REFERENCES

1. **Ingram, V.,** Abnormal haemoglobin. I. The comparison of normal human and sickle-cell haemoglobin by "fingerprinting", *Biochim. Biophys. Acta,* 28, 539, 1958.
2. **Schroeder, W. A., Jones, R. T., Cormick, J., and McCalla, K.,** Chromatographic separation of peptides on ion exchange resins: separation of peptides from enzymatic hydrolyzates of the α, β, and γ chains of human hemoglobins, *Anal. Chem.,* 34, 1570, 1962.
3. **Jones, R. T.,** Structural studies of aminoethylated hemoglobin by automatic peptide chromatography, *Cold Spring Harbor Symp. Quant. Biol.,* 29, 297, 1964.
4. **Jones, R. T.,** Automatic peptide chromatography, *Meth. Biochem. Anal.,* 18, 205, 1970.
5. **Congote, L. F., Bennett, H. P. J., and Solomon, S.,** Rapid separation of the α, β, $^{G}\gamma$, and $^{A}\gamma$ human globin chains by reversed-phase high pressure liquid chromatography, *Biochem. Biophys. Res. Commun.,* 89, 851, 1979.
6. **Schroeder, W. A., Shelton, J. B., Shelton, J. R., and Powers, D.,** Separation of peptides by high pressure liquid chromatography for the identification of a hemoglobin variant, *J. Chromatogr.,* 174, 385, 1979.
7. **Schroeder, W. A., Shelton, J. B., Shelton, J. R., and Powers, D.,** Hemoglobin Sunshine-Seth α_2(94 (G1)Asp → His)β_2, *Hemoglobin,* 3, 145, 1979.
8. **Johnson, C. S., Moyes, D., Schroeder, W. A., Shelton, J. B., Shelton, J. R., and Beutler, E.,** Hemoglobin Pasadena, $\alpha_2\beta_2$ 75(E19) Leu → Arg. Identification by high performance liquid chromatography of a new unstable variant with increased oxygen affinity, *Biochim. Biophys. Acta,* 623, 360, 1980.

9. **Schroeder, W. A., Shelton, J. B., and Shelton, J. R.,** Separation of hemoglobin peptides by high performance liquid chromatography (HPLC), *Hemoglobin,* 4, 551, 1980.
10. **Schroeder, W. A., Shelton, J. B., and Shelton, J. R.,** High performance liquid chromatography in the identification of human hemoglobin variants, in *Adv. Hemoglobin Anal. Progr. Clin. Biol. Res.,* Vol. 60, Hanash, S. M. and Brewer, G. J., Eds., Alan R. Liss, New York, 1981, 1.
11. **Schroeder, W. A., Shelton, J. B., Shelton, J. R., Powers, D., Friedman, S., Baker, J., Finklestein, J. Z., Miller, B., Johnson, C. S., Sharpsteen, J. R., Sieger, L., and Kawaoka, E.,** Identification of eleven human hemoglobin variants by high-performance liquid chromatography: additional data on functional properties and clinical expression, *Biochem. Genet.,* 20, 133, 1982.
12. **Efremov, G. D., Wilson, J. B., and Huisman, T. H. J.,** The chemical heterogeneity of human hemoglobin F. Direct evidence for the existence of three types of γ chains, the $^{G}\gamma^{I}$, $^{A}\gamma^{I}$, and $^{A}\gamma^{T}$ chains, *Biochim. Biophys. Acta,* 579, 421, 1979..
13. **Stroming, T. A., Garver, F. A., Gangarosa, M. A., Harrison, J. M., and Huisman, T. H. J.,** Separation of the $^{A}\gamma$ and $^{G}\gamma$ cyanogen bromide peptides of human fetal hemoglobin by high-pressure liquid chromatography, *Anal. Biochem.,* 96, 113, 1979.
14. **Wilson, J. B., Lam, H., Pravatmuang, P., and Huisman, T. H. J.,** Separation of tryptic peptides of normal and abnormal α, β, γ, and δ hemoglobin chains by high-performance liquid chromatography, *J. Chromatogr.,* 179, 271, 1979.
15. **Ibarra, B., Franco-Gamboa, E., Ramirez, M. L., Cantú, J. M., Wilson, J. B., Lam, H., and Huisman, T. H. J.,** Hb Chiapas $\alpha_2$114 Pro $\rightarrow$ Arg β_2: identification by high pressure liquid chromatography, *Hemoglobin,* 6, 605, 1981.
16. **Zeng, Y. T., Shu-Zheng, H., Xu, L., Gui-fang, L., Lam, H., Wilson, J. B., and Huisman, T. H. J.,** Hb Wuming or α_2 11(A9)Lys $\rightarrow$ Gln β_2, *Hemoglobin,* 5, 679, 1981.
17. **Nakatsuji, T., Wilson, J. B., Lam, H., and Huisman, T. H. J.,** Identification and quantitation of Hb Olympia [β20(B2)Val $\rightarrow$ Met] and Hb San Diego [β109(G11)Val $\rightarrow$ Met] by high performance liquid chromatography, *J. Chromatogr.,* 259, 511, 1983.
18. **Congote, L. F.,** Reverse-phase high pressure liquid chromatography of globin chains: its application of the prenatal diagnosis of β-thalassemia, *Adv. Hemoglobin Anal.; Progr. Clin. Biol. Res.,* 60, 39, 1981.
19. **Jones, R. T.,** unpublished data, 1983.
20. **Schroeder, W. A. and Huisman, T. H. J.,** The chromatography of hemoglobin, *Clin. Biochem. Anal.,* 9, 1, 1980.
21. **Anson, M. L and Mirsky, A. E.,** Protein coagulation and its reversal, *J. Gen. Physiol.,* 13, 469, 1930.
22. **Clegg, J. B., Naughton, M. A., and Weatherall, D. J.,** Abnormal human haemoglobins: separation and characterization of the α and β chains by chromatography, and the determination of two new variants, Hb Chesapeake and Hb J (Bangkok), *J. Mol. Biol.,* 19, 91, 1966.
23. **Jones, R. T., Casey, R., Brimhall, B.,** Application of glycinamidation to structural studies of hemoglobin, *Anal. Biochem.,* 75, 241, 1976.
24. **Neumann, N. P.,** Oxidation with hydrogen peroxide, *Methods Enzymol.,* 25, 393, 1972.
25. **Huisman, T. H. J. and Jonxis, J. H. P.,** *The Hemoglobinopathies: Techniques of Identification,* Marcel Dekker, New York, 1977, 214.
26. **Schroeder, W. A., Shelton, J. R., Shelton, J. B., Cormick, J., and Jones, R. T.,** The amino acid sequence of the γ chain of human fetal hemoglobin, *Biochemistry,* 2, 992, 1963.
27. **Schneider, R. G., Hightower, B., Carpentieri, U., Duerst, M. L., Shih, T. B., and Jones, R. T.,** Hemoglobin Oleander [$\alpha_2$116(GH4)Glu $\rightarrow$ Glnβ_2]: structural and functional characterization, *Hemoglobin,* 6, 465, 1982.
28. **Johnson, C. S., Schroeder, W. A., Shelton, J. B., and Shelton, J. R.,** The first example of a deletion in the human α chain: hemoglobin Boyle Heights or $\alpha_2$6(A4)Asp $\rightarrow$ oβ_2, *Hemoglobin,* 7, 125, 1983.
29. **Webber, B. B., Lam, H., Wilson, J. B., and Huisman, T. H. J.,** Hb Albany-GA or α_2 11(A9)Lys $\rightarrow$ Asn β_2, *Hemoglobin,* 7, 257, 1983.
30. **Nakatsuji, T., Abraham, B. L., Lam, H., Wilson, J. B., and Huisman, T. H. J.,** Hb Winnipeg or α_2 75(EF4)Asp $\rightarrow$ Tyr β_2 in a large caucasian family living in Georgia, USA, *Hemoglobin,* 7, 105, 1983.
31. **Headlee, M. G., Nakatsuji, T., Lam, H., Wrightstone, R. N., and Huisman, T. H. J.,** Hb Etobicoke, α85(F5) Ser $\rightarrow$ Arg found in a newborn of French-Indian-English descent, *Hemoglobin,* 7, 285, 1983.
32. **Moo-Penn, W. F., Johnson, M. H., McGuffey, J. E., Jue, D. L., and Therrell, B. L., Jr.,** Hemoglobin Rio Grande [β8 (A5) Lys $\rightarrow$ Thr], a new variant found in a Mexican-American family, *Hemoglobin,* 7, 91, 1983.
33. **Boissel, J. P., Wajcman, H., Fabritius, H., Cabannes, R., and Labie, D.,** Application of high performance liquid chromatography to abnormal hemoglobin studies. Characterization of hemoglobins D in Ivory Coast and description of a new variant Hb Cocody [β21 (B3) Asp $\rightarrow$ Asn], *Biochim. Biophys. Acta,* 670, 203, 1981.
34. **Brennen, S. O., Williamson, D., Whisson, M. E., and Carrel, R. W.,** Hemoglobin Palmerston North β23 (B5) Val $\rightarrow$ Phe, a new variant identified in a patient with polycythemia, *Hemoglobin,* 6, 569, 1982.

35. **Sciarratta, G. V., Sansone, G., Valbonesi, M., Wilson, J. B., Lam, H., Webber, B. B., Headlee, M. E., and Huisman, T. H. J.,** Hb Cheverly or $\alpha_2\beta_2$ 45 (CD4) Phe → Ser in an elderly Italian male, *Hemoglobin,* 6, 419, 1982.
36. **Honig, G. R., Shamsuddi, M., Vida, L. N., Mompoint, M., Valcourt, E., and Borders, M.,** A third American black family with Hb J Bangkok: association of Hb J Bangkok with Hb C, *Hemoglobin,* 6, 635, 1982.
37. **Boissel, J. R., Wajcman, H., Labie, D., Fabritius, H., and Cabannes, R.,** Hb J Doloa [β57(E1)Asn → Asp]: a new variant found in Ivory Coast, *Hemoglobin,* 6, 433, 1982.
38. **Honig, G. R., Seeler, R. A., Shamsuddin, M., Vida, L. N., Mompoint, M., and Valcourt, E.,** Hemoglobin Korle Bu in a Mexican family, *Hemoglobin,* 7, 185, 1983.
39. **Bogoevski, P., Efremov, G. D., Kezic, J., Lam, H., Wilson, J. B., and Huisman, T. H. J.,** Hb Sabine or $\alpha_2\beta_2$ 91(F7)Leu → Pro in a Yugoslavian boy, *Hemoglobin,* 7, 195, 1983.
40. **Ohta, Y., Saito, S., Fujita, S., Wilson, J. B., Lam, H., and Huisman, T. H. J.,** Hb F-Meinohoma or $\alpha_2\gamma_2$ (5 Glu → Gly; 75 Ile; 136 Gly), *Hemoglobin,* 5, 565, 1981.
41. **Nakatsuji, T., Webber, B., Lam, H., Wilson, J. B., Huisman, T. H. J., Sciarratta, G. V., Sansone, G., and Molaro, G. L.,** A new γ chain variant: Hb F-Pordenone [γ6(A3)Glu → Gln: 75Ile: 136Ala], *Hemoglobin,* 6, 397, 1982.
42. **Nakatsuji, T., Headlee, M., Lam, H., Wilson, J. B., and Huisman, T. H. J.,** Hb F-Bonaire-Ga or $\alpha_2{}^{A}\gamma_2$ 39(C5) Gln → Arg, characterized by high pressure liquid chromatographic and microsequencing procedures, *Hemoglobin,* 6, 599, 1982.
43. **Nakatsuji, T., Lam, H., and Huisman, T. H. J.,** Hb F-Kennestone or $\alpha_2{}^{G}\gamma_2$ (E1) 77 His → Arg observed in a caucasian baby, *Hemoglobin,* 7, 267, 1983.
44. **Nakatsuji, T., Lam, H., Carver, J., and Huisman, T. H. J.,** Hb F-Marietta or ${}^{G}\gamma^{I}$ 80 (EF4) Asp → Asn observed in a caucasian baby, *Hemoglobin,* 6, 407, 1982.
45. **Nakatsuji, T., Lam, H., Wilson, J. B., Webber, B. B., and Huisman, T. H. J.,** Hb F-Columbia-Ga or $\alpha_2{}^{G}\gamma_2$ 94(FG1)Asp → Asn, *Hemoglobin,* 6, 593, 1982.
46. **Shelton, J. B., Shelton, J. R., Espinueva, Z., Huynh, V., Schroeder, W. A., and Powers, D.,** Hemoglobin F-Caltech: $\alpha_2{}^{G}\gamma_2$ 120Lys → Glu, *Hemoglobin,* 6, 577, 1982.

THE SEPARATION OF GLOBIN CHAINS BY HIGH PERFORMANCE LIQUID CHROMATOGRAPHY

Walter A. Schroeder

INTRODUCTION

The ability to separate the globin chains of a hemoglobin (Hb) has been of much utility whether the desired information be structural, functional, or biosynthetic. The most widely used method for achieving a separation of globin chains is the chromatographic procedure of Clegg et al.,[1] which uses a phosphate gradient in 8 *M* urea at approximately neutral pH with CM-cellulose as the support (see also the chapters on chromatography in this volume for details of the method). An electrophoretic micromethod in nonionic detergent has recently been devised. The present chapter describes rapid and accurate methods for the separation and quantitation of globin chains by high performance liquid chromatography (HPLC).

Since this chapter was written, a new system has been devised. A large-pore C_4 column is substituted for the small-pore C_{18} packing which is used in the three methods that are detailed in this chapter. The new method is described briefly in the Addendum.

HISTORY

The description by Congote et al.[2] of the separation of globin chains by HPLC was quickly followed by one of Shelton et al.[3] Huisman and Wilson[4] modified the gradients of Shelton et al.[3] to achieve a better separation and, importantly, used hemoglobin rather than globin as the sample. Shelton et al. have made extensive modifications in the composition of developers.[5,6] Further changes in procedure have been reported by Huisman et al.[7] as well as by Congote[8,9] and Congote and Kendall.[10] Petrides et al.[11] have used a pyridine formate-propanol developer which required detection by fluorescence instead of detection by absorbance at 220 or 280 nm as practiced by others. The latter method will not be discussed further because fluorescence detection requires additional apparatus.

EQUIPMENT

The choice of equipment is unimportant and depends solely on what is available to the investigator. A detector and recorder are essential, but the pumping system and method of forming gradients are a matter of choice. Congote et al.[2,10] have emphasized the advantages of a simple system. Initially, their gradient was formed by siphoning a solution from one beaker into a second solution in a mixing beaker from which the gradient mixture was then withdrawn by a single pump.[2] More recently, a second pump has been used to move solution at a controlled slower flow rate into a second solution in a mixing chamber from which the gradient solution is pumped at a faster rate.[10] The simple two-vessel system of Bock and Ling[12] was chosen by Shelton et al.[3] to form reproducible gradients with a single pump; different densities of solutions did not interfere with the production of gradients by this device. At the present time, Shelton et al. and Huisman et al. use complete HPLC equipment with two pumps and electronic control of gradients.

HPLC COLUMNS

The three groups use the same type of packing in the HPLC column, namely, a 3.9 × 300 mm Waters μBondapak C_{18} column. C_{18}-Type columns from different manufacturers

Table 1
VARIOUS DETAILS OF REPORTED PROCEDURES

Authors	Guard columns	Sample	Detection	Quantitation
Congote et al.	Whatman Co-Pell ODS[9]	Globin: 0.05 to 4 mg in 0.5% TFA[2] or 0.3 mg in 150 μℓ of 25 to 65 m*M* TFA;[9] Hb: Vol. with 100 to 500 μg diluted at least 2× with 0.2% TFA[9]	280 nm	Radioactivity and absorbance
Huisman et al.	Waters μBondapak C_{18}Corasil[7]	300 μg Hb with 25 μℓ phosphate soln;[a] 50 to 300 μg in 5 to 100 μℓ;[b] 5 to 10 μℓ of lysate;[b] 10 to 2000 μg[b]	220 nm	Weight of cut-out peaks
Shelton et al.	Bio-Rad Bio-Sil ODS-10 Micro-Guard	0.2 to 0.3 mg Hb in 20 to 100 μℓ H_2O	220 nm	Planimetry

[a] See Table 2 for composition.
[b] Solvent not stated.

are not equivalent in their properties, and not all are satisfactory for the separation of globin chains. Shelton et al.[5] have examined not only different C_{18} packings but other types as well. Congote[9] also notes that the type of packing must be chosen carefully.

A guard column (i.e., a short replaceable column between the injector and main column) can significantly prolong the useful life. The type of guard column which is used by several groups is discussed in Table 1. In recent studies by Shelton et al., the main column has been dedicated to the separation of globin chains. With occasional changes of the guard column, separations showed some deterioration by the time 700 chromatograms had been run. The column may be further protected if samples are filtered with a microfilter system MF-1 with a 0.45-μm BA-85 nitrocellulose filter (Bioanalytical Systems, Inc., West Lafayette, Ind.).

There seems to be little advantage in using two or three columns in series.[9] Often, a column may be restored almost to its initial performance by removing and replacing the frit and some packing at the inlet.

THE SAMPLE

Although globin was the sample in the first experiments,[2,3] the use of hemoglobin itself by Huisman et al.[4] represented a major advance in technique. Within limits, the amount of hemoglobin, the volume of sample, and the solvent for the sample probably are unimportant. Table 1 lists various ways in which sample preparation has been described in publications.

A sample of 0.1 to 0.5 mg seems to be most satisfactory, gives excellent resolution, and is appropriate for quantitation (see next section).

DETECTION AND QUANTITATION

Shelton et al. and Huisman et al. use absorbance at 220 nm for detection of the globin chains whereas Congote et al. have chosen 280 nm. The greater sensitivity at 220 nm is to be preferred. At sample loads of 0.1 to 0.5 mg, baseline noise is minimal and recording can be done at 0.5 AUFS.

Quantitation is easily done by planimetry or by copying the recording, cutting out the peaks, and weighing them. Planimetry is the faster and more accurate procedure. In order to reduce error from the planimetry or weighing, the sensitivity of the recorder may be adjusted to the sample size so that appropriately sized peaks are produced on the record.

DEVELOPMENT

The HPLC separation of globin chains is sensitive to minor changes in development procedure, a fact which may be illustrated by a recent experience in this laboratory. Before the manufacturer upgraded the electronics in an early model of a controller for two pumps, the gradient for separating baboon globin chains was 61 to 67.5% of one component. After upgrading, elution was too rapid, and the gradient had to be changed to 59 to 65.6%. Thus, this experience points up the probability that reported gradients may require some modification in other laboratories because of different equipment.

Although, as may be seen from Table 2, the developers for HPLC separations of globin chains differ greatly, all of them (even the pyridine formate of Petrides et al.[11]) use an acid pH. The acidity presumably removes the heme when hemoglobin is the sample and probably is also necessary to retain the chains in solution.

The details of the chromatographic conditions for separation of the globin chains as given by publications of the three groups are presented in Table 2. The next section will provide examples of the separations by each of these systems and will be followed by a section of comments.

EXAMPLES

The examples to be presented for the three diverse systems are illustrative of the results when the "standard" procedure of each type is used. However, all methods are sensitive to minor changes in developmental conditions. Consequently, when the objective of a particular separation changes, conditions usually are modified somewhat.

Method of Congote et al.

Figure 1 illustrates some separations as reported by Congote and Kendall.[10] Figures 1A to C are HPL chromatograms of the designated hemoglobins after isolation on CM-Sepharose. Under these conditions, heme emerges quickly, β-chains precede, and γ-chains follow α-chains. The gradient in Figures 1B and C was slightly different from that in Figure 1A in order to improve the separation of α- and β-chains; the exact difference is not stated. In Figure 1A, the radioactivity defines the position of the $^{G}\gamma$ peak which is barely detectable by absorbance. Figure 1D is the HPL chromatogram of Hb F that had been isolated by CM-Sepharose chromatography from a large amount of Hb A. Although contamination with β-chains is evident, the separation of $^{G}\gamma$- and $^{A}\gamma$-chains is excellent. The position of $^{A}\gamma^{T}$-chains under these conditions is not known. However, $^{A}\gamma^{T}$-chains may have been observed (Reference 9, Figures 2 and 3) but interpreted as a second $^{G}\gamma$-chain.

On the basis of Figures 1B and C, the β^{A} and β^{C} chains probably would be partially separated if the whole hemoglobin from an AC heterozygote were chromatographed. Presumably, the separation of β^{A} and β^{C} chains could be improved by some modification of conditions. Thus, Congote and Kendall,[10] under standard conditions, found $\beta^{New\ York}$ only poorly separated from heme. When 1 mℓ of methanol was added to initial Solution B, all peaks emerged more slowly and $\beta^{New\ York}$ was now well separated. Increased elution time is a well-known effect of methanol in the developer. The β- and δ-chains do not separate.[9]

Table 2
DEVELOPER SYSTEMS FOR THE HPLC SEPARATION OF HUMAN GLOBIN CHAINS[a]

First solution	Second solution	Gradient	Reequilibration	Flow rate	Temp.	Total time[b]	Ref.
A[c] H_2O: Ac[d]: TFA 110:90:1 B H_2O: Ac:[d] TFA 550:450:3	C H_2O: Ac 1:1	40 mℓ B in mixer; pump C into mixer at 0.54 mℓ/min; pump from mixer at 1.7 mℓ/min	Purge with ≈15 mℓ 1:4 H_2O:Ac and reequilibrate with 25 mℓ of solution A	1.7 mℓ/min	40°	60 min	10
B 38:9.5:52.5 Ac:M:[d]P[d]	A 50:5:45 Ac:M:P	60 mℓ 10:90 A:B isocratically; 112.5 mℓ linear gradient to 35:65 A:B then 105 mℓ linear gradient to 72:28 A:B	Purge with 22.5 mℓ of 99:1 A:B and reequilibrate with 15 mℓ of 10:90 A:B	1.5 mℓ/min	Ambient	210 min	7
C 80:5:15:0.1:0.05 Pe[d]:M:Ac:Ph[d]:N[d,e]	D 20:5:75:0.1:0.05 Pe:M:Ac:Ph:N[e]	57 mℓ 39.5:60.5 C:D isocratically; then 37 mℓ linear gradient to 33.5:66.5 C:D	Purge in 3 mℓ to 100% D, then 100% D for 8 mℓ; return to 39.5:60.5 C:D in 5 mℓ and reequilibrate with 20—25 mℓ of latter	1.5 mℓ/min	Ambient	90 min	6

[a] These data derive from the most recent descriptions by the various authors.

[b] This is the total time between injection of samples.

[c] Congote et al. use Solution A for equilibration but not development.

[d] Ac, acetonitrile; M, methanol; P, phosphate buffer (49 m*M* KH_2PO_4 and 5.4 m*M* H_3PO_4 at pH 2.86); Pe, 0.15 *M* $NaClO_4$; Ph, 85% H_3PO_4; N, nonylamine.

[e] In Solutions C and D, the ratio of nonylamine to methanol is 1:100. Because of the small amount of nonylamine, these solutions can be made up most reproducibly by adding nonylamine as a 1% solution in methanol.

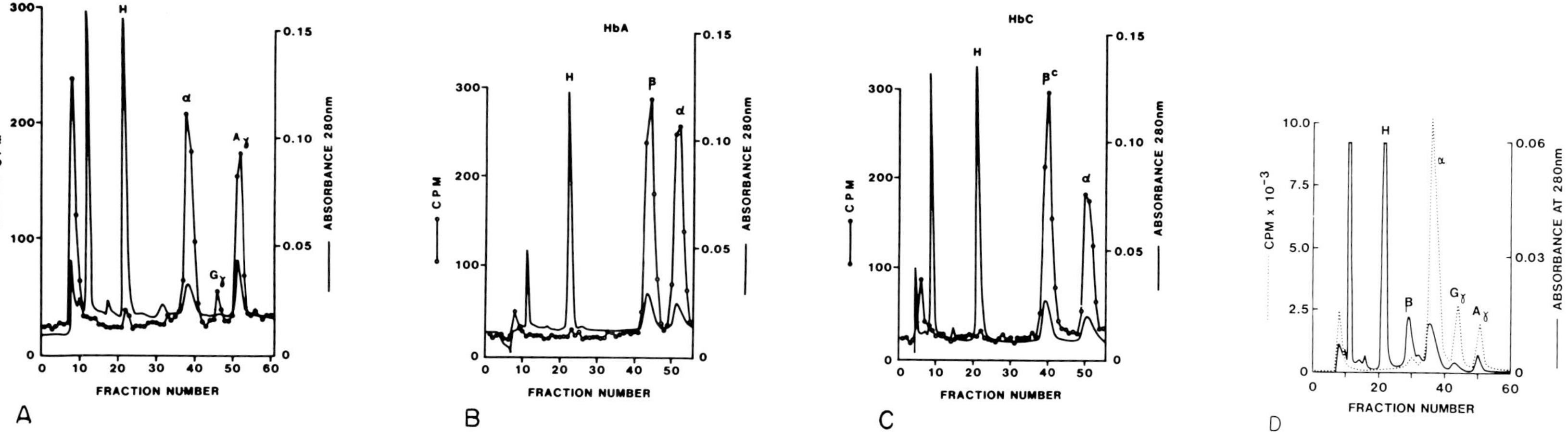

FIGURE 1. Examples of various separations by the standard method of Congote et al. Fraction size was 0.85 mℓ and fraction time was 30 sec. "H" denotes the heme peak. (From Congote, L. F. and Kendall, A. G., *Anal. Biochem.*, 123, 124, 1982. With permission.)

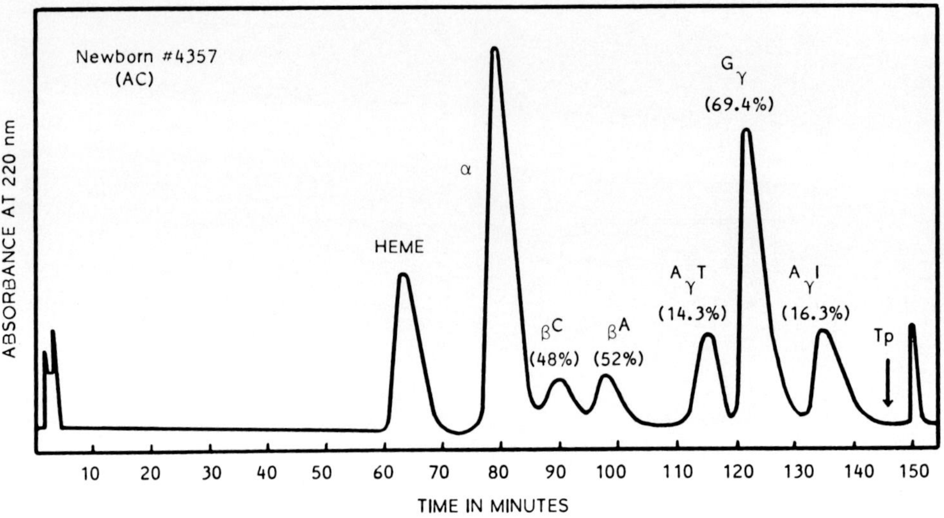

FIGURE 2. Separation of globin chains by the standard procedure of Huisman et al. Flow rate was 1.5 mℓ/min. (From Efremov, G. D. et al., *Am. J. Hematol.*, 12, 367, 1982. With permission.)

The main application of these methods[9,10] has been the study of samples from fetuses at risk for β-thalassemia. In this way, biosynthetic α- to non-α-chain ratios may be determined quickly and with a minimum of material in contrast to the Clegg-Naughton-Weatherall method.

Method of Huisman et al.

The procedure of Huisman et al. produces a rather different picture of separations (Figure 2). Heme emerges rather slowly, the β-chain here follows the α-chain, and finally the γ-chains elute. The normal $^{G}\gamma$-and $^{A}\gamma$-chains separate well from each other and from the common $^{A}\gamma^{T}$ variant. In this system, a 60-mℓ isocratic development is needed to remove heme. However, because the elution of heme is relatively little influenced by conditions, α-, β-, and γ-chains may be eluted before the heme.[14] On the other hand, if this is done, there is little room to achieve maximum separation of chains.

The β^{A}- and β^{C}-chains separate in this system (Figure 2) as do the β- and δ-chains,[7] but the β^{A}- and β^{S}-chains are reported not to separate,[15] and the δβ hybrid chain of Hb Lepore-Washington (= Hb Lepore-Boston) approximates the α-chain in mobility.[7] Nakatsuji et al. report on the HPLC behavior of several γ variants other than the $^{A}\gamma^{T}$-chain.[16]

Huisman and collaborators have applied these methods to thousands of samples in order to determine the nature of the γ-chain heterogeneity. In the results so far reported,[4,7,13-20] not only have many genetic abnormalities been detected and defined, but also the normal situation has been more correctly delimited than was possible with cruder methods.[21,22] In these applications, most of the samples were hemolysates with several hemoglobins, but sometimes, the Hb F was isolated prior to the HPL chromatogram.

Method of Shelton et al.

The current method of Shelton et al. (Reference 6 and Tables 1 and 2) is the result of several modifications.[3,5] The separations in Figure 3 are typical of what may be observed in the hemoglobins of an AA cord blood that has an $^{A}\gamma^{T}$-chain. As in the method of Congote et al., heme emerges rapidly and the sequence of β, α, and γ peaks is the same, although Congote et al. do not report on the position of the $^{A}\gamma^{T}$ peak (see also above). This chromatogram resulted before the electronics of the controller were modified, and the curve in panel D should be lowered 2% throughout (see ''Development'' section and Table 2).

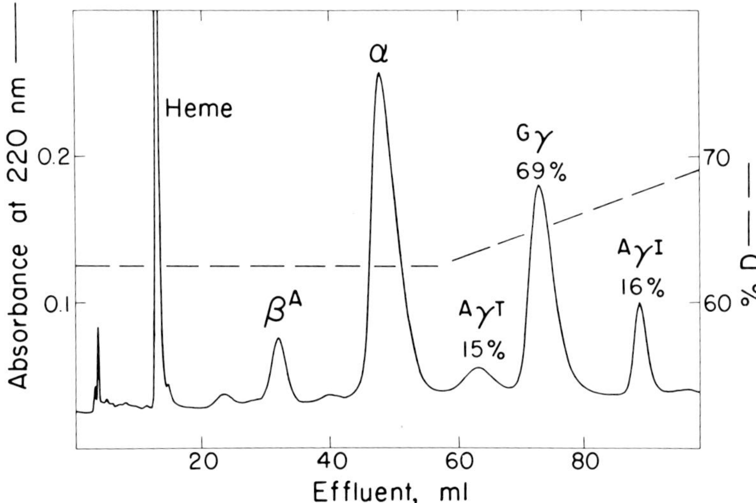

FIGURE 3. Application of the standard method of Shelton et al. to the separation of the globin chains in a cord blood sample. (From Shelton, J. B. et al., *Hemoglobin,* 6, 451, 1982. With permission.)

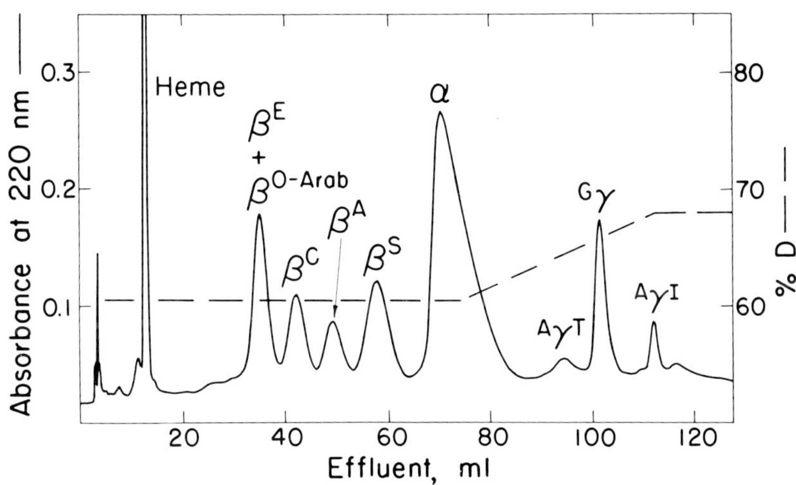

FIGURE 4. Separation of globin chains in an artificial mixture of hemoglobins by a modification of the standard method of Shelton et al. (From Shelton, J. B., et al., *Hemoglobin,* 6, 451, 1982. With permission.)

More complex mixtures of chains may also be separated as illustrated by Figure 4. Eight peaks are apparent from an artificial mixture with nine chains. The development as here shown would also have to be adjusted to reproduce these data. The behavior of several β variants in relation to the movement of the β^A-chain is as follows. More rapid than β^A: C, D-Los Angeles, E, O-Arab, Fort Gordon, Buenos Aires, Santa Ana, G-San Jose, and Malmö. Inseparable from β^A: Köln, Olympia, Hope, Shepherds Bush, and J-Baltimore (also Lepore and δ). Slower than β^A: S and N-Baltimore. Thus, there is easy distinction of β^E or $\beta^{O\text{-Arab}}$ from β^C or of $\beta^{D\text{-Los Angeles}}$ from β^S. It has not been possible to separate α variants from the normal α-chain by this procedure.[28]

This method has been most extensively used to study the heterogeneity of baboon γ-chains in fetal and postnatal samples and in older baboons that have been stressed to induce Hb F.[5,6,23,24] Although some modification of the gradient is necessary for the separation of the baboon chains, the heme, β-, α-, $^V\gamma$-, and $^I\gamma$-chains separate readily. (The $^V\gamma$- and $^I\gamma$-chains have valine and isoleucine, respectively, in residue 75). An electrophoretically silent β-chain that is "loud" by HPLC has been detected and identified,[6] and an abnormal $^V\gamma$-chain also is known.[24]

This method has not been applied in routine fashion to large numbers of human samples. Rather, the main use has been to monitor samples with variants both in the hemolysate of whole blood and after isolation as well as to determine the $^G\gamma$ to $^A\gamma$ ratio in selected samples.

COMMENTS

The three procedures differ very significantly in methodology and approach. Likewise, the three groups have been used to pursue rather different goals in their applications. A potential user would have to choose a method on the basis of his goals and would have to consider such aspects as available equipment, cost, complexity of samples, qualitative vs. quantitative data, etc.

Column Packing

Although Congote[9] notes that the choice of column packing is critical, apparently only Shelton et al.[5] have reported on the characteristics of other packings. Depending upon the objectives, another packing might be advantageous. Thus, on a DuPont Zorbax CN column as compared to a Waters μBondapak C_{18} column, the order of elution of the α- and β-chains is reversed when the same type of developer is used.[5]

With continued use, there may be some deterioration in the characteristics of the packing, although this certainly may be slowed by the use of guard columns and careful filtration of the sample before injection. Congote[9] claims to circumvent some of these problems by using two columns in series and altering the temperature. Disadvantages of such an approach are increased pressure with possible need to decrease flow rate. In addition, changes in developmental procedure are necessary.[9] As already mentioned, sometimes a mere replacement of the frit and a few millimeters of packing at the inlet of the column will solve the problem.

Detection and Quantitation

Detection at 220 rather than 280 nm is to be recommended. Although the sensitivity of the recorder may be altered in order to detect small peaks at 280 nm, the baseline simultaneously may become more erratic, and quantitation more difficult.

Although initially quantitation in this laboratory was done by weighing the cut-out peaks of duplicated copies of the recording, the procedure is not only time-consuming, but variation in duplicate or triplicate determinations introduced an unacceptable error. Planimetry is more rapid, more accurate, and more enjoyable.

Analysis vs. Isolation

The HPLC methods are superb analytical tools with which qualitative and quantitative data may be obtained with 0.1 to 0.5 mg of hemoglobin (or perhaps less). Thus, one may use the contents of a microhematocrit tube.

Isolation in much quantity, however, does pose obstacles; repeated chromatograms and final pooling of analogous zones presumably would be necessary but also expensive and time-consuming. Although HPLC columns with about twice the common diameter of about 4 mm are available, they are expensive ($700 to 800, 1985) and in our experience have provided separations of less quality at equivalent load than the smaller columns.

If isolation is desired, the method of Congote et al. may be the one of choice because of the volatility of the components in the developers. Removal of salts that are used in the other two methods by dialysis or Sephadex® chromatography might lead to large losses of hemoglobin fractions.

Time and Cost

As may be seen from Table 2, the time between successive sample injections in different systems varies by a factor of 3.5. A longer time increases the cost of the experiment — an important consideration because of the expense of HPLC-quality acetonitrile. A fast chromatogram may be as undesirable as an unduly long one, because the full separating potential of the column may not be realized. In this laboratory, we have chosen an intermediate position for routine work, but in special cases, movement of peaks may easily be speeded or slowed by modifications of isocratic or gradient development.

Modifications

Although Huisman and collaborators have shown devotion to a single type of development, both Congote et al. and we have found it useful to modify conditions to achieve improvements in specific separations. Indeed, Congote[8] studied a variety of solutions before devising his standard method. Strahler et al.[25] have achieved excellent separation of chains by a modification of Congote's procedure and have detected a ''silent'' mutation. The versatility of the HPLC of globin chains is apparent from the differences in the three methods. To achieve any goal then, the use of any one of the methods and modifications within that method must be given consideration.

Mechanisms

Much has been written about the mechanisms which bring about the separations in reversed-phase HPLC. It can hardly be denied that hydrophobicity is a major factor. Ion pairing has also been discussed in great detail. Certainly, in the acidic developers for the HPLC of globin chains, the ionization of acidic groups will be suppressed and basic groups will be neutralized (i.e., ion-paired) with probable increase in hydrophobicity. Yet it is surprising that one methylene group can be so effective in altering the hydrophobicity of a γ-chain that the excellent separation of $^{G}\gamma$- and $^{A}\gamma$-chains can be achieved. Equally unexpected and possibly related to some common unknown aspect is the electrophoretic separation of $^{G}\gamma$- and $^{A}\gamma$-chains in detergent. It is also interesting to note (Figure 4) that β^{C}- and β^{E}-chains are separable, although both have a Glu→Lys substitution and presumably the same change in hydrophobicity. The addition of nonylamine[6] to the perchlorate-phosphate-methanol-acetonitrile developers of Shelton et al.[5] has produced a dramatic effect on the separation of human globin chains (less so on baboon globin chains). By hydrophobic interaction with the C_{18} chains, nonylamine may introduce an ion exchange character to the packing. Conversely, by interacting with free silanol groups, nonylamine may increase hydrophobic character. The HPLC separation of globin chains is good, and the applications of the methods have produced significant information.

ADDENDUM

Since this chapter was written, a new system on an entirely different packing has been devised to separate globin chains.[26,27] The packing is a large-pore (330 Å) C_4 spherical material. The procedure in brief is described below.

The column is a Vydac large-pore C_4 column (Cat. #214TP54) (4.6 × 250 mm) from The Separations Group, Hesperia, Calif. Chromatograms are developed with linear gradients between mixtures of 0.1% aqueous TFA and 0.1% TFA in acetonitrile. Mixture A has 80% of the TFA-water solution and 20% of the TFA-acetonitrile solution and Mixture B has 40

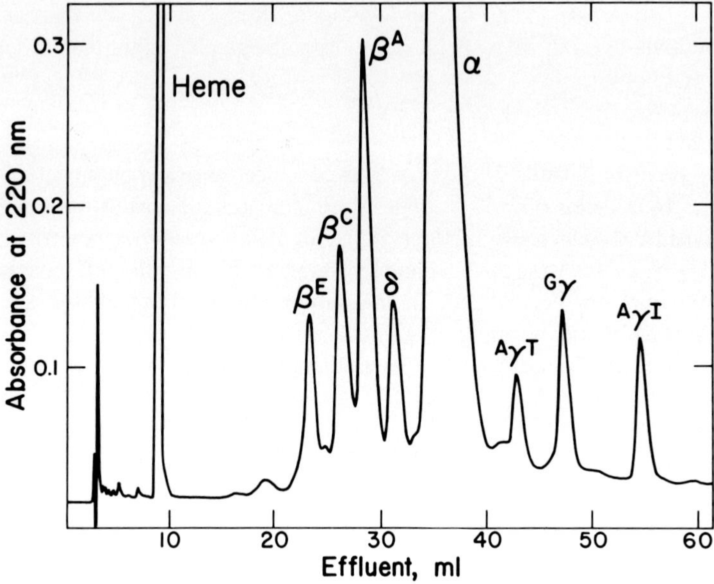

FIGURE 5. Separation of an artificial mixture of globin chains on a large-pore Vydac C_4 column. Conditions are described in the Addendum.

and 60%, respectively. The most effective gradient from human samples goes from 44 to 56.5% B in 60 min at 1 mℓ/min. Purging is done only after five or six runs: otherwise, the column is simply re-equilibrated with 25 mℓ of the initial mixture for the gradient. The purge contains only 2 to 3% of the material applied.

Figure 5 depicts the separation when an artificial mixture of isolated Hb A, Hb C, Hb A_2, Hb E, Hb N-Baltimore, and Hb F was chromatographed. Of the nine chains, distinct peaks are seen for eight. Only the $\beta^{N\text{-}Baltimore}$ peak is not apparent. In this mixture, it is overwhelmed by the massive α-peak whereas, in the HbN-Baltimore trait, the $\beta^{N\text{-}Baltimore}$ peak is very evident on the leading edge of, but incompletely separated from, the α-peak. This method separates the three common γ-chains completely. If the β^S-chain were present, it would be between β^A and δ; in a sickle cell trait sample, β^A and β^S are not completely resolved. The $\beta^{O\text{-}Arab}$ chain falls in the position of β^E. Reference 27 has other examples, and application of the method to the separation of baboon globin chains has been reported.[26]

The system has many advantages: peaks are sharp and almost symmetrical, the procedure is fast, purging need be done only infrequently, and the solvents are volatile.

Depending upon the goal of the experiment and the complexity of the mixture, changes in the starting point and/or slope of the gradient may be used to advantage to speed up or slow the separations and thus to provide adequate rapid separations for simple mixtures or improve the resolution of complex mixtures.

ACKNOWLEDGMENTS

The experiments in this laboratory as well as the writing of this chapter were supported in part by grant HL-02558 from the National Institutes of Health, U. S. Public Health Service. Joan B. Shelton and J. Roger Shelton were active in experimental design and experimentation. This is Contribution No. 6767 from the Division of Chemistry and Chemical Engineering, California Institute of Technology.

REFERENCES

1. **Clegg, J. B., Naughton, M. A., and Weatherall, D. J.,** Abnormal human hemoglobins. Separation and characterization of the α and β chains by chromatography, and the determination of two new variants, Hb-Chesapeake and Hb J(Bangkok), *J. Mol. Biol.*, 19, 91, 1966.
2. **Congote, L. F., Bennett, H. P. J., and Solomon, S.,** Rapid separation of the α, β, $^{G}\gamma$, and $^{A}\gamma$ human globin chains by reversed-phase high pressure liquid chromatography, *Biochem. Biophys. Res. Commun.*, 89, 851, 1979.
3. **Shelton, J. B., Shelton, J. R., and Schroeder, W. A.,** Preliminary experiments in the separation of globin chains by high performance liquid chromatography, *Hemoglobin*, 3, 353, 1979.
4. **Huisman, T. H. J. and Wilson, J. B.,** Recent advances in the quantitation of human fetal hemoglobins with different gamma chains, *Am. J. Hematol.*, 9, 225, 1980.
5. **Shelton, J. B., Shelton, J. R., and Schroeder, W. A.,** Further experiments in the separation of globin chains by high performance liquid chromatography, *J. Liq. Chromatogr.*, 4, 1381, 1981.
6. **Shelton, J. B., Shelton, J. R., Schroeder, W. A., and DeSimone, J.,** Detection of Hb-Papio B, a silent mutation of the baboon β chain, by high performance liquid chromatography. Improved procedures for the separation of globin chains by HPLC, *Hemoglobin*, 6, 451, 1982.
7. **Huisman, T. H. J., Webber, B., Okonjo, K., Reese, A. L., and Wilson, J. B.,** The separation of human hemoglobin chains by high pressure liquid chromatography, in *Advances in Hemoglobin Analysis*, Hanash, S. M. and Brewer, G. J., Eds., Alan R. Liss, New York, 1981, 23.
8. **Congote, L. F.,** Reversed-phase high pressure liquid chromatography of globin chains: its application for the prenatal diagnosis of β-thalassemia, in *Advances in Hemoglobin Analysis*, Hanash, S. M. and Brewer, G. J., Eds., Alan R. Liss, New York, 1981, 39.
9. **Congote, L. F.,** Rapid procedure for globin chain analysis in blood samples of normal and β-thalassemia fetuses, *Blood*, 57, 353, 1981.
10. **Congote, L. F. and Kendall, A. G.,** Rapid analysis of labeled globin chains without acetone precipitation or dialysis by high-pressure liquid chromatography and ion-exchange chromatography, *Anal. Biochem.*, 123, 124, 1982.
11. **Petrides, P. E., Jones, R. T., and Böhlen, P.,** Reverse-phase high performance liquid chromatography of proteins: the separation of hemoglobin chain variants, *Anal. Biochem.*, 105, 383, 1980.
12. **Bock, R. M. and Ling, N.-S.,** Devices for gradient elution in chromatography, *Anal. Chem.*, 26, 1543, 1954.
13. **Efremov, G. D., Ibarra, B., Gurgey, G., Sukumaran, P. K., Altay, C., and Huisman, T. H. J.,** Gamma-chain heterogeneity of fetal hemoglobin in nonblack β- and $\delta\beta$-thalassemia and HPFH heterozygotes and homozygotes, *Am. J. Hematol.*, 12, 367, 1982.
14. **Shimizu, K., Wilson, J. B., and Huisman, T. H. J.,** The determination of the percentages of the $^{G}\gamma$- and $^{A}\gamma$-chains in human fetal hemoglobin by HPLC, *Hemoglobin*, 4, 487, 1980.
15. **Huisman, T. H. J., Altay, C., Webber, B., Reese, A. L., Gravely, M. E., Okonjo, K., and Wilson, J. B.,** Quantitation of three types of γ chain of HbF by high pressure liquid chromatography; application of this method to the Hb F of patients with sickle cell anemia or the S-HPFH condition, *Blood*, 57, 75, 1981.
16. **Nakatsuji, T., Carver, J., Wilson, J. B., Lam, H., Reese, A. L., Nagle, S., Miwa, S., and Huisman, T. H. J.,** Alpha chain and gamma chain abnormal hemoglobins in newborn babies: structural and genetic aspects, *Am. J. Hematol.*, 14, 121, 1983.
17. **Huisman, T. H. J. and Altay, C.,** The chemical heterogeneity of the fetal hemoglobin of black newborn babies and adults: a reevaluation, *Blood*, 58, 491, 1981.
18. **Gardiner, M. B., Reese, A. L., Headlee, M. E., and Huisman, T. H. J.,** The heterogeneity of the γ-chain of fetal hemoglobin in Hb S heterozygotes, *Blood*, 60, 513, 1982.
19. **Huisman, T. H. J., Gravely, M. E., Webber, B., Okonjo, K., Henson, J., and Reese, A. L.,** The gamma chain heterogeneity of fetal hemoglobin in black β-thalassemia and HPFH heterozygotes, *Blood*, 58, 62, 1981.
20. **Huisman, T. H. J., Reese, A. L., Gardiner, M. B., Wilson, J. B., Lam, H., Reynolds, A., Nagle, S., Trowell, P., Zeng, Y.-T., Huang, S.-Z., Sukumaran, P. K., Miwa, S., Efremov, G. D., Petkov, G., Sciarratta, G. V., and Sansone, G.,** The occurrence of different levels of $^{G}\gamma$ chain and of the $^{A}\gamma^{T}$ variant of fetal hemoglobin in newborn babies from several countries, *Am. J. Hematol.*, 14, 133, 1983.
21. **Schroeder, W. A., Huisman, T. H. J., Shelton, J. R., Shelton, J. B., Kleihauer, E. F., Dozy, A. M., and Robberson, B.,** Evidence for multiple structural genes for the γ chain of human fetal hemoglobin, *Proc. Natl. Acad. Sci. U.S.A.*, 60, 537, 1968.
22. **Schroeder, W. A., Huisman, T. H. J., Efremov, G. D., Shelton, J. R., Shelton, J. B., Phillips, R., Reese, A., Gravely, M., Harrison, J. M., and Lam, H.,** Further studies of the frequency and significance of the $^{T}\gamma$ chain of human fetal hemoglobin, *J. Clin. Invest.*, 63, 268, 1979.

23. **Schroeder, W. A., DeSimone, J., Shelton, J. B., Shelton, J. R., Espinueva, Z., Hall, L., and Zwiers, D.,** Changes in the γ chain heterogeneity of the Hb F of the baboon (*Papio cynocephalus*) postnatally and after partial switching to Hb F production by various stimuli, *J. Biol. Chem.*, 258, 3121, 1983.
24. **Schroeder, W. A., DeSimone, J., Shelton, J. B., and Shelton, J. R.,** unpublished data.
25. **Strahler, J. R., Rosenbloom, B. B., and Hanash, S. M.,** A silent neutral substitution detected by reverse-phase high-performance liquid chromatography: hemoglobin Beirut, *Science*, 221, 860, 1983.
26. **DeSimone, J., Schroeder, W. A., Shelton, J. B., Shelton, J. R., Espinueva, Z., Huynh, V., Hall, L., and Zwiers, D.,** Speciation in the baboon and its relation to γ-chain heterogeneity and to the response to induction of Hb-F by 5-azacytidine, *Blood*, 63, 1088, 1984.
27. **Shelton, J. B., Shelton, J. R., and Schroeder, W. A.,** High performance liquid chromatographic separation of globin chains on a large-pore C_4 column, *J. Liq. Chromatog.*, 7, 1969, 1984.
28. **Schroeder, W. A.,** unpublished.

HEMOGLOBINOPATHIES

Ruth N. Wrightstone

INTRODUCTION

The following tables of hemoglobin variants are arranged according to the specific polypeptide chain, i.e., α, β, γ, δ, in which the abnormality is found and according to the type of change, i.e., substitution or deletion. Tables 1 to 4 list the hemoglobin variants resulting from a change(s) in a nucleotide of the mRNA triplet codon. A second group of variants results from deletion of one to five mRNA triplet codons. These variants are generally unstable because the deletion of a codon shortens the chain and disrupts the conformation of the molecule, breaking or changing normal bonding sites. The β-chain deleted hemoglobins are Hbs Leiden, Lyon, Freiburg, Niteroi, Tochigi, St. Antoine, Vicksburg, Tours, Gun Hill, Leslie (Deaconess), and Coventry. One α-chain variant has been reported that is the result of a deleted residue and that is Hb Boyle Heights.

The extended chains form another group of variants. These hemoglobins are formed when there is a substitution or frameshift in the mRNA strand that fails to terminate the synthesis of the polypeptide chain at the normal terminating codon. As many as 31 additional amino acids have been added to a polypeptide chain before the next terminating codon is reached. The hemoglobins with extended α-chains are Hbs Constant Spring, Icaria, Koya Dora, and Wayne. Hemoglobins with extensions of the β-chain are Hb Tak and Hb Cranston. One hemoglobin, Hb Grady, is the result of an insertion of three amino acids in the α-chain, probably due to a tandem duplication of base pairs which may have arisen by a process of mismatched intragenic crossing over.

The fusion group of hemoglobins is the result of nonhomologous crossing over of genetic material during meiosis. Fusion chains have been formed between δβ-chains in which the N-terminal part of the chain is from the δ-polypeptide chain, and the C-terminal part is from the β-polypeptide chain. The crossovers may exist anywhere in the two chains but still retain the normal number of amino acids per chain. These are known as Lepore hemoglobins. They are Lepore Hollandia, Lepore Baltimore, and Lepore Washington-Boston. There are also anti-Lepore hemoglobins. These have, as the N-terminal, amino acids found in the β-polypeptide chain, whereas the C-terminal has the sequence of the δ-chain. These are Hbs Miyada, P Congo, and P Nilotic. Hb Lincoln Park is an anti-Lepore hemoglobin in which residue δ137 has been deleted.* One fusion hemoglobin (Hb Kenya) is the result of a crossover between the γ- and β-polypeptide chains; the N-terminal follows the sequence of the γ-chain, and the C-terminal follows that of the β-chain.

The hemoglobin variants are also grouped according to their functional properties. Substitutions in certain areas of the molecule may cause either an increase or decrease in affinity for oxygen. These may occur in any of the globin chains and may cause a polycythemia or anemia.

Five hemoglobin variants are known in which there is a change in two different mRNA triplet codons appearing in two different areas of the same chain. This results in the substitution of two amino acids in a single polypeptide chain. These are Hbs C Harlem, Arlington Park, J Singapore, C Ziguinchor, and S Travis.

Included in the major tables are the contacts that each individual amino acid makes within the quaternary structure. Each of the hemoglobins are listed with appropriate reference(s).

Since hemoglobin variants are continually reported in the literature, these tables will be

* Hb Parchman is a fusion hemoglobin which is the result of a double nonhomologous crossover between the δ- and β-globin genes.

out of date by the time this volume is published. A current list of hemoglobin variants is maintained by the director of the International Hemoglobin Information Center. Anyone desiring additional information on any hemoglobinopathy or a current list of hemoglobin variants may write to Dr. Ruth N. Wrightstone, Director, International Hemoglobin Information Center, Medical College of Georgia, Augusta, Georgia, 30912.

Table 1
VARIANTS OF THE α-CHAIN

Residue	Substitution	Name	Major abnormal property	Contacts	Ref.
1(NA1)	Val			α-α	
2(NA2)	Leu			Central	
3(A1)	Ser			External	
4(A2)	Pro			External	
5(A3)	Ala→Asp	Hb J Toronto		External	1
6(A4)	Asp→Ala	Hb Sawara	↑ O_2 affinity	External	2
	Asp→Asn	Hb Dunn	↑ O_2 affinity		3
	Asp→Val	Hb Ferndown	↑ O_2 affinity		4
	Asp→Tyr	Hb Woodville	↑ O_2 affinity		478
7(A5)	Lys			External	
8(A6)	Thr			External	
9(A7)	Asn			External	
10(A8)	Val			Internal	
11(A9)	Lys→Glu	Hb Anantharaj		External	5
	Lys→Gln	Hb Wenchang-Wuming			6
	Lys→Asn	Hb Albany-Suma			479, 480
12(A10)	Ala→Asp	Hb J Paris-I,		External	7
		J Aljezur			8
13(A11)	Ala			Internal	
14(A12)	Trp→Arg	Hb Evanston		Internal	481,482
15(A13)	Gly→Asp	Hb I Interlaken,		External	9
		J Oxford,			10
		N Cosenza			11
	Gly→Arg	Hb Ottawa,		External	12
		Siam			13
16(A14)	Lys→Glu	Hb I,	Normal O_2 affinity	External	14
		I Philadelphia,			15
		I Texas,			16
		I Burlington,			17
		I Skamania			18
	Lys→Asn	Hb Beijing			483

Table 1 (continued)
VARIANTS OF THE α-CHAIN

Residue	Substitution	Name	Major abnormal property	Contacts	Ref.
17(A15)	Val			Internal	
18(A16)	Gly→Arg	Hb Handsworth		External	19
19(AB1)	Ala→Asp	Hb J Kurosh		External	20
20(B1)	His→Tyr	Hb Necker Enfants-Malades		External	21
21(B2)	Ala→Asp	Hb J Nyanza		External	22
22(B3)	Gly→Asp	Hb J Medellin		External	23
23(B4)	Glu→Gln	Hb Memphis		External	24
	Glu→Lys	Hb Chad			25
	Glu→Val	Hb G Audhali			26
24(B5)	Tyr			OH external, ring internal	
25(B6)	Gly			Internal	
26(B7)	Ala			External	
27(B8)	Glu→Gly	Hb Fort Worth		External	27
	Glu→Val	Hb Spanish Town			28
	Glu→Lys	Hb Shuangfeng	Unstable		29
28(B9)	Ala			Internal	
29(B10)	Leu			Internal	
30(B11)	Glu→Lys	Hb O Padova	Normal O_2 affinity	α_1-β_1	30
	Glu→Gln	Hb G Honolulu,			31
		G Singapore,			32
		G Chinese,			33
		G Hong Kong			33
31(B12)	Arg→Ser	Hb Prato		α_1-β_1	34
32(B13)	Met			Heme	
33(B14)	Phe			Internal	
34(B15)	Leu→Arg	Hb Queens		α_1-β_1	35
35(B16)	Ser			α_1-β_1	
36(C1)	Phe			α_1-β_1	
37(C2)	Pro			α_1-β_2	
38(C3)	Thr			α_1-β_2	
39(C4)	Thr			Heme	

40(C5)	Lys→Glu	Hb Kariya	↑ O_2 Affinity, unstable	Deoxy: α_1-β_2	484
41(C6)	Thr			α_1-β_2	
42(C7)	Tyr			α_1-β_2; Heme	
43(CE1)	Phe→Val	Hb Torino	Unstable, ↓ O_2 affinity	Heme	36
	Phe→Leu	Hb Hirosaki	Unstable		37
44(CE2)	Pro→Leu	Hb Milledgeville	↑ O_2 affinity	α_1-β_2	38
	Pro→Arg	Hb Kawachi	↑ O_2 affinity		39
45(CE3)	His→Arg	Hb Fort de France	↑ O_2 affinity	Heme	40
	His→Gln	Hb Bari	Normal O_2 affinity		41
46(CE4)	Phe			Heme	
47(CE5)	Asp→Gly	Kokura,	Unstable	External	42
		Hb Umi,			42
		Michigan-I,			
		Michigan-II,			
		Yukuhashi-II,			42
		L Gaslini,			
		Tagawa-II			42,43
		Beilinson,			44
		Mugino			42
	Asp→His	Hb Hasharon,	Unstable		45
		Sinai,			46
		Sealy,			47
		L Ferrara			48, 49
	Asp→Asn	Hb Arya	Slightly unstable		50
	Asp→Ala	Hb Cordele	Unstable		485
48(CE6)	Leu→Arg	Hb Montgomery		Surface	51
49(CE7)	Ser→Arg	Hb Savaria	Normal O_2 affinity	External	52
50(CE8)	His→Asp	Hb J Sardegna		External	53
	His→Arg	Hb Aichi			486
51(CE9)	Gly→Asp	Hb J Abidjan		External	54
	Gly→Arg	Hb Russ			55
52(E1)	Ser			External	
53(E2)	Ala→Asp	Hb J Rovigo	Unstable	External	56
54(E3)	Gln→Arg	Hb Shimonoseki, Hikoshima	Normal O_2 affinity	External	57

Table 1 (continued)
VARIANTS OF THE α-CHAIN

Residue	Substitution	Name	Major abnormal property	Contacts	Ref.
	Gln→Glu	Hb Mexico,			58
		J Paris-II,			59
		Uppsala			60
55(E4)	Val			Internal	
56(E5)	Lys→Thr	Hb Thailand	Normal O_2 affinity	External	61
	Lys→Glu	Hb Shaare Zedek			62
57(E6)	Gly→Arg	Hb L Persian Gulf		External	63
	Gly→Asp	Hb J Norfolk,			64
		Kagoshima,			65
		Nishik-I, II, III			
58(E7)	His→Tyr	HbM Boston,	↓ O_2 affinity,	Heme "distal"	66
		M Osaka,			67
		Gothenburg,			68
		M Kiskunhalas			69
59(E8)	Gly→Val	Hb Tottori	Unstable	Internal	70
60(E9)	Lys→Asn	Hb Zambia		External	71
	Lys→Glu	Hb Dagestan			72
61(E10)	Lys→Asn	Hb J Buda		External	73
62(E11)	Val			Heme	
63(E12)	Ala→Asp	Hb Pontoise	Unstable, normal O_2 affinity	Surface	74
64(E13)	Asp→Asn	Hb G Waimanalo,	Normal O_2 affinity	External	75
		Aida			76
	Asp→His	Hb Q India			77
	Asp→Tyr	Hb Perspolis			20
65(E14)	Ala			External	
66(E15)	Leu			Internal	
67(E16)	Thr			External	

68(E17)	Asn→Asp	Hb Ube-2	Normal O_2 affinity	External	78
	Asn→Lys	Hb G Philadelphia,			79
		G Knoxville-I			80
		Stanleyville-I,			81
		D Washington,			80
		D St. Louis,			82
		G Bristol,			83
		G Azakuoli,			80
		D Baltimore			80
69(E18)	Ala			Internal	
70(E19)	Val			Surface	
71(E20)	Ala→Glu	Hb J Habana		External	84
72(EF1)	His→Arg	Hb Daneskgah-Tehran		External	85
73(EF2)	Val			Surface	
74(EF3)	Asp→His	G Taichung,	Normal O_2 affinity	External	87
		Hb Mahidol,			86
		Q Thailand			88
	Asp→Asn	Hb G Pest			73
	Asp→Gly	Hb Chapel Hill			89
	Asp→Ala	Hb Lille			90
75(EF4)	Asp→His	Hb Q Iran		External	88
	Asp→Ala	Hb Duan			91
	Asp→Tyr	Hb Winnipeg			92
	Asp→Asn	Hb Matsue-Oki	Normal O_2 affinity		93
	Asp→Gly	Hb Mizushi	Normal O_2 affinity		94
76(EF5)	Met→Lys	Hb Noko		Internal	95
77(EF6)	Pro			External	
78(EF7)	Asn→Lys	Hb Stanleyville-II		External	96
	Asn→Asp	Hb J Singa			487
79(EF8)	Ala			External	
80(F1)	Leu→Arg	Hb Ann Arbor	Unstable	Surface	97, 98
81(F2)	Ser→Cys	Hb Nigeria		External	99
82(F3)	Ala→Asp	Hb Garden State		External	100
83(F4)	Leu			Heme	
84(F5)	Ser→Arg	Hb Etobicoke	↑ O_2 affinity	Internal	101,102

Table 1 (continued)
VARIANTS OF THE α-CHAIN

Residue	Substitution	Name	Major abnormal property	Contacts	Ref.
85(F6)	Asp→Asn	Hb G Norfolk	(?) ↑ O_2 affinity	External	103, 104
	Asp→Tyr	Hb Atago	↑ O_2 affinity		105, 106
	Asp→Val	Hb Inkster	↑ O_2 affinity		107, 106
86(F7)	Leu→Arg	Hb Moabit	Unstable, ↓ O_2 affinity	Heme	108
87(F8)	His→Tyr	Hb Iwate,	Ferri Hb, ↓ O_2 affinity	Heme "proximal"	109
		M Kankakee,			110
		M Oldenburg			111
	His→Arg	HbM Iwata	Unstable		112
88(F9)	Ala			Surface	
89(FG1)	His			External	
90(FG2)	Lys→Asn	Hb J Broussais,		External	113,114
		Tagawa-I			115
	Lys→Thr	Hb J Rajappen			116
	Lys→Met	Hb Handa	↑ O_2 affinity		117
91(FG3)	Leu→Pro	Hb Port Phillip	Unstable	α_1-β_2	118
92(FG4)	Arg→Gln	Hb J Cape Town	↑ O_2 affinity	α_1-β_2	119, 120
	Arg→Leu	Hb Chesapeake	↑ O_2 affinity		121, 122
93(FG5)	Val			Heme;α_1-β_1	
94(G1)	Asp→Tyr	Hb Setif	Unstable, ↓ O_2 affinity	α_1-β_2	123
	Asp→His	Hb Sunshine Seth			124
	Asp→Asn	Hb Titusville	↓ O_2 affinity, ↑ dissociation		125
95(G2)	Pro→Leu	HbG Georgia	↑ dissociation, ↑ O_2 affinity	α_1-β_2	126
	Pro→Ser	Hb Rampa	↑ dissociation, ↑ O_2 affinity		127, 128
	Pro→Ala	Hb Denmark Hill	↑ O_2 affinity		129
	Pro→Arg	Hb St. Lukes	↑ dissociation, ↑ O_2 affinity		130
96(G3)	Val			α_1-β_2	

97(G4)	Asn→Lys	Hb Dallas	↑ O_2 affinity	Heme	488
98(G5)	Phe			Heme	
99(G6)	Lys			Central	
100(G7)	Leu			Surface	
101(G8)	Leu			Heme	
102(G9)	Ser→Arg	Hb Manitoba	Slightly unstable	Central	131
103(G10)	His→Arg	Hb Contaldo	Unstable	α_1-β_1	489
104(G11)	Cys			α_1-β_1	
105(G12)	Leu			Internal	
106(G13)	Leu			α_1-β_1	
107(G14)	Val			α_1-β_1	
108(G15)	Thr			Internal	
109(G16)	Leu→Arg	Hb Suan Dok	Unstable	Internal	132
110(G17)	Ala→Asp	Hb Petah Tikva	Unstable	Internal	133
111(G18)	Ala			α_1-β_1	
112(G19)	His→Asp	Hb Hopkins-II	Unstable, ↑ O_2 affinity	External	134
	His→Arg	Hb Strumica,			135
		Serbia			136
113(GH1)	Leu			Surface	
114(GH2)	Pro→Arg	Hb Chiapas		α_1-β_1	58
115(GH3)	Ala→Asp	Hb J Tongariki		External	137
116(GH4)	Glu→Lys	Hb O Indonesia,		External	138
		Buginese-X,			139
		Oliviere			140
	Glu→Ala	Hb Ube-4	Normal O_2 affinity		141
	Glu→Gln	Hb Oleander	Normal O_2 affinity		142
117(GH5)	Phe			α_1-β_1	
118(H1)	Thr			External	
119(H2)	Pro			α_1-β_1	
120(H3)	Ala→Glu	Hb J Meerut,		External	143
		J Birmingham			144
121(H4)	Val			Surface	
122(H5)	His→Gln	Hb Westmead		α_1-β_1	145
123(H6)	Ala			α_1-β_1	
124(H7)	Ser			Surface	
125(H8)	Leu→Pro	Hb Quong Sze		Internal	146

Table 1 (continued)
VARIANTS OF THE α-CHAIN

Residue	Substitution	Name	Major abnormal property	Contacts	Ref.
126(H9)	Asp→Asn	Hb Tarrant	↑ O_2 affinity	α_1-β_1	147
127(H10)	Lys→Thr	Hb St. Claude		Central	148
	Lys→Asn	Hb Jackson			149
128(H11)	Phe			Internal	
129(H12)	Leu			Heme	
130(H13)	Ala			Central	
131(H14)	Ser			Central	
132(H15)	Val			Heme	
133(H16)	Ser			Central	
134(H17)	Thr			Central	
135(H18)	Val			Surface	
136(H19)	Leu→Pro	Hb Bibba	Unstable, ↑ dissociation	Heme	150
137(H20)	Thr			Central	
138(H21)	Ser			Central	
139(HC1)	Lys→Thr	Hb Tokoname	↑ O_2 Affinity	External	490
140(HC2)	Tyr			Deoxy: HB to FG5 same α-chain oxy: mobile, cooperativity	
141(HC3)	Arg→Pro	Hb Singapore		External, deoxy, salt bonds to H9, H10, NA1 other α-chain, oxy: mobile, Bohr	151
	Arg→His	Hb Suresnes	↑ O_2 affinity		152
	Arg→Ser	Hb J Cubujuqui	↑ O_2 affinity		153
	Arg→Leu	Hb Legnano	↑ O_2 affinity		154
	Arg→Gly	Hb J Camagüey			155

Table 2
VARIANTS OF THE β-CHAIN

Residue	Substitution	Name	Major abnormal property	Contacts	Ref.
1(NA1)	Val→Ac-Ala	Hb Raleigh	↓ O_2 affinity, ↓ dissociation	DPG Binding	156
2(NA2)	His→Arg	Hb Deer Lodge	↑ O_2 affinity	DPG Binding	157
	His→Gln	Hb Okayama	↑ O_2 affinity		491
3(NA3)	Leu			Surface	
4(A1)	Thr			External	
5(A2)	Pro			External	
6(A3)	Glu→Val	Hb S	Sickling	External	158
	Glu→Lys	Hb C			159
	Glu→Ala	Hb G Makassar			160
	Glu→Gln	Hb Machida			492
7(A4)	Glu→Gly	Hb G San José	Mildly unstable, normal O_2 affinity	External	161
	Glu→Lys	Hb Siriraj			162
8(A5)	Lys→Thr	Hb Rio Grande	Normal O_2 affinity	External	493
	Lys→Gln	Hb J Luhe			494
9(A6)	Ser→Cys	Hb Pôrto Alegre	Polymerization, ↑ O_2 affinity	External	163, 164
10(A7)	Ala→Asp	Hb Ankara		External	165
11(A8)	Val→Ile	Hb Hamilton		Internal	495
12(A9)	Thr			Surface	
13(A10)	Ala→Asp	Hb J Lens		External	166
14(A11)	Leu→Arg	Hb Sogn	Unstable, normal O_2 affinity	Surface	167
	Leu→Pro	Hb Saki	Unstable, normal O_2 affinity		168, 169
15(A12)	Trp→Arg	Hb Belfast	Unstable, ↑ O_2 affinity	Internal	170, 171

Table 2 (continued)
VARIANTS OF THE β-CHAIN

Residue	Substitution	Name	Major abnormal property	Contacts	Ref.
16(A13)	Gly→Asp	Hb J Baltimore		External	172
		J Trinidad,			173
		J Ireland,			173
		N New Haven,			174
		J Georgia			175
	Gly→Arg	Hb D Bushman			176
17(A14)	Lys→Glu	Hb Nagasaki		External	177
	Lys→Asn	Hb J Amiens			49
18(A15)	Val			Internal	
19(B1)	Asn→Lys	Hb D Ouled Rabah		External	178
	Asn→Asp	Hb Alamo			179
20(B2)	Val→Met	Hb Olympia	↑ O_2 affinity	External	180
21(B3)	Asp→Tyr	Hb Yusa	Normal O_2 affinity	External	181
	Asp→Gly	Hb Connecticut	↓ O_2 affinity		182
	Asp→Asn	Hb Cocody			183
22(B4)	Glu→Lys	Hb E Saskatoon	Unstable	External	184
	Glu→Gly	Hb G Taipei			185
	Glu→Ala	G Coushatta,			188
		Hb G Saskatoon,			186
		Hsin Chu,			187
		G Taegu			189
	Glu→Gln	Hb D Iran	Normal O_2 affinity		190
23(B5)	Val→Asp	Hb Strasbourg	↑ O_2 affinity	Internal	191,192
	Val→Gly	Hb Miyashiro	Unstable, ↑ O_2 affinity		193
	Val→Phe	Hb Palmerston North	↑ O_2 affinity, unstable		49
24(B6)	Gly→Arg	Hb Riverdale-Bronx	Unstable, ↑ O_2 affinity	Internal	194
	Gly→Val	Hb Savannah	Unstable		195
	Gly→Asp	Hb Moscva	Unstable, ↓ O_2 affinity		196

25(B7)	Gly→Arg	Hb G Taiwan Ami		External	197
26(B8)	Glu→Lys	Hb E	Unstable, thalassemia	External	198
	Glu→Val	Hb Henri Mondor	Unstable (slight)		199
27(B9)	Ala→Asp	Hb Volga,	Unstable	Internal	200
		Drenthe			201
	Ala→Ser	Hb Knossos			498
28(B10)	Leu→Gln	Hb St. Louis	Unstable, ferri Hb, ↑ O_2 affinity	Internal	202, 203
	Leu→Pro	Hb Genova	Unstable, ↑ O_2 affinity		204
29(B11)	Gly→Asp	Hb Lufkin	Unstable	Internal	205
30(B12)	Arg→Ser	Hb Tacoma	Unstable, ↓ Bohr and heme-heme, normal O_2 affinity	α_1-β_1	206
31(B13)	Leu→Pro	Hb Yokohama	Unstable	Heme	207
32(B14)	Leu→Pro	Hb Perth,	Unstable,	Internal	208
		Abraham Lincoln	normal O_2 affinity		209
	Leu→Arg	Hb Castilla	Unstable		210
33(B15)	Val			α_1-β_1	
34(B16)	Val→Phe	Hb Pitie-Salpetriere	↑ O_2 affinity	α_1-β_1	211
35(C1)	Tyr→Phe	Hb Philly	Unstable, ↑ O_2 affinity	α_1-β_1	212
36(C2)	Pro			α_1-β_2	
37(C3)	Trp→Ser	Hb Hirose	↑ O_2 affinity, ↑ dissociation	α_1-β_2	213
	Trp→Arg	Hb Rothschild	↓ O_2 affinity		214
38(C4)	Thr			Heme	
39(C5)	Gln→Lys	Hb Alabama		α_1-β_2	215
	Gln→Glu	Hb Vaasa	Unstable		216
40(C6)	Arg→Lys	Hb Athens-Ga.,	↑ O_2 affinity,	α_1-β_2	217
		Waco			218
	Arg→Ser	Hb Austin	↑ O_2 affinity, ↑ dissociation		218
41(C7)	Phe→Tyr	Hb Mequon		Heme	219
42(CD1)	Phe→Ser	Hb Hammersmith,	Unstable,	Heme	220
		Chiba	↓ O_2 affinity		221
	Phe→Leu	Hb Louisville,	Unstable,		222
		Bucuresti	↓ O_2 affinity		223

Table 2 (continued)
VARIANTS OF THE β-CHAIN

Residue	Substitution	Name	Major abnormal property	Contacts	Ref.
43(CD2)	Glu→Ala	Hb G Galveston,		External	224
		G Port Arthur,			224
		G Texas			224
	Glu→Gln	Hb Hoshida	Normal O_2 affinity		225
44(CD3)	Ser			Heme	
45(CD4)	Phe→Ser	Hb Cheverly	Unstable, ↓ O_2 affinity	Heme	226
46(CD5)	Gly→Glu	HbK Ibadan		External	227
47(CD6)	Asp→Asn	Hb G Copenhagen		External	228
	Asp→Gly	Hb Gavello	Normal O_2 affinity		229
	Asp→Ala	Hb Avicenna			230
	Asp→Tyr	Hb Maputo			499
48(CD7)	Leu→Arg	Hb Okaloosa	Unstable, ↓ O_2 affinity	Surface	231
49(CD8)	Ser			External	
50(D1)	Thr→Lys	Hb Edmonton		External	232
51(D2)	Pro→Arg	Hb Willamette	↑ O_2 affinity	α_1-β_1	233
52(D3)	Asp→Asn	Hb Osu Christiansborg		External	234
	Asp→Ala	Hb Ocho Rios			235
	Asp→His	Hb Summer Hill	Normal O_2 affinity		236
53(D4)	Ala			External	
54(D5)	Val			Internal	
55(D6)	Met			α_1-β_1	
56(D7)	Gly→Asp	Hb J Bangkok,		External	237
		J Meinung,			238
		J Korat,			238
		J Manado			239
	Gly→Arg	Hb Hamadan			240
57(E1)	Asn→Lys	Hb G Ferrara	Unstable, normal O_2 affinity	External	241
	Asn→Asp	Hb J Daloa			500

58(E2)	Pro→Arg	Hb Yukuhashi, Dhofar		External	115 242
59(E3)	Lys→Glu	Hb I High Wycombe		External	243
	Lys→Thr	Hb J Kaohsiung, J Honolulu			244 245
	Lys→Asn	Hb J-Lome	Normal O_2 affinity, ↑ auto-oxidation		246
60(E4)	Val→Leu	Hb Yatsushiro		Internal	247
	Val→Ala	Hb Collingwood	Unstable normal O_2 affinity		501
61(E5)	Lys→Glu	Hb N Seattle		External	248
	Lys→Asn	Hb Hikari	Normal O_2 affinity		249
	Lys→Met	Hb Bologna	↓ O_2 affinity		250
62(E6)	Ala→Pro	Hb Duarte	Unstable, ↑ O_2 affinity	External	251
63(E7)	His→Arg	Hb Zürich	Unstable, ↑ O_2 affinity	Heme ''distal''	252
	His→Tyr	Hb M Saskatoon, M Emory, M Kurume, M Hida M Radom, M Arhus, M Chicago, Leipzig, Hörlein-Weber, Novi Sad, M Erlangen	Ferri-Hb, ↑ O_2 affinity		253 253 254 255 256 257 258 259 260 261
	His→Pro	Hb Bicêtre	Unstable, auto-oxidizing		262
64(E8)	Gly→Asp	Hb J Calabria, J Bari, J Cosenza	Unstable, ↑ O_2 affinity	Internal	263
65(E9)	Lys→Asn	Hb J Sicilia		External	264
	Lys→Gln	Hb J Cairo	↓ O_2 affinity, auto-oxidation		265
66(E10)	Lys→Glu	Hb I Toulouse	Unstable, ferri-Hb, normal O_2 affinity	External, ? heme	266

Table 2 (continued)
VARIANTS OF THE β-CHAIN

Residue	Substitution	Name	Major abnormal property	Contacts	Ref.
67(E11)	Val→Asp	Hb Bristol	Unstable,	Heme	267
			↓ O_2 affinity		
	Val→Glu	Hb M Milwaukee-I	Ferri-Hb,		253
			↓ O_2 affinity		
	Val→Ala	Hb Sydney	Unstable		268
68(E12)	Leu→Pro	Hb Mizuho	Unstable	Internal	269
	Leu→His	Hb Brisbane,	↑ O_2 affinity,		270
		Great Lakes	(?) unstable		271
69(E13)	Gly→Asp	Hb J Cambridge,		External	228
		J Rambam			272
70(E14)	Ala→Asp	Hb Seattle	↓ O_2 affinity, unstable	Heme	273
71(E15)	Phe→Ser	Hb Christchurch	Unstable	Heme	274
72(E16)	Ser			External	
73(E17)	Asp→Tyr	Hb Vancouver	↓ O_2 affinity	External	275
	Asp→Asn	Hb Korle Bu,	↓ O_2 affinity		276
		G Accra			277
	Asp→Val	Hb Mobile	↓ O_2 affinity		278, 275
74(E18)	Gly→Val	Hb Bushwick	Unstable	External	279
	Gly→Asp	Hb Shepherds Bush	Unstable,		280
			↑ O_2 affinity		
75(E19)	Leu→Pro	Hb Atlanta	Unstable	Internal	281
	Leu→Arg	Hb Pasadena	Unstable,		282
			↑ O_2 affinity		
76(E20)	Ala→Asp	Hb J Chicago		External	283
77(EF1)	His→Asp	Hb J Iran		External	284
78(EF2)	Leu→Arg	Hb Quin-Hai		Internal	502
79(EF3)	Asp→Gly	Hb G Hsi-Tsou	↑ O_2 affinity	External	285, 286
	Asp→Tyr	Hb Tampa			287
80(EF4)	Asn→Lys	Hb G Szuhu,	Normal O_2 affinity	External	288
		Gifu			289
81(EF5)	Leu→Arg	Hb Baylor	↑ O_2 affinity, unstable	Internal	290

82(EF6)	Lys→Asn→Asp	Hb Providence	↓ O_2 affinity	DPG Binding	291, 292
	Lys→Thr	Hb Rahere	↑ O_2 affinity		293
	Lys→Met	Hb Helsinki	↑ O_2 affinity		294
83(EF7)	Gly→Cys	Hb Ta-li	Slightly unstable, polymerization	External	295
	Gly→Asp	Hb Pyrgos	(Sl.) ↓ O_2 affinity		296, 297
84(EF8)	Thr			External	
85(F1)	Phe→Ser	Buenos Aires	Unstable, ↑ O_2 affinity	Internal	299
		Hb Bryn Mawr			298
86(F2)	Ala			External	
87(F3)	Thr→Lys	HbD Ibadan		External	300
88(F4)	Leu→Arg	Hb Borås	Unstable	Heme	301
	Leu→Pro	Hb Santa Ana	Unstable		302
89(F5)	Ser→Asn	Hb Creteil	↑ O_2 affinity	Internal	303
	Ser→Arg	Hb Vanderbilt	↑ O_2 affinity		304
90(F6)	Glu→Lys	Hb Agenogi	↓ O_2 affinity	External	305
91(F7)	Leu→Pro	Hb Sabine	Unstable	Heme	306
	Leu→Arg	Hb Caribbean	Unstable, ↓ O_2 affinity		307
92(F8)	His→Tyr	Hb M Hyde Park, M Akita	Normal O_2 affinity, ferri-Hb	Heme "Proximal"	308 309
	His→Gln	Hb St. Etienne, Istanbul	Unstable, ↑ O_2 affinity, ↑ dissociation		310 311
	His→Asp	Hb J Altgeld Gardens	Normal O_2 affinity, unstable		312
	His→Pro	Hb Newcastle	Unstable		313
	His→Arg	Hb Mozhaisk	Unstable, ↑ O_2 affinity		314
93(F9)	Cys			External	
94(FG1)	Asp→His	Hb Barcelona	↑ O_2 affinity	External	315
	Asp→Asn	Hb Bunbury	↑ O_2 affinity		503
95(FG2)	Lys→Glu	Hb N Baltimore, Hopkins-I, Jenkins, N Memphis, Kenwood		External	316 317 318 319, 320
	Lys→Asn	Hb Detroit	Normal O_2 affinity		321
96(FG3)	Leu			Heme	

Table 2 (continued)
VARIANTS OF THE β-CHAIN

Residue	Substitution	Name	Major abnormal property	Contacts	Ref.
97(FG4)	His→Gln	Hb Malmö	↑ O_2 affinity	α_1-β_2	322
	His→Leu	Hb Wood	↑ O_2 affinity		323, 324
98(FG5)	Val→Met	Hb Köln,	Unstable, ↑ O_2 affinity	Heme, α_1-β_2	325
		San Francisco (Pacific),			326
		Ube I			327
	Val→Gly	Hb Nottingham	Unstable, ↑ O_2 affinity		328
	Val→Ala	Hb Djelfa	Unstable, ↑ O_2 affinity		329
99(G1)	Asp→Asn	Hb Kempsey	↑ O_2 affinity		330
	Asp→His	Hb Yakima	↑ O_2 affinity		331
	Asp→Ala	Hb Radcliffe	↑ O_2 affinity		332
	Asp→Tyr	Hb Ypsilanti	↑ O_2 affinity		333
	Asp→Gly	Hb Hotel-Dieu	↑ O_2 affinity		334
	Asp→Val	Hb Chemilly	↑ O_2 affinity		504
100(G2)	Pro→Leu	Hb Brigham	↑ O_2 affinity	α_1-β_2	335
101(G3)	Glu→Lys	Hb British Columbia	↑ O_2 affinity	α_1-β_2	336
	Glu→Gln	Hb Rush	Unstable, normal O_2 affinity		337
	Glu→Gly	Hb Alberta	↑ O_2 affinity		338
	Glu→Asp	Hb Potomac	↑ O_2 affinity		339
102(G4)	Asn→Lys	Hb Richmond	Asymmetric hybrids	Heme, α_1-β_2	340
	Asn→Thr	Hb Kansas	↓ O_2 affinity, ↑ dissociation		341
	Asn→Ser	Hb Beth Israel	↓ O_2 affinity, unstable		342
	Asn→Tyr	Hb St. Mandé	↓ O_2 affinity		343
103(G5)	Phe→Leu	Hb Heathrow	↑ O_2 affinity	Heme	344
104(G6)	Arg→Ser	Hb Camperdown	Slightly unstable, normal O_2 affinity	Central cavity	345
	Arg→Thr	Hb Sherwood Forest			346
105(G7)	Leu			Internal	
106(G8)	Leu→Pro	Hb Southampton	↑ O_2 affinity unstable	Heme	347
		Hb Casper			348
	Leu→Gln	Hb Tübingen	Unstable, ↑ O_2 affinity		349, 350

107(G9)	Gly→Arg	Hb Burke	↓ O_2 affinity, unstable	Internal	351
108(G10)	Asn→Asp	Hb Yoshizuka	↓ O_2 affinity	α_1-β_1	352
	Asn→Lys	Hb Presbyterian	↓ O_2 affinity		353
109(G11)	Val→Met	Hb San Diego	↑ O_2 affinity	Internal	354
110(G12)	Leu			Internal	
111(G13)	Val→Phe	Hb Peterborough	Unstable, ↓ O_2 affinity	Internal	355
112(G14)	Cys→Arg	Hb Indianapolis	Unstable	α_1-β_1	356
113(G15)	Val→Glu	Hb New York	Unstable, ↓ O_2 affinity	Internal	357
114(G16)	Leu			Internal	
115(G17)	Ala→Pro	Hb Madrid	Unstable	α_1-β_1	358
116(G18)	His			α_1-β_1	
117(G19)	His→Arg	Hb P Galveston		External	359
	His→Pro	Hb Saitama	Unstable		505
118(GH1)	Phe→Tyr	Hb Minneapolis-Laos	Normal O_2 affinity	Surface	506
119(GH2)	Gly→Asp	Hb Fannin-Lubbock	Unstable (slightly), normal O_2 affinity	α_1-β_1	360, 361
	Gly→Val	Hb Bougardirey-Mali	Slightly unstable		362
120(GH3)	Lys→Glu	Hb Hijiyama		External	363
	Lys→Asn	Hb Riyadh,			364
		Karatsu			365
	Lys→Gln	Hb Takamatsu			366
	Lys→Ile	Hb Jianghua			507
121(GH4)	Glu→Gln	Hb D Los Angeles,	↑ O_2 affinity	External	367
		D Punjab,			368, 369
		D North Carolina,			370
		D Portugal,			371
		Oak Ridge,			372
		D Chicago			373
	Glu→Lys	Hb O Arab,	Normal O_2 affinity		374
		Egypt			375
	Glu→Val	Hb Beograd			376
122(GH5)	Phe			α_1-β_1	
123(H1)	Thr			α_1-β_1	
124(H2)	Pro→Arg	Hb Khartoum	Unstable	α_1-β_1	377
	Pro→Gln	Hb Ty Gard	↑ O_2 affinity		378
125(H3)	Pro			α_1-β_1	

Table 2 (continued)
VARIANTS OF THE β-CHAIN

Residue	Substitution	Name	Major abnormal property	Contacts	Ref.
126(H4)	Val→Glu	Hb Hofu	Unstable	Surface	379
	Val→Ala	Hb Beirut			508
127(H5)	Gln→Glu	Hb Hacettepe		α_1-β_1	380
128(H6)	Ala→Asp	Hb J Guantanamo	Unstable	α_1-β_1	381
129(H7)	Ala→Asp	Hb J Taichung		Surface	382
	Ala→Glu or Asp	Hb K Cameroon			227
	Ala→Pro	Hb Crete	Unstable, ↑ O_2 affinity		383
130(H8)	Tyr→Asp	Hb Wien	Unstable	Internal	384
131(H9)	Gln→Glu	Hb Camden, Tokuchi	Normal O_2 affinity	α_1-β_1	385 386
132(H10)	Lys→Gln	Hb K Woolwich		Surface	227
133(H11)	Val			Internal	
134(H12)	Val→Glu	Hb North Shore	Unstable, normal O_2 affinity	Internal	387, 388
135(H13)	Ala→Pro	Hb Altdorf	Unstable, ↑ O_2 affinity	Central	389
136(H14)	Gly→Asp	Hb Hope	Unstable, ↓ O_2 affinity	Central	390
137(H15)	Val			Heme	
138(H16)	Ala→Pro	Hb Brockton	Unstable	Central	391
139(H17)	Asn→Asp	Hb Jinan		Central	509
140(H18)	Ala→Thr	Hb Saint-Jacques	↑ O_2 affinity	Central	510
141(H19)	Leu→Arg	Hb Olmsted	Unstable	Heme	322
142(H20)	Ala→Asp	Hb Ohio	↑ O_2 affinity	Central	392
	Ala→Pro	Hb Toyoake	↑ O_2 affinity, unstable		393
143(H21)	His→Arg	Hb Abruzzo	↑ O_2 affinity	DPG Binding	394
	His→Gln	Hb Little Rock	↑ O_2 affinity		395
	His→Pro	Hb Syracuse	↑ O_2 affinity		396
144(HC1)	Lys→Asn	Hb Andrew-Minneapolis	↑ O_2 affinity	External	397
145(HC2)	Tyr→His	Hb Bethesda	↑ O_2 affinity	Hydrogen bond to val FG5 same β-chain in deoxy form	398

Residue	Substitution	Name	Properties	Contact	Ref.
	Tyr→Cys	Hb Rainier	↑ O_2 affinity, alkali resistant		398
	Tyr→Asp	Hb Fort Gordon, Osler, Nancy	↑ O_2 affinity		399 400 401
	Tyr→Term	Hb McKees Rocks	↑ O_2 affinity		402
146(HC3)	His→Asp	Hb Hiroshima	↑ O_2 affinity	α_1-β_2	403, 404
	His→Pro	Hb York	↑ O_2 affinity		405
	His→Arg	Hb Cochin-Port Royal	Normal O_2 affinity		406
	His→Leu	Hb Cowtown	↑ O_2 Affinity		407

Table 3
VARIANTS OF THE δ-CHAIN

Residue	Substitution	Name	Ref.
2(NA2)	His→Arg	Hb A_2 Sphakiá	408
12(A9)	Asn→Lys	Hb A_2 NYU	409
16(A13)	Gly→Arg	Hb A_2' (B_2)	410
20(B2)	Val→Glu	Hb A_2 Roosevelt	411
22(B4)	Ala→Glu	Hb A_2 Flatbush	412
24(B6)	Gly→Asp	Hb A_2 Victoria	511
43(CD2)	Glu→Lys	Hb A_2 Melbourne	413
51(D2)	Pro→Arg	Hb A_2 Adria	414
69(E13)	Gly→Arg	Hb A_2 Indonesia	415
99(G1)	Asp→Asn	Hb A_2 Canada, ↑ O_2 affinity	512
116(G18)	Arg→His	Hb A_2 Coburg	416
121(GH4)	Glu→Val	Hb A_2 Manzanares	513
125(H3)	Gln→Glu	Hb A_2 Zagreb	514
136(H14)	Gly→Asp	Hb A_2 Babinga	417
142(H20)	Ala→Asp	Hb A_2 Fitzroy	515

Table 4
VARIANTS OF THE γ-CHAIN

Residue	Substitution	Name	Ref.
1(NA1)	Gly→Cys $({}^{G}\gamma)$	Hb F Malaysia	418
5(A2)	Glu→Lys $({}^{A}\gamma^{I})$	Hb F Texas-I	419, 420
	Glu→Gly $({}^{G}\gamma^{I})$	Hb F Meinohama	421
6(A3)	Glu→Lys	Hb F Texas-II	422
	Glu→Gly $({}^{A}\gamma^{I})$	Hb F Kotobuki	423
	Glu→Gln $({}^{A}\gamma^{I})$	Hb F Pordenone	516
7(A4)	Asp→Asn $({}^{G}\gamma)$	Hb F Auckland	424
12(A9)	Thr→Lys	Hb F Alexandra	425
	Thr→Arg $({}^{G}\gamma^{I})$	Hb F Heather	517
	Thr→Arg $({}^{A}\gamma^{I})$	Hb F Calluna	518
16(A13)	Gly→Arg $({}^{G}\gamma^{I})$	Hb F Melbourne	426
22(B4)	Asp→Gly $({}^{A}\gamma^{I})$	Hb F Kuala Lumpur	427
39(C5)	Gln→Arg $({}^{A}\gamma^{I})$	Hb F Bonaire-GA	519
44(CD3)	Ser→Arg $({}^{G}\gamma^{I})$	Hb F Lodz	520
55(D6)	Met→Arg $({}^{G}\gamma)$	Hb F Kingston	521
61(E5)	Lys→Glu $({}^{A}\gamma)$	Hb F Jamaica	428
63(E7)	His→Tyr $({}^{G}\gamma)$	Hb F M-Osaka	429
66(E10)	Lys→Arg $({}^{G}\gamma^{I})$	Hb F Shanghai	522
72(E16)	Gly→Arg $({}^{A}\gamma^{I})$	Hb F Iwata	430
75(E19)	Ile→Thr	Hb F Sardinia	431
77(EF1)	His→Arg $({}^{G}\gamma^{I})$	Hb F Kennestone	523
80(EF4)	Asp→Tyr $({}^{A}\gamma)$	Hb F Victoria Jubilee	432
	Asp→Asn $({}^{G}\gamma^{I})$	Hb F Marietta	524
	Asp→Asn $({}^{A}\gamma^{T})$	Hb F Yamaguchi	430
94(FG1)	Asp→Asn $({}^{G}\gamma^{I})$	Hb F Columbus-Ga.	525
97(FG4)	His→Arg $({}^{A}\gamma^{I})$	Hb F Dickinson	433
101(G3)	Glu→Lys $({}^{G}\gamma)$	Hb F Lagrange	526
108(G10)	Asn→Lys	Hb F Ube	434
117(G19)	His→Arg $({}^{G}\gamma)$	Hb F Malta-I	435
120(GH3)	Lys→Gln $({}^{G}\gamma)$	Hb F Caltech	527
121(GH4)	Glu→Lys $({}^{A}\gamma)$	Hb F Hull	436
	Glu→Lys $({}^{G}\gamma)$	Hb F Carlton	426
	Glu→Lys $({}^{A}\gamma^{T})$	Hb F Siena	528
125(H3)	Glu→Ala $({}^{G}\gamma^{I})$	Hb F Port Royal	437
130(H8)	Trp→Gly $({}^{G}\gamma^{I})$	Hb F Poole	438

Table 5
FUSION HEMOGLOBINS

												Ref.
	A6	A9	B4	D1	F2	F3	G18	G19	H2	H4		
	9	12	22	50	86	87	116	117	124	126		
δ-Chain →→→→→	Thr	Asn	Ala	Ser	Ser	Gln	Arg	Asn	Gln	Met		
β-Chain →→→→→	Ser	Thr	Glu	Thr	Ala	Thr	His	His	Pro	Val		
Lepore-Hollandia			δ	β								439
Lepore-Baltimore				δ	β							440
Lepore-Washington-Boston						δ	β					441
Parchman		δ	β	β		δ						442
Miyada		β	δ									443
P Congo			β				δ					444
P Nilotic			β	δ								445
Lincoln Park			β	δ							δ137 Val→0	446
	NA1		EF4	EF5	F2	F3				HC3		
	1		80	81	86	87				146		
γ-Chain →→→→→	Gly		Asp	Leu	Ala	Gln				His		
β-Chain →→→→→	Val		Asn	Leu	Ala	Thr				His		
Kenya				γ	β							447

Table 6
EXTENDED CHAINS

	Residue	Name	Major abnormal property	Ref.
α141	140 (31 additional residues) Tyr-Arg-Gln-Ala-Gly 150 Ala-Ser-Val-Ala-Val-Pro-Pro-Ala-Arg-Trp-Ala 160 Ser-Gln-Arg-Ala-Leu-Leu-Pro-Ser-Leu-His-Arg 170 Pro-Phe-Leu-Val-Phe-Glu-COOH	Hb Constant Spring	Stable	448
α141	31 additional residues — identical to Hb Constant Spring except for residue 142 which is lysine instead of glutamine	Hb Icaria		449
α141	140 (16 or 17 additional residues Tyr-Arg(Ser,Ala, 150 Gly,Ala,Ser,Val,Ala,Val,Pro,Pro,Ala)-Arg(?,Ala, Ser,Gln)-Arg-COOH	Hb Koya Dora		450
α146	150 (11 additional residues)Thr-Lys-Leu-Ala-Phe- Leu-Leu-Ser-Asn-Phe-Tyr-COOH	Hb Tak	↑ O_2 affinity, sl. unstable	451—453
α139-141	140 Thr-Ser-Asn-Thr-Val-Lys-Leu-Glu-Pro-Arg-COOH (Frameshift)	Hb Wayne,	↑ O_2 affinity	454
β145	144 150 Lys-Ser-Ile-Thr-Lys-Leu-Ala-Phe-Leu-Leu-Ser- 155 Asn-Phe-Tyr-COOH	Hb Cranston Unstable,	↑ O_2 affinity	456—458
α115-118	115 116 117 118 119 Ala-Glu-Phe-Thr-Glu-Phe-Thr-Pro(insertion)	Hb Grady, Dakar	Unstable, ↑ O_2 affinity	456—458

Table 7
DELETED RESIDUES

Residue	Substitution	Name	Major abnormal property	Ref.
β6 or 7	Glu→O	Hb Leiden	Unstable, slightly ↑ O_2 affinity	459
β17—18	(Lys-Val)→O	Hb Lyon	↑ O_2 affinity, unstable	460
β23	Val→O	Hb Freiburg	↑ O_2 affinity	461
β42—44 or 43—45	(Phe-Glu-Ser)→O or (Glu-Ser-Phe)→O	Hb Niteroi	↓ O_2 affinity, unstable	462
β56—59	(Gly-Asn-Pro-Lys)→O	Hb Tochigi	Unstable, O_2 affinity not known	463
β74—75	(Gly-Leu)→O	Hb St. Antoine	Unstable, normal O_2 affinity	464
β75	Leu→O	Hb Vicksburg	Stable	465
β87	Thr→O	Hb Tours	↑ O_2 affinity, unstable	464
β91—95	(Leu-His-Cys-Asp-Lys)→O	Hb Gun Hill	Unstable, ↑ O_2 affinity ↑ dissociation	466
β131	Gln→O	Hb Leslie, Deaconess	Unstable, normal O_2 affinity	467, 468 469
β141	Leu→O	Hb Coventry	Normal O_2 affinity	470
α6	Asp→O	Hb Boyle Heights	Unstable	471

Table 8
MORE THAN ONE POINT MUTATION IN THE SAME POLYPEPTIDE CHAIN

Residue	Substitution	Name	Major abnormal property	Ref.
β6(A3)	Glu→Val, 73Asp→Asn	Hb C Harlem, C Georgetown	Normal O_2 affinity	472 473
	Glu→Lys, 95Lys→Glu	Hb Arlington Park	Not done	474
α78—79	Asn→Asp Ala→Gly	Hb J Singapore	Not done	475
β6(A3)	Glu→Val, 58Pro→Arg	Hb C Ziguinchor	Sickling	476
β6(A3)	Glu→Val, 142Ala→Val	Hb S Travis	↑ O_2 affinity, sickling	477

Table 9
α-CHAIN VARIANTS WITH LOW OXYGEN AFFINITY

Residue	Substitution	Name	Contact
43(CE1)	Phe→Val	Hb Torino	Heme
58(E7)	His→Tyr	Hb M Boston, M Osaka, Gothenburg, M Kiskunhalas	Heme, "distal"
86(F7)	Leu→Arg	Hb Moabit	Heme
87(F8)	His→Tyr	Hb M Iwate, M Kankakee, M Oldenburg	Heme, "proximal"
94(G1)	Asp→Asn	Hb Titusville	αa_1-β_2
94(G1)	Asp→Tyr	Hb Setif	α_1-β_2

Table 10
α-CHAIN VARIANTS WITH HIGH OXYGEN AFFINITY

Residue	Substitution	Name	Contact
6(A4)	Asp→Ala	Hb Sawara	External
	Asp→Asn	Hb Dunn	
	Asp→Val	Hb Ferndown	
	Asp→Tyr	Hb Woodville	
14(A12)	Trp→Arg	Hb Evanston	Internal
40(C5)	Lys→Glu	Hb Kariya	Deoxy: α_1-β_2
44(CE2)	Pro→Leu	Hb Milledgeville	α_1-β_2
	Pro→Arg	Hb Kawachi	
45(CE3)	His→Arg	Hb Fort de France	Heme
47(CE5)	Asp→Gly	Hb Kokura	External
84(F5)	Ser→Arg	Hb Etobicoke	Internal
85(F6)	Asp→Asn	Hb G Norfolk	External
	Asp→Tyr	Hb Atago	
	Asp→Val	Hb Inkster	
90(FG2)	Lys→Met	Hb Handa	External
92(FG4)	Arg→Gln	Hb J Cape Town	α_1-β_2
	Arg→Leu	Hb Chesapeake	
95(G2)	Pro→Ala	Hb Denmark Hill	α_1-β_2
	Pro→Ser	Hb Rampa	
	Pro→Leu	Hb G Georgia	
	Pro→Arg	Hb St. Lukes	
97(G4)	Asn→Lys	Hb Dallas	Heme
112(G19)	His→Asp	Hb Hopkins-II	External
126(H9)	Asp→Asn	Hb Tarrant	α_1-β_1
139(HC2)	Lys→Thr	Hb Tokoname	External
141(HC3)	Arg→His	Hb Suresnes	External, deoxy, salt bonds to H9, H10, NA1 other α-chain, oxy: Mobile, Bohr
	Arg→Leu	Hb Legnano	
	Arg→Ser	Hb J Cubujuqui	

Table 11
α-CHAINS (UNSTABLE)

Residue	Substitution	Name	Contact
26(B7)	Ala→Glu	Hb Shenyang	External
27(B8)	Glu→Lys	Hb Shuangfeng	External
31(B12)	Arg→Ser	Hb Prato	α_1-β_1
40(C5)	Lys→Glu	Hb Kariya	Deoxy: α_1-β_2
43(CE1)	Phe→Val	Hb Torino	Heme
	Phe→Leu	Hb Hirosaki	
47(CE5)	Asp→His	Hb Hasharon, Sinai, Sealy, L Ferrara	External
	Asp→Gly	Hb Umi, Kokura, Beilinson, Tagawa-II	
	Asp→Asn	Hb Arya	
	Asp→Ala	Hb Cordele	
53(E2)	Ala→Asp	Hb J Rovigo	External
59(E8)	Gly→Val	Hb Tottori	Internal
63(E12)	Ala→Asp	Hb Pontoise	Surface
80(F1)	Leu→Arg	Hb Ann Arbor	Surface
86(F7)	Leu→Arg	Hb Moabit	Heme
87(F8)	His→Arg	Hb M Iwata	Heme
91(FG3)	Leu→Pro	Hb Port Phillip	α_1-β_2
94(G1)	Asp→Tyr	Hb Setif	α_1-β_2
102(G9)	Ser→Arg	Hb Manitoba	Central
103(G10)	His→Arg	Hb Contaldo	α_1-β_1
109(G16)	Leu→Arg	Hb Suan-dok	Internal
110(G17)	Ala→Asp	Hb Petah Tikva	Internal
112(G19)	His→Asp	Hb Hopkins-II	External
136(H19)	Leu→Pro	Hb Bibba	Heme

Table 12
β-CHAIN VARIANTS WITH LOW OXYGEN AFFINITY

Residue	Substitution	Name	Contact
1(NA1)	Val-Ac-Ala	Hb Raleigh	DPG Binding
21(B3)	Asp→Gly	Hb Connecticut	External
24(B6)	Gly→Asp	Hb Moscva	Internal
37(C3)	Trp→Arg	Hb Rothschild	α_1-β_1
42(CD1)	Phe→Ser	Hb Hammersmith, Chiba	Heme
	Phe→Leu	Hb Louisville, Bucuresti	
45(CD4)	Phe→Ser	Hb Cheverly	Heme
48(CD7)	Leu→Arg	Hb Okaloosa	Surface
61(E5)	Lys→Met	Hb Bologna	External
65(E9)	Lys→Gln	Hb J Cairo	External
67(E11)	Val→Glu	Hb M Milwaukee-I	Heme
	Val→Asp	Hb Bristol	
70(E14)	Ala→Asp	Hb Seattle	Heme
73(E17)	Asp→Tyr	Hb Vancouver	External
	Asp→Asn	Hb Korle Bu	
	Asp→Val	Hb Mobile	
82(EF6)	Lys→Asn→Asp	Hb Providence	DPG Binding
83(EF7)	Gly→Asp	Hb Pyrgos	External
90(F6)	Glu→Lys	Hb Agenogi	External
91(F7)	Leu→Arg	Hb Caribbean	Heme
102(G4)	Asn→Thr	Hb Kansas	Heme, α_1-β_2
	Asn→Ser	Hb Beth Israel	
	Asn→Tyr	Hb St. Mande	
107(G9)	Gly→Arg	Hb Burke	Internal
108(G10)	Asn→Asp	Hb Yoshizuka	α_1-β_1
	Asn→Lys	Hb Presbyterian	
111(G13)	Val→Phe	Hb Peterborough	Internal
113(G15)	Val→Glu	Hb New York	Internal
136(H14)	Gly→Asp	Hb Hope	Central

Table 13
β-CHAIN VARIANTS WITH HIGH OXYGEN AFFINITY

Residue	Substitution	Name	Contact
2(NA2)	His→Arg	Hb Deer Lodge	DPG Binding
	His→Gln	Hb Okayama	
9(A6)	Ser→Cys	Hb Pôrto Alegre	External
15(A12)	Trp→Arg	Hb Belfast	Internal
20(B2)	Val→Met	Hb Olympia	External
23(B5)	Val→Asp	Hb Strasbourg	Internal
	Val→Gly	Hb Miyashiro	
	Val→Phe	Hb Palmerston North	
24(B6)	Gly→Arg	Hb Riverdale-Bronx	Internal
28(B10)	Leu→Gln	Hb St. Louis	Internal
	Leu→Pro	Hb Genova	
34(B16)	Val→Phe	Hb Pitie-Salpetriere	α_1-β_1
35(C1)	Tyr→Phe	Hb Philly	α_1-β_1
37(C3)	Trp→Ser	Hb Hirose	α_1-β_2
40(C6)	Arg→Lys	Hb Athens-Ga., Waco	α_1-β_2
	Arg→Ser	Hb Austin	
51(D2)	Pro→Arg	Hb Willamette	α_1-β_1
62(E6)	Ala→Pro	Hb Duarte	External
63(E7)	His→Arg	Hb Zürich	Heme, "distal"
	His→Tyr	Hb M Saskatoon, M Emory, K Kurume, M Hida, M Radom, M Århus, M Chicago, Leipzig Hörlein-Weber, Novi Sad, M Erlangen	
64(E8)	Gly→Asp	Hb J Calabria	Internal
68(E12)	Leu→His	Hb Brisbane, Great Lakes	Internal
74(E18)	Gly→Asp	Hb Shepherds Bush	External
75(E19)	Leu→Arg	Hb Pasadena	
79(EF3)	Asp→Gly	Hb G Hsi-Tsou	External
81(EF5)	Leu→Arg	Hb Baylor	Internal
82(EF6)	Lys→Thr	Hb Rahere	DPG Binding
	Lys→Met	Hb Helsinki	
85(F1)	Phe→Ser	Hb Bryn Mawr, Buenos Aires	Internal
89(F5)	Ser→Asn	Hb Creteil	Internal
	Ser→Arg	Hb Vanderbilt	
92(F8)	His→Gln	Hb St. Etienne, Istanbul	Heme, "Proximal"
	His→Arg	Hb Mozhaisk	
94(FG1)	Asp→His	Hb Barcelona	External
	Asp→Asn	Hb Bunbury	
97(FG4)	His→Gln	Hb Malmö	α_1-β_2
	His→Leu	Hb Wood	
98(FG5)	Val→Met	Hb Köln, San Francisco (Pacific)	Heme, α_1-β_2
	Val→Gly	Hb Nottingham	
	Val→Ala	Hb Djelfa	
99(G1)	Asp→Asn	Hb Kempsey	α_1-β_2
	Asp→His	Hb Yakima	
	Asp→Tyr	Hb Ypsilanti	

Table 13 (continued)
β-CHAIN VARIANTS WITH HIGH OXYGEN AFFINITY

Residue	Substitution	Name	Contact
	Asp→Ala	Hb Radcliffe	
	Asp→Gly	Hb Hotel-Dieu	
	Asp→Val	Hb Chemilly	
100(G2)	Pro→Leu	Hb Brigham	α_1-β_2
101(G3)	Glu→Lys	Hb British Columbia	α_1-β_2
	Glu→Gly	Hb Alberta	
	Glu→Asp	Hb Potomac	
103(G5)	Phe→Leu	Hb Heathrow	Heme
106(G8)	Leu→Pro	Hb Southampton, Casper	Heme
	Leu→Gln	Hb Tübingen	
109(G11)	Val→Met	Hb San Diego	Internal
121(GH4)	Glu→Gln	Hb D Los Angeles, D Punjab D Chicago, D Punjab, D North Carolina, D Portugal, Oak Ridge	External
124(H2)	Pro→Gln	Hb Ty Gard	α_1-β_1
129(H7)	Ala→Pro	Hb Crete	Surface
135(H13)	Ala→Pro	Hb Altdorf	Central
140(H18)	Ala→Thr	Hb Saint Jacques	Central
142(H20)	Ala→Asp	Hb Ohio	Central
	Ala→Pro	Hb Toyoake	
143(H21)	His→Arg	Hb Abruzzo	DPG Binding
	His→Gln	Hb Little Rock	
	His→Pro	Hb Syracuse	
144(HC1)	Lys→Asn	Hb Andrew-Minneapolis	External
145(HC2)	Tyr→His	Hb Bethesda	Hydrogen bond to Val FG5, same β-chain in deoxy form
	Tyr→Cys	Hb Rainier	
	Tyr→Asp	Hb Fort Gordon, Osler, Nancy	
	Tyr→Term	Hb McKees Rocks	
146(HC3)	His→Asp	Hb Hiroshima	α_1-β_2
	His→Pro	Hb York	
	His→Leu	Hb Cowtown	

Table 14
β-CHAINS (UNSTABLE)

Residue	Substitution	Name	Contact
7(A4)	Glu→Gly	Hb G San José	External
14(A11)	Leu→Pro	Hb Saki	Surface
	Leu→Arg	Hb Sogn	Internal
15(A12)	Trp→Arg	Hb Belfast	Internal
22(B4)	Glu→Lys	Hb E Saskatoon	External
23(B5)	Val→Gly	Hb Miyashiro	Internal
	Val→Phe	Hb Palmerston North	Internal
24(B6)	Gly→Arg	Hb Riverdale-Bronx	Internal
	Gly→Val	Hb Savannah	
	Gly→Asp	Hb Moscva	
26(B8)	Glu→Val	Hb Henri Mondor	External
27(B9)	Ala→Asp	Hb Volga, Drenthe	Internal
28(B10)	Leu→Gln	Hb St. Louis	Internal
	Leu→Pro	Hb Genova	
29(B11)	Gly→Asp	Hb Lufkin	Internal
30(B12)	Arg→Ser	Hb Tacoma	α_1-β_1
31(B13)	Leu→Pro	Hb Yokohama	Heme
32(B14)	Leu→Pro	Hb Perth, Abraham Lincoln	Internal
	Leu→Arg	Hb Castilla	
35(C1)	Tyr→Phe	Hb Philly	α_1-β_1
39(C5)	Gln→Glu	Hb Vaasa	α_1-β_2
42(CD1)	Phe→Ser	Hb Hammersmith, Chiba	Heme
	Phe→Leu	Hb Louisville, Bucuresti	
45(CD4)	Phe→Ser	Hb Cheverly	Heme
48(CD7)	Leu→Arg	Hb Okaloosa	Surface
57(E1)	Asn→Lys	Hb G-Ferrara	External
60(E4)	Val→Ala	Hb Collingwood	Internal
62(E6)	Ala→Pro	Hb Duarte	External
63(E7)	His→Arg	Hb Zürich	Heme, "distal"
	His→Pro	Hb Bicêtre	
64(E8)	Gly→Asp	Hb J Calabria, J Bari, J Cosenza	Internal
66(E10)	Lys→Glu	Hb I Toulouse	External, ? heme
67(E11)	Val→Asp	Hb Bristol	Heme
	Val→Ala	Hb Sydney	
68(E12)	Leu→Pro	Hb Mizuho	Internal
	Leu→His	Hb Brisbane, Great Lakes	
70(E14)	Ala→Asp	Hb Seattle	Heme
71(E15)	Phe→Ser	Hb Christchurch	Heme
74(E18)	Gly→Asp	Hb Shepherds Bush	External
	Gly→Val	Hb Bushwick	
75(E19)	Leu→Pro	Hb Atlanta	Internal
	Leu→Arg	Hb Pasadena	
81(EF5)	Leu→Arg	Hb Baylor	Internal
83(EF7)	Gly→Cys	Hb Ta-Li	External
85(F1)	Phe→Ser	Hb Bryn Mawr, Buenos Aires	Internal
88(F4)	Leu→Arg	Hb Borås	Heme
	Leu→Pro	Hb Santa Ana	
91(F7)	Leu→Pro	Hb Sabine	Heme
	Leu→Arg	Hb Caribbean	
92(F8)	His→Gln	Hb St. Etienne, Istanbul	Heme, "proximal"
	His→Pro	Hb Newcastle	
	His→Arg	Hb Mozhaisk	
	His→Asp	Hb J Altgeld Gardens	
98(FG5)	Val→Met	Hb Köln, San Francisco (Pacific), Ube I	Heme, α_1-β_2

Table 14 (continued)
β-CHAINS (UNSTABLE)

Residue	Substitution	Name	Contact
	Val→Gly	Hb Nottingham	
	Val→Ala	Hb Djelfa	
101(G3)	Glu→Gln	Hb Rush	α_1-β_2
102(G4)	Asn→Ser	Hb Beth Israel	Heme, α_1-β_2
104(G6)	Asp→Ser	Hb Camperdown	Central, cavity
106(G8)	Leu→Gln	Hb Tübingen	Heme
	Leu→Pro	Hb Southampton, Casper	
107(G9)	Gly→Arg	Hb Burke	Internal
111(G13)	Val→Phe	Hb Peterborough	Internal
112(G14)	Cys→Arg	Hb Indianapolis	α_1-β_1
113(G15)	Val→Glu	Hb New York	Internal
115(G17)	Ala→Pro	Hb Madrid	α_1-β_1
117(G19)	His→Pro	Hb Saitama	External
119(GH2)	Gly→Asp	Hb Fannin-Lubbock	α_1-β_1
	Gly→Val	Hb Bougardirey-Mali	
124(H2)	Pro→Arg	Hb Khartoum	α_1-β_1
126(H4)	Val→Glu	Hb Hofu	Surface
128(H6)	Ala→Asp	Hb Guantanamo	α_1-β_1
129(H7)	Ala→Pro	Hb Crete	Surface
130(H8)	Tyr→Asp	Hb Wien	Internal
134(H12)	Val→Glu	Hb North Shore	Internal
135(H13)	Ala→Pro	Hb Altdorf	Central
136(H14)	Gly→Asp	Hb Hope	Central
138(H16)	Ala→Pro	Hb Brockton	Central
141(H19)	Leu→Arg	Hb Olmsted	Heme
142(H20)	Ala→Pro	Hb Toyoake	Central

Addendum
UPDATED CHAIN VARIANTS

Variants of the α-Chain

Residue	Substitution	Name	Major Abnormal Property	Contacts	Ref.
2(NA2)	Leu→Arg	Hb Chongqing	↑ O_2 affinity, unstable	Central	529
6(A4)	Asp→Gly	Hb Swan River		External	530
16(A14)	Lys→Met	Hb Harbin	↑ O_2 affinity, slightly unstable	External	529
19(AB1)	Ala→Glu	Hb Tashikuergan		External	531
20(B1)	His→Gln	Hb Le Lamentin		External	532
26(B7)	Ala→Glu	Hb Shenyang	Unstable	External	533
76(EF5)	Met→Thr	Hb Aztec		Internal	534
77(EF6)	Pro→Arg	Hb GuiZhou		External	535
113(GH1)	Leu→His	Hb Twin Peaks		Surface	536
121(H4)	Val→Met	Hb Owari	Normal O_2 affinity	Surface	537
136(H19)	Leu→Met	HB Chicago		Heme	538
141(HC3)	Arg→Cys	Hb Nunobiki	↑ O_2 affinity	External, deoxy, salt bonds to H9, H10, NA1 other α-chain oxy: Mobile, Bohr	539

UPDATED CHAIN VARIANTS (continued)

Variants of the α-Chain

Residue	Substitution	Name	Major Abnormal Property	Contacts	Ref.
		Variants of the β-Chain			
5(A2)	Pro→Arg	Hb Warwickshire			540
36(C2)	Pro→Thr	Hb Linkoping	Unstable, ↑ O_2 affinity	$\alpha_1\beta_2$	541
	Pro→Ser	Hb North Chicago	↑ O_2 affinity	$\alpha_1\beta_2$	542
38(C4)	Thr→Pro	Hb Hazenbrouck	Unstable, ↓ O_2 affinity	Heme	543
44(CD3)	Ser→Cys	Hb Mississippi		Heme	544
46(CD5)	Gly→Arg	Hb Gainesville		External	545
65(39)	Lys→Met	Hb J-Antakya		External	546
69(E13)	Gly→Ser	Hb City of Hope		External	547
	Gly→Arg	Hb Kenitra			548
84(EF8)	Thr→Ile	Hb Kofu	Normal O_2 affinity	External	549
90(F6)	Glu→Gly	Hb Rouseau-Poite a Pitre	Unstable, ↓ O_2 affinity	External	550
93(F9)	Cys→Arg	Hb Okazaki	↑ O_2 affinity, unstable	External	551
96(FG3)	Leu→Val	Hb Regina	↑ O_2 affinity	Heme	552
97(FG4)	His→Pro	Hb Nagoya	↑ O_2 affinity, unstable	$\alpha_1\beta_2$	553
127(G5)	Gln→Glu	Hb Complutense		$\alpha_1\beta_1$	546
131(H9)	Gln→Lys	Hb Shelby	Unstable, normal O_2 affinity	$\alpha_1\beta_1$	554
139(H17)	Asn→Asp	Hb Geelong	Unstable	Central	555
140(H18)	Ala→Asp	Hb Himeji	Unstable, ↓ O_2 affinity	Central	556
144(HC1)	Lys→Glu	Hb Mito	↑ O_2 affinity	External	557
		Variants of the δ-Chain			
25(B7)	Gly→Asp	Hb A_2 Yokoshima			558
90(F6)	Glu→Val	Hb Honai			559
		Variants of the γ-Chain			
22(B4)	Asp→Gly $^G\gamma^I$	Hb F Urumqi			560
34(B16)	Val→Ile $^G\gamma^I$	Hb F Tokyo			561
36(C2)	Pro→Arg $^A\gamma^I$	Hb F Pendergrass			562
37(C3)	Trp→Gly $^A\gamma^I$	Hb F Cobb			563
53(D4)	Ala→Asp $^A\gamma^I$	Hb F Beech Island			564
73(E17)	Asp→Asn $^A\gamma^T$	Hb F Forest Park			565
79(EF3)	Asp→Asn $^A\gamma^I$	Hb F Dammam			566

Extended Chains

β143	Pro-Ser-Ile-Thr-Lys-Leu-Ala-Phe-Leu-Leu-Ser-Asn-Phe-Tyr-COOH	Hb Saverne	↑ O_2 affinity, unstable	567
β1	Met-Val-Pro-Leu- (−1 +1 +2)	Hb Long Island-Marseille		568, 569
β1	Met-Glu-His-Leu- (−1 +1 +2)	Hb Doha		570
β1	Met-Met-His-Leu (−1 +1 +2)	Hb South Florida		571

UPDATED CHAIN VARIANTS (continued)

Variants of the α-Chain

Residue	Substitution	Name	Major Abnormal Property	Contacts	Ref.
	More Than One Point Mutation in the Same Polypeptide Chain				
β26	Glu→Lys 121 Glu→Gln	Hb T-Cambodia			572
β56	Gly→Arg 86 Ala→Pro	Hb Poissy	Unstable		573

REFERENCES

1. **Crookston, J. H., Beale, D., Irvine, D., and Lehmann, H.,** A new haemoglobin J Toronto (α5 Alanine→Aspartic acid), *Nature (London),* 208, 1059, 1965.
2. **Sumida, I., Ohta, Y., Imamura, T., and Yanase, T.,** Hemoglobin Sawara: α6(A4) Aspartic acid→Alanine, *Biochim. Biophys. Acta,* 322, 23, 1973.
3. **Jue, D. L., Johnson, M. H., Patchen, L. C., and Moo-Penn, W. F.,** Hemoglobin Dunn: α6(A4) Aspartic acid→Asparagine, *Hemoglobin,* 3, 137, 1979.
4. **Lee-Potter, J. P., Deacon-Smith, R. A., Lehmann, H., and Robb, L.,** Haemoglobin Ferndown (α6[A4] Aspartic acid→Valine), *FEBS Lett.,* 126, 117, 1981.
5. **Pootrakul, S., Kematorn, B., Na-Nakorn, S., and Suanpan, S.,** A new haemoglobin variant: Haemoglobin Anantharaj alpha 11 (A9) Lysine→Glutamic acid, *Biochim. Biophys. Acta,* 405, 161, 1975.
6. **Zeng, Y.-T., Huang, S.-Z., Liang, X., Long, G.-F., Lam, H., Wilson, J. B., and Huisman, T. H. J.,** Hb Wuming or α_2 11(A9) Lys→Gln β_2, *Hemoglobin,* 5, 679, 1981.
7. **Rosa, J., Maleknia, N., Vergoz, D., and Dunet, R.,** Une nouvelle hémoglobine anormale: l'hémoglobin J α Paris 12 Ala→Asp, *Nouv. Rev. Fr. Hematol.,* 6, 423, 1965.
8. **Trincao, C., Martins De Melo, J., Lorkin, P. A., and Lehmann, H.,** Haemoglobin J Paris in the South of Portugal (Algarve), *Acta Haematol.,* 39, 291, 1968.
9. **Marti, H. R., Pik, C., and Mosimann, P.,** Eine neue hämoglobin I variante: Hb I Interlaken, *Acta Haematol.,* 32, 9, 1964.
10. **Liddell, J., Brown, D., Beale, D., Lehmann, H., and Huntsman, R. G.,** A new haemoglobin — Jα Oxford found during a survey of an English population, *Nature (London),* 204, 269, 1964.
11. **Silvestroni, E., Bianco, I., Tentori, L., Vivaldi, G., Carta, S., Sorcini, M., and Brancati, C.,** *Proc. 10th Congr. Eur. Soc. Hematol.,* Strasbourg, 1965. Part II, Karger, Basel/New York, 1967, 232.
12. **Vella, F., Casey, R., Lehmann, H., Labossiere, A., and Jones, T. G.,** Haemoglobin Ottawa: α_2 15(A13) Gly→Arg β_2, *Biochim. Biophys. Acta,* 336, 25, 1974.
13. **Pootrakul, S., Stichiyanont, S., Wasi, P., and Suanpan, S.,** Hemoglobin Siam (α_2 15 Arg β_2): a new chain variant, *Humangenetik,* 23, 199, 1974.
14. **Beale, D. and Lehmann, H.,** Abnormal haemoglobins and the genetic code, *Nature (London),* 207, 259, 1965.
15. **Schneider, R. G., Alperin, J. B., Beale, D., and Lehmann, H.,** Hemoglobin I in an American Negro family: structural and hematologic studies, *J. Lab. Clin. Med.,* 68, 940, 1966.
16. **Bowman, B. H. and Barnett, D. R.,** Amino-acid substituion in Haemoglobin I (Texas variant), *Nature (London),* 214, 499, 1967.
17. **O'Brien, C., Gray, M. J., and Jacobs, A. S.,** A survey of cord blood for abnormal hemoglobin with further observations on Hemoglobin I Burlington, *Am. J. Obstetr. Gynecol.,* 88, 816, 1964.
18. **Baur, E. W.,** Hb α_2 glu β_2 (Hb I) in a Caucasian family: independent mutation or common origin?, *Humangenetik,* 6, 368, 1968.
19. **Griffiths, K. D., Lang, A., Lehmann, H., Mann, J. R., Plowman, D., and Raine, D. N.,** Haemoglobin Handsworth α18 (A16) Glycine→Arginine, *FEBS Lett.,* 75, 93, 1977.
20. **Rahbar, S., Ala, F., Akhavan, E., Nowzari, G., Shoa'i, I., and Zamanianpoor, M. H.,** Two new haemoglobins: Haemoglobin Perspolis [α64 (E13) Asp→Tyr] and Haemoglobin J-Kurosh [α19 (AB1) Ala→Asp], *Biochim. Biophys. Acta,* 427, 119, 1976.
21. **Wajcman, H., Elion, J., Boissel, J. P., Labie, D., Jos, J., and Girot, R.,** A silent hemoglobin variant: Hemoglobin Necker Enfants-Malades α20(B1) His→Tyr, *Hemoglobin,* 4, 177, 1980.

22. **Kendall, A. G., Barr, R. D., Lang, A., and Lehmann, H.,** Haemoglobin J Nyanza: α21 (B2) Ala→Asp, *Biochim. Biophys. Acta,* 310, 357, 1973.
23. **Gottlieb, A. J., Restrepo, A., and Itano, H. A.,** Hemoglobin J Medellin. Chemical and genetic study, *Fed. Proc.,* 23, 172, 1964.
24. **Kraus, A. P., Miyaji, T., Iuchi, I., and Kraus, L. M.,** Memphis. A new variety of sickle cell anemia with clinically mild symptoms due to an α-chain variant of hemoglobin (α23 Glu NH2), *J. Lab. Clin. Med.,* 66, 886, 1965.
25. **Boyer, S. H., Crosby, E. F., Fuller, G. F., Ulenurm, L., and Buck, A. A.,** A survey of hemoglobins in the Republic of Chad and characterization of Hemoglobin Chad. α_2 23Glu→Lys β_2, *Am. J. Hum. Genet.,* 20, 570, 1968.
26. **Marengo-Rowe, A. J., Beale, D., and Lehmann, H.,** New human haemoglobin variant from southern Arabia: G-Audhali (α23 (B4) Glutamic acid→Valine) and the variability of B4 in human haemoglobin, *Nature (London),* 219, 1164, 1968.
27. **Schneider, R. G., Brimhall, B., Jones, R. T., Bryant, R., Mitchell, C. B., and Goldberg, A. I.,** Hb Fort Worth: α27 Glu→Gly (B8) a variant present in unusually low concentration, *Biochim. Biophys. Acta,* 243, 164, 1971.
28. **Ahern, E., Ahern, V., Holder, W., Palomino, E., Serjeant, G. R., Serjeant, B. E., Forbes, M., Brimhall, B., and Jones, R. T.,** Haemoglobin Spanish Town α27 Glu→Val (B8), *Biochim. Biophys. Acta,* 427, 530, 1976.
29. **Liang, C., Tao, H., Lo, H., Huang, S., Li, R., and Wang, B.,** Hemoglobin Shuangfeng (α27(B8) Glu→Lys): a new unstable hemoglobin variant, *Hemoglobin,* 5, 691, 1981.
30. **Vettore, L., DeSandre, G., Dilorio, E. E., Winterhalter, K. H., Lang, H., and Lehmann, H.,** A new abnormal hemoglobin O Padova, α30 (B11) Glu→Lys and a dyserythropoietic anemia with erythroblastic multinuclearity coexisting in the same patient, *Blood,* 44, 869, 1974.
31. **Schneider, R. G. and Jim, R. T. S.,** A new haemoglobin variant (the 'Honolulu Type') in a Chinese, *Nature (London),* 190, 454, 1961.
32. **Vella, F., Ager, J. A. M., and Lehmann, H.,** An abnormal haemoglobin in a Chinese: Haemoglobin G, *Nature (London),* 182, 460, 1958.
33. **Swenson, R. T., Hill, R. L., Lehmann, H., and Jim, R. T. S.,** A chemical abnormality in Hemoglobin G from Chinese individuals, *J. Biol. Chem.,* 237, 1517, 1962.
34. **Marinucci, M., Mavilio, F., Massa, A., Gabbianelli, M., Fontanarosa, P. P., Camagna, A., Ignesti, C., and Tentori, L.,** A new abnormal human hemoglobin: Hb Prato ($\alpha_2$31(B12) Arg→Ser β_2), *Biochim. Biophys. Acta,* 578, 534, 1979.
35. **Tatsis, B.,** Hemoglobin Queens (α34(B15) Leu→Arg): a new variant at the $\alpha_1\beta_1$ contact, *Blood,* 54(Suppl. 1), 61a, 1979.
36. **Beretta, A., Prato, V., Gallo, E., and Lehmann, H.,** Haemoglobin Torino — α43 (CD1) Phenylalanine→Valine, *Nature (London),* 217, 1016, 1968.
37. **Ohba, Y., Miyaji, T., Matsuoka, M., Yokoyama, M., Numakura, H., Nagata, K., Takebe, Y., Izumi, Y., and Shibata, S.,** Hemoglobin Hirosaki (α43 [CE 1] Phe→Leu), a new unstable variant, *Biochim. Biophys. Acta,* 405, 155, 1975.
38. **Honig, G. R., Vida, L. N., Shamsuddin, M., Mason, R. G., Schlumpf, H. W., and Luke, R. A.,** Hemoglobin Milledgeville (α44(CD2) Pro→Leu) a new variant with increased oxygen affinity, *Biochim. Biophys. Acta,* 626, 424, 1980.
39. **Harano, T., Harano, K., Ueda, S., Shibata, S., Imai, K., Ohba, Y., Shinohara, T., Horio, S., Nishioka, K., and Shirotani, H.,** Hemoglobin Kawachi [α44(CE2)Pro→Arg]: a new hemoglobin variant of high oxygen affinity with amino acid substitution at $\alpha_1\beta_1$ contact, *Hemoglobin,* 6, 43, 1982.
40. **Braconnier, F., Gacon, G., Thillet, J., Wajcman, H., Soria, J., Maigret, P., Labie, D., and Rosa, J.,** Hemoglobin Fort de France (α_2^{45}(CD3) His→Arg β_2) a new variant with increased oxygen affinity, *Biochim. Biophys. Acta,* 493, 228, 1977.
41. **Marinucci, M., Mavilio, F., Tentori, L., D'Erasmo, F., Colapietro, A., De Stasio, G., and Di Fonzo, S.,** A new human hemoglobin variant: Hb Bari (α_2 45(CD3) His→Gln β_2), *Biochim. Biophys. Acta,* 622, 315, 1980.
42. **Sumida, I.,** Studies of abnormal hemoglobins in Western Japan. Frequency of visible hemoglobin variants, and chemical characterization of Hemoglobin Sawara ($\alpha_2$6Alaβ_2) and Hemoglobin Mugino (Hb L Ferrara: $\alpha_2$47Glyβ_2), *Jpn. J. Hum. Genet.,* 19, 343, 1975.
43. **Fujimura, T., Kawasaki, K., Imamura, T., Ohta, Y., Hanada, M., and Yamaoka, K.,** Two kindreds of abnormal hemoglobins: Hb Tagawa I and Hb Tagawa II, *Jpn. J. Clin. Hematol.,* 6, 71, 1964.
44. **DeVries, A., Joshua, H., Lehmann, H., Hill, R. L., and Fellows, R. E.,** The first observation of an abnormal haemoglobin in a Jewish family: Haemoglobin Beilinson, *Br. J. Haematol.,* 9, 484, 1963.
45. **Halbrecht, I., Isaacs, W. A., Lehmann, H., and Ben-Porat, F.,** Hemoglobin Hasharon (α47 Aspartic acid→Histidine), *Isr. J. Med. Sci.,* 3, 827, 1967.

46. **Ostertag, W. and Smith, E. W.**, Hb Sinai: a new α chain mutant α47 His, *Humangenetik*, 6, 377, 1968.
47. **Schneider, R. G., Ueda, S., Alperin, J. B., Brimhall, B., and Jones, R. T.**, Hemoglobin Sealy ($\alpha_2$47Hisβ_2): a new variant in a Jewish family, *Am. J. Hum. Genet.*, 20, 151, 1968.
48. **Bianco, I., Modiano, G., Bottini, E., and Lucci, R.**, Alteration in the α-chain of Haemoglobin L Ferrara, *Nature (London)*, 198, 395, 1963.
49. **Tentori, L.**, Hemoglobin L Ferrara = Hemoglobin Hasharon, *Hemoglobin*, 1, 602, 1977.
50. **Rahbar, S., Mahdavi, N., Nowzari, G., and Mostafavi, I.**, Hemoglobin Arya: $\alpha_2$47(CD5) Aspartic acid→Asparagine, *Biochim. Biophys. Acta*, 386, 525, 1975.
51. **Brimhall, B., Jones, R. T., Schneider, R. G., Hosty, T. S., Tomlin, G., and Atkins, R.**, Two new hemoglobins: Hemoglobin Alabama (β39(C5)Gln→Lys) and Hemoglobin Montgomery (α48(CD6) Leu→Arg), *Biochim. Biophys. Acta*, 379, 28, 1975.
52. **Szelényi, J. G., Horányi, M., Földi, J. Hudacsek, J., István, L., and Hollán, S. R.**, A new hemoglobin variant in Hungary: Hb Savaria — α 49 (CE7) Ser→Arg, *Hemoglobin*, 4, 27, 1980.
53. **Tangheroni, W., Zorcolo, G., Gallo, E., and Lehmann, H.**, Haemoglobin J Sardegna: α50 (CD8) Histidine→Aspartic acid, *Nature (London)*, 218, 470, 1968.
54. **Cabannes, R., Renaud, R., Mauran, A., Pennors, H., Charlesworth, D., Price, B. G., and Lehmann, H.**, Deux hémoglobines rapides an Cote-D'Ivoire: l'Hb K Woolwich et une nouvelle hémoglobine, l'Hb J Abidjan (α51 Gly→Asp), *Nouv. Rev. Fr. Hematol.*, 12, 289, 1972.
55. **Reynolds, C. A. and Huisman, T. H. J.**, Hemoglobin Russ or $\alpha_2$51Argβ_2, *Biochim. Biophys. Acta*, 130, 541, 1966.
56. **Alberti, R., Mariuzzi, G. M., Artibani, L., Bruni, E., and Tentori, L.**, A new haemoglobin variant: J-Rovigo alpha 53 (E-2) Alanine→Aspartic acid, *Biochim. Biophys. Acta*, 342, 1, 1974.
57. **Miyaji, T., Iuchi, I., Takeda, I., and Shibata, S.**, Hemoglobin Shimonoseki ($\alpha_2$54Argβ_2A), a slow-moving hemoglobin found in a Japanese family, with special reference to its chemistry, *Acta Haematol. Jpn.*, 26, 531, 1963.
58. **Jones, R. T., Brimhall, B., and Lisker, R.**, Chemical characterization of Hemoglobin Mexico and Hemoglobin Chiapas, *Biochim. Biophys. Acta*, 154, 488, 1968.
59. **Rosa, J., Labie, D., Maleknia, N., and Blum, N.**, Sur quelques hémoglobines anormales nouvelles recemment isolées en France, International Symposium on Comparative Hemoglobin Structure, Thessaloniki, April 11, 1966.
60. **Phessas, Ph., Kaltsoya, A., Loukopoulos, D., and Nilsson, L.-O.**, On the chemical structure of Haemoglobin Uppsala, *Hum. Hered.*, 19, 152, 1969.
61. **Pootrakul, S., Boonyarat, D., Kematorn, B., Suanpan, S., and Wasi, P.**, Hemoglobin Thailand [α56 (E5) Lys→Thr]: a new abnormal human hemoglobin, *Hemoglobin*, 1, 781, 1977.
62. **Abramov, A., Lehmann, H., and Robb, L.**, Hb Shaare Zedek (α56 E5 Lys→Glu), *FEBS Lett.*, 113, 235, 1980.
63. **Rahbar, S., Kinderlerer, J. L., and Lehmann, H.**, Haemoglobin L Persian Gulf: α57 (E6) Glycine→Arginine, *Acta Haematol.*, 42, 169, 1969.
64. **Baglioni, C.**, A chemical study of Hemoglobin Norfolk, *J. Biol. Chem.*, 237, 69, 1962.
65. **Imamura, T.**, Hemoglobin Kagoshima: an example of Hemoglobin Norfolk in a Japanese family, *Am. J. Hum. Genet.*, 18, 584, 1966.
66. **Gerald, P. S. and Efron, M. L.**, Chemical studies of several varieties of Hb M, *Proc. Natl. Acad. Sci. U.S.A.*, 47, 1758, 1961.
67. **Shimizu, A., Hayashi, A., Yamamura, Y., Tsugita, A., and Kitayama, K.**, The structural study on a new hemoglobin variant, Hb M Osaka, *Biochim. Biophys. Acta*, 97, 472, 1965.
68. **Hansen, H. A., Jagenburg, O. R., and Johansson, B. G.**, Studies on an abnormal hemoglobin causing hereditary congenital cyanosis, *Acta Paediatr.*, 49, 503, 1960.
69. **Hollán, S. R., Szelényi, J. G., Lehmann, H., and Beale, D.**, A Boston-type Haemoglobin M in Hungary: Haemoglobin M Kiskunhalas, *Haematologia*, 1, 11, 1967.
70. **Nakatsuji, T., Miwa, S., Ohba, Y., Miyaji, T., Matsumoto, N., and Matsuoka, I.**, Hemoglobin Tottori (α59[E8] Glycine→Valine) a new unstable hemoglobin, *Hemoglobin*, 5, 427, 1981.
71. **Barclay, G. P. T., Charlesworth, D., and Lehmann, H.**, Abnormal haemoglobin in Zambia. A new Haemoglobin Zambia α60 (E9) Lysine→Asparagine, *Br. Med. J.*, 4, 595, 1969.
72. **Spivak, V. A., Molchanova, T. P., Ermakov, N. V., Tokarev, Y. N., Martinez, G., Szelényi, J., Horányi, M., Földi, J., Hollán, S., Kazieva, H., and Shamov, I. A.**, A new hemoglobin variant: Hb Dagestan α60(E9) Lys→Glu, *Hemoglobin*, 5, 133, 1981.
73. **Brimhall, B., Duerst, M., Hollán, S. R., Stenzel, P., Szelényi, J., and Jones, R. T.**, Structural characterizations of Hemoglobins J. Buda (α61 (E10) Lys→Asn) and G Pest (α74 (EF3) Asp→Asn), *Biochim. Biophys. Acta*, 336, 344, 1974.
74. **Thillet, J., Blouquit, Y., Perron, F., and Rosa, J.**, Hemoglobin Pontoise α63Ala→Asp (E12). A new fast moving variant, *Biochim. Biophys. Acta*, 491, 16, 1977.

75. **Blackwell, R. Q., Jim, R. T. S., Tan, T. G. H., Weng, M.-I., Liu, C.-S., and Wang, C.-L.,** Hemoglobin G Waimanalo: α64 Asp→Asn, *Biochim. Biophys. Acta,* 322, 27, 1973.
76. **Ramot, B., Kinderlerer, J. B., and Lehmann, H.,** Cited in WHO Technical Report Series No. 509, Annex 1, Geneva, 1972.
77. **Sukumaran, P. K., Merchant, S. M., Desai, M. P., Wiltshire, B. G., and Lehmann, H.,** Haemoglobin Q India (α64(E13) Aspartic acid→Histidine) associated with β-thalassemia observed in three Sindhi families, *J. Med. Genet.,* 9, 436, 1972.
78. **Miyaji, T., Iuchi, I., Yamamoto, K., Ohba, Y., and Shibata, S.,** Amino acid substitution of Hemoglobin Ube 2 ($\alpha_2$68Asp β_2): an example of successful application of partial hydrolysis of peptide with 5% acetic acid, *Clin. Chim. Acta,* 16, 347, 1967.
79. **Baglioni, C. and Ingram, V. M.,** Abnormal human haemoglobins. V. Chemical investigation of Haemoglobins A, G, C, X from one individual, *Biochim. Biophys. Acta,* 48, 253, 1961.
80. **Chernoff, A. I. and Pettit, N., Jr.,** The amino acid composition of hemoglobin. VI. Separation of the tryptic peptides of Hemoglobin Knoxville No. 1 on Dowex-1 X-2 and Sephadex, *Biochim. Biophys. Acta,* 97, 47, 1965.
81. **Bowman, B., Barnett, D. R., Hodgkinson, K. T., and Schneider, R. G.,** Chemical characterization of Haemoglobin G St-1, *Nature (London),* 211, 1305, 1966.
82. **Minnich, V., Cordonnier, J. K., Williams, W. J., and Moore, C. V.,** Alpha, beta and gamma hemoglobin polypeptide chains during the neonatal period with description of a fetal form of Hemoglobin D St. Louis, *Blood,* 19, 137, 1962.
83. **Dance, N., Huehns, E. R., and Shooter, E. M.,** The chemical investigation of Haemoglobin G Bristol and G Bristol/C, *Biochim. Biophys. Acta,* 86, 144, 1964.
84. **Colombo, B., Vidal, H., Kamuzora, H., and Lehmann, H.,** A new Haemoglobin J-Habana α71 (E20) Alanine→Glutamic acid, *Biochim. Biophys. Acta,* 351, 1, 1974.
85. **Rahbar, S., Nowzari, G., and Daneshmand, P.,** Hemoglobin Daneshgah-Tehran α_2 72 (EF1) Histidine Arginine β_2A. *Nature (New Biol.),* 245, 268, 1973.
86. **Pootrakul, S. and Dixon, G. H.,** Hemoglobin Mahidol: a new hemoglobin α-chain mutant, *Can. J. Biochem.,* 48, 1066, 1970.
87. **Blackwell, R. Q. and Liu, C.-S.,** Hemoglobin G Taichung: α74 Asp→His, *Biochim. Biophys. Acta,* 200, 70, 1970.
88. **Lorkin, P. A., Charlesworth, D., Lehmann, H., Rahbar, S., Tuchinda, S., and Lie-Injo, L. E.,** Two Haemoglobins Q, α74 (EF3) and α75 (EF4) Aspartic acid→Histidine, *Br. J. Haematol.,* 19, 117, 1970.
89. **Orringer, E. P., Wilson, J. B., and Huisman, T. H. J.,** Hemoglobin Chapel Hill or $\alpha_2$74Asp→Gly β_2, *FEBS Lett.,* 65, 297, 1976.
90. **Djoumessi, S., Rousseaux, J., Descamps, J., Goudemand, M., and Dautrevaux, M.,** Hemoglobin Lille, α_2 [74(EF3) Asp→Ala] β_2, *Hemoglobin,* 5, 475, 1981.
91. **Liang, C.-C., Chen, S.-S., Jia, P.-C., Wang, L.-F., Luo, H.-Y., Liu, G.-Y., Liang, S., Lung, G.-F., Yu, C.-M., Zhuang, L.-Z., Liang, B.-L., and Tang, Z.-N.,** Hemoglobin Duan, α75(EF4) Asp→Ala, a new variant found in China, *Hemoglobin,* 5, 481, 1981.
92. **Vella, F., Wiltshire, B., Lehmann, H., and Galbraith, P.,** Hemoglobin Winnipeg α_2 75 Asp→Tyr β_2, *Clin. Biochem.,* 6, 66, 1973.
93. **Ohba, Y., Miyaji, T., Matsuoka, M., Takeda, I., Fukuba, Y., Shibata, S., and Ohkura, K.,** Hemoglobin Matsue-Oki: alpha 75 (EF4) Aspartic acid → Asparagine, *Hemoglobin,* 1, 383, 1977.
94. **Iuchi, I., Shimasaki, S., Hidaka, K., Harano, T., Ueda, S., Shibata, S., Mizushima, J., and Kubo, N.,** Hemoglobin Mizushi (α75[EF4] Asp→Gly): a new hemoglobin variant observed in a Japanese family, *Hemoglobin,* 4, 209, 1980.
95. **Shibata, S., Ueda, S., Miyaji, T., and Imamura, T.,** Hemoglobinopathies in Japan, *Hemoglobin,* 5, 509, 1981.
96. **Van Ros, G., Beale, D., and Lehmann, H.,** Haemoglobin Stanleyville-II (α78 Asparagine→Lysine), *Br. Med. J.,* 4, 92, 1968.
97. **Rucknagel, D. L., Brandt, N. J., and Spencer, H. H.,** α-Chain mutants of human hemoglobin contributing to the genetics of the α-chain locus, Proc. 1st Inter-American Symposium on Hemoglobins, Caracas, 1969.
98. **Adams, J. G., III, Winter, W. P., Rucknagel, D. L., and Spencer, H. H.,** Biosynthesis of Hemoglobin Ann Arbor: evidence for catabolic and feedback regulation, *Science,* 176, 1427, 1972.
99. **Honig, G. R., Shamsuddin, M., Tremaine, L. M., Mason, R. G., Vida, L. N., Sarnwick, R., and Shahidi, N. T.,** Hemoglobin Nigeria (α81 Ser→Cys), a new variant having an inhibitory effect on the gelation of sickle hemoglobin, *Blood,* 52 (Suppl. 1), 113, 1978.
100. **Winter, W. P., Rucknagel, D. L., and Fielding, J.,** Identification of several rare hemoglobin variants discovered in a population survey including a new variant Hb Garden State α82 Ala→Asp, *Clin. Res.,* 26, 22A, 1978.

101. **Crookston, J. H., Farquharson, H. A., Beale, D., and Lehmann, H.,** Hemoglobin Etobicoke: α84 (F5) serine replaced by Arginine, *Can. J. Biochem.*, 47, 143, 1969.
102. **Huehns, E. R.,** The unstable hemoglobins, *Bull. Soc. Chim. Biol.*, 52, 1131, 1970.
103. **Lorkin, P. A., Huntsman, R. G., Ager, J. A. M., Lehmann, H., Vella, F., and Darbre, P. D.,** Haemoglobin G Norfolk: α85 (F6) Asp→Asn, *Biochim. Biophys. Acta*, 379, 22, 1975.
104. **Cohen-Solal, M., Manasse, B., Thillet, J., and Rosa, J.,** Haemoglobin G Norfolk α86 (F6) Asp→Asn. Structural characterization by sequenator analysis and functional properties of a new variant with high oxygen affinity, *FEBS Lett.*, 50, 163, 1975.
105. **Fujiwara, N., Maekawa, T., and Matsuda, G.,** Hemoglobin Atago (α_2 85 Tyr β_2) a new abnormal human hemoglobin found in Nagasaki, *Int. J. Prot. Res.*, 3, 35, 1971.
106. **Benesch, R.,** personal communication.
107. **Reed, R. E., Winter, W. P., and Rucknagel, D. L.,** Haemoglobin Inkster ($\alpha_2$85 Aspartic acid→Valine β_2) coexisting with β-thalassemia in a Caucasian family, *Br. J. Haematol.*, 26, 475, 1974.
108. **Knuth, A., Pribilla, W., Marti, H. R., and Winterhalter, K. H.,** Hemoglobin Moabit: alpha 86 (F7) Leu→Arg. A new unstable abnormal hemoglobin, *Acta Haematol.*, 61, 121, 1979.
109. **Miyaji, T., Iuchi, I., Shibata, S., Takeda, I., and Tamura, A.,** Possible amino acid substitution in the α-chain (α87 Tyr) of Hb M Iwate, *Acta Haematol. Jpn.*, 26, 538, 1963.
110. **Heller, P., Weinstein, H. G., Yakulis, V. J., and Rosenthal, I. M.,** Hemoglobin M Kankakee, a new variant of Hemoglobin M, *Blood*, 20, 287, 1962.
111. **Pik, C. and Tönz, O.,** Nature of Haemoglobin M Oldenburg, *Nature (London)*, 210, 1182, 1966.
112. **Ohba, Y., Miyaji, T., Hattori, Y., Fuyuno, K., and Matsuoka, M.,** Unstable hemoglobins in Japan, *Hemoglobin*, 4, 307, 1980.
113. **De Traverse, P. M., Lehmann, H., Coquelet, M. L., Beale, D., and Isaacs, W. A.,** Etude d'une hémoglobine J α non encore décrite, dans une famille Française, *C. R. Seances Soc. Biol.*, 160, 2270, 1966.
114. **Vella, F., Charlesworth, D., Lorkin, P. A., and Lehmann, H.,** Hemoglobin Broussais α90 Lys→Asn, *Can. J. Biochem.*, 48, 908, 1970.
115. **Yanase, T., Hanada, M., Seita, M., Ohya, I., Ohta, Y., Imamura, T., Fujimura, T., Kawasaki, K., and Yamaoka, K.,** Molecular basis of morbidity — from a series of studies of hemoglobinopathies in Western Japan, *Jpn. J. Hum. Genet.*, 13, 40, 1968.
116. **Hyde, R. D., Kinderlerer, J. L., Lehmann, H., and Hall, M. D.,** Haemoglobin J Rajappen: α90 (FG2) Lys→Thr, *Biochim. Biophys. Acta*, 243, 515, 1971.
117. **Harano, T., Harano, K., Shibata, S., Ueda, S., Imai, K., and Seki, M.,** Hb Handa [α90(FG2)Lys→Met]: structure and biosynthesis of a new slightly higher oxygen affinity variant, *Hemoglobin*, 6, 379, 1982.
118. **Brennan, S. O., Tauro, G. P., Melrose, W., and Carrell, R. W.,** Haemoglobin Port Phillip α91 (FG3) Leu→Pro. A new unstable haemoglobin, *FEBS Lett.*, 81, 115, 1977.
119. **Botha, M. C., Beale, D., Isaacs, W. A., and Lehmann, H.,** Haemoglobin J Cape Town α_2 92 Arginine→Glutamine β_2, *Nature (London)*, 212, 792, 1966.
120. **Lines, J. G. and McIntosh, R.,** Oxygen binding by Haemoglobin J Cape Town (α_2 92 Arg→Gln), *Nature (London)*, 215, 297, 1967.
121. **Clegg, J. B., Naughton, M. A., and Weatherall, D. J.,** Abnormal human haemoglobins. Separation and characterization of the α and β chains by chromatography, and the determination of two new variants, Hb Chesapeake and Hb J (Bangkok), *J. Mol. Biol.*, 19, 91, 1966.
122. **Charache, S., Weatherall, D. J., and Clegg, J. B.,** Polycythemia associated with a hemoglobinopathy, *J. Clin. Invest.*, 45, 813, 1966.
123. **Wajcman, H., Belkhodja, O., and Labie, D.,** Hb Setif: G1 (94) αAsp→Tyr. A new α chain hemoglobin variant with substitution of the residue involved in a hydrogen bond between unlike subunits, *FEBS Lett.*, 27, 298, 1972.
124. **Schroeder, W. A., Shelton, J. B., Shelton, J. R., and Powars, D.,** Hemoglobin Sunshine Seth — α_2 (94(G1) Asp→His) β_2, Hemoglobin, 3, 145, 1979.
125. **Schneider, R. G., Atkins, R. J., Hosty, T. S., Tomlin, G., Casey, R., Lehmann, H., Lorkin, P. A., and Nagai, K.,** Haemoglobin Titusville: α94 Asp→Asn, a new haemoglobin with a lowered affinity for oxygen, *Biochim. Biophys. Acta*, 400, 365, 1975.
126. **Huisman, T. H. J., Adams, H. R., Wilson, J. B., Efremov, G. D., Reynolds, C. A., and Wrightstone, R. N.,** Hemoglobin G Georgia or $\alpha_2$95Leu (G2) β_2, *Biochim. Biophys. Acta*, 200, 578, 1970.
127. **Smith, L. L., Plese, C. L., Barton, B. P., Charache, S., Wilson, J. B., and Huisman, T. H. J.,** Subunit dissociation of the abnormal Hemoglobin G Georgia ($\alpha_2$95Leu (G2) β_2) and Rampa ($\alpha_2$95Ser (G2) β_2), *J. Biol. Chem.*, 247, 1433, 1972.
128. **De Jong, W. W. W., Bernini, L. F., and Meera Khan, P.,** Haemoglobin Rampa: α95 Pro→Ser, *Biochim. Biophys. Acta*, 236, 197, 1971.

129. **Wiltshire, B. G., Clark, K. G. A., and Lorkin, P. A., and Lehmann, H.,** Haemoglobin Denmark Hill α95 (G2) Pro→Ala, a variant with unusual electrophoretic and oxygen binding properties, *Biochim. Biophys. Acta,* 278, 459, 1972.
130. **Bannister, W. H., Grech, J. L., Plese, C. F., Smith, L. L., Barton, B. P., Wilson, J. B., Reynolds, C. A., and Huisman, T. H. J.,** Hemoglobin St. Luke's or $\alpha_2$95Arg (G2) β_2, *Eur. J. Biochem.,* 29, 301, 1972.
131. **Crookston, J. H., Farquharson, H. A., Kinderlerer, J. L., and Lehmann, H.,** Hemoglobin Manitoba: α102 (G9) Serine replaced by Arginine, *Can. J. Biochem.,* 48, 911, 1970.
132. **Sanguansermsri, T., Matragoon, S., Changloah, L., and Flatz, G.,** Hemoglobin Suan-Dok (α_2 109 (G16) Leu→Arg β_2): an unstable variant associated with α-thalassemia, *Hemoglobin,* 3, 161, 1979.
133. **Honig, G. R., Shamsuddin, M., Zaizov, R., Steinherz, M., Solar, I., and Kirschmann, C.,** Hemoglobin Petah Tikva (α110 Ala→Asp): a new unstable variant with α-thalassemia-like expression, *Blood,* 57, 705, 1981.
134. **Clegg, J. B. and Charache, S.,** The structure of Hemoglobin Hopkins-2, *Hemoglobin,* 2, 85, 1978.
135. **Niazi, G. A., Efremov, G. D., Nikolov, N., Hunter, E., Jr., and Huisman, T. H. J.,** Hemoglobin Strumica or α_2 112(G19) His→Arg β_2. (With an addendum: Hemoglobin J Paris-I α_2 12(A10) Ala→Asp β_2, in the same population), *Biochim. Biophys. Acta,* 412, 181, 1975.
136. **Beksedic, D., Rajevska, T., Lorkin, P. A., and Lehmann, H.,** Hb Serbia (α112(G19) His→Arg), a new haemoglobin variant from Yugoslavia, *FEBS Lett.,* 58, 226, 1975.
137. **Gajdusek, D. C., Guiart, J., Kirk, R. L., Carrell, R. W., Irvine, D., Kynoch, P. A. M., and Lehmann, H.,** Haemoglobin J Tongariki (α115 Alanine → Aspartic acid): the first new haemoglobin variant found in a Pacific (Melanesian) population, *J. Med. Genet.,* 4, 1, 1967.
138. **Baglioni, C. and Lehmann, H.,** Chemical heterogeneity of Haemoglobin O, *Nature (London),* 196, 229, 1962.
139. **Lie-Injo, L. E. and Sadono,** Haemoglobin O (Buginese X) in Sulawesi, *Br. Med. J.,* 1, 1461, 1958.
140. **Sansone, G., Centa, A., Sciarratta, V., Gallo, E., and Lehmann, H.,** Haemoglobin O Indonesia (α116 Glu→Lys) in an Italian family, *Acta Haematol.,* 43, 40, 1970.
141. **Ohba, Y., Miyaji, T., Matsuoka, M., Morito, M., and Iuchi, I.,** Characterization of Hb Ube-4: alpha 116 (GH4) Glu→Ala, *Hemoglobin,* 2, 181, 1978.
142. **Schneider, R. G., Hightower, B., Carpentieri, U., Duerst, M. L., Shih, T. B., and Jones, R. T.,** Hemoglobin Oleander [$\alpha_2$116(GH4)Glu→Gln β_2]: structural and functional characterization, *Hemoglobin,* 6, 465, 1982.
143. **Blackwell, R. Q., Wong Hock Boon, Wang, C.-L., Weng, M.-I., and Liu, C.-S.,** Hemoglobin J Meerut: α120 Ala→Glu, *Biochim. Biophys. Acta,* 351, 7, 1974.
144. **Kamuzora, H., Lehmann, H., Griffiths, K. D., Mann, J. R., and Raine, D. N.,** A new haemoglobin variant Haemoglobin J Birmingham α120 (H3) Ala→Glu, *Ann. Clin. Biochem.,* 11, 53, 1974.
145. **Fleming, P. J., Hughes, W. G., Farmilo, R. K., Wyatt, K., and Cooper, W. N.,** Hemoglobin Westmead α_2 122(H5) His→Gln β_2: a new hemoglobin variant with the substitution in the $\alpha_1\beta_1$ contact area, *Hemoglobin,* 4, 39, 1980.
146. **Goossens, M., Lee, K. Y., Liebhaber, S. A., and Kan, Y. W.,** Globin structural mutant α125Leu→Pro is a novel cause of α-thalassemia, *Nature (London),* 296, 864, 1982.
147. **Moo-Penn, W. F., Jue, D. L., Johnson, M. H., Wilson, S. M., Therrel, B., Jr., and Schmidt, R. M.,** Hemoglobin Tarrant: α126 (H9) Asp→Asn. A new hemoglobin variant in the $\alpha_1\beta_1$ contact region showing high oxygen affinity and reduced cooperativity, *Biochim. Biophys. Acta,* 490, 443, 1977.
148. **Vella, F., Galbraith, P., Wilson, J. B., Wong, S. C., Folger, G. C., and Huisman, T. H. J.,** Hemoglobin St. Claude or α_2 (H10) Lys→Thr β_2, *Biochim. Biophys. Acta,* 365, 318, 1974.
149. **Moo-Penn, W. F., Bechtel, K. C., Johnson, M. H., Jue, D. L., Holland, S., Huff, C., and Schmidt, R. M.,** Hemoglobin Jackson, α127 (H10) Lys→Asn, *Am. J. Clin. Pathol.,* 66, 453, 1976.
150. **Kleihauer, E. F., Reynolds, C. A., Dozy, A. M., Wilson, J. B., Moores, R. R., Berenson, M. P., Wright, C.-S., and Huisman, T. H. J.,** Hemoglobin Bibba or α_2 136 Pro β_2, an unstable α-chain abnormal hemoglobin, *Biochim. Biophys. Acta,* 154, 220, 1968.
151. **Clegg, J. B., Weatherall, D. J., Wong Hock Boon, and Mustafa, D.,** Two new haemoglobin variants involving proline substitutions, *Nature (London),* 222, 379, 1969.
152. **Poyart, C., Krishnamoorthy, R., Bursaux, E., Gacon, G., and Labie, D.,** Structural and functional studies of Haemoglobin Suresnes or $\alpha_2$141 (HC3) Arg→His β_2, a new high oxygen affinity mutant, *FEBS Lett.,* 69, 103, 1976.
153. **Saenz, G. F., Elizondo, J., Alvarado, M. A., Atmetlla, F., Arroys, G., Martinez, G., Lima, F., and Colombo, B.,** Chemical characterization of a new haemoglobin variant Haemoglobin J Cubujuqui (α_2 141 (HC3) Arg→Ser β_2), *Biochim. Biophys. Acta,* 494, 48, 1977.
154. **Mavilio, F., Marinucci, M., Tentori, L., Fontanarosa, P. P., Rossi, U., and Biagiotti, S.,** Hemoglobin Legnano (α_2 141 (HC3) Arg→Leu β_2): a new abnormal hemoglobin with high oxygen affinity, *Hemoglobin,* 2, 249, 1978.

155. **Martinez, G., Lima, F., Residenti, C., and Colombo, B.,** Hb J Camagüey α_2 141 (HC3) Arg→Gly β_2. A new abnormal human hemoglobin, *Hemoglobin,* 2, 47, 1978.
156. **Moo-Penn, W. F., Bechtel, K. C., Schmidt, R. M., Johnson, M. H., Jue, D. L., Schmidt, D. E., Jr., Dunlap, W. M., Opella, S. J., Bonaventura, J., and Bonaventura, C.,** Hemoglobin Raleigh (β1 Valine→Acetylalanine). Structural and functional characterization, *Biochemistry,* 16, 4872, 1977.
157. **Labossiere, A., Vella, F., Hiebert, J., and Galbraith, P.,** Hemoglobin Deer Lodge: $\alpha_2\beta_2$ 2 His→Arg, *Clin. Biochem.,* 5, 46, 1972.
158. **Ingram, V. M.,** Abnormal human haemoglobins. III. The chemical differences between normal and sickle cell haemoglobins, *Biochim. Biophys. Acta,* 36, 402, 1959.
159. **Hunt, J. A. and Ingram, V. M.,** Abnormal human haemoglobins. IV. The chemical differences between normal human haemoglobins and Haemoglobin C, *Biochim. Biophys. Acta,* 42, 409, 1960.
160. **Blackwell, R. Q., Oemijati, S., Pribadi, W., Weng, M.-I., and Liu, C.-S.,** Hemoglobin G Makassar: β6 Glu→Ala, *Biochim. Biophys. Acta,* 214, 396, 1970.
161. **Hill, R. L., Swenson, R. T., and Schwartz, H. C.,** Characterization of a chemical abnormality in Hemoglobin G, *J. Biol. Chem.,* 235, 3182, 1960.
162. **Tuchinda, S., Beale, D., and Lehmann, H.,** A new haemoglobin in a Thai family. A case of Haemoglobin Siriraj-β-thalassaemia, *Br. Med. J.,* 1, 1583, 1965.
163. **Bonaventura, J. and Riggs, A.,** Polymerization of hemoglobins of mouse and man. Structural basis, *Science,* 158, 800, 1967.
164. **Tondo, C. V., Bonaventura, J., Bonaventura, C., Brunori, M., Amiconi, G., Antonini, E.,** Functional properties of Hemoglobin Pôrto Alegre $\alpha_2{}^A\beta_2 9$ Ser→Cys) and the reactivity of its extra cysteinyl residue, *Biochim. Biophys. Acta,* 342, 15, 1974.
165. **Arcasoy, A., Casey, R., Lehmann, H., Cavdar, A. O., and Berki, A.,** A new Haemoglobin J from Turkey — Hb Ankara (β10 (A7) Ala→Asp), *FEBS Lett.,* 42, 121, 1974.
166. **Djoumessi, S., Rousseaux, J., and Dautrevaux, M.,** Structural studies of a new hemoglobin: Hb J Lens, β13(A10) Ala→Asp, *FEBS Lett.,* 136, 145, 1981.
167. **Monn, E., Gaffney, P. J., and Lehmann, H.,** Haemoglobin Sogn (β14 Arginine). A new haemoglobin variant, *Scand. J. Haematol.,* 5, 353, 1968.
168. **Beuzard, Y., Basset, P., Braconnier, F., El Gammel, H., Martin, L., Oudard, J. L., and Thillet, J.,** Haemoglobin Saki $\alpha_2\beta_2$ 14 Leu→Pro (A11) structure and function, *Biochim. Biophys Acta,* 393, 182, 1975.
169. **Milner, P. F., Corley, C. C., Pomeroy, W. L., Wilson, J. B., Gravely, M., and Huisman, T. H. J.,** Thalassemia intermedia caused by heterozygosity for both β-thalassemia and Hemoglobin Saki (β14 (11) Leu→Pro), *Am. J. Hematol.,* 1, 283, 1976.
170. **Kennedy, C. C., Blundell, G., Lorkin, P. A., Lang, A., and Lehmann, H.,** Haemoglobin Belfast 15(A12) Tryptophan→Arginine: a new unstable haemoglobin variant, *Br. Med. J.,* 4, 324, 1974.
171. **Gacon, G., Wajcman, H., Labie, D., Varet, B., and Christoforov, B.,** A second case of Haemoglobin Belfast (β^{15}[A12]Trp→Arg) observed in a French patient, *Acta Haematol.,* 55, 313, 1976.
172. **Baglioni, C. and Weatherall, D. J.,** Abnormal human hemoglobins. IX. Chemistry of Hemoglobin J Baltimore, *Biochim. Biophys. Acta,* 78, 637, 1963.
173. **Weatherall, D. J.,** Hemoglobin J (Baltimore) coexisting in a family with Hemoglobin S, *Johns Hopkins Hosp. Bull.,* 114, 1, 1964.
174. **Chernoff, A. I. and Perillie, P. E.,** The amino acid composition of HGB New Haven #2 (HGB N New Haven), *Biochem. Biophys. Res. Commun.,* 16, 368, 1964.
175. **Wong, S. C., Bouver, N., Wilson, J. B., and Huisman, T. H. J.,** Hb J Georgia = Hb J Baltimore = $\alpha_2\beta_2$16Gly→Asp, *Clin. Chim. Acta,* 35, 521, 1971.
176. **Wade, P. T., Jenkins, T., and Huehns, E. R.,** Haemoglobin variant in a Bushman: Haemoglobin Dβ-Bushman $\alpha\beta_{22}$16Gly→Arg, *Nature (London),* 216, 688, 1967.
177. **Maekawa, M., Maekawa, T., Fujiwara, N., Tabara, K., and Matsuda, G.,** Hemoglobin Nagasaki: $\alpha_2{}^A\beta_2$ 17 Glu. A new abnormal human hemoglobin found in one family in Nagasaki, *Int. J. Prot. Res.,* II, 147, 1970.
178. **Elion, J., Belkhodja, O., Wajcman, H., and Labie, D.,** Two variants of Hemoglobin D in the Algerian population: Hemoglobin D Ouled Rabah β19(B1) Asn→Lys and Hemoglobin D Iran β22(B4) Glu→Gln, *Biochim. Biophys. Acta,* 310, 360, 1973.
179. **Lam, H., Wilson, J. B., Harris, H., Gravely, M., and Huisman, T. H. J.,** Hemoglobin Alamo [$\alpha_2\beta_2$ 19 (B1) Asn→Asp], *Hemoglobin,* 1, 703, 1977.
180. **Stamatoyannopoulos, G., Nute, P. E., Adamson, J. W., Bellingham, A. J., Funk, D., and Hornung, S.,** Hemoglobin Olympia (β20 Valine→Methionine): an electrophoretically silent variant associated with high oxygen affinity and erythrocytosis, *J. Clin. Invest.,* 52, 342, 1973.
181. **Harano, T., Harano, K., Ueda, S., Shibata, S., and Iuchi, I.,** Hemoglobin Yusa (β21(B3) Asp→Tyr), a new abnormal hemoglobin found in Japan, *Hemoglobin,* 5, 121, 1981.

182. **Moo-Penn, W. F., McPhedran, P., Bobrow, W., Johnson, M. H., Jue, D. L., and Olsen, K. W.,** Hemoglobin Connecticut (β21 (B3) Asp→Gly): a hemoglobin variant with low oxygen affinity, *Am. J. Hematol.,* 11, 137, 1981.
183. **Boissel, J. P., Wajcman, H., Fabritius, H., Cabannes, R., and Labie, D.,** Application of high-performance liquid chromatography to abnormal hemoglobin studies. Characterization of hemoglobin D in Ivory Coast and description of a new variant Hb Cocody (beta 21 (B3) Asp leads to Asn), *Biochim. Biophys. Acta,* 670, 203, 1981.
184. **Vella, F., Lorkin, P. A., Carrell, R. W., and Lehmann, H.,** A new hemoglobin variant resembling Hemoglobin E. Hemoglobin E Saskatoon: β22 Glu→Lys, *Can. J. Biochem.,* 45, 1385, 1967.
185. **Blackwell, R. Q., Yang, H. J., and Wang, C. C.,** Hemoglobin G Taipei: $\alpha_2\beta_2$ 22 Glu→Gly, *Biochim. Biophys. Acta,* 175, 237, 1969.
186. **Vella, F., Isaacs, W. A., and Lehmann, H.,** Hemoglobin G Saskatoon: β22 Glu→Ala, *Can. J. Biochem.,* 45, 351, 1967.
187. **Blackwell, R. Q., Liu, C. S., Yang, H. J., Wang, C. C., and Huang, J. T. H.,** Hemoglobin variant common to Chinese and North American Indians: $\alpha_2\beta_2$ 22 Glu→Ala, *Science,* 161, 381, 1968.
188. **Bowman, B. H., Barnett, D. R., and Hite, R.,** Hemoglobin G Coushatta: a beta variant with a delta-like substitution, *Biochem. Biophys. Res. Commun.,* 26, 466, 1967.
189. **Blackwell, R. Q., Ro, I. H., Liu, C. S., Yang, H. J., Wang, C. C., and Huang, J. T. H.,** Hemoglobin variant found in Koreans, Chinese, and North American Indians. $\alpha_2\beta_2$ 22 Glu→Ala, *Am. J. Phys. Anthropol.,* 30, 389, 1969.
190. **Rahbar, S.,** Haemoglobin D Iran: β22 Glutamic acid→Glutamine (B4), *Br. J. Haematol.,* 24, 31, 1973.
191. **Garel, M. C., Blouquit, Y., Arous, N., and Rosa, J.,** Hb Strasbourg $\alpha_2\beta_2$ 20(B2) Val→Asp: a variant at the same locus as Hb Olympia β^{20}Val→Met, *FEBS Lett.,* 72, 1, 1976.
192. **Forget, B. G.,** Nucleotide sequence of human β globin messenger RNA, *Hemoglobin,* 1, 879, 1977.
193. **Nakatsuji, T., Miwa, S., Ohba, Y., Hattori, Y., Miyaji, T., Miyata, H., Shinohara, T., Hori, T., and Takayama, J.,** Hemoglobin Miyashiro (β23[B5]Val→Gly) an electrophoretically silent variant discovered by the isopropanol test, *Hemoglobin,* 6, 653, 1981.
194. **Ranney, H. M., Jacobs, A. S., Udem, L., and Zalusky, R.,** Hemoglobin Riverdale-Bronx, an unstable hemoglobin resulting from the substitution of arginine for glycine at helical residue B6 of the β polypeptide chain, *Biochim. Biophys. Acta,* 33, 1004, 1968.
195. **Huisman, T. H. J., Brown, A. K., Efremov, G. D., Wilson, J. B., Reynolds, C. A., Uy, R., and Smith, L. L.,** Hemoglobin Savannah (B6(24)β-Glycine→Valine): an unstable variant causing anemia with inclusion bodies, *J. Clin. Invest.,* 50, 650, 1971.
196. **Idelson, L. I., Didkowsky, N. A., Casey, R., Lorkin, P. A., and Lehmann, H.,** New unstable haemoglobin (Hb Moscva, β24(B6) Gly→Asp) found in the U.S.S.R., *Nature (London),* 249, 768, 1974.
197. **Blackwell, R. Q. and Liu, C.-S.,** Hemoglobin G Taiwan-Ami $\alpha_2\beta_2$ 25 Gly→Arg, *Biochem. Biophys. Res. Commun.,* 30, 690, 1968.
198. **Hunt, J. A. and Ingram, V. M.,** Abnormal human haemoglobins. VI. The chemical difference between Haemoglobins A and E, *Biochim. Biophys. Acta,* 49, 520, 1961.
199. **Blouquit, Y., Arous, N., Machado, P. E. A., and Garel, M. C.,** Hb Henri Mondor: β^{26}(B8) Glu→Val: a variant with a substitution localized at the same position as that of Hb E β^{26} Glu→Lys, *FEBS Lett.,* 72, 5, 1976.
200. **Idelson, L. I., Didkovsky, N. A., Filippova, A. V., Casey, R., Kynoch, P. A. M., and Lehmann, H.,** Haemoglobin Volga, β27 (B9) Ala→Asp, a new highly unstable haemoglobin with a suppressed charge, *FEBS Lett.,* 58, 122, 1975.
201. **Kuis-Reerink, J. D., Jonxis, J. H. P., Niazi, G. A., Wilson, J. B., Bolch, K. C., Gravely, M., and Huisman, T. H. J.,** Hb Volga or $\alpha_2\beta_2$ 27(B9) Ala→Asp: an unstable hemoglobin variant in three generations of a Dutch family, *Biochim. Biophys. Acta,* 439, 63, 1976.
202. **Cohen-Solal, M., Seligmann, M., Thillet, J., and Rosa, J.,** Haemoglobin Saint Louis β28(B10) Leucine→Glutamine. A new unstable haemoglobin only present in a ferri form. Abstr. 408, XIV Int. Congr. Hematol., Sao Paulo, 1972, *FEBS Lett.,* 33, 37, 1973.
203. **Thillet, J., Cohen-Solal, M., Selilgmann, M., and Rosa, J.,** Functional and physicochemical studies of Hemoglobin St. Louis β^{28} (B10) Leu→Gln, *J. Clin. Invest.,* 58, 1098, 1976.
204. **Sansone, G., Carrell, R. W., and Lehmann, H.,** Haemoglobin Genova: β28 (B10) Leucine→Proline, *Nature (London),* 214, 877, 1967.
205. **Schmidt, R. M., Bechtel, K. C., Johnson, M. H., Therrell, B. J., Jr., and Moo-Penn, W. F.,** Hemoglobin Lufkin: β29 (B11) Gly→Asp: an unstable hemoglobin variant involving an internal amino acid residue, *Hemoglobin,* 1, 799, 1977.
206. **Brimhall, B., Jones, R. T., Baur, E. W., and Motulsky, A. G.,** Structural characterization of Hemoglobin Tacoma, *Biochemistry,* 8, 2125, 1969.

207. **Nakatsuji, T., Miwa, S., Ohba, Y., Hattori, Y., Miyaji, T., Hino, S., and Matsumoto, N.,** A new unstable hemoglobin, Hb Yokohama β31(B13) Leu→Pro, causing hemolytic anemia, *Hemoglobin,* 5, 667, 1981.
208. **Jackson, J. M., Yates, A., and Huehns, E. R.,** Haemoglobin Perth: β32 (B14) Leu→Pro. An unstable haemoglobin causing haemolysis, *Br. J. Haematol.,* 25, 607, 1973.
209. **Honig, G. R., Green, D., Shamsuddin, M., Vida, L. N., Mason, R. G., Gnarra, D. J., and Maurer, H. S.,** Hemoglobin Abraham Lincoln, β32(B14) Leucine→Proline. An unstable variant producing severe hemolytic anemia, *J. Clin. Invest.,* 52, 1746, 1973.
210. **Garel, M. C., Blouquit, Y., and Rosa, J.,** Hemoglobin Castilla B32(B14) Leu→Arg: a new unstable variant producing severe hemolytic disease, *FEBS Lett.,* 58, 145, 1975.
211. **Blouquit, Y., Braconnier, F., Cohen-Solal, M., Foldi, J., Arous, N., Ankri, A., Binet, J. L., and Rosa, J.,** Hemoglobin Pitie-Salpetriere β34 (B16) Val→Phe a new high oxygen affinity variant associated with familial erythrocytosis, *Biochim. Biophys. Acta,* 624, 473, 1980.
212. **Rieder, R. F., Oski, F. A., and Clegg, J. B.,** Hemoglobin Philly (β35 Tyrosine→Phenylalanine): studies in the molecular pathology of hemoglobin, *J. Clin. Invest.,* 48, 1627, 1969.
213. **Yamaoka, K.,** Hemoglobin Hirose: $\alpha_1\beta_2$ 37(C3) Tryptophan yielding Serine, *Blood,* 38, 730, 1971.
214. **Gacon, G., Belkhodja, O., Wajcman, H., and Labie, D.,** Structural and functional studies of Hb Rothschild β37 (C3) Trp→Arg. A new variant of the $\alpha_1\beta_2$ contact, *FEBS Lett.,* 82, 243, 1977.
215. **Brimhall, B., Jones, R. T., Schneider, R. G., Hosty, T. S., Tomlin, G., and Atkins, R.,** Two new hemoglobins: Hemoglobin Alabama (β39 (C5) Gln→Lys) and Hemoglobin Montgomery (α48 (CD6) Leu→Arg), *Biochim. Biophys. Acta,* 379, 28, 1975.
216. **Kendall, A. G., Pas, A. T., Wilson, J. B., Cope, N., Bolch, K., and Huisman, T. H. J.,** Hb Vaasa or $\alpha_2\beta_2$ (39(C5) Gln→Glu), a mildly unstable variant found in a Finnish family, *Hemoglobin,* 1, 292, 1977.
217. **Brown, W. J., Niazi, G. A., Jayalakshmi, M., Abraham, E. C., and Huisman, T. H. J.,** Hemoglobin Athens-Georgia, or $\alpha_2\beta_2$ 40(C6) Arg→Lys, a hemoglobin variant with an increased oxygen affinity, *Biochim. Biophys. Acta,* 439, 70, 1976.
218. **Moo-Penn, W. F., Johnson, M. H., Bechtel, K. C., Jue, D. L., Therrell, B. L., and Schmidt, R. M.,** Hemoglobins Austin and Waco: two hemoglobins with substitutions in the $\alpha_1\beta_2$ contact region, *Arch. Biochem. Biophys.,* 179, 86, 1977.
219. **Burkett, L. B., Sharma, V. S., Pisciotta, A. V., Ranney, H. M., and Bruckheimer, S.,** Hemoglobin Mequon β41 (C7) Phenylalanine→Tyrosine, *Blood,* 48, 645, 1976.
220. **Dacie, J. V., Shinton, N. K., Gaffney, P. J., Jr., Carrell, R. W., and Lehmann, H.,** Haemoglobin Hammersmith (β42(CD1) Phe→Ser), *Nature (London),* 216, 663, 1967.
221. **Ohba, Y., Miyaji, T., Matsuoka, M., Yamaguchi, K., Yonemitsu, H., Ishii, T., and Shibata, S.,** Hemoglobin Chiba: Hb Hammersmith in a Japanese girl, *Acta Haematol. Jpn.,* 38, 53, 1975.
222. **Keeling, M. M., Ogdon, L. L., Wrightstone, R. N., Wilson, J. B., Reynolds, C. A., Kitchens, J. L., and Huisman, T. H. J.,** Hemoglobin Louisville (β42(CD1) Phe → Leu): an unstable variant causing mild hemolytic anemia, *J. Clin. Invest.,* 50, 2395, 1971.
223. **Bratu, V., Lorkin, P. A., Lehmann, H., and Predescu, C.,** Haemoglobin Bucuresti β42(CD1) Phe→Leu, a cause of unstable haemoglobin haemolytic anaemia, *Biochim. Biophys. Acta,* 251, 1, 1971.
224. **Bowman, B. H., Oliver, C. P., Barnett, D. R., Cunningham, J. R., and Schneider, R. G.,** Chemical characterization of three Hemoglobins G, *Blood,* 23, 193, 1964.
225. **Iuchi, I., Ueda, S., Hidaka, K., and Shibata, S.,** Hemoglobin Hoshida (β43 (CD-2) Glu→Gln), a new hemoglobin variant discovered in Japan, *Hemoglobin,* 2, 235, 1978.
226. **Yeager, A. M., Zinkham, W. H., Jue, D. L., Winslow, R. M., Johnson, M. H., McGuffey, J. E., and Moo-Penn, W. F.,** Hemoglobin Cheverly: β45 (CD4) Phe→Ser an unstable hemoglobin associated with chronic mild anemia, *Pediatr. Res.,* 17, 503, 1983.
227. **Allan, N., Beale, D., Irvine, D., and Lehmann, H.,** Three haemoglobins K: Woolwich, an abnormal, Cameroon and Ibadan, two unusual variants of human Haemoglobin A, *Nature (London),* 208, 658, 1965.
228. **Sick, K., Beale, D., Irvine, D., Lehmann, H., Goodall, P. T., and MacDougall, S.,** Haemoglobin G Copenhagen and Haemoglobin J Cambridge. Two new β-chain variants of Haemoglobin A, *Biochim. Biophys. Acta,* 140, 231, 1967.
229. **Marinucci, M., Mavilio, F., Tentori, L., and Alberti, R.,** Hemoglobin Gavello $\alpha_2\beta_2$ 47(CD6) Asp→Gly, a new hemoglobin variant from Polesine (Italy), *Hemoglobin,* 1, 771, 1977.
230. **Rahbar, S., Nowzari, G., and Ala, F.,** Haemoglobin Avicenna (β47 (CD6) Asp→Ala), a new abnormal haemoglobin, *Biochim. Biophys. Acta,* 576, 466, 1979.
231. **Charache, S., Brimhall, B., Milner, P., and Cobb, L.,** Hemoglobin Okaloosa (β48(CD7) Leucine→Arginine). An unstable hemoglobin with decreased oxygen affinity, *J. Clin. Invest.,* 52, 2858, 1973.
232. **Labossiere, A., Hill, J. R., and Vella, F.,** A new βTp V hemoglobin variant: Hb Edmonton, *Clin. Biochem.,* 4, 114, 1971.
233. **Jones, R. T., Koler, R. D., Duerst, M. L., and Dhindsa, D. S.,** Hemoglobin Willamette [$\alpha_2\beta_2$ 51 Pro→Arg (D2)] a new abnormal human hemoglobin, *Hemoglobin,* 1, 45, 1976.

234. **Konotey-Ahulu, F. I. D., Kinderlerer, J. L., Lehmann, H., and Ringelhann, B.,** Haemoglobin Osu-Christiansborg: a new β-chain variant of Haemoglobin A (β52(D3) Aspartic acid→Asparagine) in combination with Haemoglobin S, *J. Med. Genet.*, 8, 302, 1971.
235. **Beresford, C. H., Clegg, J. B., and Weatherall, D. J.,** Haemoglobin Ocho Rios (β52(D3) Aspartic acid→Alanine); a new β-chain variant of Haemoglobin A found in combination with Haemoglobin S, *J. Med. Genet.*, 9, 151, 1972.
236. **Wilkinson, T., Brennan, S. O., Carrell, R. W., Wells, R. M., Como, P., and Kronenberg, H.,** Hemoglobin Summer Hill β52 (D3) Asp→His a new variant from Sydney, Australia, *Hemoglobin*, 4, 185, 1980.
237. **Clegg, J. B., Naughton, M. A., and Weatherall, D. J.,** Abnormal human haemoglobins. Separation and characterization of the α and β chains by chromatography, and the determination of two new variants, *J. Mol. Biol.*, 19, 91, 1966.
238. **Blackwell, R. Q. and Liu, C.-S.,** The identical structural anomalies of Hemoglobin J Meinung and J Korat, *Biochem. Biophys. Res. Commun.*, 24, 732, 1966.
239. **Blackwell, R. Q., Liu, C.-S., Lie-Injo, L. E., and Pribadi, W.,** Fast hemoglobin variant in Minahassan people of Sulawesi, Chinese and Thais: $\alpha_2\beta_2$ 56 Gly→Asp, *Am. J. Phys. Anthropol.*, 32, 147, 1970.
240. **Rahbar, S., Nowzari, G., Haydari, H., and Daneshmand, P.,** Haemoglobin Hamadan $\alpha_2{}^A\beta_2$ 56 Glycine→Arginine (D7), *Biochim. Biophys. Acta*, 379, 645, 1975.
241. **Giardina, B., Brunori, M., Antonini, E., and Tentori, L.,** Properties of Hemoglobin G Ferrara (β_{57} (E1) Asn→Lys), *Biochim. Biophys. Acta*, 534, 1, 1978.
242. **Marengo-Rowe, A. J., Lorkin, P. A., Gallo, E., and Lehmann, H.,** Haemoglobin Dhofar — a new variant from Southern Arabia, *Biochim. Biophys. Acta*, 168, 58, 1968.
243. **Boulton, F. E., Huntsman, R. G., Lehmann, H., Lorkin, P., and Romero Herrera, A.,** Myoglobin variants, *Br. J. Haematol.*, 20, 671, 1971.
244. **Blackwell, R. Q., Liu, C.-S., and Shigh, T.-B.,** Hemoglobin J Kaohsiung: β59 Lys→Thr, *Biochim. Biophys. Acta*, 229, 343, 1971.
245. **Blackwell, R. Q., Jim, R. T. S., Liu, C.-S., Weng, M.-I., Wang, C.-L., and Shih, T.-B.,** Fast hemoglobin variant found in Hawaiian-Chinese-Caucasian family in Hawaii and a Chinese subject in Taiwan, *Vox Sang.*, 22, 469, 1972.
246. **Wajcman, H., Amegnizin, K. P. E., Belkhodja, O., and Labie, D.,** Hemoglobin J Lome 59(E3) Lys→Asn. A new fast moving variant found in a Togolese, *FEBS Lett.*, 84, 372, 1977.
247. **Kagimoto, T., Morino, Y., and Kishimoto, S.,** A new hemoglobin variant Hb Yatsushiro $\alpha_2^A\beta_2^{60}$ Val→Leu, *Biochim. Biophys. Acta*, 532, 195, 1978.
248. **Jones, R. T., Brimhall, B., Huehns, E. R., and Motulsky, A. G.,** Structural characterization of Hemoglobin N Seattle: $\alpha_2{}^A\beta_2$ 61 Lys→Glu, *Biochim. Biophys. Acta*, 154, 278, 1968.
249. **Shibata, S., Miyaji, T., Iuchi, I., Ueda, S., and Takeda, I.,** Hemoglobin Hikari ($\alpha_2{}^A\beta_2$ 61 AspNH2): a fast moving hemoglobin found in two unrelated Japanese families, *Clin. Chim. Acta*, 10, 101, 1964.
250. **Marinucci, M., Giuliani, A., Maffi, D., Massa, A., Giampaolo, A., Mavilio, F., Zannotti, M., and Tentori, L.,** Hemoglobin Bologna ($\alpha_2\beta_2$ 61(E5) Lys→Met) an abnormal human hemoglobin with low oxygen affinity, *Biochim. Biophys. Acta*, 668, 209, 1981.
251. **Beutler, E., Lang, A., and Lehmann, H.,** Hemoglobin Duarte: $\alpha_2\beta_2$ 62(E6) Ala→Pro: a new unstable hemoglobin with increased oxygen affinity, *Blood*, 43, 527, 1974.
252. **Muller, C. J. and Kingma, S.,** Haemoglobin Zürich $\alpha_2{}^A\beta_2$63 Arg, *Biochim. Biophys. Acta*, 50, 595, 1961.
253. **Gerald, P. S. and Efron, M. L.,** Chemical studies of several varieties of Hb M, *Proc. Natl. Acad. Sci. U.S.A.*, 47, 1758, 1961.
254. **Shibata, S., Miyaji, T., Iuchi, I., and Ueda, S.,** A comparative study of Hemoglobin M Iwate and Hemoglobin M Kurume by means of electrophoresis, chromatography and analysis of peptide chains, *Acta Haematol. Jpn.*, 24, 486, 1961.
255. **Murawski, K., Szymanowska, Z., and Kozlowska, J.,** A new variant of abnormal methaemoglobin: Hb M Radom, *Biochim. Biophys. Acta*, 69, 442, 1963.
256. **Hobolth, N.,** Haemoglobin M Arhus: I. Clinical family study, *Acta Paediatr. Scand.*, 54, 357, 1965.
257. **Josephson, A. M., Weinstein, H. G., Yakulis, V. J., Singer, L., and Heller, P.,** A new variant of Hemoglobin M disease: Hemoglobin M Chicago, *J. Lab. Clin. Med.*, 59, 918, 1962.
258. **Betke, K., Gröschner, E., and Bock, K.,** Properties of a further variant of Haemoglobin M, *Nature (London)*, 188, 864, 1960.
259. **Hörlein, H. and Weber, G.,** Über chronishe familiäre Methämoglobinämie und eine neue Modifikation des Methämoglobins, *Dtsch. Med. Wochenschr.*, 74, 476, 1948.
260. **Efremov, G. D., Huisman, T. H. J., Stanulovic, M., Zurovec, M., Duma, H., Wilson, J. B., and Jeremic, V.,** Haemoglobin M Saskatoon and Haemoglobin M Hyde Park in two Yugoslavian families, *Scand. J. Haematol.*, 13, 48, 1974.

261. **Kohne, E., Grosze, H. P., Versmold, H., Kley, H. P., and Kleihauer, E.,** Hb M Erlangen: $\alpha_2\beta_2$ 63 (E7) Tyr. Eine neue Mutation mit Hämolyse und Diaphorasemangel, *Kinderheilk,* 120, 69, 1975.
262. **Wajcman, H., Krishnamoorthy, R., Gacon, G., Elion, J., Allard, C., and Labie, D.,** A new hemoglobin variant involving the distal histidine: Hb Bicetre (β63(E7) His→Pro), *J. Mol. Med.,* 1, 187, 1976.
263. **Tentori, L.,** Three examples of double heterozygosis beta-thalassemia and rare hemoglobin variants. Intl. Symp. Abnormal Hemoglobin and Thalassemia, Istanbul, Turkey, Abstract 68, 1974.
264. **Ricco, G., Pich, P. G., Mazza, U., Rossi, G., Ajmar, F., Arese, P., and Gallo, E.,** Hb J Sicilia: β65(E9) Lys→Asn, a beta homologue of Hb Zambia, *FEBS Lett.,* 39, 200, 1974.
265. **Garel, M. C., Hassan, W., Coquelet, M. T., Goossens, M., and Rosa, J.,** Hemoglobin J Cairo: β65(E9) Lys→Gln, a new hemoglobin variant discovered in an Egyptian family, *Biochim. Biophys. Acta,* 420, 97, 1976.
266. **Rosa, J., Labie, D., Wajcman, H., Boigne, J. M., Cabannes, R., Bierme, R., and Ruffie, J.,** Haemoglobin I Toulouse: β66 (E10) Lys→Glu: a new abnormal haemoglobin with a mutation localized on the E10 porphyrin surrounding zones, *Nature (London),* 223, 190, 1969.
267. **Steadman, J. H., Yates, A., and Huehns, E. R.,** Idiopathic Heinz body anemias: Hb-Bristol (β67(E11) Val→Asp), *Br. J. Haematol.,* 18, 435, 1970.
268. **Carrell, R. W., Lehmann, H., Lorkin, P. A., Raik, E., and Hunter, E.,** Haemoglobin Sydney: β67(E11) Valine→Alanine: an emerging pattern of unstable haemoglobins, *Nature (London),* 215, 626, 1967.
269. **Ohba, Y., Miyaji, T., Matsuoka, M., Sugiyama, K., Suzuki, T., and Sugiura, T.,** Hemoglobin Mizuho or beta 68(E12) Leucine→Proline, a new unstable variant associated with severe hemolytic anemia, *Hemoglobin,* 1, 467, 1977.
270. **Brennan, S. O., Wells, R. M., Smith, H., and Carrell, R. W.,** Hemoglobin Brisbane: β68 Leu→His. A new high oxygen affinity variant, *Hemoglobin,* 5, 325, 1981.
271. **Rahbar, S., Winkler, K., Louis, J., Rea, C., Blume, K., and Beutler, E.,** Hemoglobin Great Lakes (β68[E12] Leucine→Histidine): a new high-affinity hemoglobin, *Blood,* 58, 813, 1981.
272. **Salomon, H., Tatarski, I., Dance, N., Huehns, E. R., and Shooter, E. M.,** A new hemoglobin variant found in a Bedouin tribe: Hemoglobin "Rambam", *Isr. J. Med. Sci.,* 1, 836, 1965.
273. **Kurachi, S., Hermodson, M., Hornung, S., and Stamatoyannopoulos, G.,** Structure of Haemoglobin Seattle, *Nature (New Biol.),* 243, 275, 1973.
274. **Carrell, R. W. and Owen, M. C.,** A new approach to haemoglobin variant identification. Haemoglobin Christchurch β71(E15) Phenylalanine→Serine, *Biochim. Biophys. Acta,* 236, 507, 1971.
275. **Jones, R. T., Brimhall, B., Pootrakul, S., and Gray, G.,** Hemoglobin Vancouver [$\alpha_2\beta_2$ 73(E17) Asp→Tyr]: its structure and function, *J. Mol. Evol.,* 9, 37, 1976.
276. **Konotey-Ahulu, F. I. D., Gallo, E., Lehmann, H., and Ringelhann, B.,** Haemoglobin Korle-Bu (β73 Aspartic acid→Asparagine) showing one of the two amino acid substitutions of Haemoglobin C Harlem, *J. Med. Genet.,* 5, 107, 1968.
277. **Bio-Doku, F. S., Kinderlerer, J., and Lehman, H.,** *Atlas of Protein Sequence and Structure,* Vol. 5, Dayhoff, M. O., Ed., Natl. Biomedical Res. Found., Washington, D.C., 1972, 73.
278. **Schneider, R. G., Hosty, T. S., Tomlin, G., Atkins, R., Brimhall, B., and Jones, R. T.,** Hb Mobile [$\alpha_2\beta_2$ 73(E17) Asp→Val]: a new variant, *Biochem. Genet.,* 13, 411, 1975.
279. **Rieder, R. F., Wolf, D. J., Clegg, J. B., and Lee, S. L.,** Rapid post-synthetic destruction of unstable Haemoglobin Bushwick, *Nature (London),* 254, 725, 1975.
280. **White, J. M., Brain, M. C., Lorkin, P. A., Lehmann, H., and Smith, M.,** Mild "unstable haemoglobin haemolytic anaemia" caused by Haemoglobin Shepherds Bush (β74 (E18) Gly→Asp), *Nature (London),* 225, 939, 1970.
281. **Hubbard, M., Winton, E. F., Lindeman, J. G., Dessauer, P. L., Wilson, J. B., Wrightstone, R. N., and Huisman, T. H. J.,** Hemoglobin Atlanta or $\alpha_2\beta_2$ 75 Leu→Pro (E19): an unstable variant found in several members of a Caucasian family, *Biochim. Biophys. Acta,* 386, 538, 1975.
282. **Johnson, C. S., Moyes, D., Schroeder, W. A., Shelton, J. B., Shelton, J. R., and Beutler, E.,** Hemoglobin Pasadena, $\alpha_2\beta_2$ 75(E19) Leu→Arg: identification by high performance liquid chromatography of a new unstable variant with increased oxygen affinity, *Biochim. Biophys. Acta,* 623, 360, 1980.
283. **Romain, P. L., Schwartz, A. D., Shamsuddin, M., Adams, J. G., III, Mason, R. G., Vida, L. N., and Honig, G. R.,** Hemoglobin J-Chicago (β76 (E20) Ala→Asp): a new hemoglobin variant resulting from a substitution of an external residue, *Blood,* 45, 387, 1975.
284. **Rahbar, S., Beale, D., Isaacs, W. A., and Lehmann, H.,** Abnormal haemoglobins in Iran. Observation of a new variant — Haemoglobin J Iran ($\alpha_2\beta_2$ 77 His→Arg), *Br. Med. J.,* 1, 674, 1967.
285. **Blackwell, R. Q., Shih, T.-B., Wang, C.-L., and Liu, C.-S.,** Hemoglobin G-Hsi-Tsou: β79 Asp→Gly, *Biochim. Biophys. Acta,* 257, 49, 1972.
286. **Benesch, R., Edilji, R., and Benesch, R. W.,** Oxygenation properties of hemoglobin variants with substitutions near the polyphosphate binding site, *Biochim. Biophys. Acta,* 393, 368, 1975.

287. **Johnson, M. H., Jue, D. L., Patchen, L. C., Hartwig, E. C., Jr., Schneider, N. J., and Moo-Penn, W. F.,** Hemoglobin Tampa: β79 (EF3) Aspartic acid→Tyrosine, *Biochim. Biophys. Acta,* 623, 119, 1980.
288. **Blackwell, R. Q., Yang, H. T., and Wang, C. C.,** Hemoglobin G-Szuhu: β80 Asn→Lys, *Biochim. Biophys. Acta,* 188, 59, 1969.
289. **Imai, K., Morimoto, H., Kotani, M., Shibata, S., Miyaji, T., and Matsumoto, K.,** Studies on the function of abnormal hemoglobins. II. Oxygen equilibrium of abnormal hemoglobins: Shimonoseki, Ube II, Hikari, Gifu, and Agenogi, *Biochim. Biophys. Acta,* 200, 197, 1970.
290. **Schneider, R. G., Hettig, R. A., Bilunos, M., and Brimhall, B.,** Hemoglobin Baylor [$\alpha_2\beta_2$ 81 (EF5) Leu→Arg] — an unstable mutant with high oxygen affinity, *Hemoglobin,* 1, 85, 1976.
291. **Moo-Penn, W. F., Jue, D. L., Bechtel, K. C., Johnson, M. H., Schmidt, R. M., McCurdy, P. R., Fox, J., Bonaventura, J., Sullivan, B., and Bonaventura, C.,** Hemoglobin Providence. A human hemoglobin variant occurring in two forms *in vivo, J. Biol. Chem.,* 251, 7557, 1976.
292. **Bonaventura, J., Bonaventura, C., Sullivan, B., Ferruzzi, G., McCurdy, P. R., Fox, J., and Moo-Penn, W. F.,** Hemoglobin Providence. Functional consequences of two alterations of the 2,3-diphosphoglycerate binding site at position β82, *J. Biol. Chem.,* 251, 7563, 1976.
293. **Lorkin, P. A., Stephens, A. D., Beard, M. E. J., Wrigley, P. F. M., Adams, L., and Lehmann, H.,** Haemoglobin Rahere (β82 Lys→Thr): a new high affinity haemoglobin associated with decreased 2,3-diphosphoglycerate binding and relative polycythaemia, *Br. Med. J.,* 4, 200, 1975.
294. **Ikkala, E., Koskela, J., Pikkarainen, P., Rahiala, E.-L., El-Hazmi, M. A. F., Nagai, K., Lang, A., and Lehmann, H.,** Hb Helsinki: a variant with a high oxygen affinity and a substitution at a 2,3-DPG binding site (β^{82}[EF6]Lys→Met), *Acta Haematol.,* 56, 257, 1976.
295. **Blackwell, R. Q., Liu, C.-S., and Wang, C.-L.,** Hemoglobin Ta-li: β83 Gly→Cys, *Biochim. Biophys. Acta,* 243, 467, 1971.
296. **Tatsis, B., Sofroniadou, K., and Stergiopoulos, C. I.,** Hemoglobin Pyrogos ($\alpha_2\beta_2$ 83(EF7) Gly→ Asp). A new hemoglobin (Hb) variant. Annual Meeting of the American Society of Hematology, Miami, Abstract 168, 1972.
297. **Tatsis, B., Sofroniadou, K., and Stergiopoulos, C. I.,** Hemoglobin Pyrogos $\alpha_2\beta_2$ 83(EF7) Gly→Asp: a new hemoglobin variant in double heterozygosity with Hemoglobin S, *Blood,* 47, 827, 1976.
298. **Bradley, T. B., Wohl, R. C., Murphy, S. B., Oski, F. A., and Bunn, H. F.,** Properties of Hemoglobin Bryn Mawr, β85 Phe→Ser, a new spontaneous mutation producing an unstable hemoglobin with high oxygen affinity. Annual Meeting of the American Society of Hematology, Miami, Abstract 40, 1972.
299. **de Weinstein, B. I., White, J. M., Wiltshire, B. G., and Lehmann, H.,** A new unstable haemoglobin: Hb Buenos Aires, β85(F1) Phe→Ser, *Acta Haematol.,* 50, 357, 1973.
300. **Watson-Williams, E. J., Beale, D., Irvine, D., and Lehmann, H.,** A new haemoglobin, D Ibadan (β87 Threonine→Lysine), producing no sickle cell Haemoglobin D disease with Haemoglobin S, *Nature (London),* 205, 1237, 1965.
301. **Hollender, A., Lorkin, P. A., Lehmann, H., and Svensson, B.,** New unstable Haemoglobin Borås: β88(F4) Leucine→Arginine, *Nature (London),* 222, 953, 1969.
302. **Opfell, R. W., Lorkin, P. A., and Lehmann, H.,** Hereditary non-spherocytic haemolytic anaemia with post-splenectomy inclusion bodies and pigmenturia caused by an unstable Haemoglobin Santa Ana-β88(F4) Leucine→Proline, *J. Med. Genet.,* 5, 292, 1968.
303. **Thillet, J., Blouquit, Y., Garel, M. C., Dreyfus, B., Reyes, F., Cohen-Solal, M., Beuzard, Y., and Rosa, J.,** Hemoglobin Creteil β89(F5) Ser→Asn: high oxygen affinity variant of hemoglobin frozen in a quaternary R-structure, *J. Mol. Med.,* 1, 135, 1976.
304. **Paniker, N. V., Kuang-Tzu Davis Lin, Krantz, S. B., Flexner, J. M., Wasserman, B. K., and Puett, D.,** Haemoglobin Vanderbilt ($\alpha_2\beta_2$ 89 Ser→Arg): a new haemoglobin with high oxygen affinity and compensatory erythrocytes, *Br. J. Haematol.,* 39, 249, 1978.
305. **Miyaji, R., Suzuki, H., Ohba, Y., and Shibata, S.,** Hemoglobin Agenogi ($\alpha_2\beta_2$ 90 Lys), a slow moving hemoglobin of a Japanese family resembling Hb-E, *Clin. Chim. Acta,* 14, 624, 1966.
306. **Schneider, R. G., Satoshi, U., Alperin, J. B., Brimhall, B., and Jones, R. T.,** Hemoglobin Sabine, β91(F7) Leu→Pro. An unstable variant causing severe anemia with inclusion bodies, *N. Engl. J. Med.,* 280, 739, 1969.
307. **Ahern, E., Ahern, C., Hilton, T., Serjeant, G. R., Serjeant, B. E., Seakins, M., Lang, A., Middleton, A., and Lehmann, H.,** Haemoglobin Caribbean β91(F7) Leu→Arg: a mildly unstable haemoglobin with low oxygen affinity, *FEBS Lett.,* 69, 99, 1976.
308. **Heller, P., Coleman, R. D., and Yakulis, V.,** Hemoglobin M Hyde Park: a new variant of abnormal methemoglobin, *J. Clin. Invest.,* 45, 1021, 1966.
309. **Shibata, S., Yamamoto, K., Ohba, Y., Miyaji, R., Karita, K., and Iuchi, I.,** Hemoglobin M Akita disease, *Acta Haematol. Jpn.,* 32, 311, 1969.
310. **Beuzard, Y., Courvalin, J.Cl., Cohen-Solal, M., Garel, M. C., Rosa, J., Brizard, C. P., and Gibaud, A.,** Structural studies of Hemoglobin Saint Etienne β92(F8) His→Gln: a new abnormal hemoglobin with loss of β proximal histidine and absence of heme on the β chains, *FEBS Lett.,* 27, 76, 1972.

311. **Aksoy, M., Erdem, S., Efremov, G. D., Wilson, J. B., Huisman, T. H. J., Schroeder, W. A., Shelton, J. R., Shelton, J. B., Ulitin, O. N., and Müftuglü, A.,** Hemoglobin Istanbul: substitution of Glutamine for Histidine in a proximal Histidine (F8(92)β), *J. Clin. Invest.*, 51, 2380, 1972.
312. **Adams, J. G., III, Przywara, K. P., Shamsuddin, M., and Heller, P.,** Hemoglobin J Altgeld Gardens (β92(F8) His→Asp): a new hemoglobin variant involving a substitution of the proximal histidine, Am. Soc. Hematol. 18th Annual Meeting, Dallas, Texas, 1975.
313. **Finney, R., Casey, R., Lehmann, H., and Walker, W.,** Hb Newcastle: β92(F8) His→Pro, *FEBS Lett.*, 60, 435, 1975.
314. **Spivak, V. A., Molchanova, T. P., Postnikov, Y. V., Aseeva, E. A., Lutsenko, I. N., and Tokarev, Y. N.,** A new abnormal hemoglobin: Hb Mozhaisk β92(F8)His→Arg, *Hemoglobin*, 6, 169, 1982.
315. **Wajcman, H., Aguilar, J. L., Bascompte, I., Labie, D., Poyart, C., and Bohn, B.,** Structural and functional studies of Hemoglobin Barcelona ($\alpha_2\beta_2$ 94Asp(FG_1)→His), *J. Mol. Biol.*, 156, 185, 1982.
316. **Clegg, J. B., Naughton, M. A., and Weatherall, D. J.,** An improved method for the characterization of human haemoglobin mutants: identification of $\alpha_2\beta_2$ 95 Glu, Haemoglobin N (Baltimore), *Nature (London)*, 207, 945, 1965.
317. **Gottlieb, A. J., Robinson, E. A., and Itano, H. A.,** Primary structure of Hopkins-I haemoglobin, *Nature (London)*, 214, 189, 1967.
318. **Dobbs, N. B., Jr., Simmons, J. W., Wilson, J. B., and Huisman, T. H. J.,** Hemoglobin Jenkins or Hemoglobin N-Baltimore or $\alpha_2\beta_2$ 95 Glu, *Biochim. Biophys. Acta*, 117, 492, 1966.
319. **Bayrakci, C., Josephson, A., Singer, L., Heller, P., and Coleman, R. D.,** A new fast hemoglobin, Xth Congress of the International Society of Haematology, Stockholm, Sweden, 1964.
320. **Hamilton, H. H., Iuchi, I., Miyaji, T., and Shibata, S.,** Hemoglobin Hiroshima (β^{143} Histidine→Aspartic acid): a newly identified fast moving beta chain variant associated with increased oxygen affinity and compensatory erythremia (personal communication, P. Heller), *J. Clin. Invest.*, 48, 525, 1969.
321. **Moo-Penn, W. F., Schneider, R. G., Andrian, S., and Das, D. K.,** Hemoglobin Detroit: β95 (FG2) Lysine→Asparagine, *Biochim. Biophys. Acta*, 536, 283, 1978.
322. **Lorkin, P. A., Lehmann, H., Fairbanks, V. F., Berglund, G., and Leonhardt, T.,** Two new pathological haemoglobins: Olmsted β141 (H19) Leu→Arg and Malmö: β97 (FG4) His→Gln, *Biochem. J.*, 119, 68, 1970.
323. **Taketa, F., Huang, Y. P., Libnoch, J. A., and Dessell, B. H.,** Hemoglobin Wood β97(FG4) His→Leu: a new high-oxygen-affinity hemoglobin associated with familial erythrocytosis, *Biochim. Biophys. Acta*, 400, 348, 1975.
324. **Taketa, F., Antholine, W. E., Mauk, A. G., and Libnoch, J. A.,** Nitrosyl-hemoglobin Wood: effects of inositol hexaphosphate on thiol reactivity and electron paramagnetic resonance spectrum, *Biochemistry*, 14, 3229, 1975.
325. **Carrell, R. W., Lehmann, H., and Hutchison, H. E.,** Haemoglobin Köln (β98 Valine→Methionine): an unstable protein causing inclusion-body anaemia, *Nature (London)*, 210, 915, 1966.
326. **Woodson, R. D., Heywood, J. D., and Lenfant, C.,** Oxygen transport in Hemoglobin San Francisco, *Clin. Res.*, 18, 134, 1970.
327. **Ohba, Y., Miyaji, T., and Shibata, S.,** Identical substitution in Hb Ube-1 and Hb Köln, *Nature (New Biol.)*, 243, 205, 1973.
328. **Gordon-Smith, E. C., Dacie, J. V., Blecher, T. E., French, E. A., Wiltshire, B. G., and Lehmann, H.,** Haemoglobin Nottingham, β98(FG5) Val→Gly: a new unstable haemoglobin producing severe haemolysis, *Proc. R. Soc. Med.*, 66, 507, 1973.
329. **Gacon, G., Wajcman, H., and Labie, D.,** A new unstable hemoglobin mutated in β98(FG5) Val→Ala: Hb Djelfa, *FEBS Lett.*, 58, 238, 1975.
330. **Reed, C. S., Hampson, R., Gordon, S., Jones, R. T., Novy, M. J., Brimhall, B., Edwards, M. J., and Koler, R. D.,** Erythrocytosis secondary to increased oxygen affinity of a mutant hemoglobin, Hemoglobin Kempsey, *Blood*, 31, 623, 1968.
331. **Jones, R. T., Osgood, E. E., Brimhall, B., and Koler, R. D.,** Hemoglobin Yakima. I. Clinical and biochemical studies, *J. Clin. Invest.*, 46, 1840, 1967.
332. **Weatherall, D. J., Clegg, J. B., Callender, S. T., Wells, R. M. G., Gale, R. E., Huehns, E. R., Perutz, M. F., Viggiano, G., and Ho, C.,** Haemoglobin Radcliffe ($\alpha_2\beta_2$ 99(G1)Ala): a high oxygen-affinity variant causing familial polycythaemia, *Br. J. Haematol.*, 35, 177, 1977.
333. **Rucknagel, D. L., Glynn, K. P., and Smith, J. R.,** Hemoglobin Ypsilanti characterized by increased oxygen affinity, abnormal polymerization and erythremia, *Clin. Res.*, 15, 270, 1967.
334. **Blouquit, Y., Braconnier, F., Galacteros, F., Arous, N., Soria, J., Zittoun, R., and Rosa, J.,** Hemoglobin Hotel-Dieu β99 Asp→Gly (G1). A new abnormal hemoglobin with high oxygen affinity, *Hemoglobin*, 5, 19, 1981.
335. **Lokich, J. J., Mahoney, C. W., Bunn, H. F., Bruckheimer, S. M., and Ranney, H. M.,** Hemoglobin Brigham ($\alpha_2{}^A\beta_2$ 100 Pro→Leu). Hemoglobin variant associated with familial erythrocytosis, *J. Clin. Invest.*, 52, 2060, 1973.

336. **Jones, R. T., Brimhall, B., and Gray, G.,** Hemoglobin British Columbia [$\alpha_2\beta_2$ 101(G3) Glu→Lys]: a new variant with high oxygen affinity, *Hemoglobin,* 1, 171, 1976.
337. **Adams, J. B., Winter, W. P., Tausk, K., and Heller, P.,** Hemoglobin Rush [β-101(G3) Glutamine]: a new unstable hemoglobin causing mild hemolytic anemia, *Blood,* 45, 261, 1974.
338. **Mant, M. J., Salkie, M. L., Cope, N., Appling, F., Bolch, K., Jayalakshmi, M., Gravely, M., Wilson, J. B., and Huisman, T. H. J.,** Hb Alberta or $\alpha_2\beta_2$ (101 (G3) Glu→Gly), a new high-oxygen-affinity hemoglobin variant causing erythrocytosis, *Hemoglobin,* 1, 183, 1976-77.
339. **Charache, S., Jacobson, R., Brimhall, B., Murphy, E. A., Hathaway, P., Winslow, R., Jones, R., Rath, C., and Simkovich, J.,** Hb Potomac (β101 Glu→Asp): speculations on placental oxygen transport in carriers of high-affinity hemoglobins, *Blood,* 51, 331, 1978.
340. **Efremov, G. D., Huisman, T. H. J., Smith, L. L., Wilson, J. B., Kitchens, J. L., Wrightstone, R. N., and Adams, H. R.,** Hemoglobin Richmond, a human hemoglobin which forms asymmetric hybrids with other hemoglobins, *J. Biol. Chem.,* 244, 6105, 1969.
341. **Bonaventura, J. and Riggs, A.,** Hemoglobin Kansas, a human hemoglobin with a neutral amino acid substitution and an abnormal oxygen equilibrium, *J. Biol. Chem.,* 243, 980, 1968.
342. **Nagel, R. L., Joshua, L., Johnson, J., Landau, L., Bookchin, R. M., and Harris, M. B.,** Hemoglobin Beth Israel: a mutant causing clinically apparent cyanosis, *N. Engl. J. Med.,* 295, 125, 1976.
343. **Arous, N., Braconnier, F., Thillet, J., Blouquit, Y., Galacteros, F., Chevrier, M., Bordahandy, C., and Rosa, J.,** Hemoglobin Saint Mandé β102(G4)Asn→Tyr: a new low oxygen affinity variant, *FEBS Lett.,* 126, 114, 1981.
344. **White, J. M., Szur, L., Gillies, I. D. S., Lorkin, P. A., and Lehmann, H.,** Familial polycythaemia caused by a new haemoglobin variant. Hb Heathrow β103(G5) Phenylalanine→Leucine, *Br. Med. J.,* 3, 665, 1973.
345. **Wilkinson, T., Ching Geh Chua, Carrell, R. W., Robin, H., Exner, T., Kit Ming Lee, and Kronenberg, H.,** A new haemoglobin variant, Haemoglobin Camperdown β104(G6) Arginine→Serine, *Biochim. Biophys. Acta,* 393, 195, 1975.
346. **Ryrie, D. R., Plowman, D., and Lehmann, H.,** Haemoglobin Sherwood Forest β104(G6) Arg→Thr, *FEBS Lett.,* 83, 260, 1977.
347. **Hyde, R. D., Hall, M. D., Wiltshire, B. G., and Lehmann, H.,** Haemoglobin Southampton, β106(G8) Leu→Pro: an unstable variant producing severe haemolysis, *Lancet,* 2, 1170, 1972.
348. **Koler, R. D., Jones, R. T., Bigley, R. H., Litt, M., Lovrien, E., Brooks, R., Lahey, M. E., and Fowler, R.,** Hemoglobin Capser: β106(G8) Leu→Pro, a contemporary mutation, *Am. J. Med.,* 55, 549, 1973.
349. **Kleihauer, E., Waller, H. D., Benöhr, H. C., Kohne, E., and Gelinsky, P.,** Hb Tübingen, eine neue β-kettenvariante (βTp 10-12) mit erhöhter spontanoxydation, *Klin. Wochenschr.,* 48, 651, 1971.
350. **Kohne, E., Kley, H. P., Kleihauer, E., Versmold, H., Benöhr, H. C., and Braunitzer, G.,** Structural and functional characteristics of the Hb Tübingen: β^{106}(G8) Leu→Gln, *FEBS Lett.,* 64, 443, 1976.
351. **Turner, J. W., Jr., Jones, R. T., Brimhall, B., Du Val, M. C., and Koler, R. D.,** Characterization of Hemoglobin Burke [β107(G9)Gly→Arg], *Biochem. Genet.,* 14, 577, 1976.
352. **Imamura, T., Fujita, S., Ohta, Y., Hanada, M., and Yanase, T.,** Hemoglobin Yoshizuka (G10(108) β Asparagine→Aspartic acid): a new variant with a reduced oxygen affinity from a Japanese family, *J. Clin. Invest.,* 48, 2341, 1969.
353. **Moo-Penn, W. F., Wolff, J. A., Simon, G., Vacek, M., Jue, D. L., and Johnson, M. H.,** Hemoglobin Presbyterian: β108(G10) Asparagine→Lysine. A hemoglobin variant with low oxygen affinity, *FEBS Lett.,* 92, 53, 1978.
354. **Nute, P. E., Stamatoyannopoulos, G., Hermodson, M. A., Roth, D., and Hornung, S.,** Hemoglobinopathic erythrocytosis due to a new electrophoretically silent variant, Hemoglobin San Diego (β109(G11) Val→Met), *J. Clin. Invest.,* 53, 320, 1974.
355. **King, M. A. R., Wiltshire, G. B., Lehmann, H., and Morimoto, H.,** An unstable haemoglobin with a reduced oxygen affinity: Haemoglobin Peterborough, β111(G13) Valine→Phenylalanine, its interaction with normal haemoglobin and with Haemoglobin Lepore, *Br. J. Haematol.,* 22, 125, 1972.
356. **Adams, J. G., Boxer, L. A., Baehner, R. L., Forget, B. G., Tsistrokis, G. A., and Steinberg, M. H.,** Hemoglobin Indianapolis: post-translational degradation of an unstable β-chain variant producing a phenotype of severe heterozygous β-thalassemia, *Clin. Res.,* 26, 501A, 1978.
357. **Ranney, H. M., Jacobs, A. S., and Nagel, R. L.,** Haemoglobin New York, *Nature (London),* 213, 876, 1967.
358. **Outeirino, J., Casey, R., White, J. M., and Lehmann, H.,** Haemoglobin Madrid, β115(G17) Alanine→Proline: an unstable variant associated with haemolytic anaemia, *Acta Haematol.,* 52, 53, 1974.
359. **Schneider, R. G., Alperin, J. B., Brimhall, B., and Jones, R. T.,** Hemoglobin P ($\alpha_2\beta_2$ 117Arg): structure and properties, *J. Lab. Clin.,* 73, 616, 1969.
360. **Schneider, R. G., Berkman, N. L., Brimhall, B., and Jones, R. T.,** Hemoglobin Fannin-Lubbock [$\alpha_2\beta_2^{119}$ (GH2) Gly→Asp]: A slightly unstable mutant, *Biochim. Biophys. Acta,* 453, 478, 1976.

361. **Moo-Penn, W. F., Bechtel, K. C., Johnson, M. H., Jue, D. L., Therrell, B. L., Jr., Morrison, B. Y., and Schmidt, R. M.**, Hemoglobin Fannin-Lubbock [$\alpha_2\beta_2^{119}$ (GH2) Gly→Asp]: a new hemoglobin variant at the $\alpha_1\beta_1$ contact, *Biochim. Biophys. Acta,* 453, 472, 1976.
362. **Chen-Marotel, J., Braconnier, F., Blouquit, Y., Martin-Caburi, J., Kammerer, J., and Rosa, J.**, Hemoglobin Bougardirey-Mali β119 (GH2) Gly→Val. An electrophoretically silent variant migrating in isoelectrofocusing as Hb F, *Hemoglobin,* 3, 253, 1979.
363. **Miyaji, T., Ohba, Y., Yamamoto, K., Shibata, S., Iuchi, I., and Hamilton, H. B.**, Hemoglobin Hijiyama: a new fast-moving hemoglobin in a Japanese family, *Science,* 159, 204, 1968.
364. **El-Hazmi, M. A. F. and Lehmann, H.**, Hemoglobin Riyadh [$\alpha_2\beta_2$120(GH3) Lys→Asn] — a new variant found in association with α-thalassemia and iron deficiency, *Hemoglobin,* 1, 59, 1976.
365. **Miyaji, T., Ohba, Y., Matsuoka, M., Kudoh, H., Asano, M., Yamamoto, K., and Satoh, H.**, Hemoglobin Karatsu: beta 120(GH3) Lysine→Asparagine. An example of Hb Riyadh in Japan, *Hemoglobin,* 1, 461, 1977.
366. **Iuchi, I., Hidaka, K., Harano, T., Ueda, S., Shibata, S., Shimasaki, S., Mizushima, J., Kubo, N., Miyake, T., and Uchida, T.**, Hemoglobin Takamatsu (β120 (GH3) Lys→Gln): a new abnormal hemoglobin detected in three unrelated families in the Takamatsu area of Shikoku, *Hemoglobin,* 4, 165, 1980.
367. **Baglioni, C.**, Abnormal human haemoglobins. VIII. Chemical studies on Haemoglobin D, *Biochim. Biophys. Acta,* 59, 437, 1962.
368. **Özsoylu, S.**, Homozygous Hemoglobin D Punjab, *Acta Haematol.,* 42, 353, 1970.
369. **Ramot, B., Rotem, J., Rahbar, S., Jacobs, A. S., Uden, L., and Ranney, H. M.**, Hemoglobin D Punjab in a Bulgarian Jewish family, *Isr. J. Med. Sci.,* 6, 1066, 1969.
370. **Smith, E. W. and Conley, C. L.**, Sickle cell-Hemoglobin D disease, *Ann. Intern. Med.,* 50, 94, 1959.
371. **Wasi, P., Pootrakul, S., Na-Nakorn, S., Beale, D., and Lehmann, H.**, Haemoglobin D β Los Angeles (D Punjab, $\alpha_2\beta_2$ 121 $GluNH_2$) in a Thai family, *Acta Haematol.,* 39, 151, 1968.
372. **Imamura, T. and Riggs, A.**, Identification of Hemoglobin Oak Ridge with Hemoglobin D Punjab (Los Angeles), *Biochem. Genet.,* 7, 127, 1972.
373. **Bowman, B. and Ingram, V. M.**, Abnormal human haemoglobins. VII. The comparison of normal human Haemoglobin D Chicago, *Biochim. Biophys. Acta,* 53, 569, 1961.
374. **Baglioni, C. and Lehmann, H.**, Chemical heterogeneity of Haemoglobin O, *Nature (London),* 196, 229, 1962.
375. **Kamel, K., Hoerman, K., and Awny, A.**, Ethnological significance of hemoglobin $\alpha_2\beta_2$ 121 Lys, *Am. J. Phys. Anthropol.,* 26, 107, 1970.
376. **Efremov, G. D., Duma, H., Rudivic, R., Rolovic, Z., Wilson, J. B., and Huisman, T. H. J.**, Hemoglobin Beograd or $\alpha_2\beta_2$ 121 Glu→Val (GH4), *Biochim. Biophys. Acta,* 328, 81, 1973.
377. **Clegg, J. B., Weatherall, D. J., Wong Hock Boon, and Mustafa, D.**, Two new haemoglobin variants involving proline substitutions, *Nature (London),* 22, 379, 1969.
378. **Bursaux, E., Blouquit, Y., Poyart, C., Rosa, J., Arous, N., and Bohn, B.**, Hemoglobin Ty Gard ($\alpha_2^A\beta_2$124(H2) Pro→Gln): a stable high O_2 affinity variant at the $\alpha_1\beta_1$ contact, *FEBS Lett.,* 88, 155, 1978.
379. **Miyaji, T., Ohba, Y., Yamamoto, K., Shibata, S., Iuchi, I., and Takenaka, H.**, Japanese haemoglobin variant, *Nature (London),* 217, 89, 1968.
380. **Altay, C., Altinöz, N., Wilson, J. B., Bolch, K. C., and Huisman, T. H. J.**, Hemoglobin Hacettepe or $\alpha_2\beta_2$ 127 (H5) Gln→Glu, *Biochim. Biophys. Acta,* 434, 1, 1976.
381. **Martinez, G., Lima, F., and Colombo, B.**, Haemoglobin J Guantanamo ($\alpha_2\beta_2$ 128 (H6) Ala→Asp). A new fast unstable haemoglobin found in a Cuban family, *Biochim. Biophys. Acta,* 491, 1, 1977.
382. **Blackwell, R. Q., Yang, Y.-J., and Wang, C.-C.**, Hemoglobin J Taichung: β 129 Ala→Asp, *Biochim. Biophys. Acta,* 194, 1, 1969.
383. **Maniatis, A., Bousios, T., Nagel, R. L., Balazs, T., Ueda, Y., Bookchin, R. M., and Maniatis, G. M.**, Hemoglobin Crete (β129 Ala→Pro): a new high-affinity variant interacting with β^0- and $\delta\beta^0$-thalassemia, *Blood,* 54, 54, 1979.
384. **Lorkin, P. A., Pietschmann, H., Braunsteiner, H., and Lehmann, H.**, Structure of Haemoglobin Wien β130 (H8) Tyrosine→Aspartic acid: an unstable haemoglobin variant, *Acta Haematol.,* 51, 351, 1974.
385. **Wade Cohen, P. T., Yates, A., Bellingham, A. J., and Huehns, E. R.**, Amino-acid substitution on the $\alpha_1\beta_1$ intersubunit contact of Haemoglobin Camden β131 (H9) Gln→Glu, *Nature (New Biol.),* 243, 467, 1973.
386. **Ohba, Y., Miyaji, T., Matsuoka, M., Ueda, S., Iuchi, I., and Shibata, S.**, Hemoglobin Tokuchi: β131 Glutamine → Glutamic acid, an example of Hb Camden in Japan, *Acta Haematol. Jpn.,* 38, 1, 1975.
387. **Brennan, S. O., Arnold, B., Fleming, P., and Carrell, R. W.**, A new unstable haemoglobin, β134 Val→Glu, *Proc. N.Z. Med. J.,* 85, 398, 1977.
388. **Arends, T., Lehmann, H., Plowman, D., and Stathopoulou, R.**, Haemoglobin North Shore-Caracas β134 (H12) Valine→Glutamic acid, *FEBS Lett.,* 80, 261, 1977.

389. **Marti, H. R., Winterhalter, K. H., Di Iorio, E. E., Lorkin, P. A., and Lehmann, H.,** Hb Altdorf $\alpha_2\beta_2$ 135(H13) Ala→Pro: a new electrophoretically silent unstable haemoglobin variant from Switzerland, *FEBS Lett.*, 63, 193, 1976.
390. **Minnich, V., Hill, R. J., Khuri, P. D., and Anderson, M. E.,** Hemoglobin Hope: a beta chain variant, *Blood,* 25, 830, 1965.
391. **Moo-Penn, W. F., Jue, D. L., Johnson, M. H., Bechtel, K. C., and Patchen, L. C.,** Hemoglobin variants and methods used for their characterization during 7 years of screening at the Center for Disease Control, *Hemoglobin,* 4, 347, 1980.
392. **Moo-Penn, W. F., Schneider, R. G., Shih, T.-B., Jones, R. T., Govindarajan, S., Govindarajan, P. G., and Patchen, L. C.,** Hemoglobin Ohio (β142 Ala→Asp): a new abnormal hemoglobin with high oxygen affinity and erythrocytosis, *Blood,* 56, 246, 1980.
393. **Hirano, M., Ohba, Y., Imai, K., Ino, T., Morishita, Y., Matsui, T., Shimizu, S., Sumi, H., Yamamoto, K., and Miyaji, T.,** Hb Toyoake: β142 (H20) Ala→Pro. A new unstable hemoglobin with high oxygen affinity, *Blood,* 57, 697, 1981.
394. **Tentori, L., Carta Sorcini, M., and Bucella, C.,** Hemoglobin Abruzzo: beta 143 (H21) His→Arg, *Clin. Chim. Acta,* 38, 258, 1972.
395. **Bromberg, P. A., Alben, J. O., Bare, G. H., Balcerzak, S. P., Jones, R. T., Brimhall, B., and Padilla, F.,** Hemoglobin Little Rock (β143 His→Gln: (H21). A high oxygen affinity haemoglobin variant with unique properties, *Nature (New Biol.),* 243, 177, 1973.
396. **Jensen, M., Oski, F. A., Nathan, D. G., and Bunn, H. F.,** Hemoglobin Syracuse ($\alpha_2\beta_2$ 143 (H21) His→Pro), a new high-affinity variant detected by special electrophoretic methods, *J. Clin. Invest.,* 55, 469, 1975.
397. **Zak, S. J., Brimhall, B., Jones, R. T., and Kaplan, M. E.,** Hemoglobin Andrew-Minneapolis $\alpha_2{}^A\beta_2$ 144 Lys→Asn: a new high-oxygen-affinity mutant human hemoglobin, *Blood,* 44, 543, 1974.
398. **Hayashim, A., Stamatoyannopoulos, G., Yoshida, A., and Adamson, J.,** Haemoglobin Rainier: β145(HC2) Tyrosine→Cysteine and Haemoglobin Bethesda: β145(HC2) Tyrosine→Histidine, *Nature (New Biol.),* 230, 264, 1971.
399. **Kleckner, H. B., Wilson, J. B., Lindeman, J. G., Stevens, P. D., Niazi, G., Hunter, E., Chen, C. J., and Huisman, T. H. J.,** Hemoglobin Fort Gordon or $\alpha_2\beta_2$ 145 Tyr→Asp, a new high-oxygen-affinity hemoglobin variant, *Biochim. Biophys. Acta,* 400, 343, 1975.
400. **Charache, S., Brimhall, B., and Jones, R. T.,** Polycythemia produced by Hemoglobin Osler (β145(HC2) Tyr→Asp), *Johns Hopkins Med. J.,* 136, 132, 1975.
401. **Gacon, G., Wajcman, H., and Labie, D.,** Structural and functional study of Hb Nancy β145 (HC2) Tyr→Asp: A high oxygen affinity hemoglobin, *FEBS Lett.,* 56, 39, 1975.
402. **Winslow, R. M., Swenberg, M.-L., Gross, E., Chervenick, P. A., Buchman, R. R., and Anderson, W. F.,** Hemoglobin McKees Rocks ($\alpha_2\beta_2$ 145 Tyr→Term): a human "nonsense" mutation leading to a shortened β-chain, *J. Clin. Invest.,* 57, 772, 1976.
403. **Imai, K.,** Oxygen-equilibrium characteristics of abnormal Hemoglobin Hiroshima ($\alpha_2\beta_2$ 143 Asp), *Arch. Biochem. Biophys.,* 127, 543, 1968.
404. **Perutz, M. F., del Pulsinelli, P., Ten Eyck, L., Kilmartin, J. V., Shibata, S., Iuchi, I., Miyaji, T., and Hamilton, H. B.,** Haemoglobin Hiroshima and the Mechanism of the Alkaline Bohr Effect, *Nature (New Biol.),* 232, 147, 1971.
405. **Barem, G. H., Bromberg, P. A., Alben, J. O., Brimhall, B., Jones, R. T., Mintz, S., and Rother, I.,** Altered C-terminal salt bridges in Haemoglobin York cause high oxygen affinity, *Nature (London),* 259, 155, 1976.
406. **Wajcman, H., Kilmartin, J. V., Najman, A., and Labie, D.,** Hemoglobin Cochin-Port Royal — consequences of the replacement of the β chain C-terminal by an arginine, *Biochim. Biophys. Acta,* 400, 354, 1975.
407. **Schneider, R. G., Bremner, J. E., Brimhall, B., Jones, R. T., and Shih, T.-B.,** Hemoglobin Cowtown (β146 HC3 His→Leu): a mutant with high oxygen affinity and erythrocytosis, *Am. J. Clin. Pathol.,* 72, 1028, 1979.
408. **Jones, R. T., Brimhall, B., Huehns, E. R., and Barnicot, N. A.,** Hemoglobin Sphakiá: a delta chain variant of Hemoglobin A_2 from Crete, *Science,* 151, 1406, 1966.
409. **Ranney, H. M., Jacobs, A. S., Ramot, B., and Bradley, T. B., Jr.,** Hemoglobin NYU, a delta chain variant, $\alpha_2\delta_2$ 12 Lys, *J. Clin. Invest.,* 48, 2057, 1969.
410. **Ball, E. W., Meynell, M. J., Beale, D., Kynoch, P., Lehmann, H., and Stretton, A. O. W.,** Haemoglobin A_2': $\alpha_2\delta_2$ 16 Glycine → Arginine, *Nature (London),* 209, 1217, 1968.
411. **Rieder, R. F., Clegg, J. B., Weiss, H. J., Christy, N. P., and Rabinowitz, R.,** Hemoglobin A_2-Roosevelt: $\alpha_2\delta_2$ 20 Val→Glu, *Biochim. Biophys. Acta,* 439, 501, 1976.
412. **Jones, R. T. and Brimhall, B.,** Structural characterization of two δ chain variants, *J. Biol. Chem.,* 242, 5141, 1967.

413. **Sharma, R. S., Harding, D. L., Wong, S. C., Wilson, J. B., Gravely, M. E., and Huisman, T. H. J.,** A new δ chain variant Haemoglobin A_2 — Melbourne or $\alpha_2\delta_2$ 43Glu→Lys(CD2), *Biochim. Biophys. Acta,* 359, 233, 1974.
414. XIII Meeting Gruppo di Studio Dell'Entrocita, Torino, June 12, 1977.
415. **Lie Injo, L. E., Pribada, W., Boerma, F. W., Efremov, G. D., Wilson, J. B., Reynolds, C. A., and Huisman, T. H. J.,** Hemoglobin A_2-Indonesia or $\alpha_2\delta_2$ 69(E13) Gly→Arg, *Biochim. Biophys. Acta,* 229, 335, 1971.
416. **Sharma, R. S., Williams, L., Wilson, J. B., and Huisman, T. H. J.,** Hemoglobin A_2-Coburg or $\alpha_2\delta_2$ 116 Arg→His (G18), *Biochim. Biophys. Acta,* 393, 379, 1975.
417. **DeJong, W. W. W. and Bernini, L. f.,** Haemoglobin Babinga (δ136 Glycine → Aspartic acid): a new delta chain variant, *Nature (London),* 219, 1360, 1968.
418. **Lie-Injo, L. E., Kamuzora, H., and Lehmann, H.,** Haemoglobin F Malaysia: $\alpha_2\gamma_2$ 1(NA1) Glycine→Cysteine: 136 Glycine, *J. Med. Genet.,* 11, 25, 1974.
419. **Jenkins, G. C., Beale, D., Black, A. J., Huntsman, G. R., and Lehmann, H.,** Haemoglobin F Texas I ($\alpha_2\gamma_2$ 5 Glu→Lys): a variant of Haemoglobin F, *Br. J. Haematol.,* 13, 252, 1967.
420. **Ahern, E. J., Wiltshire, B. G., and Lehmann, H.,** Further characterization of Haemoglobin F. Texas I γ5 Glutamic acid→Lysine: γ136 Alanine, *Biochim. Biophys. Acta,* 271, 61, 1972.
421. **Ohta, Y., Saito, S., Fujita, S., Wilson, J. B., Lam, H., and Huisman, T. H. J.,** Hb F-Meinohama or $\alpha_2\gamma_2$ (5 Glu→Gly; 75Ile; 136Gly), *Hemoglobin,* 5, 565, 1981.
422. **Larkin, I. L. M., Baker, T., Lorkin, P. A., Lehmann, H., Black, A. J., and Huntsman, R. G.,** Haemoglobin F Texas II ($\alpha_2\gamma_2$ 6Glu→Lys). The second of the Haemoglobin F Texas variants, *Br. J. Haematol.,* 14, 233, 1968.
423. **Yoshinaka, H., Ohba, Y., Hattori, Y., Matsuoka, M., Miyaji, T., and Fuyuno, K.,** A new γ chain variant, Hb F Kotobuki or $^{A}\gamma^{I}6$ (A3) Glu→Gly, *Hemoglobin,* 6, 37, 1982.
424. **Carrell, R. W., Owen, M. C., Anderson, R., and Berry, E.,** Haemoglobin F Auckland $^{G}\gamma$ 7 Asp→Asn — further evidence for multiple genes for the gamma chain, *Biochim. Biophys. Acta,* 365, 323, 1974.
425. **Loukopoulos, D., Kaltsoya, A., and Fessas, Ph.,** On the chemical abnormality of Hb "Alexandra" a fetal hemoglobin variant, *Blood,* 33, 114, 1969.
426. **Brennan, S. O., Smith, Merran, B., and Carrell, R. W.,** Haemoglobin F Melbourne $^{G}\gamma$ 16 Gly→Arg and Haemoglobin F Carlton $^{G}\gamma$ 121 Glu→Lys, *Biochim. Biophys. Acta,* 490, 452, 1977.
427. **Lie-Injo, L. E., Wiltshire, B. G., and Lehmann, H.,** Structural identification of Haemoglobin F Kuala Lumpur ($\alpha_2\gamma_2$ 22(B4) Asp→Gly: (136Ala), *Biochim. Biophys. Acta,* 322, 224, 1973.
428. **Ahern, E. J., Jones, R. T., Brimhall, B., and Gray, R. H.,** Haemoglobin F Jamaica ($\alpha_2\gamma_2$ 61 Lys→Glu: 136Ala), *Br. J. Haematol.,* 18, 369, 1970.
429. **Hayashi, A., Fujita, T., Fujimura, M., and Titani, K.,** A new abnormal fetal hemoglobin, Hb F M-Osaka ($\alpha_2\gamma_2$ 63 His→Tyr), *Hemoglobin,* 4, 447, 1980.
430. **Fuyuno, K., Torigoe, T., Ohba, Y., Matsuoka, M., and Miyaji, T.,** Survey of cord blood hemoglobin in Japan and identification of two new γ chain variants, *Hemoglobin,* 5, 139, 1981.
431. **Ricco, G., Mazza, U., Turi, R. M., Pich, P. G., Camaschella, C., Saglio, G., and Bernini, L. F.,** Significance of a new type of human fetal hemoglobin carrying a replacement isoleucine→threonine at position 75 (E19) of the γ chain, *Hum. Genet.,* 32, 305, 1976.
432. **Ahern, E., Holder, W., Ahern, V., Serjeant, G. R., Serjeant, B. E., Forbes, M., Brimhall, B., and Jones, R. T.,** Haemoglobin F Victoria Jubilee ($\alpha_2{}^{A}\gamma_2$ 80 Asp→Tyr), *Biochim. Biophys. Acta,* 393, 188, 1975.
433. **Schneider, R. G., Haggard, M. E., Gustavson, L. P., Brimhall, B., and Jones, R. T.,** Genetic haemoglobin abnormalities in about 9,000 Black and 7,000 White newborns: Haemoglobin F Dickinson (A97 His→Arg), a new variant, *Br. J. Haematol.,* 28, 515, 1974.
434. **Omura, H., Miyaji, T., and Shibata, S.,** Hemoglobin F Ube (108 Asn→Lys), a new abnormal fetal hemoglobin found in a Japanese baby, *Chem. Abstr.,* 83, 266, 1975.
435. **Cauchi, M. N., Clegg, J. B., and Weatherall, D. J.,** Haemoglobin F (Malta) a new foetal haemoglobin variant with a high incidence in Maltese infants, *Nature (London),* 223, 311, 1969.
436. **Sacker, L. S., Beale, D., Black, A. J., Huntsman, R. G., Lehmann, H., and Lorkin, P. A.,** Haemoglobin F Hull (γ121 Glutamic acid → Lysine), homologous with Haemoglobins O and O Indonesia, *Br. Med. J.,* 3, 531, 1967.
437. **Brimhall, B., Vedvick, T. S., Jones, R. T., Ahern, E., Palomino, E., and Ahern, V.,** Haemoglobin F Port Royal ($\alpha_2{}^{G}\gamma$ 125 Glu→Ala), *Br. J. Haematol.,* 27, 313, 1973.
438. **Lee-Potter, J. P., Deacon-Smith, R. A., Simpkiss, M. J., Kamuzora, H., and Lehmann, H.,** A new cause of haemolytic anaemia in the newborn. A description of an unstable fetal haemoglobin: F Poole, $\alpha_2{}^{G}\gamma_2$ 130 Tryptophan→Glycine, *J. Clin. Pathol.,* 28, 317, 1975.
439. **Barnabas, J. and Muller, C. J.,** Haemoglobin Lepore Hollandia, *Nature (London),* 194, 931, 1962.
440. **Ostertag, W. and Smith, E. W.,** Hemoglobin-Lepore Baltimore, a third type of a δβ crossover (δ50, β86), *Eur. J. Biochem.,* 10, 371, 1969.

441. **Baglioni, C.,** The fusion of two peptide chains in Hemoglobin Lepore and its interpretation as a genetic deletion, *Proc. Natl. Acad. Sci. U.S.A.*, 48, 1880, 1962.
442. **Adams, J. G., III, Morrison, W. T., and Steinberg, M. H.,** Hemoglobin Parchman: Double crossover within a single human gene, *Science*, 218, 291, 1982.
443. **Ohta, Y., Yamaoka, K., Sumida, I., and Yanase, T.,** Hemoglobin Miyada, a β-δ fusion peptide (anti-Lepore) type discovered in a Japanese family, *Nature (New Biol.)*, 234, 218, 1977.
444. **Lehmann, H. and Charlesworth, D.,** Observation on Haemoglobin P (Congo type), *Biochem. J.*, 119, 43, 1970.
445. **Badr, F. M., Lorkin, P. A., and Lehmann, H.,** Haemoglobin P-Nilotic: containing a β-δ chain, *Nature (New Biol.)*, 242, 107, 1973.
446. **Honig, G. R., Shamsuddin, M., Mason, R. G., and Vida, L. N.,** Hemoglobin Lincoln Park: A δβ fusion (anti-Lepore) variant with an amino acid deletion in the δ chain-derived segment, *Proc. Natl. Acad. Sci.*, 75, 1475, 1978.
447. **Huisman, T. H. J., Wrightstone, R. N., Wilson, J. B., Schroeder, W. A., and Kendall, A. G.,** Hemoglobin Kenya, the product of fusion of γ and β polypeptide chains, *Arch. Biochem. Biophys.*, 153, 850, 1972.
448. **Clegg, J. B., Weatherall, D. J., and Milner, P. F.,** Haemoglobin Constant Spring — a chain termination mutant, *Nature (London)*, 234, 337, 1971.
449. **Clegg, J. B., Weatherall, D. J., Contopolou-Griva, I., Caroutsos, K., Poungouras, P., and Tsevrenis, H.,** Haemoglobin Icaria, a new chain-termination mutant which causes α thalassemia, *Nature (London)*, 251, 245, 1974.
450. **DeJong, W. W. W., Meera Khan, P., and Bernini, L. F.,** Hemoglobin Koya Dora: high frequency of a chain termination mutant, *Am. J. Hum. Genet.*, 27, 81, 1975.
451. **Flatz, G., Kinderlerer, J. L., Kilmartin, J. V., and Lehmann, H.,** Haemoglobin Tak: a variant with additional residues at the end of the β-chains, *Lancet*, 10, 732, 1971.
452. **Imai, K. and Lehmann, H.,** The oxygen affinity of Haemoglobin Tak, a variant with an elongated β chain, *Biochim. Biophys. Acta*, 412, 288, 1975.
453. **Lehmann, H., Casey, R., Lang, A., Stathopoulou, R., Imai, K., Tuchinda, S., Vinai, P., and Flatz, G.,** Haemoglobin Tak: a β-chain elongation, *Br. J. Haematol.*, 31(Suppl), 119, 1975.
454. **Seid-Akhavan, M., Winter, W. P., Abramson, R. K., and Rucknagel, D. L.,** Hemoglobin Wayne: a frameshift mutation detected in human hemoglobin alapha chains, *Proc. Natl. Acad. Sci. U.S.A.*, 73, 882, 1976.
455. **Bunn, H. F., Schmidt, G. J., Haney, D. N., and Dluhy, R. G.,** Hemoglobin Cranston, an unstable variant having an elongated β chain due to a nonhomologous crossover between two normal β chain genes, *Proc. Natl. Acad. Sci. U.S.A.*, 72, 3609, 1975.
456. **Huisman, T. H. J., Wilson, J. B., Gravely, M., and Hubbard, M.,** Hemoglobin Grady: the first example of a variant with elongated chains due to an insertion of residues, *Proc. Natl. Acad. Sci. U.S.A.*, 71, 3270, 1974.
457. **Tentori, L.,** personal communication, International Committee for Standardization in Hematology, Kyoto, Japan, 1976.
458. **Garel, M. C., Goossens, M., Oudart, J. L., Blouquit, Y., Thillet, J., and Rosa, J.,** Hemoglobin Dakar = Hemoglobin Grady: demonstration by a new approach to the analysis of the tryptic core region of the α chain and oxygen equilibrium properties, *Biochim. Biophys. Acta*, 453, 459, 1976.
459. **DeJong, W. W. W., Went, L. N., and Bernini, L. F.,** Haemoglobin Leiden: deletion of β6 or 7 glutamic acid, *Nature(London)*, 220, 788, 1968.
460. **Cohen-Solal, M., Blouquit, Y., Garel, M. C., Thillet, J., Gaillard, L., Creyssel, R., Gibaud, A., and Rosa, J.,** Haemoglobin Lyon (β17-18(A14-15) Lys-Val→O) determination of sequenator analysis, *Biochim. Biophys. Acta*, 351, 306, 1974.
461. **Jones, R. T., Brimhall, B., Huisman, T. H. J., Kleihauer, E., and Betke, K.,** Hemoglobin Freiburg: abnormal hemoglobin due to deletion of a single amino acid residue, *Science*, 154, 1024, 1966.
462. **Praxedes, H. and Lehmann, H.,** Haemoglobin Niteroi — a new unstable variant, Proc. 14th International Congress of Hematology, Sao Paulo, Brazil, 1972.
463. **Shibata, S., Miyaji, T., Ueda, S., Matsuoka, M., Iuchi, I., Yamada, K., and Shinkai, N.,** Hemoglobin Tochigi (beta 56-59 deleted). A new unstable hemoglobin discovered in a Japanese family, *Proc. Jpn. Acad.*, 46, 440, 1970.
464. **Wajcman, H., Labie, D., and Schapira, G.,** Two new hemoglobin variants with deletion. Hemoglobin Tours: Thr β87(F3) deleted and Hemoglobin St. Antoine: Gly→Leu β74-75 (E18-19) deleted. Consequences for oxygen affinity and protein stability, *Biochim. Biophys. Acta*, 295, 495, 1973.
465. **Adams, J. G., III, Steinberg, M. H., Newman, M. V., Morrison, W. T., Benz, E. J., Jr., and Iyer, R.,** β-Thalassemia present *in cis* to a new β-chain structural variant, Hb Vicksburg [β75(E19)Leu→O], *Proc. Natl. Acad. Sci. U.S.A.*, 78, 469, 1981.

466. **Bradley, T. B., Wohl, R. C., and Rieder, R. F.,** Hemoglobin Gun Hill: deletion of five amino acid residues and impaired heme-globin binding, *Science*, 157, 1581, 1967.
467. **Lutcher, C. L. and Huisman, T. H. J.,** Hb-Leslie, an unstable variant due to deletion of Gln β131, occurring in combination with β^0-thalassemia, Hb-S, and Hb-C, *Clin. Res.*, 23, 278A, 1975.
468. **Lutcher, C. L., Wilson, J. B., Gravely, M. E., Stevens, P. D., Chen, C. J., Linderman, J. G., Wong, S. C., Miller, A., Gottlieb, M., and Huisman, T. H. J.,** Hb Leslie, an unstable hemoglobin due to deletion of glutaminyl residue β131(H9) occurring in association with β^0-thalassemia, Hb-C, and Hb-S, *Blood*, 47, 99, 1976.
469. **Moo-Penn, W. F., Jue, D. L., Bechtel, K. C., Johnson, M. H., Bemis, E., Brosious, E., and Schmidt, R. M.,** Hemoglobin Deaconess, a new deletion mutant: β131(H9) Glutamine deleted, *Biochem. Biophys. Res. Commun.*, 65, 8, 1975.
470. **Casey, R., Kynoch, P. A. M., Lang, A., Lehmann, H., Nozari, G., and Shinton, N. K.,** Double heterozygosity for two unstable haemoglobins: Hb Sydney (β67[E11] Val→Ala) and Hb Coventry (β141[H19] Leu deleted), *Br. J. Haematol.*, 38, 195, 1978.
471. **Johnson, C. S., Schroeder, W. A., Shelton, J. B., and Shelton, J. R.,** Hemoglobin Boyle Heights: the first example of a deletion in the α chain, *Blood*, 58(Suppl. 1), #5 1981.
472. **Bookchin, R. M., Nagel, R. L., and Ranney, H. M.,** Structure and properties of Hemoglobin C Harlem, a human hemoglobin variant with amino acid substitutions in 2 residues of the β-polypeptide chain, *J. Biol. Chem.*, 242, 248, 1967.
473. **Lang, A., Lehmann, H., McCurdy, P. R., and Pierce, L.,** Identification of Haemoglobin C Georgetown, *Biochim. Biophys. Acta*, 278, 57, 1972.
474. **Adams, J. G. and Heller, P.,** Hemoglobin Arlington Park (β6 Glu→Lys 95 Lys→Glu): electrophoretically "silent" hemoglobin variant with two amino acid substitutions in the polypeptide chain, *Blood*, 42, 990, 1973.
475. **Blackwell, R. Q., Wong Hock Boon, Liu, C.-S., and Weng, M. I.,** Hemoglobin J Singapore: α78 Asn→Asp: α79 Ala→Gly, *Biochim. Biophys. Acta*, 278, 482, 1972.
476. **Goossens, M., Garel, M. C., Auvinet, J., Basset, P., Gomes, P. F., and Rosa, J.,** Hemoglobin C Ziguinchor $\alpha_2{}^A\beta_2$ 6(A3) Glu→Val β58 (E2) Pro→Arg: The second sickling variant with amino acid substitutions in 2 residues of the β polypeptide chain, *FEBS Lett.*, 58, 149, 1975.
477. **Moo-Penn, W. F., Schmidt, R. M., Jue, D. L., Bechtel, K. C., Wright, J. M., Horne, M. K., III, Haycraft, G. L., Roth, E. F., and Nagel, R. L.,** Hemoglobin S Travis. A sickling hemoglobin with two amino acid substitutions [β6(A3) Glutamic acid → Valine and β142(H20) Alanine → Valine], *Eur. J. Biochem.*, 77, 561, 1977.
478. **Wilkinson, T.,** Abstract present at the AGM Haematology Society Meeting of Australia, 1983.
479. **Webber, B. B., Lam, H., Wilson, J. B., and Huisman, T. H. J.,** Hb Albany-GA or $\alpha_2$11(A9)Lys→Asn β_2, *Hemoglobin*, 7, 257, 1983.
480. **Shimasaki, S., Iuchi, I., Hidaka, K., and Mizuta, W.,** The survey of abnormal hemoglobin in Kobe district, *Jpn. J. Hum. Genet.*, 28, 127, 1983.
481. **Honig, G. R., Shamsuddin, M., Vida, L. N., Mompoint, M., Bowie, L., Jones, E., and Weil, S.,** Hb Evanston (α14 Trp→Arg): a new variant with thalassemia-like hematologic expression, *Blood*, 60(Suppl. 1), 53a, 1982.
482. **Moo-Penn, W. F., Baine, R. M., Jue, D. L., Johnson, M. H., McGuffey, J. E., and Benson, J. M.,** Hemoglobin Evanston: α14 (A12) Trp→Arg, a variant hemoglobin associated with α-thalssemia-2, *Biochim. Biophys. Acta*, 747, 65, 1983.
483. **Liang, C-C., Chen, S., Yang, K., Jia, P., Ma, Y., Li, T., Ni, X., Wang, X., Deng, Q., and Yao, S.,** Hemoglobin Beijing [α16(A14)Lys→Asn]: a new fast-moving hemoglobin variant, *Hemoglobin*, 6, 629, 1982.
484. **Harano, T., Harano, K., Shibata, S., Ueda, S., Imai, K., Tsuneshige, A., Yamada, H., Seki, M., and Fukui, H.,** Hemoglobin Kariya [α40(C5)Lys→Glu]: a new hemoglobin variant with an increased oxygen affinity, *FEBS Lett.*, 153, 332, 1983.
485. **Nakatsuji, T., Wilson, J. B., and Huisman, T. H. J.,** Hb Cordele $\alpha_2$47(CE5) Asp→Alaβ_2 a mildly unstable variant observed in Black twins, *Hemoglobin*, 8, 37, 1984.
486. **Harano, T., Harano, K., Shibata, S., Ueda, S., Mori, H., and Seki, M.,** Hemoglobin Aichi [α50(CE8)His→Arg]: a new slightly unstable hemoglobin variant discovered in Japan, *FEBS Lett.*, 169, 297, 1984.
487. **Wong, S. C., Ali, M. A. M., Pond, J. R., Rubin, S. M., Johnson, S. E. N., Wilson, J. B., and Huisman, T. H. J.,** Hb J-Singa (α-78 Asn→Asp), a newly discovered hemoglobin variant with the same amino acid substitution as one of the two present in Hb J-Singapore (α-78 Asn→Asp, α-79 Ala→Gly), *Biochim. Biophys. Acta*, 784, 187, 1984.
488. **Dysert, P. A., II, Head, C. G., Shih, T. B., Jones, R. T., and Schneider, R. G.,** Hb Dallas $\alpha_2$97(G4)Asn→Lysβ_2: a new abnormal hemoglobin with high oxygen affinity, *Blood*, 60(Suppl. 1), 53a, 1982.

489. **Sciarratta, G. V., Ivaldi, G., Parodi, M. I., Sansone, G., Molaro, G. L., Salkie, M. L., Wilson, J. B., Reese, A. L., and Huisman, T. H. J.,** The characterization of Hemoglobin Manitoba or $\alpha_2 102(G9)Ser \rightarrow Arg\beta_2$ and Hemoglobin Contaldo or $\alpha_2 103(G10)His \rightarrow Arg\beta_2$ by high performance liquid chromatography, *Hemoglobin,* 8, 169, 1984.

490. **Harano, T., Harano, K., Shibata, S., Ueda, S., Imai, K., and Seki, M.,** Hemoglobin Tokoname [α139 (HC 1) Lys → Thr]: a new hemoglobin variant with a slightly increased oxygen affinity, *Hemoglobin,* 7, 85, 1983.

491. **Harano, T., Harano, K., Shibata, S., Ueda, S., Mori, H., and Arimasa, N.,** Hemoglobin Okayama [β2 (NA2) His→Gln]: a new 'silent' hemoglobin variant with substituted amino acid residue at the 2,3 diphosphoglycerate binding site, *FEBS Lett.,* 156, 20, 1983.

492. **Harano, T., Harano, K., Ueda, S., Shibata, S., Imai, K., and Seki, M.,** Hemoglobin Machida [β6 (A3) Glu → Gln], a new abnormal hemoglobin discovered in a Japanese family: structure, function, and biosynthesis, *Hemoglobin,* 6, 531, 1982.

493. **Moo-Penn, W. F., Johnson, M. H., McGuffey, J. E., Jue, D. L., and Therrell, B. L., Jr.,** Hemoglobin Rio Grande [β8 (A5) Lys→Thr] a new variant found in a Mexican-American family, *Hemoglobin,* 7, 91, 1983.

494. **Cai, Y.-l., Wang, H.-b., Yang, X-y., Liu, Z.-h., Ao, Z.-f., Gong, D.-h., Ma, J.-p., Wang, M.-j., Ma, D.-r., Xu, Y.-q., and Chen, E.-h.,** A new fast-moving hemoglobin variant, Hb J Luhe β8 (A5) Lys→Gln, *Chin. Hematol. J.,* 3, 263, 1982.

495. **Wong, S. C., Ali, M. A. M., Lam, H., Webber, B. B., Wilson, J. B., and Huisman, T. H. J.,** Hemoglobin Hamilton or $\alpha_2\beta_2 11(A8)Val \rightarrow Ile$, a silent β-chain variant detected by Triton X-100 acid-urea polyacrylamide gel electrophoresis, *Am. J. Hematol.,* 16, 47, 1984.

496. **Elion, J., Wajcman, H., Belkhodja-Dunda, O., Lapoumeroulie, C., Labie, D., Messerschmitt, J., Staal, A. M., and Desableno, B.,** Hemoglobin J Amiens Beta 17 (A14) Lys replaced by Asn. Coincidence of a functionally silent new abnormal hemoglobin and a polycythemia vera, *Nouv. Rev. Fr. Hematol.,* 21, 347, 1979.

497. **Brennan, S. O., Williamson, D., Whisson, M. E., and Carrell, R. W.,** Hemoglobin Palmerston North β23 (B5) Val→Phe: a new variant identified in a patient with polycythemia, *Hemoglobin,* 6, 569, 1982.

498. **Arous, N., Galacteros, F., Fessas, Ph., Loukopoulos, D., Blouquit, Y., Komis, G., Sellaye, M., Boussiou, M., and Rosa, J.,** Structural study of Hemoglobin Knossos, β27 (B9) Ala→Ser. A new abnormal hemoglobin present as a silent β-thalassemia, *FEBS Lett.,* 147, 247, 1982.

499. **Marinucci, M., Boissel, J. P., Massa, A., Wajcman, H., Tentori, L., and Labie, D.,** Hemoglobin Maputo: a new β-chain variant ($\alpha_2\beta_2$ 47 (CD6) Asp→Tyr) in combination with Hemoglobin S, identified by high performance liquid chromatography (HPLC), *Hemoglobin,* 7, 423, 1983.

500. **Boissel, J. P., Wajcman, H., Labie, D., Fabritius, H., and Cabannes, R.,** Hb J Daloa (β57 (E1) Asn→Asp): a new variant found in Ivory Coast, *Hemoglobin,* 6, 433, 1982.

501. **Williamson, D., Brennan, S. O., Muir, H., and Carrell, R. W.,** Hemoglobin Collingwood β60 (E4) Val→Ala a new unstable hemoglobin, *Hemoglobin,* 7, 511, 1983.

502. **Jen, P. C., Chen, L. C., Chen, P. F., Wong, Y., Chen, L. F., Guo, Y. Y., Chang, F. Q., Chow, Y. C., and Chiu, Y.,** Hemoglobin Quin-Hai, β78 (EF2) Leu→Arg, a new abnormal hemoglobin found in Guangdong, China, *Hemoglobin,* 7, 407, 1983.

503. **Como, P. F., Kennett, D., Wilkinson, T., and Kronenberg, H.,** A new hemoglobin with high oxygen affinity — Hemoglobin Bunbury: $\alpha_2\beta_2$[94 (FG1) Asp→Asn], *Hemoglobin,* 7, 413, 1983.

504. **Rochette, J., Poyart, C., Varet, B., and Wajcman, H.,** A new hemoglobin variant altering the $\alpha_1\beta_2$ contact: Hb Chemilly $\alpha_2\beta_2$ 99 (G1) Asp→Val, *FEBS Lett.,* 166, 8, 1984.

505. **Ohba, Y., Hasegawa, Y., Amino, H., Miwa, S., Nakatsuji, T., Hattori, Y., and Miyaji, T.,** Hemoglobin Saitama or β117 (G19) His→Pro, a new variant causing hemolytic disease, *Hemoglobin,* 7, 47, 1983.

506. **Hedlund, B., Paine, S., Smith, C. M., II, Raines, J., Morrison, W. T., and Adams, J., III,** Hemoglobin Minneapolis-Laos [β-118 (GH1) Phe→Tyr] a new hemoglobin variant with normal functional properties, *Hemoglobin,* 8, 75, 1984.

507. **Lu, Y.-Q., Fan, J.-L., Liu, J. F., Hu, H.-L., Peng, X.-H., Huang, C.-H., Huang, P.-Y., Chen, S.-S., Jia, P.-C., Yang, K.-G., Liang, C.-C., Ren, X.-D., Zuo, C.-R.,** Hemoglobin Jianghua [β120(GH3) Lys→Ile]: a new fast-moving variant found in China, *Hemoglobin,* 7, 321, 1983.

508. **Strahler, J. R., Rosenbloom, B. B., and Hanash, S. M.,** A silent, neutral substitution detected by reverse-phase high-performance liquid chromatography: Hemoglobin Beirut, *Science,* 221, 860, 1983.

509. **Yang, K., Chen, S., Jia, P., Ma, Y., Wu, S., Liang, C., Chen, X., Zhang, M., Tu, Z., and Gong, S.,** Hemoglobin Jinan [β139(H17)Asn→Asp], a new abnormal hemoglobin found in China, *Hemoglobin,* 8, in press, 1985.

510. **Rochette, J., Varet, B., Boissel, J. P., Clough, K., Labie, D., Wajcman, H., Bohn, B., Magne, P., and Poyart, C.,** Structure and function of Hb Saint-Jacques ($\alpha_2\beta_2 140(H18)Ala \rightarrow Thr$): a new high-oxygen-affinity variant with altered bisphosphoglycerate binding, *Biochim. Biophys. Acta,* 785, 14, 1984.

511. **Brennan, S. O., Williamson, D., Smith, M. B., Cauchi, M. N., Macphee, A., and Carrell, R. W.,** HbA_2 Victoria $\delta 24$ (B6) Gly $\rightarrow$ Asp a new δ chain variant occurring with β-thalassemia, *Hemoglobin,* 8, 163, 1984.
512. **Salkie, M. L., Gordon, P. A., Rigal, W. M., Lam, H., Wilson, J. B., Headlee, M. E., and Huisman, T. H. J.,** Hb A_2-Canada or $\alpha_2\delta_2$ 99(G1) Asp $\rightarrow$ Asn, a newly discovered delta chain variant with increased oxygen affinity occurring *in cis* to β-thalassemia, *Hemoglobin,* 6, 223, 1982.
513. **Garcia, R. C., Navarro, J. L., Lam, H., Webber, B. B., Headlee, M. G., Wilson, J. B., and Huisman, T. H. J.,** Hb A_2-Manzanares or $\alpha_2\delta_2$ 121(GH4) Glu$\rightarrow$Val, an unstable δ chain variant observed in a Spanish family, *Hemoglobin,* 7, 435, 1983.
514. **Juricic, D., Crepinko, I., Efremov, G. D., Lam, H., Webber, B. B., Headlee, M. G., and Huisman, T. H. J.,** Hb A_2-Zabreg or $\alpha_2\delta_2$125(H3)Gln$\rightarrow$Glu, a new chain variant in association with $\delta\beta$-thalassemia, *Hemoglobin,* 7, 443, 1983.
515. **Williamson, D., Brennan, S. O., Strosberg, H., Whitty, J., and Carrell, R. W.,** Hemoglobin A_2 Fitzroy δ142 Ala $\rightarrow$ Asp: a new delta-chain variant, *Hemoglobin,* 8, 325, 1984.
516. **Nakatsuji, T., Webber, B., Lam, H., Wilson, J. B., Huisman, T. H. J., Sciarratta, G. V., Sansone, G., and Molaro, G. L.,** A new γ chain variant: Hb F-Pordenone [γ6(A3) Glu $\rightarrow$ Gln: 75Ile: 136Ala], *Hemoglobin,* 6, 397, 1982.
517. **Bradley, T. B.,** personal communication, 1982.
518. **Nakatsuji, T., Lam, H., and Huisman, T. H. J.,** Hb F-Calluna or $\alpha_2\gamma_2$(12 Thr$\rightarrow$Arg; 75Ile; 136Ala) in a Caucasian baby, *Hemoglobin,* 7, 563, 1983.
519. **Nakatsuji, T., Headlee, M., Lam, H., Wilson, J. B., and Huisman, T. H. J.,** Hb F-Bonaire-Ga or $\alpha_2{}^A\gamma_2$39(C5) Gln$\rightarrow$Arg, characterized by high pressure liquid chromatographic and microsequencing procedures, *Hemoglobin,* 6, 599, 1982.
520. **Honig, G. R., Koshy, M., Schroeder, W. A., Shelton, J. B., and Shelton, J. R.,** Hemoglobin F Lodz (${}^G\gamma^I$ 44 Ser$\rightarrow$Arg); a newly identified variant from an American infant of Polish descent, *Biochim. Biophys. Acta,* 707, 213, 1982.
521. **Serjeant, G. R., Serjeant, B. E., Lehmann, H., Dukes, M., and Robb, L.,** Hb F Kingston [${}^G\gamma$55 (D6) Met$\rightarrow$Arg], *FEBS Lett.,* 150, 77, 1982.
522. **Zeng, Y.-t., Huang, S.-z., Nakatsuji, T., and Huisman, T. H. J.,** -${}^G\gamma{}^A\gamma$-Thalassemia and γ-chain variants in Chinese newborn babies, *Am. J. Hematol.,* submitted, 1985.
523. **Nakatsuji, T., Lam, H., and Huisman, T. H. J.,** Hb F-Kennestone or $\alpha_2{}^G\gamma_2$ (EF1)77 His$\rightarrow$Arg observed in a Caucasian baby, *Hemoglobin,* 7, 267, 1983.
524. **Nakatsuji, T., Lam, H., Carver, J., and Huisman, T. H. J.,** Hb F-Marietta or ${}^G\gamma^I$ 80[EF4] Asp $\rightarrow$ Asn, observed in a Caucasian baby, *Hemoglobin,* 6, 407, 1982.
525. **Nakatsuji, T., Lam, H., Wilson, J. B., Webber, B. B., and Huisman, T. H. J.,** Hb F-Columbus-Ga or α_2 ${}^G\gamma_2$ 94(FG1)Asp $\rightarrow$ Asn, *Hemoglobin,* 6, 593, 1982.
526. **Nakatsuji, T., Shimizu, K., and Huisman, T. H. J.,** Hb F-La Grange or $\alpha_2\gamma_2$101(G3)Glu$\rightarrow$Lys; 75Ile; 136Gly; a high oxygen affinity fetal hemoglobin variant observed in a Caucasian newborn, *Biochim. Biophys. Acta,* 789, 224, 1984.
527. **Shelton, J. B., Shelton, J. R., Espinueva, Z., Huynh, V., Schroeder, W. A., and Powars, D.,** Hemoglobin F-Caltech: $\alpha_2{}^G\gamma_2$120Lys$\rightarrow$Gln, *Hemoglobin,* 6, 577, 1982.
528. **Care, A., Marinucci, M., Massa, A., Maffi, D., Sposi, N. M., Improta, T., and Tentori, L.,** Hb F-Siena ($\alpha_2{}^A\gamma^T{}_2$121 (GH4) Glu$\rightarrow$Lys). A new fetal hemoglobin variant, *Hemoglobin,* 7, 79, 1983.
529. **Zing, Y.-T., Huang, S.-Z., Qiu, X.-K., Cheng, G.-C., Ren, Z.-R., Jin, Q.-C., Chen, C.-Y., Jiao, C.-T., Tang, Z.-G., Liu, R.-H., Bao, X.-H., Zeng, L.-Z., Duan, Y.-Q., and Zhang, G.-Y.,** Hemoglobin Chongqing (α2 (NA2) Leu$\rightarrow$Arg) and Hemoglobin Harbin (α16 (A14) Lys$\rightarrow$Met) found in China, *Hemoglobin,* 8, 569, 1984.
530. **Como, P. F., Raven, J. L., Wilkinson, T., and Kronenberg, H.,** Comparison of the Six Hemoglobin Variants Occurring at the α6 (A4) Position with Particular Reference to the α6 Asp$\rightarrow$Gly Substitution Found in Perth, Western Australia, Haematology Society of Australia, Perth, Western Australia, October, 1984.
531. **Houjun, L., Dexiang, L., Zhiguo, L., Ping, L., Ly, L., Ji, C., and Shaozhi, H.,** A new fast-moving hemoglobin variant, Hb J-Tashikuergan α19 (AB1) Ala$\rightarrow$Glu, *Hemoglobin,* 8, 391, 1984.
532. **Sellaye, M., Blouquit, Y., Galacteros, F., Arous, N., Monplaisir, N., Rhoda, M. D., Braconnier, F., and Rosa, J.,** A new silent hemoglobin variant in a Black family from French West Indies. Hemoglobin Le Lamentin α20 His$\rightarrow$Gln, *FEBS Lett.,* 145(1), 128, 1983.
533. **Zeng, Y.-T., Huang, S.-Z., Zhou, X.-D., Qui, X.-K., Dong, Q.-Y., Li, M.-Y., and Bai, J.-H.,** Hb Shenyang [α26 (B7) Ala$\rightarrow$Glu]: a new unstable variant found in China, *Hemoglobin,* 6(6), 625, 1982.
534. **Shelton, J. B., Shelton, J. R., Schroeder, W. A., and Powars, D. R.,** Hb Aztec or $\alpha_2{}^{76}$ (EF5) MET$\rightarrow$THR$_{\beta_2}$ detection of a silent mutant by high performance liquid chromatography, *Hemoglobin,* 9, 325, 1985.

535. **Chih-chuan, L., Fei, X., Kegong, Y., Songsen, C., Peichen, J., Maoqi, Z., and Zhiheng, Z.,** Hemoglobin Guizhou or α_2 77 (EF6) PRO→ARG β_2, a new slow-moving hemoglobin variant observed in China, *Hemoglobin,* 8, 387, 1984.
536. **Guis, M., Mentzer, W. C., Jue, D. L., Johnson, M. H., McGuffey, J. E., and Moo-Penn, W. F.,** Hemoglobin Twin Peaks α113 (Gh1) Leu→His, *Hemoglobin,* 9, 175, 1985.
537. **Harano, T., Harano, K., and Ueda, S.,** Hb Owari [α121 (H4) Val→Met]: a new hemoglobin variant with a neutral-to-neutral amino acid substitution detected by isoelectric focusing, *Hemoglobin,* 10, in press, 1986.
538. **Bowman, J. E., Bloom, R., Chen, S.-S., Webber, B. B., Wilson, J. B., Kutlar, A., and Huisman, T. H. J.,** Hb Chicago or $\alpha_2$136 (H19) Leu→Met β_2, *Hemoglobin,* submitted, 1986.
539. **Shimasaki, S.,** A new hemoglobin variant, hemoglobin Nunobiki [α141 (HC3) Arg→Cys]. Notable influence of the carboxy-terminal cysteine upon various physico-chemical characteristics of hemoglobin, *J. Clin. Invest.,* 75, 695, 1985.
540. **Wilson, C. I. D., Cave, R. J., Lehmann, H., Close, M., and Imai, K.,** Haemoglobin Warwickshire (β5 [A2] Pro→Arg): a possible 'fine tuning' of 2,3-DPG affinity by β5 Pro (FEBS 1918), *FEBS Lett.,* 176, 331, 1984.
541. **Jeppson, J. O., Kallman, L., Lindgren, G., and Fagerstam, L. G.,** Hb Linkoping (β36 Pro→Thr): a new hemoglobin mutant characterized by reversed-phase high performance liquid chromatography, *J. Chromatogr.,* 297, 31, 1984.
542. **Rahbar, S., Louis, J., Lee, T., and Asmerom, Y.,** Hemoglobin North Chicago (β36 [C2] proline→serine): a new high affinity hemoglobin, *Hemoglobin,* 9, 559, 1985.
543. **Blouquit, Y., Delanoe-Garin, J., Lacombe, C., Arous, N., Cayre, Y., Peduzzi, J., Braconnier, F., and Galacteros, F.,** Structural study of hemoglobin Hazebrouck, β38 (C4) Thr→Pro: a new abnormal hemoglobin with instability and low oxygen affinity (FEBS 1563), *FEBS Lett.,* 172, 155, 1984.
544. **Adams, J. G., III, Morrison, W. T., Pullen, D. J., Abney, R. L., III, and Steinberg, M. H.,** Hemoglobin Mississippi (MS): a new hemoglobin variant with three distinct electrophoretic mobilities, *Clin. Res,* 33, 603A, 1985.
545. **Chen, S. S., Webber, B. B., Wilson, J. B., and Huisman, T. H. J.,** Hb Gainesville-GA or $\alpha_2\beta_2$ 46 (CD5) Gly→Arg, *Hemoglobin,* 9, 179, 1985.
546. **Huisman, T. H. J., Wilson, J. B., Kutlar, A., Yang, K.-G., Chen, S.-S., Webber, B. B., Altay, C., and Martinez, A. V.,** Hb J-Antakya or $\alpha_2\beta_2$ 65 (E9) Lys→Met in a Turkish family and Hb Complutense or $\alpha_2\beta_2$ 127 (H5) Gln→Glu in a Spanish family; correction of a previously published identification, *Biochim. Biophys. Acta,* submitted, 1986.
547. **Rahbar, S., Asmerom, Y., and Blume, K. G.,** A silent hemoglobin variant detected by HPLC: Hemoglobin City of Hope β69 (E13) GLY→SER, *Hemoglobin,* 8, 333, 1984.
548. **Delanoe-Garin, J., Arous, N., Blouquit, Y., Hafsia, R., Bardakdjian, J., Lacombe, C., Rosa J., and Galacteros, F.,** Hemoglobin Kenitra $\alpha_2\beta_2$ 69 (E13) Gly→Arg. A new β variant of elevated expression associated with α-thalassemia, found in a Moroccan woman, *Hemoglobin,* 9, 1, 1985.
549. **Harano, T., Harano, K., Ueda, S., Imai, N., and Kitazumi, T.,** A new hemoglobin variant with a neutral to neutral amino acid substitution: Hemoglobin Kofu or $\alpha_2\beta_2$ 84 (EF8) Thr→Ile, *Hemoglobin,* 10, in press, 1986.
550. **Merault, G., Keclard, L., Saint-Martin, C., Jasmin, K., Campier, A., Delanoe-Garin, J., Arous, N., Fortune, R., Theodore, M., Seytor, S., Rosa, J., Blouquit, Y., and Galacteros, F.,** Hemoglobin Roseau-Pointe a Pitre $\alpha_2\beta_2$ 90 (F6) Glu→Gly: a new hemoglobin variant with slight instability and low oxygen affinity, *FEBS Lett.,* 184, 10, 1985.
551. **Harano, K., Harano, T., Shibata, S., Ueda, S., Mori, H., and Siki, M.,** Hb Okazaki [β93 (F8) Cys→Arg], a new hemoglobin variant with increased oxygen affinity and instability, *FEBS Lett.,* 173, 45, 1984.
552. **Devaraj, R., Wilson, J. B., and Huisman, T. H. J.,** Hb Regina or $\alpha_2\beta_2$ 96 (FG3) Leu→Val, a high oxygen affinity variant discovered by cation-exchange HPLC, *Am. J. Hematol.,* 19, 195, 1985.
553. **Ohba, Y., Imanaka, M., Matsuoka, M., Hattori, Y., Miyaji, T., Funaki, C., Shibata, K., Shimokata, H., Kuzuya, F., and Miwa, S.,** A new unstable, high oxygen affinity hemoglobin: Hb Nagoya or β97 (FG4) His→Pro, *Hemoglobin,* 9, 11, 1985.
554. **Moo-Penn, W. F., Johnson, M. H., McGuffey, J. E., and Jue, D. L.,** Hemoglobin Shelby [β131 (H9) GLN→LYS]: a correction to the structure of Hemoglobin Deaconess and Hemoglobin Leslie, *Hemoglobin,* 8, 583, 1984.
555. **Como, P. F., Hockey, D., Trent, R. J., and Kronenberg, H.,** Hb Geelong: β_2 139 (H17) Asn→Asp. A New Hemoglobin with Thalassemia-Like Characteristics, presented as abstract at February meeting of N.S.W. Thalassemia Society, 1985.
556. **Ohba, Y., Miyaji, T., Murakami, M., Kadowaki, S., Fujita, T., Oimomi, M., Hatanaka, H., Ishikawa, K., Baba, S., Hitaka, K., and Imai, K.,** Hb Himeji or β140 (H18) Ala→Asp a slightly unstable hemoglobin with increased βN-terminal glycation, *Hemoglobin,* 10, in press, 1986.

557. **Harano, K., Harano, T., Ueda, S., Ohkushi, T., and Imai, K.,** A new hemoglobin variant, Hb Mito [β144 (HC1) Lys$\rightarrow$Glu], with increased oxygen affinity, *FEBS Lett.*, 192, 75, 1985.

558. **Ohba, Y., Igarashi, M., Tsukahara, M., Nakashima, M., Sanada, C., Ami, M., Arai, Y., and Miyaji, T.,** Hb A Yokoshima, $\alpha_2\delta_2^{25\ (B7)\ GLY\rightarrow ASP}$, a new δ chain variant found in a Japanese family, *Hemoglobin*, 9, 613, 1985.

559. **Fujita, S., Ohta, Y., Saito, S., Kobayashi, Y., Naritomi, Y., Kawaguchi, T., Imamura, T., Wada,Y., and Hayashi, A.,** Hemoglobin A_2 Honai ($\alpha_2\delta_2$90 (F6) Glu$\rightarrow$Val): a new delta chain variant, *Hemoglobin*, 9, 597, 1985.

560. **Hu, H. and Ma, M.,** Hb F-Urumqi $^G\gamma^I$ 22 (B4) Asp$\rightarrow$Gly: a new fetal hemoglobin variant found in an Uygur baby, *Hemoglobin*, 10, in press, 1986.

561. **Chen, S. S., Wilson, J. B., Webber, B. B., Huisman, T. H. J., Miwa, S., and Amenomori, Y.,** Hb F-Tokyo or $\alpha_2{}^G\gamma_2$ 34 (B16) Val$\rightarrow$Ile, a silent γ chain variant detected by reverse phase high performance liquid chromatography, *Hemoglobin*, 9, 25, 1985.

562. **Chen, S. S., Wilson, J. B., and Huisman, T. H. J.,** Hb F-Pendergrass, and $^A\gamma^I$ variant with a Pro$\rightarrow$Arg substitution at position γ36 (C2), *Hemoglobin*, 9, 73, 1985.

563. **Chen, S.-S., Webber, B. B., Kutlar, A., Wilson, J. B., and Huisman, T. H. J.,** Hb F-Cobb or $\alpha_2{}^A\gamma_2{}^{37}$ (C3) Trp$\rightarrow$Gly, *Hemoglobin*, 9, 617, 1985.

564. **Chen, S.-S., Wilson, J. B., Webber, B. B., and Huisman, T. H. J.,** Hb F-Beech Island or $\alpha_2{}^A\gamma_2$53 (D4) Ala$\rightarrow$Asp, *Hemoglobin*, 9, 525, 1985.

565. **Chen, S. S., Webber, B. B., Wilson, J. B., and Huisman, T. H. J.,** Hb F-Forest Park, a new $^A\gamma$ variant with two amino acid substitutions, 75(E19) Ile$\rightarrow$Thr and 73(E17) Asp$\rightarrow$Asn, which can be identified in adults by gene-mapping analysis, *Biochim. Biophys. Acta*, 832, 242, 1985.

566. **Al-Awamy, B. H., Niazi, G. A., Al-Mouzan, M. I., Chen, S. S., Wilson, J. B., Webber, B. B., and Huisman, T. H. J.,** Hb F-Damman or $\alpha_2{}^A\gamma_2$ 79 (EF3) Asp$\rightarrow$Asn, *Hemoglobin*, 9, 171, 1985.

567. **Delano, J., North, M. L., Arous, N., Bardakjian, J., Pflumio, F., Brunagel, M. L., Lacombe, C., Poyart, C., Galacteros, F., Rosa, J., and Blouquit, Y.,** Hb Saverne: a new variant having an elongated β chain, *Blood*, 64(1), 56a, 1984.

568. **Jones, R. T., Barwick, R. C., Head, C. G., Shih, F. C., and Shih, T. B.,** Hemoglobin Long Island, Abstract #151, 20th Congr. Int. Soc. Haematology, Buenos Aires, Argentina, 1984.

569. **Blouquit, Y., Lena-Russo, D., Delanoe, J., Arous, N., Bardakjian, J., Lacombe, C., Vovan, L., Orsini, A., Rosa, J., and Galacteros, F.,** Hb Marsielle $\alpha_2{}^A\beta_2$ 1 (A1) NH_2-Met, 2 (A2) His 3 (A3) Pro: first variant having a N-terminal elongated β chain, *Blood*, 64(1), 55a, 1984.

570. **Kamel, K., El-Najjar, A., Webber, B. B., Chen, S. S., Wilson, J. B., Kutlar, A., and Huisman, T. H. J.,** Hb Doha or $\alpha_2\beta_2$ [X-N-Met-1 (NA1) Val$\rightarrow$Glu]; a new β chain abnormal hemoglobin observed in a Qatari female, *Biochem. Biophys. Acta*, 831, 257, 1985.

571. **Boissel, J.-P., Kasper, T. J., Shah, S. C., Malone, J. I., and Bunn, H. F.,** Amino-terminal processing of proteins: hemoglobin South Florida, a variant with retention of initiator methionine and N^α-acetylation, *Proc. Natl. Acad. Sci. U.S.A.*, 82, 8448, 1985.

572. **Barwick, R. C., Head, C. G., Shih, M.F.-C., Block, S. H., and Jones, R. T.,** Hb T-Cambodia [Beta 26 (B8) Glu$\rightarrow$Lys, Beta 121 (GH4) Glu$\rightarrow$Gln]: a new doubly substituted beta globin variant found in a Cambodian family, *Blood*, 66(1), 68a, 1985.

573. **Lacombe, C., Craescu, C. T., Blouquit, Y., Kister, J., Poyart, C., Delanoe-Garin, J., Arous, N., Bardakdjian, J., Riou, J., Rosa, J., Schaeffer, C., and Galacteros, F.,** Structural and functional studies of hemoglobin Poissy $\alpha_2\beta_2{}^{56}$ (D7) Gly$\rightarrow$Arg and 86 (F2) Ala$\rightarrow$Pro, *Eur. J. Biochem.*, 153, 655.

MOLECULAR BASIS OF THE THALASSEMIA SYNDROMES

Stylianos E. Antonarakis and Haig H. Kazazian, Jr.

INTRODUCTION

The thalassemias are genetic disorders characterized by absent or deficient synthesis of the globin polypeptide chains. Adult hemoglobin A (Hb A) consists of two α- and two β-globin chains. The α-thalassemias are characterized by diminished or absent α-globin synthesis, while the β-thalassemias are characterized by diminished or absent β-globin synthesis. Recent advances in recombinant DNA technology have led to the elucidation of the molecular etiology of most of the α- and β-thalassemias in different human populations. In this chapter the various molecular defects producing thalassemias will be discussed.

HEMOGLOBIN GENES

Hemoglobin is a tetramer that consists of two α- and two β-like globin subunits. These subunits are encoded by two clusters of genes, each of which is expressed sequentially during development. The α-genes are clustered on the short arm of chromosome 16 in a 25-kb (25,000 base pair) region.[1] In the cluster there are two expressed α-globin structural genes (α_1 and α_2) located less than 3 kb apart. Three other genes belong to this cluster: the embryonic ζ-gene and the pseudogenes $\psi\alpha_1$ and $\psi\zeta$.[2] Pseudogenes are genes that have sequence homology with the active genes but contains mutations that prevent their expression.[3] The locations of the α-like globin genes are shown in Figure 1. The β-globin gene cluster is found on the short arm of chromosome 11 in a 50-kb region.[4,5] The arrangement for the gene for the embryonic ε-globin gene, the fetal $^G\gamma$- and $^A\gamma$-globin genes, the δ- and β-(adult) globin genes, as well as the pseudogene $\psi\beta_1$ is shown in Figure 1B.

Every expressed globin gene has three exons (sequences which mostly code for the globin chains) and two intervening sequences. The intervening sequences are transcribed in erythroid cells into a single RNA that is a mosaic of coding and intervening sequences. Within the nucleus, RNA processing enzymes excise the intervening sequences and ligate the coding blocks together to assemble the final mRNA molecule. The detailed structures of the α- and β-globin genes are shown in Figure 1.

The precise DNA sequences of the human α- and β-globin genes as well as all the other genes of the clusters have been determined.[6,7] Appendix I shows the nucleotide composition of one normal α-globin gene and the normal β-gene.

β-THALASSEMIAS DUE TO POINT MUTATIONS

β-Thalassemias are caused by deficient (β^+) or absent (β^0) production of β-globin. This is a very heterogeneous disorder caused by many different defects in the β-globin gene. Recombinant DNA technology and DNA polymorphisms in the β-globin gene cluster have enabled many laboratories to clone and sequence a number of different β-thalassemia genes. The methodology and the strategy for the detection of the various β-thalassemia mutants can be found elsewhere.[8,9] To date a total of 21 different point mutations have been found in the globin gene that produce reduced or absent production of β-globin. The mutations are generally different in different ethnic groups even when the DNA polymorphisms surrounding the β-globin gene are the same.

Table 1 shows all the point mutations producing either β^+- or β^0-thalassemias. Of the 21 mutations that produce β-thalassemia so far analyzed, 9 (43%) represent mutations that block

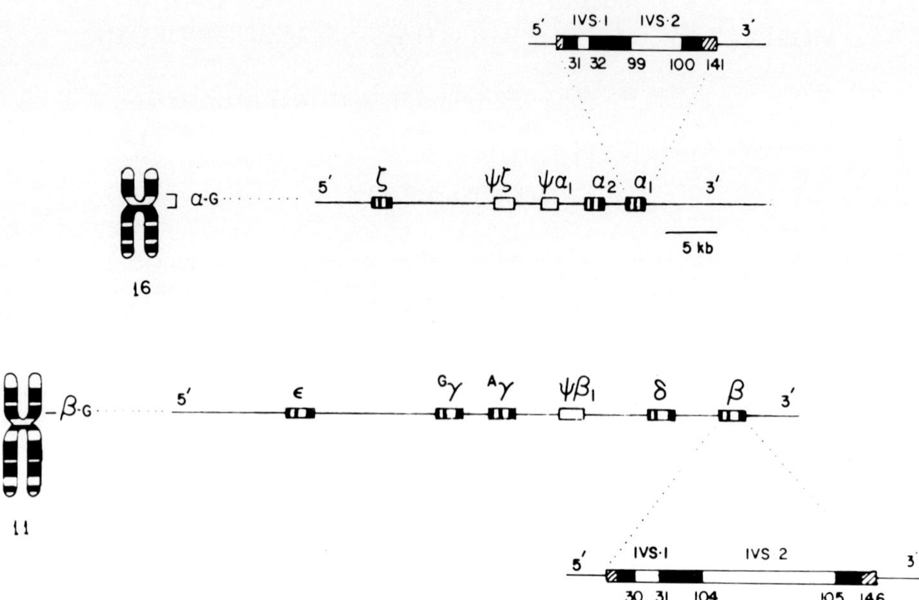

FIGURE 1. Arrangement of the human globin genes. For every gene, black boxes represent coding regions, white boxes represent intervening sequences, and hatched boxes are the 5′ and 3′ untranslated regions; α-G = alpha globin genes, β-G = beta globin genes, IVS-1 = first intervening sequence, IVS-2 = second intervening sequence. The numbers below the bars represent the corresponding amino acid residue numbers in the globin chain that are coded by the particular sequence of DNA.

translation into protein (frameshifts and nonsense codons), 10 (47%) represent mutations that affect the RNA splicing mechanism, and only 2 (10%) are mutations that affect transcription.

It is of interest that in certain cases abnormal β-globins secondary to single nucleotide substitutions can also produce mild thalassemia syndromes. For example, the β^E (β^{26}Glu→Lys)[15,16] and the $\beta^{Knossos}$ ($\beta^{27\ Ala \to Ser}$)[11,17,18] mutations produce β-thalassemia because the nucleotide change responsible for the amino acid substitution is also responsible for activation of a cryptic donor RNA splicing site. This new splicing site affects the RNA splicing mechanism and produces an abnormal RNA molecule which cannot be translated into normal β-globin.

Analysis of the mutations that produce β-thalassemia shows that they are similar to the point mutations that produce abnormal hemoglobins. We therefore no longer distinguish β-thalassemias from β-hemoglobinopathies at the DNA level.

Because there are so many mutations that produce the same final result, i.e., reduced or absent β-globin synthesis, there are many combinations of genes which produce the phenotype of β-thalassemia major. The frequency of genetic compounds, i.e., β-thalassemia individuals with two different β-thalassemia alleles, is much greater than was initially appreciated. For example, among β-thalassemics of Italian, Greek, and Indian origins, 85, 50, and 50%, respectively, are genetic compounds.[8,29] Thus, genetic compounds rather than homozygotes are the rule in this disorder.

Only a small percentage of the point mutations of Table 1 can be directly detectable by restriction analysis because most of them do not alter the recognition site of any restriction endonuclease known to date.[8,29] Therefore, prenatal diagnosis using DNA from amniotic cells has to rely on analysis of the linkage between the β-globin gene and DNA polymorphisms in the β-globin gene cluster.[30] Use of oligonucleotide probes specific for each mutation may soon provide a definitive method of prenatal diagnosis using fetal DNA.[31,32]

Table 1
POINT MUTATIONS PRODUCING β-THALASSEMIA

Mutation	Mechanism	Type of thalassemia	Ethnic group	Prevalence	Direct detection	Ref.
NT-87 C→G	Transcription defect	β^+	Mediterraneans	Rare mutation	Avr II	8
NT-28 A→C	Transcription defect, mutation in the TATA box	β^+	Kurdish Jews	Frequency unknown	No	10
Deletion of NT 70 Codon #6	Frameshift	β^+	Mediterraneans	Rare in Italians	Mst II	11
Deletion of NT 75 and 76 Codon #8	Frameshift	β^0	Mediterraneans	Rare mutation	No	12
Insertion of G between NTS 77 and 78 Codons #8 and 9	Frameshift	β^0	Asiatic Indians	About 10% of β-thal. in India	No	11
Deletion of NT 101 Codon #16	Frameshift	β^0	Asiatic Indians	Rare mutation	No	11
NT 102 A→T, Codon #17	Nonsense	β^0	Chinese	Frequency unknown	No	13
NT 125, T→A, Codon #24	Splicing defect: activation of a cryptic donor splicing site in exon-1	β^+	American blacks	Frequency unknown	No	14
NT 129 G→A Codon #26	Splicing defect: activation of a cryptic donor splicing site in exon-1	β^{26} Glu-Lys β^E	Southeast Asia	Only common β-chain hemoglobin variant in Southeast Asia	No	15, 16

Table 1 (continued)
POINT MUTATIONS PRODUCING β-THALASSEMIA

Mutation	Mechanism	Type of thalassemia	Ethnic group	Prevalence	Direct detection	Ref.
NT 133 G→T Codon #27	Splicing defect: activation of a cryptic donor splicing site in exon-1	$\beta^{Knossos}$, $\beta^{27\ Ala}$ Ser	Mediterraneans	Found only in one family in Greece	No	11, 17, 18
NT 143 G→A	Splicing defect: mutation in the donor splicing site of IVS-1	β^0	Mediterraneans	About 12% of β-thal. in Mediterraneans	No	8
NT 147 G→C	Splicing defect: mutation in the donor splicing site of IVS-1	β^+	Asiatic Indians	The most common mutation in India ~70% of β-thal.	No	19
NT 148 T→C	Splicing defect: mutation in the donor splicing site of IVS-1	β^+	Mediterraneans	About 6% of β-thal. in Mediterraneans	No	8
NT 252 G→A	Splicing defect: new acceptor splicing site in IVS-1	β^+	Mediterraneans	Most common in Mediterraneans; approximately 50% of β-thal.	No	20, 21, 22
Deletion of NTS 251—275	Splicing defect and frameshift	β^0	Asiatic Indians	Rare mutation in India	Fnu 4H	11
NT 298 C→T Codon #39	Nonsense	β^0	Mediterraneans	Fairly common mutation in Mediterraneans ~18% of β-thal.	No	12, 23, 24
Deletion of NTS 306—309 Codons #41, 42	Frameshift	β^0	Asiatic Indians	About 13% of β-thal. in India	No	11

Deletion of NT 315 Codon #44	Frameshift	β^0	Kurdish Jews	Common mutation in Kurdish, ~70% of β-thal.	No	25
NT 496 G→A	Splicing defect: mutation in the donor splicing site of IVS-2	β^0	Mediterraneans	About 8% of β-thal. in Mediterraneans	HphI	8, 26, 27
NT 1200 T→G	Splicing defect: ?	β^+	Mediterraneans	Frequency unknown	No	28
NT 1240 C→G	Splicing defect: new donor splicing site in IVS-2	β^+	Mediterraneans	About 6% of β-thal. in Mediterraneans	RsaI	8

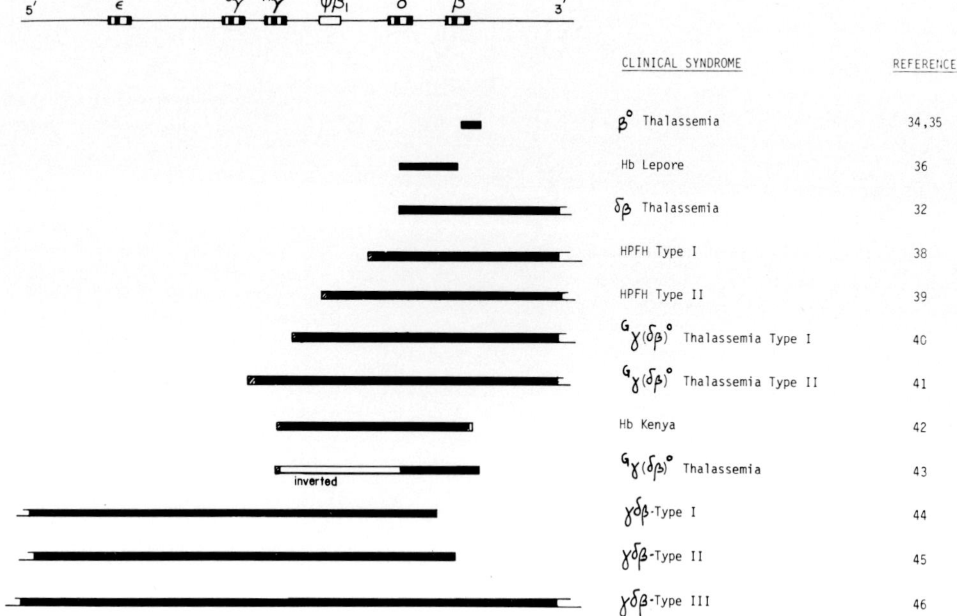

FIGURE 2. Deletions in the β-globin gene cluster. The locations of various deletions within the gene cluster are represented below the map. Filled boxes represent areas known to be deleted. Open areas indicate that the end point of the deletion has not been determined. Boxes with diagonal lines indicate that there is uncertainty in the extent of the deletion.

SYNDROMES DUE TO DELETIONS IN THE β-GLOBIN GENE CLUSTER

Deletions of different sizes involving the β-globin gene cluster produce different syndromes: β^0-thalassemias, hereditary persistence of fetal hemoglobin syndromes (HPFH — pancellular type), δβ-thalassemias, γδβ-thalassemias, and hemoglobins due to hybrid genes (Lepore, Kenya). Figure 2 shows the various deletions found in the β-globin gene cluster, all of which can be detected by restriction endonuclease analysis.[33] While nearly all of these deletions are rare, the deletion of 624 nucleotides which involve the 3′ region of the β-globin gene accounts for almost 25% of the β-thalassemia genes in Asiatic Indians.[34,35]

THE α-THALASSEMIAS

In α-thalassemias there is decreased or absent production of the α-globin chains. In contrast to β-thalassemias, most of the defects that produce α-thalassemia are due to gene deletions in the α-globin gene cluster.

α-THALASSEMIAS DUE TO POINT MUTATIONS

Table 2 shows all the point mutations in the α-globin genes that produce α-thalassemia. The chain termination mutants have the phenotype of α-thalassemia because the mRNA is very unstable.[51] In the case of Hb Quong Sze,[49] the mutation in codon 125 in the α-globin gene impedes α-β dimer formation. Recently, one splicing defect has been identified due to deletion of five nucleotides in the donor splice junction of the α_2-globin gene.[47] Many nondeletion forms of α-thalassemia remain to be discovered. In Saudi Arabians with Hb H disease, for example, α-thalassemia chromosomes with no detectable deletions in the α-globin gene cluster are as common as the deletion-type thalassemia chromosomes.[53] In Chinese Hb H disease almost 40% of α-thalassemia chromosomes have a nondeletion lesion.[54]

Table 2
POINT MUTATIONS PRODUCING α-THALASSEMIA

Mutation	Mechanism	Ethnic group	Direction detection with endonucleases	Ref.
Deletion of NTS 134—138[a]	Splicing defect: mutation in the donor splicing site of IVS-1 of α_2 gene	Mediterraneans (Italians)	No	47, 48
Hb Quong Sze 125 Leu→Pro NT 671 T→C	Impeded α-β dimer formation	Chinese	No	49
Hemoglobin Constant Spring NT 720 T→C 142 TER→Lys	Mutation in the chains termination codon UAA of α_2-gene New termination results in chain of 172 amino acids	Southeast Asia	No	50
Hb Icaria NT 720 T→A 142 TER→Lys	Mutation in the chain termination codon UAA of α_2-gene		No	51
Hb Seal Rock NT 720 T→G 142 TER→Glu	Mutation in the chain termination codon UAA of α_2-gene		No	52
Hb Koya-Dora NT 721 A→C 142 TER→Ser	Mutation in the chain termination codon UAA of α_2-gene		No	52

[a] Abnormal mature mRNA detected.

α-THALASSEMIA DUE TO GENE DELETION

Figure 3 shows the various deletions found in the α-globin gene cluster. The mechanism for the leftward and rightward deletions leaving one α-gene intact is thought to be an unequal crossing over event. In the rightward deletions the α_2-gene is deleted; in the leftward deletion the cross-over probably occurred within the structural gene and the single α-gene of this chromosome should be a Lepore-like fusion product of the 5′ end of α_2- and the 3′ end of the α_1-globin gene. Both of the reciprocal chromosomes with three α-globin genes as a result of the rightward or the leftward unequal crossing over have been recently observed[64,65] in Southeast Asian and Mediterranean populations.

All of the deletions are detectable using restriction endonuclease mapping techniques. Prenatal diagnosis is also available using fetal DNA isolation from the amniocytes after amniocentesis.

The question of why deletions in the α-globin gene complex are so common is unanswered. Part of the answer seems to lie in the physical makeup of the α-globin complex. The α-globin genes are highly homologous in their DNA sequences. What is more striking is that the homology is not limited to the genes themselves, but extends into the 5′ flanking region for about 1 kb and then after some interruptions is maintained for short stretches.[66] Overall, nearly 4 kb of DNA within the α-globin complex are highly homologous and duplicated. This is in marked contrast with the β-globin cluster in which homologous regions are limited to portions of the exons. The high degree of broad homology in the complex provides a large target size for recombinations of crossing-over events in the DNA.

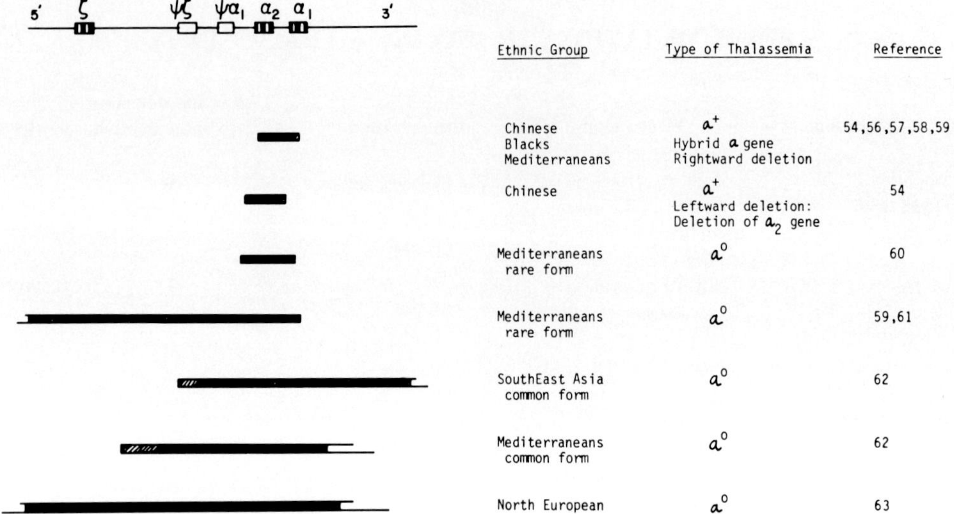

FIGURE 3. Deletions in the α-globin gene cluster. Diagrammatic details are the same as those in Figure 2. The nucleotide sequence of the α_2-globin gene is shown 5′ (left) to 3′ (right). Upper case letters represent sequences in the exons. Intervening sequences are represented by underlined lower case letters. Gene flanking sequences are in lower case.[7]

SUMMARY

Recombinant DNA technology enables us to elucidate the molecular basis of many β- and α-thalassemia syndromes. A large variety of different molecular defects account for the same phenotype: reduced or absent production of the β- or α-globin polypeptides. The elucidation of more and more natural mutations will help us to understand not only the thalassemias, but also, and more importantly, the nature of normal gene expression and function.

Appendix 1A
NUCLEOTIDE SEQUENCE OF THE HUMAN α_2-GLOBIN GENE

```
      -90       -80       -70       -60       -50       -40       -30       -20       -10
aggccgcgccccgggctccgcgccagccaatgagcgccgcccggccgggcgtgcccccgcgccccaagcataaaccctggcgcgctcgcggcccggcACT

       10        20        30        40        50        60        70        80        90       100
                                   INIValLeuSerProAlaAspLysThrAsnValLysAlaAlaTrpGlyLysValGlyAlaHisAl
CTTCTGGTCCCCACAGACTCAGAGAGAACCCACCATGGTGCTGTCTCCTGCCGACAAGACCAACGTCAAGGCCGCCTGGGGTAAGGTCGGCGCGCACGC

      110       120       130       140       150       160       170       180       190       200
aGlyGluTyrGlyAlaGluAlaLeuGluArg
TCGCGAGTATGGTGCGGAGGCCCTGGAGAGGtgaggctccctcccctgctccgacccgggctcctcgcccgccggacccacaggccaccctcaaccgtc

      210       220       230  240           250       260       270       280       290       300
                                                 MetPheLeuSerPheProThrThrLysThrTyrPheProHisPheAspLeuS
ctggccccgaacccaaaccccacccctcactctgcttctccccgcaggATGTTCCTGTCCTTCCCCACCACCAAGACCTACTTCCCGCACTTCGACCTGA

      310       320       330       340       350       360       370       380       390       400
erHisGlySerAlaGlnValLysGlyHisGlyLysLysValAlaAspAlaLeuThrAsnAlaValAlaHisValAspAspMetProAsnAlaLeuSerAl
GCCACGGCTCTGCCCAAGTTAAGGGCCACGCCAAGAAGGTGGCCGACGCGCTGACCAACGCCGTCGCGCACGTGGACGACATGCCCAACGCGCTGTCCGC

      410       420       430       440       450       460       470       480       490       500
aLeuSerAspLeuHisAlaHisLysLeuArgValAspProValAsnPheLys
CCTGAGCGACCTGCACGCCCACAAGCTTCGGGTCGACCCGGTCAACTTCAAGgtgagcggcgggccgggagcgatcttggtcgaggggcgagatggcgcc

      510       520       530       540       550       560       570       580       590       600
                                                                                            LeuLeuSe
ttcctctcagggcagaggatcacgcgggttgcgggaggtgtagcgcaggcggcggcgcggcttgggccgcactgaccctcttctctgcacagCTCCTAAG
                                                                                            100

      610       620       630       640       650       660       670       680       690       700
rHisCysLeuLeuValThrLeuAlaAlaHisLeuProAlaGluPheThrProAlaValHisAlaSerLeuAspLysPheLeuAlaSerValSerThrVal
CCACTGCCTGCTGGTGACCCTGGCCGCCCACCTCCCCGCCGAGTTCACCCCTGCGGTGCACGCTTCCCTGGACAAGTTCCTGGCTTCTGTGAGCACCGTG

      710       720       730       740      750        760       770       780      790        800
LeuThrSerLysTyrArgTER
CTGACCTCCAAATACCGTTAACCTGGAGCCTCGGTAGCCGTTCCTCCTGCCCGCTGGGCCTCCCAACGGGCCCTCCTCCCCTCCTTGCACCGGCCCTTCC

      810       820       830       840       850       860       870       880       890       900
TGTCTTTGAATAAACTCTGACTGGCCGCagcctgtgtgtgcctgggttctctctgtcccggaatgtgccaacaatggaggtgtttacctgtctcagacca

      910       920       930       940       950       960       970       980       990      1000
aggacctctctgcagctgcatggggctggggagggagaactgcagggagtatgggaggggaagctgaggtgggcctgctcaagagaaggtgctgaaccat

     1010      1020      1030
cccctgtcctgagaggtgccagcctgcaggcagtggc
```

Note: The nucleotide sequence of the α_2-globin gene is shown 5′ (left) to 3′ (right). Upper case letters represent sequences in the exons. Intervening sequences are represented by underlined lower case letters. Gene flanking sequences are in lower case.

(From Liebhaber, S. A., Goossens, M. J., and Kan, Y. W., *Proc. Natl. Acad. Sci. U.S.A.*, 77, 7054, 1980. With permission.)

Appendix 1B
NUCLEOTIDE SEQUENCE OF THE HUMAN β-GLOBIN GENE

```
 -100       -90        -80        -70        -60        -50        -40        -30        -20        -10
ccctgtggagccacaccctagggttggccaatctactcccaggagcagggagggcaggagccagggctgggcataaaagtcagggcagagccatctattg

   1         10         20         30         40         50         60         70         80         90
                                                      INIValHisLeuThrProGluGluLysSerAlaValThrAlaLeuTr
cttACATTTGCTTCTGACACAACTGTGTTCACTAGCAACCTCAAACAGACACCATGGTGCACCTGACTCCTGAGGAGAAGTCTGCCGTTACTGCCCTGTG

 100        110        120        130        140        150        160        170        180        190
pGlyLysValAsnValAspGluValGlyGlyGluAlaLeuGlyArg
GGGCAAGGTGAACGTGGATGAAGTTGGTGGTGAGGCCCTGGGCAGGttggtatcaaggttacaagacaggtttaaggagaccaatagaaactgggcatgt

 200        210        220        230        240        250        260        270        280        290
                                                                                LeuLeuValValTyrProTrpThr
ggagacagagaagactcttgggtttctgataggcactgactctctctgcctattggtctattttcccacccttaggCTGCTGGTGGTCTACCCTTGGACC

 300        310        320        330        340        350        360        370        380        390
GlnArgPhePheGluSerPheGlyAspLeuSerThrProAspAlaValMetGlyAsnProLysValLysAlaHisGlyLysLysValLeuGlyAlaPheS
CAGAGGTTCTTTGAGTCCTTTGTGGATCTGTCCACTCCTGATGCTGTTATGGGCAACCCTAAGGTGAAGGCTCATGGCAAGAAAGTGCTCGGTGCCTTTA

 400        410        420        430        440        450        460        470        480        490
erAspGlyLeuAlaHisLeuAspAsnLeuLysGlyThrPheAlaThrLeuSerGluLeuHisCysAspLysLeuHisValAspProGluAsnPheArg
GTGATGGCCTGGCTCACCTGGACAACCTCAAGGGCACCTTTGCCACACTGAGTGAGCTGCACTGTGACAAGCTGCACGTGGATCCTGAGAACTTCAGGgt

 500        510        520        530        540        550        560        570        580        590
gagtctatgggacccttgatgttttctttccccttcttttctatggttaagttcatgtcataggaaggggagaagtaacagggtacagtttagaatggga

 600        610        620        630        640        650        660        670        680        690
aacagacgaatgattgcatcagtgtggaagtctcaggatcgttttagtttcttttatttgctgttcataacaattgttttcttttgtttaattcttgctt

 700        710        720        730        740        750        760        770        780        790
tctttttttttcttctccgcaatttttactattatacttaatgccttaacattgtgtataacaaaaggaaatatctctgagatacattaagtaacttaaa

 800        810        820        830        840        850        860        870        880        890
aaaaaactttacacagtctgcctagtacattactatttggaatatatgtgtgcttatttgcatattcataatctccctactttattttcttttatttta

 900        910        920        930        940        950        960        970        980        990
attgatacataatcattatacatatttatgggttaaagtgtaatgttttaatatgtgtacacatattgaccaaatcagggtaattttgcatttgtaattt

 1000       1010       1020       1030       1040       1050       1060       1070       1080       1090
taaaaaatgctttcttcttttaatatacttttttgtttatcttatttctaatactttccctaatctctttctttcagggcaataatgatacaatgtatca

 1100       1110       1120       1130       1140       1150       1160       1170       1180       1190
tgcctctttgcaccattctaaagaataacagtgataatttctgggttaaggcaatagcaatatttctgcatataaatatttctgcatataaattgtaact

 1200       1210       1220       1230       1240       1250       1260       1270       1280       1290
gatgtaagaggtttcatattgctaatagcagctacaatccagctaccattctgcttttattttatggttgggataaggctggattattctgagtccaagc

 1300       1310       1320       1330       1340       1350       1360       1370       1380       1390
                                                LeuLeuGlyAsnValLeuValCysValLeuAlaHisHisPheGlyLysGluP
taggccctttttgctaatcatgttcatacctcttatcttcctcccacagCTCCTGGGCAACGTGCTGGTCTGTGTGCTGGCCCATCACTTTGGCAAAGAAT

 1400       1410       1420       1430       1440       1450       1460       1470       1480       1490
heThrProProValGlnAlaAlaTyrGlnLysValValAlaGlyValAlaAsnAlaLeuAlaHisLysTyrHisTER
TCACCCCACCAGTGCAGGCTGCCTATCAGAAAGTGGTGGCTGGTGTGGCTAATGCCCTGGCCCACAAGTATCACTAAGCTCGCTTTCTTGCTGTCCAATT

 1500       1510       1520       1530       1540       1550       1560       1570       1580       1590
TCTATTAAAGGTTCCTTTGTTCCCTAAGTCCAACTACTAAACTGGGGGATATTATGAAGGGCCTTGAGCATCTGGATTCTGCCTAATAAAAAACATTTAT

 1600       1610       1620       1630       1640       1650       1660       1670       1680       1690
TTTCATTGCaatgatgtatttaaattatttctgaatattttactaaaaagggaatgtgggaggtcagtgcatttaaaacataaagaaatgatgagctgtt

 1700       1710       1720       1730       1740       1750       1760       1770       1780       1790
ccaaaccttgggaaaatacactatatcttaaactccatgaaagaaggtgaggctgcaaccagctaatgcacattggcaacagcccctgatgcctatgcct

 1800       1810       1820       1830       1840       1850       1860       1870       1880       1890
tattcatccctcagaaaaggattcttgtagaggcttgatttgcaggttaaagttttgctatgctgtatttacattacttattgttttagctgtcctcat

 1900       1910       1920       1930       1940
gaatgtcttttcactacccatttgcttatcctgcatctctctcagccttgact
```

Note: The nucleotide sequence of the β-globin gene, shown 5′ (left) to 3′ (right). Upper case letters represent sequences in the exons. Intervening sequences are represented by underlined lower case letters. Gene flanking sequences are in lower case. In the 5′ flanking region, underlined lower case letters represent the "cat box" (ccaat) and the "tata box" (cataaaa), between positions −80 to −70 and −34 to −28, respectively. These are regions that are involved in initiation of transcription. Numbering refers to the encoded amino acids indicated above their respective codons. INI is the initiation codon; TER is the termination codon. (From Lawn, R. M., Efstratiadis, A., O'Connell, C., and Maniatis, T., *Cell,* 21, 647-651, 1980. With permission.)

ACKNOWLEDGMENTS

We thank Mrs. Theresa Gegorek and Melissa Garfield for the preparation of this manuscript. Haig H. Kazazian and S. E. Antonarakis are supported by grants from the NIH and the National Foundation-March of Dimes.

REFERENCES

1. **Deisseroth, A., Nienhuis, A., Turner, P., Velez, R., Anderson, W. F., Ruddle, F., Lawrence, J., Creagan, R., and Kucherlapati, R.,** Localization of the human α-globin structural gene to chromosome 16 in somatic cell hybrids by molecular hybridization assay, *Cell,* 12, 205, 1977.
2. **Maniatis, T., Fritsch, E. F., Lauer, J., and Lawn, R. M.,** The molecular genetics of human hemoglobins, *Annu. Rev. Genet.,* 14, 145, 1980.
3. **Proudfoot, N. J., Shander, M. H. M., Manley, J. L., Gefter, M. L., and Maniatis, T.,** Structure and in nitro transcription of the human globin genes, *Science,* 209, 1329, 1980.
4. **Deisseroth, A., Nienhuis, A., Lawrence, J., Giles, R., Turner, P., and Ruddle, F.,** Chromosomal localization of human β-globin gene on human chromosome 11 in somatic cell hybrids, *Proc. Natl. Acad. Sci. U.S.A.,* 75, 456, 1978.
5. **Fritsch, E. F., Lawn, R. M., and Maniatis, T.,** Molecular cloning and characterization of the human β-like globin gene cluster, *Cell,* 19, 959, 1980.
6. **Lawn, R. M., Efstratiadis, A., O'Connell, C., and Maniatis, T.,** The nucleotide sequence of the human β-globin gene, *Cell,* 21, 647, 1980.
7. **Liebhaber, S. A., Goossens, M. J., and Kan, Y. W.,** Cloning and complete sequence of human 5′ α-globin gene, *Proc. Natl. Acad. Sci. U.S.A.,* 77, 7054, 1980.
8. **Orkin, Sh., Kazazian, H. H., Jr., Antonarakis, S. E., Goff, S. C., Boehm, C. D., Sexton, J. P., Waber, P. G., and Giardina, P. J. V.,** Linkage of β-thalassemia mutations and β-globin gene polymorphisms with DNA polymorphisms in human β-globin gene cluster, *Nature (London),* 296, 627, 1982.
9. **Antonarakis, S. E., Kazazian, H. H., Jr., Orkin, S. H., Boehm, C. D., and Waber, P. G.,** DNA polymorphisms in the β-globin gene cluster: use in clinical, molecular, and evolutionary studies, in Distribution and Evolution of Hemoglobins and the Globin Loci, Bowman, J., Ed., Elsevier, New York, 1983.
10. **Poncz, M., Ballantine, M., Solowiejczyk, D., Barak, I., Schwartz, E., and Surrey, S.,** β-Thalassemia in a Kurdish Jew: single base change in the T-A-T-A-box, *J. Biol. Chem.,* 257, 5994, 1982.
11. **Antonarakis, S. E., Orkin, S. H., and Kazazian, H. H. K.,** DNA polymorphism and pathology of the human globin gene clusters, *Hum. Genet.,* 69, 1, 1985.
12. **Orkin, S. H. and Goff, S. C.,** Nonsense and frameshift mutations in β^0-thalassemia detected in cloned β-globin genes, *J. Biol. Chem.,*
13. **Chang, J. C. and Kan, Y. W.,** β^0-Thalassemia: a nonsense mutation in man, *Proc. Natl. Acad. Sci. U.S.A.,* 76, 2886, 1979.
14. **Humphries, R. K., Ley, T. J., Goldsmith, M. E., Cline, A., Kantor, J. A., and Nienhuis, A. W.,** Silent nucleotide substitution in β^+ thalassemia gene activates a cryptic splice site in β globin RNA coding sequence, *Blood,* Suppl. 60, 54A, 1982.
15. **Antonarakis, S. E., Orkin, S. H., Kazazian, H. H., Goff, S. C., Boehm, C. D., Waber, P. G., Sexton, J. P., Ostrer, H., Fairbanks, V. F., and Chakravarti, A.,** Evidence for multiple origin of the β^E globin gene in Southeast Asia, *Proc. Natl. Acad. Sci. U.S.A.,* 79, 6608, 1982.
16. **Orkin, S. H., Kazazian, H. H., Antonarakis, S. E., Ostrer, H., Goff, S. C., and Sexton, J. P.,** Abnormal RNA processing due to the exon mutation of the β^E globin gene, *Nature (London),* 300, 768, 1982.
17. **Arous, N., Galacteros, F., Fessas, P. H., Loucopoulos, D., Blouguit, Y., Komis, G., Sellaye, M., Boussion, M., and Rosa, J.,** Structural study of hemoglobin Knossos $\beta^{27\ Ala \rightarrow Ser}$. A new abnormal hemoglobin presenting as a silent thalassemia, *FEBS Lett.,* 1982.
18. **Fessas, P. H., Loucopoulos, D., Loutradi-Anagnostou, A., and Komis, G.,** "Silent" β thalassemia excused by a "Silent" β-chain mutant. The pathogenesis of a syndrome of thalassemia intermedia, *Br. J. Hematol.,* 51, 577, 1982.
19. **Kazazian, H. H., Boehm, C. D., Orkin, S. H., Sexton, J. P., and Antonarakis, S. E.,** β-Thalassemia due to deletion of the nucleotide which is substituted in sickle cell anemia, *Am. J. Hum. Genet.,* 35, 1028, 1983.

20. **Spritz, R. A., Jagadeeswaran, P., Choudary, P. V., Biro, P. A., Elder, J. T., deRiel, J. K., Manely, J. L., Gefter, M. L., Forget, B. G., and Weissman, S. M.,** Base substitution in an IVS of a β^+ thal human globin gene, *Proc. Natl. Acad. Sci. U.S.A.,* 78, 2455, 1981.
21. **Fakumaki, Y., Ghosh, P. K., Benz, E. J., Reddy, V. B., Lebowitz, P., Forget, B. G., and Weissman, S. M.,** Abnormal spliced messenger RNA in erythroid cells from patients with β^+ thalassemia and monkey cells expressing a cloned β^+ thal gene, *Cell,* 28, 585, 1982.
22. **Busslinger, M., Moschonas, N., and Flavell, R. A.,** β^+ Thalassemia: aberrant splicing results from a single point mutation in an intron, *Cell,* 27, 289, 1982.
23. **Trecartin, R. F., Liebhaber, S. A., Chang, J. C., Lee, K. Y., Kan, Y. W., Furbetta, M., Angius, A., and Cao, A.,** β^0-Thalassemia in Sardinia is caused by a nonsense mutation, *J. Clin. Invest.,* 68, 1012, 1981.
24. **Moschonas, N., deBoer, E., Grosveld, F. L., Dahl, H. H. M., Wright, S., Shewmaker, C. K.,** Structure and expression of a cloned β^0-thalassemia globin gene, *Nucl. Acid Res.,* 9, 4391, 1981.
25. **Kinniburgh, A. J., Maguat, L. E., Schedl, T., Rachmilewitz, E., and Ross, J.,** mRNA deficient β^0 thalassemia results from a single nucleotide deletion, *Nucl. Acid Res.,* 10, 5421, 1982.
26. **Baird, M., Driscoll, C., Schreiner, H., Sciarrata, G. V., Sansone, G., Niazi, G., Ramirez, F., and Bank, A.,** A nucleotide change at a splice junction in the human β globin gene is associated with β^0-thalassemia, *Proc. Natl. Acad. Sci. U.S.A.,* 78, 4218, 1981.
27. **Treisman, R., Proudfoot, N. J., Shander, M., and Maniatis, T.,** A single base change at a splice site in β^0-thalassemia gene causes abnormal RNA splicing, *Cell,* 29, 903, 1982.
28. **Spence, S. E., Pergolizzi, R. A., Donovan-Peluso, M., Kosche, K. A., Dobkin, C. S., and Bank, A.,** Five nucleotide changes in the large intervening sequence of the β globin gene in a β^+-thalassemia patient, *Nucl. Acid Res.,* 10, 1283, 1982.
29. **Antonarakis, S. E., Orkin, S. H., Kazazian, H. H., Goff, S. C., Boehm, C. D., Sexton, J. P., and Waber, P. G.,** β-Thalassemia: direct detection of mutations of restriction analysis and frequency of genetic compounds, *Pediatr. Res.,* 16, 189A, 1982.
30. **Boehm, C. D., Antonarakis, S. E., Phillips, J. A., Stetten, G., and Kazazian, H. H., Jr.,** Prenatal diagnosis using polymorphic restriction sites: report on 95 pregnancies at risk for sickle cell disease or β-thalassemia, *N. Engl. J. Med.,* 308, 1054, 1983.
31. **Pirastu, M., Kan, Y. W., Cao, A., Conner, B. J., and Wallace, R. B.,** Direct analysis of point mutations by hybridization with synthetic oligomers: applicability to prenatal diagnosis of β thalassemia, *Blood,* Suppl. 60, 56A, 1982.
32. **Orkin, S. H., Markham, A. F., and Kazazian, H. H., Jr.,** Direct detection of the common Mediterranean β-thalassemia gene with synthetic DNA probes: an alternative approach for prenatal diagnosis, *J. Clin. Invest.,* 71, 775, 1983.
33. **Antonarakis, S. E., Phillips, J. A., and Kazazian, H. H., Jr.,** Genetic diseases: diagnosis by restriction endonuclease analysis, *J. Pediatr.,* 100, 845, 1982.
34. **Orkin, S. H., Old, J. M., Weatherall, D. J., and Nathan, D. G.,** Partial deletion of globin gene DNA in certain patients with β^0 thalassemia, *Proc. Natl. Acad. Sci. U.S.A.,* 76, 2400, 1979.
35. **Spritz, R. A. and Orkin, S. H.,** Complex deletion/duplication rearrangement in a human β^0-thalassemic globin gene, *Am. J. Hum. Genet.,* 33, 167A, 1982.
36. **Flavell, R. A., Kooter, J. M., deBoer, E., Little, P. F. R., and Williamson, R.,** Analysis of the β-δglobin gene loci in normal and Hb Lepore DNA. Direct determination of gene linkage and intergene distance, *Cell,* 15, 25, 1978.
37. **Bernards, R., Kooter, J. M., and Flavell, R. A.,** Physical mapping of the globin gene deletion in $\delta\beta$-thalassemia, *Gene,* 6, 265, 1979.
38. **Fritsch, E. F., Lawn, R. M., and Maniatis, T.,** Characterization of deletions which affect the expression of fetal globin genes in man, *Nature (London),* 279, 598, 1979.
39. **Bernards, R. and Flavell, R. A.,** Physical mapping of the globin gene deletion in hereditary persistance of foetal hemoglobin (HPFH), *Nucl. Acid. Res.,* 8, 1521, 1980.
40. **Orkin, S. H., Blanche, P. S., and Cigdem, A.,** Deletion of the ${}^A\gamma$-globin gene in ${}^G\gamma\delta\beta$-thalassemia, *J. Clin. Invest.,* 64, 866, 1979.
41. **Jones, R. W., Old, J. M., Trent, R. J., Clegg, J. B., and Weatherall, D. J.,** Restriction mapping of a new deletion responsible for ${}^G\gamma(\delta\beta^0)$thalassemia, *Nucl. Acid. Res.,* 9, 6813, 1982.
42. **Huisman, T. H. J., Wrightstone, R. N., Wilson, J. B., Schroeder, W. A., and Kendall, A. G.,** Hemoglobin kenya, the product of fusion of γ and β polypeptide chains, *Arch. Biochem. Biophys.,* 153, 850, 1972.
43. **Jones, R. W., Old, J. M., Trent, R. J., Clegg, J. B., and Weatherall, D. J.,** Major rearrangement in the human β-globin gene cluster, *Nature (London),* 291, 39, 1981.
44. **Vander Ploeg, L. H. T., Kinings, A., Oort, M., Roos, D., Bernini, L., and Flavell, R. A.,** $\gamma\delta\beta$-Thalassemia studies showing that deletion of the γ and δ genes influences globin gene expression in man, *Nature (London),* 283, 637, 1980.

45. **Orkin, S. H., Goff, S. C., and Nathan, D. G.,** Heterogeneity of DNA deletion in γδβ-thalassemia, *J. Clin. Invest.*, 67, 878, 1981.
46. **Kazazian, H. H., Fearon, E. R., Waber, P. G., Lee, J. I., Antonarakis, S. E., Orkin, S. H., Vanin, E. F., Henthorn, P. A., Grosveld, F. G., Buchanan, G. R.,** γδβ-Thalassemia: deletion of the entire globin gene cluster, *Blood*, Suppl. 60, 54A, 1982.
47. **Orkin, S. H., Goff, S. C., and Hechtman, R. L.,** Mutation in an intervening sequence splice junction in man, *Proc. Natl. Acad. Sci. U.S.A.*, 78, 5041, 1981.
48. **Felber, B. K., Orkin, S. H., and Hamer, D. H.,** Abnormal RNA splicing causes one form of α thalassemia, *Cell*, 29, 895, 1982.
49. **Goossens, M., Lee, K. Y., Liebhaber, S. A., and Kan, Y. W.,** Globin structural variant $\alpha^{125\ Leu \rightarrow Pro}$ is a novel cause of α-thalassemia, *Nature (London)*, 296, 864, 1981.
50. **Clegg, J. B., Weatherall, D. J., and Milner, P. F.,** Hemoglobin Constant Spring — a chain termination mutation, *Nature (London)*, 234, 337, 1971.
51. **Clegg, J. B. and Weatherall, D. J.,** Hemoglobin Constant Spring, an unusual α-chain variant involved in the etiology of hemoglobin H disease, *Ann. N.Y. Acad. Sci.*, 232, 168, 1974.
52. **Weatherall, D. J. and Clegg, J. B.,** Molecular Genetics of human hemoglobin, *Annu. Rev. Genet.*, 10, 157, 1976.
53. **Pressley, L., Higgs, D. R., Clegg, J. B., Perrine, R. P., Pembrey, M. E., and Weatherall, D. J.,** A new genetic basis for Hemoglobin H disease, *N. Engl. J. Med.*, 303, 1383, 1980.
54. **Embury, S. H., Miller, J. A., Dozy, A. M., Kan, Y. W., Chan, V., and Todd, D.,** Two different molecular organizations account for the single α-globin gene of the α-thalassemia-2 genotype, *J. Clin. Invest.*, 66, 1314, 1980.
55. **Weatherall, D. J. and Clegg, J. B.,** Thalassemia revisited, *Cell*, 29, 7, 1982.
56. **Kan, Y. W., Dozy, A. M., Stamatoyannopoulos, G., Hadjiminas, M. G., Zachariadis, Z., Furbetta, M., and Cao, A.,** Molecular basis of hemoglobin H disease in the Mediterranean population, *Blood*, 54, 1434, 1979.
57. **Davis, J. R., Dozy, A. M., Lubin, B., Koenig, H. M., Pierce, H. I., Stamatoyannopoulos, G., and Kan, Y. W.,** Alpha thalassemia in Blacks is due to gene deletion, *Am. J. Hum. Genet.*, 31, 569, 1979.
58. **Ottolenghi, S., Lanyon, W. G., Paul, J., Williamson, R., Weatherall, D. J., Clegg, J. B., Pritchard, J., Pootrakul, S., and Boon, W. H.,** The severe form of α-thalassemia is caused by hemoglobin gene deletion, *Nature (London)*, 251, 389, 1974.
59. **Orkin, S. H., Old, J., Lazarus, H., Altay, C., Gurgey, A., Weatherall, D. J., and Nathan, D. G.,** The molecular basis of alpha thalassemia: frequent occurrence of dysfunctional alpha loci detected by restriction endonuclease mapping, *Cell*, 17, 33, 1979.
60. **Pressley, L., Higgs, D. R., Aldridge, B., Metaxotou-Mavromati, A., Clegg, J. B., and Weatherall, D. J.,** Characterization of a new alpha-thalassemia-1 defect due to a partial deletion of the α-globin gene complex, *Nucl. Acid Res.*, 8, 4889, 1980.
61. **Orkin, S. H. and Michelson, A.,** Partial deletion of the α-globin structural gene in human α-thalassemia, *Nature (London)*, 286, 538, 1980.
62. **Pressley, L., Higgs, D. R., Clegg, J. B., and Weatherall, D. J.,** Gene deletions in alpha thalassemia prove that the 5′ zeta locus is functional, *Proc. Natl. Acad. Sci. U.S.A.*, 77, 3586, 1980.
63. **Weatherall, D. J., Higgs, D. R., Bunch, C., Old, J. M., Hunt, D. M., Pressley, L., Clegg, J. B., Bethlenfalvay, N. C., Sjolin, S., Kiler, R. D., Magenis, E., Francis, J. L., and Bebbington, D.,** Hemoglobin H disease and mental retardation: a new syndrome on a remarkable coincidence?, *N. Engl. J. Med.*, 30, 607, 1981.
64. **Goossens, M., Dozy, A. M., Embury, S. H., Zachariades, Z., Hadjiminas, M. C., Stamatoyannopoulos, G., and Kan, Y. W.,** Triplicated α-globin loci in human, *Proc. Natl. Acad. Sci. U.S.A.*, 77, 518, 1980.
65. **Lie-Injo, L. E., Herrera, A. R., and Kan, Y. W.,** Two types of triplicated α-globin loci in humans, *Nucl. Acid Res.*, 9, 3707, 1981.
66. **Lauer, J., Shen, C. K. J., and Maniatis, T.,** The chromosomal arrangement of human α-like globin genes: sequence homology and α-globin gene deletions, *Cell*, 20, 119, 1980.

IRON METABOLISM

Chaim Hershko, Gabriel Izak*, and Avraham M. Konijn

INTRODUCTION

Iron is one of the most abundant elements in nature, but its solubility at a neutral pH is low, and iron deficiency is one of the most common causes of anemia. In order to facilitate the storage and internal transport of this important element, living organisms have developed highly specialized molecules to fulfill these functions. The surprising similarity in amino acid composition of the iron storage molecule ferritin, obtained from plants, fungi, and mammals, indicates its early evolution and widespread functional importance.[1,2]

In man, iron metabolism is characterized by a limited external exchange and an efficient reutilization of iron from internal sources. Normally, about two thirds of the total body iron, or 2100 to 2500 mg, are bound to hemoglobin in circulating red blood cells, 30%, or 800 to 1500 mg, are in iron stores, 3 to 5% in myoglobin, and trace amounts in iron-containing enzymes (Table 1). Only 3 mg of iron are bound to transferrin in the circulation, but this small proportion of body iron is an extremely active one which is normally replaced and lost ten times daily. Most of the daily plasma iron turnover is utilized for erythropoiesis, and erythrocytes are reprocessed at the end of their lifespan by reticuloendothelial (RE) cells in the spleen, liver, and bone marrow. The sojourn of erythrocyte iron through the RE cells is unidirectional, since RE cells can release iron derived from hemoglobin into the plasma, but cannot take up iron directly from transferrin (Figure 1). A second and less active cycle of internal iron exchange is between transferrin and parenchymal cells represented mainly by the liver. The latter exchange is bidirectional and is determined largely by the level of transferrin iron saturation.[3]

INTESTINAL ABSORPTION OF IRON

The Mechanism of Iron Absorption

The observations available to date suggest a common mechanism for the absorption of iron ingested as iron salts, iron in vegetables, in eggs, and in ferritin; it is different from the absorption process operative in heme, hemoglobin, and, probably, muscle iron absorption. The main difference between these two absorption mechanisms is that in the latter, iron absorption is unaffected by blocking substances in food, reducing agents, ascorbic acid, hydrochloric acid, and synthetic chelating agents which bind ionic iron.[4-10] This difference will be discussed in greater detail later in this chapter.

The process of absorption starts with mastication. In the stomach, iron is split from nonheme complexes by peptic digestion and liberated into a pool of miscible iron, where it may become reduced or, alternatively, chelated and rendered insoluble. Some of the iron-binding compounds such as ascorbic acid, fructose, amino acids, and mucoprotein of the gastric juice may act as carriers, while others may act as blocking substances by forming insoluble compounds with iron, such as phosphates and phytates. Protein has a potentiating effect on iron absorption, probably as a result of the formation of low molecular weight digestive products, which form soluble compounds with iron.[11]

Iron is absorbed through the jejunal mucosa in two phases: a rapid phase starting within seconds of reaching the brush borders and rising to a peak in 30 to 60 min and a slow phase extending over about 24 hr.[12-14] Once iron is absorbed into the epithelial cell, it has to pass

* Deceased.

Table 1
APPROXIMATE COMPOSITION OF IRON-CONTAINING COMPOUNDS IN THE ADULT MALE

Compound	Iron (mg)	Percentage of total
Hemoglobin	2100—2500	65
Myoglobin	130	3—5
Iron-containing enzymes	8	0.2
Transferrin	4	0.1
Ferritin and hemosiderin	800—1500	30
Total body iron	3000—4000	100

Modified from Bothwell, T. M. and Finch, C. A., *Iron Metabolism,* Little, Brown, Boston, 1962, 4.

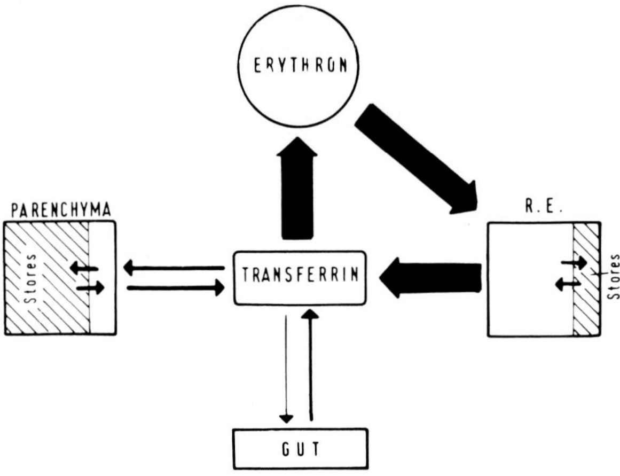

FIGURE 1. General outline of iron transport. In the normal state most of the circulating transferrin iron is utilized by the erythropoietic tissues. Iron in senescent or nonviable erythrocytes is catabolized by cells of the RE system. Parenchymal cells acquire iron directly from circulating transferrin and are also able to release iron in accordance with requirements. Only a minor fraction of the daily plasma iron turnover is supplied by intestinal absorption. Most of the iron derived from hemoglobin catabolism in RE cells is released promptly, and in consequence a smaller fraction of iron is retained in RE stores than in parenchymal stores. (From Hershko, C., *Progress in Hematology,* Vol. 10, Brown, E. B., Ed., Grune & Stratton, New York, 1977, 105. With permission.)

through its cytoplasm, after which it is released into the circulating plasma where it is bound and carried away by transferrin. These are active processes that are dependent upon oxidative metabolism.[15,16]

Evidence has been presented to show that there are specific iron receptors on the surface of mucosal cells. Brush borders isolated from jejunal epithelial cells bind more iron than those from ileal cells. This binding is much more pronounced for iron than for other metals.[17,18] It has been further demonstrated that brush borders isolated from iron-loaded animals bind substantially less iron than those isolated from normal or iron-deficient animals.[17] It has also been observed that brush borders derived from ileal epithelium, which bind small quantities of iron in normal animals, increase their uptake significantly in iron deficiency.[17] Once the iron enters the epithelial cell, it is found either in metabolically active cell components or bound to intracellular ligands. After homogenization and differential centrifugation of rat jejunal epithelium, the mitochondrial fraction contains the largest iron concentration[19] in normal, iron-deficient, and iron-loaded animals. A substantial amount of iron is also found in the particle-free soluble fraction in the normal and iron-loaded animals, but not in the iron-deficient animals, where the absolute amount of iron in the epithelial cells is greatly reduced.

Iron can penetrate the epithelial cell not only from the intestinal lumen, but also from the circulating plasma;[20] much of this latter iron can be recovered in the mitochondria,[21] where it remains throughout the lifespan of the epithelial cell. Iron entering the mucosal cell from the intestinal lumen is mostly concentrated in the soluble cell fraction with the major portion of iron bound to ferritin in the normal animal, while very little of the freshly absorbed iron in the soluble fraction is ferritin bound in the iron-deficient animal.[21-26] This makes it unlikely that ferritin is an important component of the absorptive mechanism of iron in conditions with enhanced iron absorption. Several iron-binding fractions have been isolated from the soluble mucosal cell supernatant;[27-29] however, there is still no agreement concerning the number of these fractions and their nature. Several investigators have reported iron-binding fractions have been isolated from the soluble mucosal cell supernatant;[27-29] however, there is still no agreement concerning the number of these fractions and their nature. Several investigators have reported an iron-binding protein in the soluble cell fraction of the mucosal cell of iron-deficient animals which closely resembled transferrin.[26,28,30,31]

The role of intestinal epithelial ferritin in the regulation of iron absorption was first suggested in 1946. It was proposed that ferritin synthesized in the mucosal cell in response to iron acted as a block to further absorption.[32] This theory was supported by several investigators.[20,25,33-35] However, a number of observations made the mucosal block theory untenable. Thus it was shown that mucosal ferritin synthesis is stimulated by iron in both normal and iron-deficient rats, although their mucosal cells have accumulated a normal amount of ferritin.[36,37] In rats with turpentine abscesses, the incorporation percentage of absorbed iron into mucosal ferritin is the same as in control animals, indicating that the reduction in absorption in inflammation is not due to diversion of iron into ferritin.[38] Finally, the rate of release of iron from ferritin is far too slow for ferritin to function as a transcellular carrier during the rapid phase of absorption.[39] The most plausible interpretation of the data available to date is that iron entering the mucosa in excess of what can be bound by the "carrier system" becomes bound to ferritin. Some of this iron is absorbed during the slow phase of absorption, while the remainder is lost into the intestinal lumen with the desquamating epithelial cells.

The mechanism of iron uptake by the intestinal epithelium from heme differs from that described above in several respects. Heme iron enters the mucosal cell without being released from the porphyrin ring; in the guinea pig, the absorbed heme passes into the circulating blood to be taken up by the liver.[7] In man, heme is broken down in the mucosa,[9,40] and the absorbed iron is recovered in the plasma bound to transferrin.[5,41,42] The breakdown of absorbed heme is faster in iron deficiency, and the amount absorbed appears to be limited by the transfer capacity of the cell rather than by the uptake of heme into the cell.[9] After iron is liberated from the porphyrin ring, it enters the same pool as absorbed ionic iron and is probably transferred by the same carrier. The liberation of iron from the porphyrin ring is accomplished by xanthine oxidase.[43]

Regulation of Iron Absorption

It has been universally accepted that iron absorption responds to even small changes in storage iron and to the demands of tissues, particularly of the erythroid marrow. It is also well known that the control over the amount of iron absorbed is exercised by the epithelial cell in the jejunum. The unsolved problem is how these cells receive the message of need for iron and how they react to this need. Several mechanisms have been suggested.

The binding of variable amounts of iron to components of gastric juice has been suggested to have a role in the regulation of iron absorption, but this possibility has been discarded in the light of accumulating evidence to the contrary.[44-46] Similarly, the possible role of changes in pancreatic secretion has been shown to be an unlikely factor.[47] On the other hand, exposure of the jejunal mucosa to substances present in gastric and intestinal secretions was shown to affect absorption of iron by the exposed mucosal cells. Thus, gastric and intestinal juices of iron-deficient rats or from human subjects after venesections markedly augmented iron uptake by the mucosal cells of the normal rat.[48-51]

The role of mucosal cell iron in the regulation of iron absorption has been the subject of continuous interest during the past 25 years since Conrat et al.[20,52] proposed that the absorptive capacity of the mucosal cell is determined by its iron content, which is derived partly from the diet and partly from the plasma. According to the concept put forward by these workers, mucosal iron is decreased in iron deficiency and increased in iron overload. Strong support for this hypothesis was furnished by the inverse correlation between the amount of iron absorbed and the fraction of intravenous transferrin-bound iron taken up by the duodenal mucosal cells.[53,54] Bleeding was found to augment iron absorption, prior iron loading notwithstanding,[53] and the delay observed under the latter experimental conditions was attributed to the time required for the iron-containing epithelial cells to be replaced by new iron-depleted cells.[55,56] These observations were confirmed by several investigators.[57-59] Other workers reached the conclusion that the changes in iron absorption may not be related to the nonheme iron content of the mucosal cells themselves, but rather to the amount of iron in the subepithelial layer of the jejunum.[60] In still other studies performed in guinea pigs, no correlation was found between iron absorption and the iron content of the mucosal epithelium.[61]

Recently, several groups of workers studied the total nonheme iron content in the epithelial cells and its distribution among different protein fractions, some of them functionally defined, such as succinic dehydrogenase, cytochrome oxidase, ferritin, and mitochondrial iron. A marked reduction in the iron content of these fractions was associated with iron depletion, but no increase was produced by iron overload.[62] It has been suggested that the mitochondrial iron in the intestinal epithelium is a true reflection of the body iron status, and it might be a factor in determining the uptake of iron from the intestinal lumen. In accordance with this theory, increased iron uptake was noted in animals with decreased mitochondrial iron and diminished iron-containing enzyme activity.[63] It was also confirmed that the epithelial cell obtains its iron at least partly from the plasma and is taken up largely by mitochondria.[63,64] The mitochondria have shown increased avidity for both parenterally or orally administered iron; it appears to be bound to this fraction within 30 min after it is administered.[65] There seems to be an inverse correlation between the transferrin saturation of plasma and the mitochondrial iron content of the intestinal epithelium;[66] however, increase in absorption can also be seen in patients with diminished iron stores in whom the hemoglobin concentration and plasma iron and iron-binding capacity are normal.[67-69] Furthermore, iron absorption may be decreased in patients with increased iron stores, although their plasma iron is normal.[67] Absorption of iron correlates well with the amount of stainable iron in the bone marrow reticuloendothelial cells,[70,71] presumably because the latter value varies in proportion to total storage iron. It is plausible that this correlates with a similar pool in the mitochondria of the mucosal cells, but this assumption has to be investigated.

The increased iron absorption associated with enhanced marrow activity, such as that observed in thalassemia,[72,73] in hemolytic anemia,[74] and in sideroblastic anemia,[75] cannot be explained on the basis of information available today. A tentative hypothesis has been put forward to account for this phenomenon;[76] one assumes that one of the binding sites of transferrin is more oriented to uptake of iron from the mucosa and its delivery to the marrow, while the other is more oriented to the delivery of iron to stores. Accordingly, the mucosal cell may receive a message of the need for iron without an obvious abnormality in the plasma iron or transferrin saturation. This hypothesis is built on experimental observations suggesting the existence of functional differences between the two iron-binding sites of the transferrin molecule.[76] No clinical or experimental evidence has been presented to support the concept, and it has been challenged by some subsequent studies.[77]

Attempts were made in the past to search for humoral factors affecting iron absorption, most of which were unsuccessful.[78,79] Erythropoietin was found to augment the intestinal absorption of iron through its stimulating effect on the bone marrow.[80] A similar mechanism was probably operative in cases of hypoxia-associated increase in iron absorption.[81] A plasma factor was isolated from pregnant women that increased iron uptake by the epithelial cells when introduced into the lumen, but was ineffective when given parenterally.[82] There is no solid evidence to support the existence of humoral factors stimulating intestinal iron absorption.

Food Iron Absorption

The accurate estimation of food iron absorption became possible recently, when it was shown that suitable iron salts in tracer quantities are absorbed in a similar fashion to food iron. By using such extrinsic tags, it was demonstrated that assimilation of dietary iron occurs from two independent pools, namely heme and nonheme iron.[83,84] Dietary iron must be converted into one of these two forms in order to be absorbed. Heme iron is derived from hemoglobin, myoglobin, and other heme proteins in foodstuffs of animal origin. Nonheme iron is supplied mainly by vegetables and fruit.

The amount of iron absorbed daily from food in a normal man and in nonmenstruating women is about 1.0 mg (0.6 to 1.6 mg),[85] whereas about twice this amount is absorbed by menstruating women.[86,97] In pregnant women, the "iron loss" is about 3.5 times that of a normal man, and the absorption of iron from food increases accordingly. The average amount of iron ingested daily in a normal balanced diet is about 6 mg/1000 cal or between 10 to 30 mg of iron daily.[88] About 5 to 10% of this iron is absorbed daily under physiological conditions. The amount of iron absorbed rises four- to sixfold in iron deficiency and is diminished in cases of iron overload.[89-91] While the values given here are correct for developed countries, marked variations exist in various parts of the world in the dietary iron intake both below and above the values given here.[92]

Almost all of the mucosal iron destined for absorption enters the portal blood, while less than 5% enters the lymphatics.[93,94] The unsaturated iron-binding capacity of the plasma is probably the single most important factor that determines the rate of release of intraepithelial iron into the circulation.[95-97] Iron entering the circulation is immediately taken up by the iron-carrying protein transferrin.

TRANSFERRIN METABOLISM

The following discussion deals with the transport of iron in the circulating plasma. This function is performed under physiological circumstances by the specific iron-binding protein transferrin. A brief summary of its structure, physicochemical properties, kinetics, and functions will be followed by the description of methods for its quantitative estimation in the plasma and/or serum.

Transferrin Structure

Despite the large effort invested in characterizing transferrin since it was first isolated and recognized in 1947,[98] there are still differences of opinion on many points. Thus while it is generally accepted that transferrin is a β_1-globulin, various authors have suggested a rather wide range for its molecular weight ranging from 68,000 to 88,000.[98-102,106] Transferrin is a glycoprotein with a single polypeptide chain, which contains one N-terminal amino acid residue per molecule (valine).[103] It has no free sulfhydryl groups.[104] Its total carbohydrate content is 5.3%, which is arranged in the form of two identical branched side chains, each branch ending in a sialic acid molecule. Hence, four sialic acid molecules are present per molecule of transferrin.[105] Its sedimentation constant (S_{20}, W) is 5.1 ± 0.2,[107] and its isoelectric point is at pH 5.8.[108]

The amino acid sequence of the transferrin molecule is still unknown. Among the numerous unresolved questions regarding this protein, one of the most important concerns the composition and nature of its iron-binding sites, of which there are two per transferrin molecule. Whether these sites are structurally and functionally identical, whether they bind Fe^{2+} in addition to Fe^{3+}, and whether there is or is not an interaction between these binding sites are some of the unanswered questions.[99,109] Two regions of internal homology were recently identified in the transferrin molecule, supporting the gene duplication-fusion hypothesis for its evolution, which suggested that the structure of the specific binding sites may depend on the three-dimensional configuration of the transferrin molecule contributing to the ligands involved in metal binding. The two sites may then have similar structures despite the absence of internal homology in the molecule.[110]

A more extensive discussion of the accumulated and often conflicting data concerning the many unknown properties of the transferrin molecule exceeds the scope of the present discussion. The reader is referred to the numerous detailed reviews devoted to this subject that have been published recently.[99,109] It should be noted, however, that the binding of iron to transferrin produced several changes in the properties of the protein which are relevant to the following discussion.

The first of these is the acquisition of a pink color by the apotransferrin-iron complex at the time of iron attachment to the protein. The net charge of the molecule is changed by m^1 for each iron atom bound with a consequent change in electrophoretic mobility[111] and behavior on ion exchange chromatography.[112,113] Iron binding does not induce a significant change in the molecular weight of transferrin,[114] but it causes the molecule to become more compact and more spherical in shape.[115] Iron-transferrin binding makes the transferrin molecule more stable than apoferritin, and this is manifested by its increased resistance to heat, urea, organic solvents, disulfide-breaking reagents, iodination, and resistance to proteolytic enzymes.[116-120] The conformational change in the transferrin molecule consequent to iron binding may be responsible for making certain antigenic sites on the molecule inaccessible;[121] this change of the antigenic reactivity of transferrin, however, does not significantly affect its quantitative estimation by radial immunodiffusion.[122]

Synthesis

A large variety of tissues have been shown to synthesize transferrin. The methods employed in these studies consisted mostly of culturing cells from various tissues and demonstrating the incorporation of labeled amino acids into transferrin by immunoelectrophoresis and autoradiography. Although this method is useful in proving the ability of cells to produce transferrin, it does not allow for its quantitative estimation or for the assessment of the rate of its elaboration; neither does it answer the question of whether the transferrin synthesized by the cells is secreted by them or not.

The accumulated evidence suggests that in adult animals, only the liver — and in rabbits and rats, the lactating mammary gland — synthesize and secrete quantitatively important amounts of transferrin.[123-128] In human subjects, transferrin synthesis has been demonstrated in the liver and in peripheral blood lymphocytes,[129] the latter source being quantitatively unimportant. Transferrin synthesis has recently been found in the yolk sac of early human and rat fetuses.[130,131] Increased production of transferrin was found in childhood, during pregnancy, and in iron-deficiency anemia. Estrogen administration was also found to stimulate transferrin synthesis.[132,133] On the other hand, fasting and protein depletion lead to markedly diminished rates of transferrin synthesis.[134] The diminished transferrin levels seen in kwashiorkor are probably due to a diminished synthetic rate, which rapidly returns to normal on an adequate diet.[135-136]

Distribution, Turnover, and Catabolism

Transferrin, like many other plasma proteins, is distributed throughout most of the extracellular fluid of the body with continuous circulation from the plasma to the interstitial space and back into the circulation via the lymph vessels. Its presence has been demonstrated in the interstitial fluid,[137] lymph,[138] edema fluid,[139] cerebrospinal fluid,[140-141] and in the urine.[142] The rate of exchange of transferrin between the plasma and extravascular space is similar to that of albumin. In humans, 50 to 60% of the total body transferrin is in the extravascular compartments, while 60 to 70% of this protein is extravascular in rats and rabbits.[143-144] Between 70 to 100% of the plasma transferrin pool passes through the extravascular compartments daily both in man and rabbits.[145-146] The rate of extravascular circulation varies between the different tissues, dependent largely upon the structure of the capillaries determining the permeability of the capillary walls. As a result of structural differences in the capillary network of various tissues, plasma transferrin has an almost unrestricted access to liver cells, spleen, and bone marrow. In contrast, transferrin circulates much more slowly through the interstitial fluid surrounding muscle and skin.[147,148] The functional significance of these differences in the availability of transferrin to the different tissues of the body is obvious.

About 15 to 16% of the total body transferrin pool is catabolized daily. The rate of catabolism in rabbits and rats is much higher (about 70%). The site of transferrin catabolism has not been established with certainty, although evidence has been presented to show that a substantial portion of the daily breakdown of transferrin is accomplished by the liver.[149] Transferrin may also be lost into the stomach and intestines,[150] and insignificant quantities are excreted in the urine.[151] The mechanism of degradation of transferrin has not been elucidated, but this protein seems to be taken up by cells via pinocytosis and broken down within the cells.[150] Increased transferrin catabolism was noted in patients with hemolytic anemia, infection, and nephrosis.[137,152-154] An inverse relationship was found between the fractional catabolic rate of transferrin on the one hand and the plasma transferrin concentration on the other. This finding would indicate that the amount of transferrin catabolized daily remains constant, irrespective of the plasma transferrin concentration; it follows that if the fractional catabolic rate increases, plasma transferrin concentration falls.[155]

Most of the transferrin iron turnover is directed to developing erythroid cells for incorporation into hemoglobin. This involves the binding of transferrin to cell membrane receptors[295,296] followed by endocytosis[297] (Figure 2). Within the endocytotic vesicles, pH is low, possibly because of fusion with lysosomes. This results in the release of iron from the iron-transferrin complex, and its subsequent reduction and incorporation into heme, or storage of iron in ferritin.[298] It is assumed that both the transferrin and its receptor are recycled, as transferrin is not catabolized as a result of its iron-donating function.[299] The binding of transferrin to the receptor probably protects it from proteolysis during the intracellular phase of its cycle. As the cells do not lose their transferrin-binding ability following treatment with cycloheximide, an inhibitor of protein synthesis, it appears that the transferrin receptors may also be recycled.

Studies related to the intracellular transport of iron have been reviewed extensively by Romslo.[303] Within the last two decades, a large number of potential iron-binding ligands have been described, but no coherent picture of cytosolic iron transport has emerged from

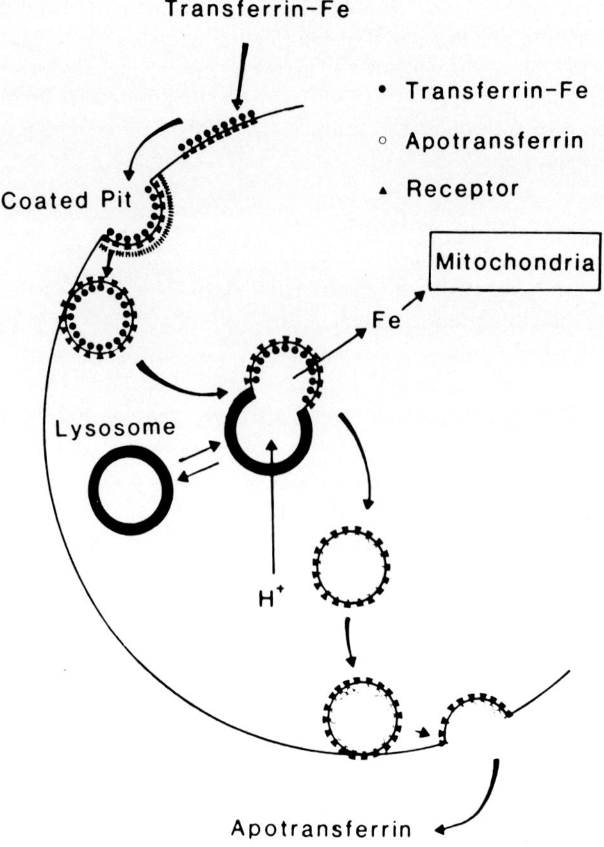

FIGURE 2. Model for the uptake and recycling of transferrin following endocytosis of the transferrin-transferrin-receptor complex by erythroid precursors. (From Armstrong, N. J. and Morgan, E. H., *Biochemistry and Physiology of Iron,* Saltman, P. and Hegenauer, J., Eds., Elsevier/North-Holland, Amsterdam, 1982, 149—157.)

these studies. A transferrin-like protein has been detected in the particular fraction of mucosal homogenates. This protein is located at the surface of the microvilli and is believed to be responsible for the absorption of alimentary iron.[304-306] The finding of similar iron-binding protein in tissues other than the mucosa and significant differences in amino acid composition of plasma and mucosal transferrin make it unlikely that mucosal transferrin is a proteolytically altered plasma transferrin.

Quantitative Estimation of Serum Iron and Unsaturated Iron-Binding Capacity

Numerous methods have been published and are employed in various laboratories for the estimation of the concentrations of the serum iron (SI) and unsaturated iron-binding capacity (UIBC) of circulating transferrin. We shall describe the method recommended by the Iron Panel of International Committee for Standardization in Hematology (ICSH) as a reference method. Other available procedures will be mentioned briefly.

Measurement of Serum Iron[156-158]

The reagents include:

1. Protein precipitant: aqueous solution containing 0.6 mol trichloroacetic acid, 0.3 mol thioglycollic acid, and 1 mol hydrochloric acid per liter (stored in dark).

2. Chromogen solution: sodium acetate (1.6 mol/ℓ) containing disodium, 4,7-diphenyl-1,10-phenantroline disulfonate (0.5 nmol/ℓ).
3. Iron standard solution containing 40 μmol/ℓ (2.24 μg/mℓ). Iron-free glassware must be used throughout.

The procedure is as follows:

1. The protein precipitating solution (2 mℓ) is added to 2 mℓ serum mixed thoroughly for 60 sec, then heated at 56°C for 15 min, followed by centrifugation to obtain an optically clear supernatant.
2. The iron standard solution (2 mℓ) is mixed with the protein precipitant solution.
3. A reagent blank is prepared by substituting the iron-free water for the iron standard used above.
4. The supernatant solution (2 mℓ) is mixed each with 2 mℓ of chromogen, mixed thoroughly, and allowed to stand for 5 min.
5. The absorbance of the chromogen-treated solutions is measured against a blank of distilled water in a spectrophotometer at a wavelength of 535 nm.
6. The iron concentration of the serum specimen is calculated from the formula (serum iron in micromoles per liter):

$$\frac{\text{Absorbance serum specimen — absorbance blank}}{\text{Absorbance standard iron — absorbance blank}} \times 40$$

The absorbance of the blank should not exceed 0.015, read against distilled water in a 1-cm pathway.

Measurement of Serum-Unsaturated Iron-Binding Capacity (UIBC)[146-148]

Iron-free water and glassware are to be used throughout. The reagents include:

1. Stock ferric chloride solution 1 mmol/ℓ in HCl, 50 nmol/ℓ. Weigh 0.27 g ferric chloride ($FeCl_2 \cdot 6H_2O$ AR), dissolve immediately in 50 mℓ HCl, 1 mol/ℓ and dilute with iron-free distilled water to 1 ℓ in 1 volumetric flask.
2. Saturating iron solution for total iron-binding capacity (TIBC), 100 μmol/ℓ in HCl, 5 nmol/ℓ. Into a 250-m volumetric flask, pipette one tenth of its volume of stock ferric chloride solution and dilute to volume with iron-free distilled water.
3. Saturating radioiron solution for UIBC, 100 μmol/ℓ containing sufficient $^{59}FeCl_3$ to give about 100,000 counts/min/μmol Fe. Into a 250-mℓ volumetric flask, pipette one tenth of its volume of stock ferric chloride solution, add a volume of $^{59}FeCl_3$ solution sufficient to give about 10,000 counts/min/mℓ in the final solution, and dilute to volume with iron-free distilled water.
4. Light magnesium carbonate reagent grade, approximate formula 3 $MgCO_3(OH)_2 \cdot 3H_2O$.
5. Standard iron solution 40 μmol/ℓ (see above).

The procedure is as follows:

1. To 2 mℓ serum in an iron-free tube add 2 mℓ saturating radioiron solution, mix well, and incubate for 15 min at room temperature.
2. Add 0.4 g of light magnesium carbonate, close tube with parafilm, and place on an angled turntable; rotate for 30 min.
3. Centrifuge for 30 min at 1000 × g, remove supernatant carefully, centrifuge supernatant again as above.

4. Pipette 2 mℓ of supernatant into an iron-free tube.
5. Prepare counting standard — 1 mℓ of saturating radioiron solution and 1 mℓ of water — in another tube.
6. Count each specimen in a gamma counter. The counting time should be such that the total counts recorded for each radioiron-containing specimen exceed 10,000 after subtraction of background.
7. Estimate iron content of saturating radioiron solution as described above.
8. Calculate UIBC according to the formula:

$$\text{UIBC } \mu\text{mol}/\ell \text{ Fe} = \frac{\text{counts/min (serum specimen)}}{\text{counts/min (counting standard)}} \times \frac{\text{absorbance (counting standard)}}{\text{absorbance (Fe standard)}} \times 80$$

TIBC can be calculated indirectly as the sum of UIBC and SI. TIBC may also be estimated directly by a slight modification of the UIBC method. The same reagents may be used as above, but no ^{59}FeCl is required. The procedure is as follows:

1. To 2 mℓ serum in an iron-free tube, add 2 mℓ saturating solution. Mix well, and leave 15 min at room temperature.
2. Add 0.4 g light magnesium carbonate, stopper the tube, and rotate on an angled turntable for 30 min.
3. Centrifuge for 30 min at 1000 × g, remove supernatant, and centrifuge again.
4. Assay the iron content of the supernatant as for the serum iron assay, by the procedure described above, using 2 mℓ supernatant instead of 2 mℓ serum. Calculate as follows:

$$\text{TIBC } (\mu\text{mol Fe}/\ell) = \frac{\text{absorbance supernatant — absorbance blank}}{\text{absorbance standard iron — absorbance blank}} \times 80$$

$$\text{Percent saturation of transferrin is calculated as } \frac{\text{SI}}{\text{TIBC}} \times 100$$

Other methods for the quantitative estimation of serum transferrin include wet digestion,[157] atomic absorption spectroscopy,[157] immunodiffusion, and more recently, spectrofluorometry.[159]

STORAGE IRON

Storage Iron Regulation

Studies of the primary structure of ferritin subunits by Crichton et al.[291,292] and X-ray crystallographic analyses by the Sheffield group[293,294] have contributed significantly to the understanding of structure-function relationships of the ferritin molecule. The ferritin protein consists of 24 subunits forming a hollow sphere of external diameter 120 Å and central cavity 70 Å. Up to 4500 iron atoms can be sequestered in one ferritin molecule. The movement of iron into and out of the central cavity is made possible by six intersubunit channels of roughly 10 Å in diameter. The ferritin subunits are cylindrical in shape. Each subunit contains four long, nearly parallel helical regions, and a shorter helix perpendicular to the others. The amino acid sequence of the 174 residues of the horse spleen apoferritin subunit has been resolved completely. Its molecular weight is 19,824. Amino acid residues within the protein shell are largely hydrophobic, whereas charged residues occupy positions on the external surface. Comparison of human and horse spleen and liver ferritin shows a

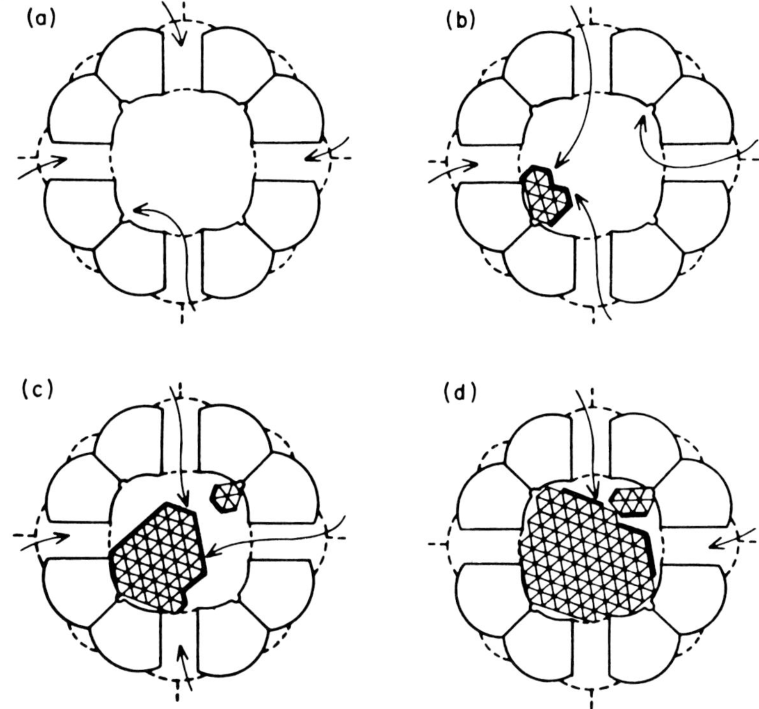

FIGURE 3. Model for iron uptake by the ferritin molecule. (a) Fe(II) enters the shell through channels and is bound to sites of oxidation (arrows). (b) Formation of Fe(III)-OOH iron-core nucleus. (c and d) Available surface for Fe deposition (thick line) first increases, and then decreases as the molecule fills. (From Harrison, P. M., Clegg, G. A., and May, K., *Iron in Biochemistry and Medicine*, Vol. 2, Jacobs, A. and Worwood, M., Eds., Academic Press, New York, 1980, 131—171.)

high degree of similarity in amino acid sequence. Most of the residues at internal positions or at interfaces are conserved, whereas a number of substitutes are found at surface positions. These surface amino acid substitutes may account for differences in isoelectric points and in antigenicity.

Oxidation and reduction of iron are essential steps in its storage and mobilization. It was proposed by Mazur et al.[160] that xanthine oxidase is responsible for ferritin iron reduction, but this theory was abandoned when it was shown that allopurinol, the potent xanthine oxidase inhibitor, does not affect iron metabolism.[161,162] An alternative enzyme system, which is more likely to be involved in ferritin iron mobilization, is ferrireductase,[163] which is capable of catalyzing the anaerobic reduction of ferritin iron by the following sequence of reactions:

$$\begin{array}{ccccc} \text{NADH} \searrow & & \swarrow \text{FMN} & & \nearrow \text{FE(II)} \\ & \text{Enzyme} & & & \\ \text{NAD} \swarrow & & \searrow \text{FMNH}_2 & & \nwarrow \text{Fe(III)} \end{array}$$

Oxidation of ferrous iron is catalyzed by apoferritin[164] and is followed by the production of microcrystalline particles within the interior of the apoferritin shell through the formation of hydroxyl and oxo bridges[1] (Figure 3). More iron can be added directly to these growing nuclei without the necessity of passing through specific oxidation sites on the protein. Because iron accumulation in ferritin occurs within the protein shell, the surface available for iron deposition first increases, then decreases as more iron is added, because the crystals are covered with protein and some channels are blocked. Furthermore, in any solid, the ratio of surface area to volume decreases as the volume increases, and this change alone would account for slowing in the rate of crystal growth.

The capacity of tissues to store iron is increased by their ability to enhance ferritin synthesis in response to increasing rates of iron deposition.[165] This effect cannot be inhibited by actinomycin D; it can be demonstrated in cell-free systems derived entirely from cytoplasmic components,[166] indicating its post-transcriptional nature. It has been proposed that iron may promote the aggregation of subunits into ferritin, thus releasing adhering ferritin subunits from mRNA, which in turn becomes available for translation.[167] An alternative explanation for increased ferritin synthesis following iron administration is a post-translational effect on subunit release, stabilization, or assembly into the multimeric protein shell.[166]

At the cellular level, iron release is facilitated by ceruloplasmin, which by virtue of its extracellular ferroxidase activity produces a steep concentration gradient between intra- and extracellular ferrous iron.[163] The role of ceruloplasmin in iron release is permissive and not regulatory, since its effect is maximal at serum levels corresponding to 10% of normal.[168] Ascorbic acid deficiency interferes with iron release from RE cells but does not affect parenchymal release.[169,170] This difference in ascorbic acid dependence of iron release may be explained by the apparent absence of ferrireductase from RE cells and its presence in parenchymal cells,[163] which provides an alternative mechanism for iron reduction. Other factors involved in the control of iron release from cells are the rate of plasma iron turnover and the amount of cellular exchangeable iron available for binding by transferrin (Figure 4).

As mentioned above, RE cells acquire iron from senescent erythrocytes and the wastage iron of erythropoiesis. The ferritin stores are relatively small and the turnover rate of storage iron is consequently fast.[171-177] In contrast, parenchymal cells acquire iron mainly from plasma transferrin and are able to incorporate the iron contained in circulating hemoglobin-haptoglobin, heme-hemopexin, and ferritin by pinocytosis.[174,178-181] Parenchymal ferritin stores are relatively large, and their rates of turnover are slow.[176,177] The known differences in the handling of iron by RE and parenchymal cells are summarized in Table 2.

Clinical Evaluation of Iron Stores

Most of the iron in the body is bound to hemoglobin, but iron stores of ferritin and hemosiderin exist in addition in the liver, spleen, and bone marrow. In conditions characterized by a negative balance between body requirements and food iron absorption, the storage compartment is depleted in order to maintain normal levels of functional iron in hemoglobin, myoglobin, and iron-containing enzymes. Conversely, when dietary iron absorption exceeds body requirements, iron stores increase. Thus the size of iron stores provides an important indicator of the balance between iron absorption and body iron requirements. Several clinical methods for assessing iron stores are in common use.

Examination of bone marrow fragments for stainable iron is one of the most commonly used procedures.[182] The slides are fixed in methyl alcohol and treated with a mixture of freshly prepared 2% potassium ferrocyanide and 2% hydrochloric acid.[183] Hemosiderin granules are stained blue, and the preparations are scored arbitrarily from 0 to 6. A composite figure of reported hemosiderin scorings summarized by Bothwell and Finch[28] is given in Table 3. As a rule, scores are low in iron deficiency and high in iron overload because of idiopathic hemochromatosis or transfusional hemosiderosis. A shift of iron from the red cell mass to reticuloendothelial cells may be found in conditions characterized by ineffective erythropoiesis, such as in pernicious anemia, or in inflammation where the release of hemoglobin iron from RE cells is blocked. In general, stainable marrow iron reflects the amount of total body iron stores. However, there are some exceptions to this rule. Since marrow iron is a reflection of RE iron deposits, in clinical states with predominantly parenchymal

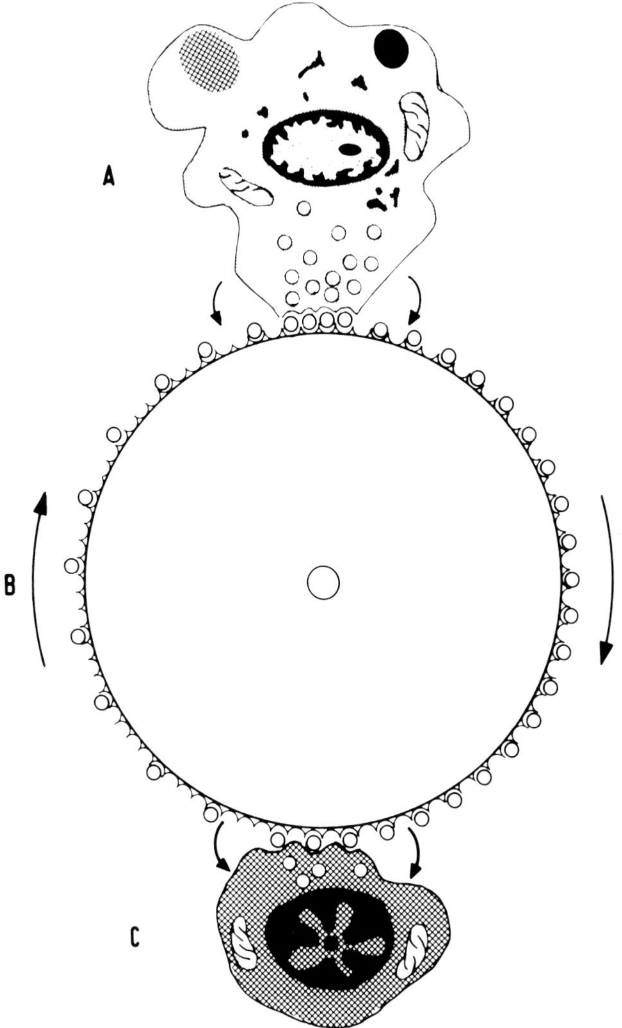

FIGURE 4. Regulation of RE iron release. Plasma iron turnover is described here as a wheel with a constant number of binding sites (B). It is driven by the active uptake of transferrin iron by erythroid precursor cells (C). The clearance of iron by erythroid precursors provides additional free binding sites which become available for interaction with RE iron (A). The amount of exchangeable RE iron is determined by the magnitude of its "prerelease" iron pool derived from RBC catabolism, or ferritin mobilization, and the number of transferrin binding sites on the cell membrane. Exchangeable iron from other cell types (intestinal mucosa, hepatocyte) may compete for available binding sites of transferrin and limit RE iron release. (From Hershko, C., *Progress in Hematology*, Vol. 10, Brown, E. B., Ed., Grune & Stratton, New York, 1977, 105. With permission.)

iron overload, such as idiopathic hemochromatosis, marrow iron may not reflect the true magnitude of iron overload. Conversely, in patients receiving parenteral iron complexes or blood transfusions, stainable iron in the marrow may be increased in the face of iron deficiency.[184]

Chelating agents such as desferrioxamine (DF) or diethylenetriamine pentaacetic acid (DTPA) can be used to estimate body iron stores.[185-188] When iron excretion following the injection of DF at a dose of 10 mg/kg is compared to the total nonheme iron concentration

Table 2
COMPARISON OF RE AND PARENCHYMAL CELL FUNCTION IN STORAGE IRON METABOLISM

Source of iron	Reticuloendothelial cells	Parenchymal cells	Ref.
	Wastage iron of erythropoiesis;	Transferrin	174, 178—181
	senescent erythrocytes;	Hemoglobin-haptoglobin	191, 214
	colloidal iron preparations	Heme-hemopexin	
^{59}Fe turnover	Rapid	Slow	171—175
Ferritin pool	Small	Large	176, 177
Dependence on ascorbic acid	Pronounced	Questionable	169
Ferrireductase activity	Absent	Present	163

From Hershko, C., *Progress in Hematology*, Vol. 10, Brown, E. B., Ed., Grune & Stratton, New York, 1977, 105. With permission.

Table 3
COMPOSITE FIGURE OF REPORTED RESULTS OF STAINABLE MARROW IRON

Condition	Amount of iron 0	1—2	3—4	5—6
Normal	6	57	19	0
Infection	6	13	31	11
Iron deficiency anemia	132	38	0	0
Pernicious anemia	6	20	69	7
Idiopathic hemochromatosis	0	0	11	13
Transfusional hemosiderosis	0	0	0	13

From Bothwell, T. M. and Finch, C. A., *Iron Metabolism*, Little, Brown, Boston, 1962, 287. With permission.

of liver biopsies obtained from the same subjects, a positive linear correlation is found (Figure 5; $r = 0.83$).[179] Studies in which the amount of stainable iron in RE and parenchymal cells is correlated to urinary excretion of chelated iron, or animal studies employing selective radioiron labels of RE and parenchymal cells indicate that iron chelated by DF is mainly obtained from parenchymatous tissues.[190,191] DF-induced iron excretion is enhanced by ascorbic acid and inhibited by vitamin E.[192,193] In patients with cirrhosis, DF-induced excretion is much higher than in control subjects with similar liver iron concentrations.[189] These complicating factors may limit the diagnostic value of DF-induced urinary iron excretion in the assessment of body iron stores. In addition, the need for drug injection and subsequent urine collection require a high degree of cooperation on the part of the subjects studied.

Serial phlebotomies of about 400 mℓ at weekly intervals are probably the most accurate method for measuring iron stores, since no assumptions have to be made as to the quantitative relation between the amount of iron removed by phlebotomy and the amount mobilized from stores. Phlebotomy is continued until hemoglobin is reduced to less than 11 g/dℓ and transferrin saturation is below 15%, indicating depletion of iron stores. The total amount of iron removed is calculated by measuring the volume and hemoglobin content of each vene-

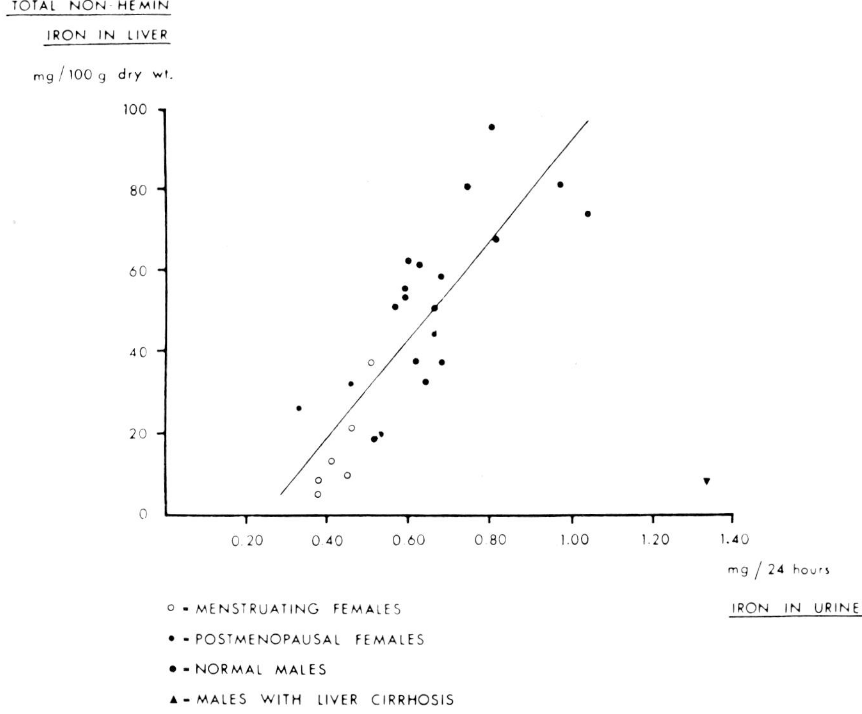

FIGURE 5. Relationship between desferrioxamine-induced urinary iron excretion and total non-heme iron concentration determined in liver biopsy specimens of the same individuals. The two subjects with liver cirrhosis are not included in the correlation study. $r = 0.83$; $p < 0.001$. (From Hallberg, L., Hedenberg, L., and Weinfeld, A., *Scand. J. Haematol.*, 3, 85, 1966. With permission.)

section. The difference between the total amount of iron removed by phlebotomy and the amount of iron lost in reducing the hemoglobin level of the subject represents the total amount of mobilizable storage iron.[194] Minor corrections are also made for the amount of iron absorbed during the study, which is about 2 to 3 mg/day. Published values of total mobilizable iron estimations obtained by quantitative phlebotomy in healthy adult males, females, and blood donors were summarized by Walters et al.[195] and are given in Table 4. At present, serial phlebotomies are still the most accurate method for the assessment of total mobilizable iron stores. However, the method is lengthy and inconvenient and is not suitable for routine clinical use.

Chemical determination of hepatic iron may be useful in specimens obtained by biopsy or at necropsy, in assessing the iron nutrition of a population, although it does not yield a direct estimate of total body iron stores. Charlton et al. have analyzed the iron content of 3983 liver specimens obtained by necropsy in 18 different countries.[196] They found no difference between individuals dying of cardiovascular disease and those killed by acute trauma. On the other hand, figures were higher in patients dying from neoplastic disease, presumably due to the trapping of iron in reticuloendothelial cells. Age had no effect on liver iron content, except for reduced iron stores in young women because of the increased iron demands of the reproductive period and a progressive increase in liver iron in the Bantu caused by an extremely high dietary intake. After excluding conditions that might have distorted hepatic iron stores by disease or excessive demand, a comparison was made between different countries (Table 5). The lowest iron concentrations were found in subjects from India and New Guinea, and the highest were found in the South African Bantu. There were significant differences between the iron stores of groups from different Western countries.

Table 4
PUBLISHED VALUES OF STORAGE IRON DETERMINATIONS BY QUANTITATIVE PHLEBOTOMY

Author	No.	Males	No.	Females	No.	Blood donors	Ref.
Olsson (1972)	11	750	—	—	14	110	219
Balcerzak (1968)	11	687	—	—	—	—	175
Pritchard (1964)	3	819	10	254	—	—	220
Haskins (1952)	2	844	—	—	2	93	184
Walters (1973)	7	900	10	210	5	400	185
Mean of all series	34	767	20	232	—	—	—

Modified from Walters, G. O., Miller, F. M., and Worwood, M., *J. Clin. Pathol.*, 26, 770, 1973. With permission.

Table 5
MEDIAN HEPATIC STORAGE IRON CONCENTRATIONS (μg/g)[a]

		Lower quartile		Median		Upper quartile	
Location	Race	Males	Females	Males	Females	Males	Females
Great Britain							
London							
St. George's Hospital	—	65	67	113	119	188	189
Middlesex Hospital	—	107	142	166	177	199	270
West Middlesex Hospital	—	98	103	143	156	243	258
St. Margaret's Hospital	—	132	—	152	285	199	—
Sweden							
Malmö	—	81	73	126	120	207	183
Czechoslovakia							
Prague	—	118	84	230	170	329	243
U.S.							
Seattle	—	103	86	186	133	266	178
Boston	—	114	73	174	115	353	187
Wisconsin	—	161	127	242	205	390	238
South Africa							
Johannesburg	White	121	46	258	128	423	253
	Bantu	373	—	946	128	2068	—
Durban	Bantu	341	203	776	496	1753	1822
	Indian	113	103	183	173	301	290
Rhodesia	Bantu	268	—	633	321	2120	—
Nigeria	Bantu	113	—	133	126	291	—
India							
Unspecified	—	76	—	83	79	185	—
New Delhi	—	48	—	93	116	166	—
Bombay	—	46	—	131	202	238	—
New Guinea							
Rabaul	—	73	—	109	—	167	—
Venezuela							
Caracas	Mestizos	90	108	165	179	270	253
	White	164	—	255	303	267	—
	Negro	56	—	128	66	210	—
Brazil							
Sao Paulo	—	85	—	173	140	259	—
Rio de Janeiro	—	185	—	268	—	350	—
Mexico							
Mexico City	Mestizos	101	—	196	159	274	—
	White	43	—	258	—	310	—

Table 5 (continued)
MEDIAN HEPATIC STORAGE IRON CONCENTRATIONS (μg/g)[a]

		Lower quartile		Median		Upper quartile	
Location	**Race**	**Males**	**Females**	**Males**	**Females**	**Males**	**Females**
Colombia	—	74	—	117	—	198	—
Taiwan							
Taipeh	—	136	131	181	233	364	393
Japan							
Tokyo	—	52	—	126	226	158	—
Israel							
Jerusalem	—	145	146	204	165	244	239
Mozambique	—	221	—	376	565	1025	—
Costa Rica	—	226	—	243	28	326	—

[a] Excluding patients dying from neoplastic, miscellaneous, and unknown causes, and females under 50 years of age.

Modified from Charlton, R. W., Hawkins, D. M., Mavor, W. O., and Bothwell, T. H., *Am. J. Clin. Nutr.*, 23, 358, 1970.

SERUM FERRITIN MEASUREMENT

Although isolated reports related to the presence of ferritin in the serum in various diseases have been published since 1956,[197,198] it was only in 1972 that the introduction of a sensitive immunoradiometric assay has made the routine measurement of serum ferritin available for clinical use.[199] The original serum ferritin assay, which resulted from a collaborative effort led by Jacobs and Hales at the Welsh National School of Medicine in Cardiff, has been largely superseded by the two-site immunoradiometric assay (IRMA) introduced by Miles et al. in 1974.[200] A detailed description of the IRMA method for the clinical measurement of serum ferritin, including recommendations for the purification of human ferritin, determination of its protein content, preparation of the immunosorbent, the production of anti-human spleen ferritin, iodination of the antibody, and the assay procedure has been published in a recent review by Worwood.[201] A great number of variations on the procedure for measuring serum ferritin are presently available. Ferritin may be labeled instead of labeling the antibody. This procedure is designated radioimmunoassay (RIA) to distinguish it from immunoradiometric methods employing labeled antibody.[202-205] Human liver or tumor ferritin may be used instead of spleen ferritin[200,206-210] as the antigen. Recently, a basic isoferritin isolated from human term placenta was shown to be comparable to spleen ferritin as an antigen.[282] ^{125}I has been used initially for labeling antiferritin. More recently, IRMA is gradually being replaced by the more stable and inexpensive enzyme-linked immunosorbent assays (ELISA) employing alkaline phosphatase, horseradish peroxidase, or β-galactosidase.[207-209,211,284] For a detailed and critical review of existing serum ferritin assays, References 201, 212, and 213 are recommended.

Although a systematic survey of methodology is out of the scope of this chapter, some of the advantages, limitations, and pitfalls of existing methods should be emphasized. The original assay of Addison et al.[199] requires long counting times, includes two incubation stages, and is more tedious than the two-site IRMA method. The latter is easier to perform, has higher counting rates, and an apparently greater working range. However, these apparent advantages of the two-site IRMA are somewhat offset by a decrease in the amount of labeled antibody bound to the tube at very high concentrations of ferritin, the so called "high-dose-hook effect". Thus, sera containing high concentrations of ferritin may be falsely interpreted as representing lower ferritin concentrations. This error can be avoided by testing each serum

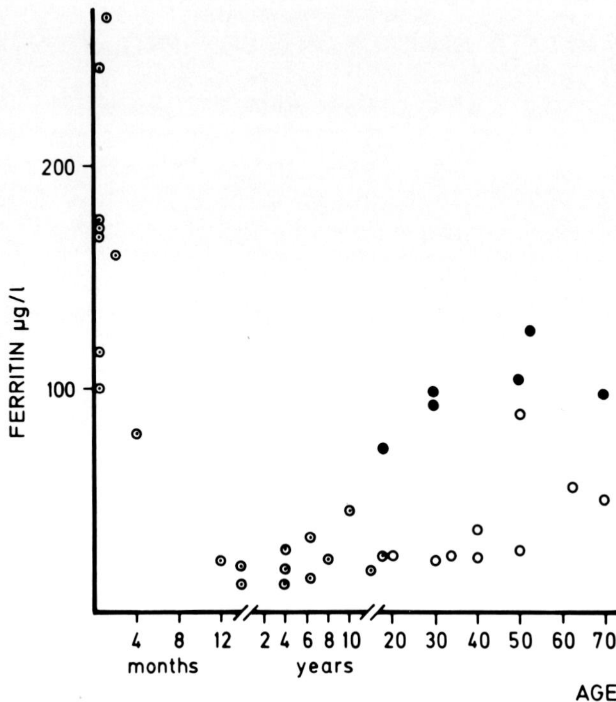

FIGURE 6. Relation between age, sex, and mean serum ferritin in normal subjects. Data derived from review by Worwood[212] of studies published prior to 1979. ●, Normal males, ○, normal females, ⊙, both males and females.

at two dilutions. Another potential source of inaccuracy of the two-site IRMA is the effect of protein composition of the test sample on the binding of ferritin to the solid phase antibody. Miles et al.[200] have recommended a way of overcoming this problem by diluting standards in 1:20 rabbit serum, and diluting unknown serum 1:20 in buffer.

Radioimmunoassays (RIAs) are generally less sensitive than IRMA but have a more extensive working range. In performance, there is no significant difference in the time and labor involved in either test.

A great number of commercial kits are available for the measurement of serum ferritin. Marechal et al.[283] have compared eight commercial radioimmunological procedures and found up to 15-fold differences in the ferritin content of control sera. Differences in the specificity of labeled antibodies might have been responsible for some of the variation. In addition, use of a universal standard reference ferritin such as the one presently in preparation by the ICSH may help in reducing interlaboratory variations. Ghielmi et al.[285] compared two RIA, one IRMA, and two ELISA methods using the same antiferritin antibody and the same ferritin standards. All tests showed the same cross-reactivity for spleen and HeLa cell ferritin. When compared to IRMA, RIA overestimated serum ferritin by about 50% whereas ELISA underestimated it by about 15%.

Figure 6 depicts mean serum ferritin concentration in healthy males and females in a large number of studies published prior to 1979 and reviewed by Worwood.[212] At birth, serum ferritin concentration is relatively high, and a further rise may be observed within the first 2 months of life due to the short lifespan of fetal erythrocytes. Thereafter, serum ferritin is reduced, and remains low during the period of rapid growth until about 18 years of age. Mean serum ferritin concentration in adult males is about 90 µg/ℓ and in females of the

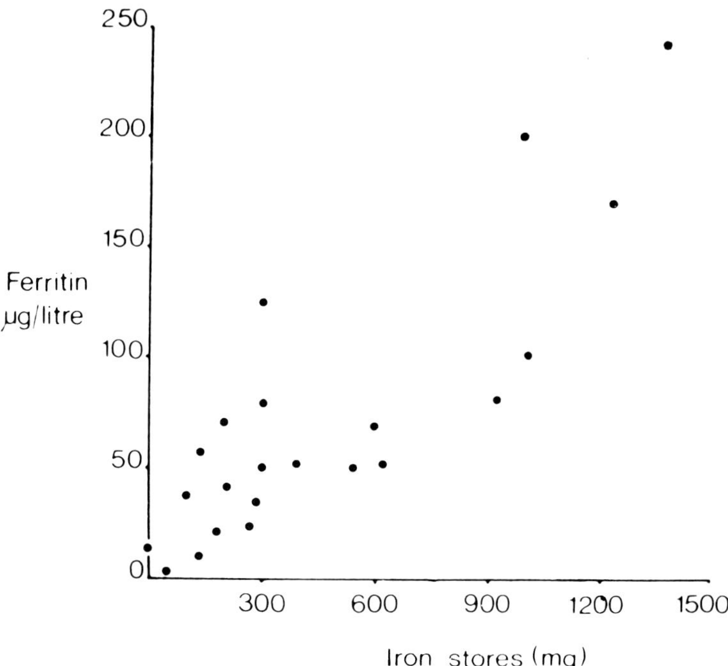

FIGURE 7. Relationship between serum ferritin concentration and mobilizable iron stores determined by serial phlebotomies. r = 0.83; $p < 0.001$. (From Walters, G. O., Miller, F. M., and Worwood, M., *J. Clin. Pathol.*, 26, 770, 1973. With permission.)

reproductive age between 25 and 50 µg/ℓ. There is some increase with age in both adult men and women, and this is more pronounced in postmenopausal females.

It is generally held that serum ferritin levels are directly proportional to the amount of iron stored in tissues. A direct linear relation between serum ferritin concentration and iron stores measured by quantitative phlebotomy has been shown by Walters et al.[195] (Figure 7). Similarly, a close correlation between serum ferritin concentration and nonheme marrow iron (r = 0.84) has been demonstrated[214] (Figure 8). Likewise, several investigators have shown a close direct relationship between serum ferritin concentration and radioiron absorption.[215-217] All of these observations indicate that the serum ferritin concentration is suitable for estimating iron stores. Every 1 µg/ℓ increment of serum ferritin is approximately equivalent to an increment of storage iron of 8 mg.[195] The following is a discussion of the clinical application of serum ferritin measurement in various abnormal states.

Iron Deficiency

A unique advantage of serum ferritin is its ability to reflect iron reserves and therefore to allow recognition of iron deficiency prior to the development of anemia. An additional advantage is the small volume of blood needed for the assay, which makes it suitable for screening populations by capillary blood samplings. This is particularly helpful in the pediatric age group. A serum ferritin concentration of 12 µg/ℓ or less is generally accepted as the best cutoff point for diagnosing iron deficiency.[218] Because low serum ferritin concentration is an earlier sign of iron deficiency than anemia, it is a particularly useful test for identifying populations at risk of iron-deficiency anemia. For instance, in one large population survey, iron-deficiency anemia was rare (2%), but low serum ferritin concentration was found in about 30% of young women, children, adolescents and 60% of women in the last trimester of pregnancy.[219] Serum ferritin assay can also be used to determine the effectiveness of preventive iron supplementation. In a study of low birth weight infants, a

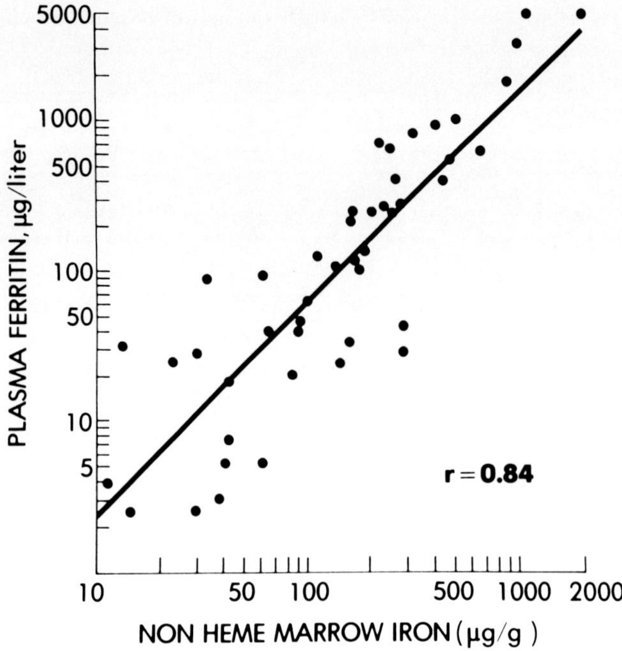

FIGURE 8. Relation between plasma ferritin and nonheme marrow iron. (From Bezwoda, W. R., Bothwell, T. H., Torrance, J. D., MacPhail, A. P., Charlton, R. W., Kay, G., and Levin, J., *Scand. J. Haematol.*, 22, 113, 1979. With permission.)

difference in serum ferritin levels was detectable at 2 months of age, 1 month earlier than the difference in transferrin saturation or hemoglobin concentration in the treated and untreated groups of infants.[20] Similarly, serum ferritin measurement was useful in assessing the effect of preventive iron supplementation in pregnant women,[221] and in studying the relation between the frequency of blood donations and the development of iron deficiency.[222] In monitoring response to the treatment of iron-deficiency anemia, assay of serum ferritin is useful in determining the endpoint of oral iron therapy. Bentley and Jacobs[223] have found that by the time hemoglobin concentration has returned to normal, serum ferritin concentration rose to 30 µg/ℓ, and after 2 months of treatment mean serum ferritin concentration was 60 µg/ℓ. Thus, in the absence of continued blood loss, 2 months of oral iron treatment appear to be sufficient to replete iron stores once anemia is corrected.

Although low serum ferritin concentration is an excellent indicator of iron depletion, there are several limitations to its use for the diagnosis of iron-deficiency anemia. It does not indicate severity of iron deficiency. Thus, in an anemic patient, low serum ferritin concentration may indicate storage iron depletion, without identifying the real cause of anemia. In such patients additional tests, such as transferrin saturation, red cell protoporphyrin concentration, and red cell indices, are helpful in establishing the diagnosis of iron-deficiency anemia. Another factor complicating the interpretation of serum ferritin concentration is the nonspecific increase in serum ferritin concentration associated with infection. Thus, in a rural population of children with a high prevalence of respiratory infections about 30% of children with iron-deficiency anemia documented by two or more abnormal laboratory parameters had serum ferritin concentration within the normal range.[224] Similarly, in a group of anemic infants receiving oral iron therapy, most subjects responding with an increase in hemoglobin of 1 g/dℓ or more had normal initial ferritin values.[225] Thus, although low serum ferritin concentration is an excellent indicator of iron depletion, normal values do not exclude iron deficiency. The latter finding is particularly common in infants and children and may be explained by coexistent minor infections.

Anemia of Inflammation

This is probably the most common type of anemia encountered in hospitalized patients. It is associated with inflammation caused by infection such as tuberculosis, connective tissue disorders such as rehumatoid arthritis, or malignancy such as Hodgkin's disease. In many respects, anemia of inflammation simulates iron-deficiency anemia. Thus, similar to iron-deficiency anemia, it is characterized by low serum iron concentration, reduced mean corpuscular volume, and increased red cell protoporphyrin. Total iron-binding capacity (TIBC) tends to be high in iron deficiency and low in inflammation, but there is considerable overlap in values encountered in the two conditions. An important difference is the amount of storage iron in macrophages by stain of hemosiderin in bone marrow aspirates: it is absent or low in iron deficiency and normal or increased in inflammation, because of a block in storage iron release.[226,227] In view of the close correlation between serum ferritin concentration and iron stores, serum ferritin assay is eminently suitable for distinguishing iron-deficiency anemia from the anemia of inflammation. In a study of 39 patients with inflammation, Lipschitz et al.[228] found that the mean serum ferritin concentration was 305 μg/ℓ and ranged from 10 to 1650 μg/ℓ (Figure 9). Correlation of serum ferritin with marrow hemosiderin stains showed that for each level of marrow hemosiderin, serum ferritin concentration in inflammation was about three times higher than in normal controls with identical levels of marrow hemosiderin. Thus, measurement of serum ferritin is useful in distinguishing iron-deficiency anemia from anemia of inflammation with increased marrow iron, but may be difficult to interpret when the two conditions coexist.

Several studies indicate that when iron deficiency documented by absent marrow hemosiderin coexists with inflammation in rheumatoid arthritis, the majority of patients have serum ferritin concentration above 12 μg/ℓ, but rarely more than 100 μg/ℓ.[229,230] When ability to respond to oral iron therapy by an increase in hemoglobin of at least 1 g/dℓ was examined in patients with rheumatoid arthritis, patients with serum ferritin below 25 μg/ℓ had a positive response, but so did many of the patients with higher ferritin levels.[231] In consequence, it has been proposed that in patients with inflammation and suspected iron-deficiency anemia, a therapeutic trial of oral iron is warranted when serum ferritin concentration is below 50 μg/ℓ. If ferritin is about 100 μg/ℓ, a positive response to iron therapy is unlikely.[218] These recommendations leave a "diagnostic gray zone" between 50 to 100 μg/ℓ.

Chronic Hemodialysis

Interest in the use of serum ferritin assay for the evaluation of iron stores in patients on chronic hemodialysis is reflected in the number of studies related to this subject published in recent years.[232-239] These studies have shown an excellent correlation between serum ferritin levels and marrow hemosiderin. When correlation with bone marrow hemosiderin is used as a guide for the selection of the single most reliable laboratory test for the assessment of iron stores, ferritin assay is clearly the most useful diagnostic aid ($r = 0.805$), followed by measurement of transferrin saturation ($r = 0.599$), and mean corpuscular volume ($r = 0.512$). Red cell protoporphyrins are increased in most patients with uremia and cannot be used for the diagnosis of iron-deficiency anemia in such patients.[240] As in the anemia of inflammation, most patients with iron deficiency coexisting with chronic hemodialysis have serum ferritin concentration about 12 μg/ℓ, and it has been proposed that in such patients a serum ferritin below 50 μg/ℓ is suggestive of iron deficiency.[218] Monitoring of serum ferritin concentration in patients receiving oral iron therapy indicated that in most subjects on chronic hemodialysis, 60 mg elemental iron daily is sufficient to maintain adequate iron stores.[236]

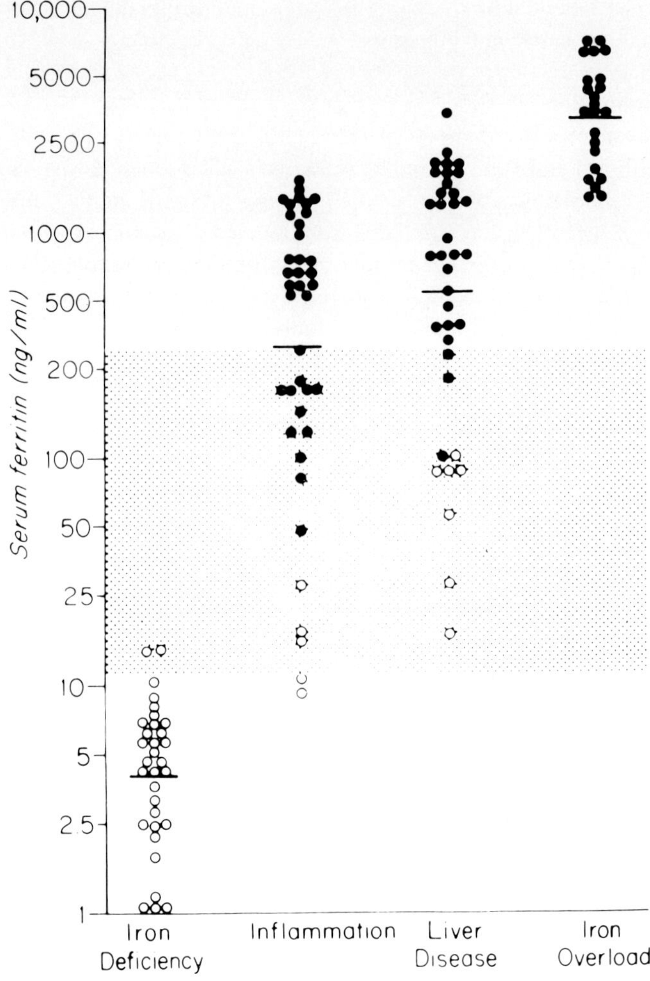

FIGURE 9. Measurements of serum ferritin in uncomplicated iron deficiency, inflammation, liver disease, and iron overload. The shaded area represents the normal range. Patients with iron deficiency defined by a low transferrin saturation or absent marrow iron are represented by open circles. (From Lipschitz, D. A,, Cook, J. D., and Finch, C. A., *N. Engl. J. Med.*, 290, 1213, 1974. With permission.)

Iron Overload

In untreated idiopathic hemochromatosis, serum ferritin concentrations usually range between 100 to 1000 μg/ℓ.[212,213,217,241] During treatment with phlebotomy, serum ferritin concentration falls gradually until values of less than 12 μg/ℓ are reached.[242] Although serum ferritin levels are above normal in the vast majority of relatives with increased iron stores,[241] several families have been reported in whom affected members with documented iron overload had normal serum ferritin concentrations.[243-246] It has been proposed that in such patients iron overload is restricted to parenchymal cells, and that serum ferritin concentration becomes elevated only when there is reticuloendothelial cell iron accumulation. In spite of its usefulness in the majority of patients with idiopathic hemochromatosis, serum ferritin should be regarded as only one of a number of available tests for the documentation of iron overload. Very useful for the screening of subjects for homozygous idiopathic hemochromatosis is the measurement of both serum ferritin and transferrin saturation. In one large study, all male homozygotes had transferrin saturation about 80% and serum ferritin above 500 μg/ℓ.[287] Serum ferritin concentration in female homozygotes overlap somewhat with normal ferritin values, but a clear distinction still exists if transferrin saturation above 80% is used for screening. Further documentation of iron overload may be made by the measurement of 24-hr urinary iron excretion after desferrioxamine and by the direct assessment of hepatic iron concentration in biopsy specimens by morphologic and chemical methods.[287] The demonstration of linkage of the locus that determines susceptibility to hemochromatosis with the HLA locus has been of central importance in resolving the mode of genetic transmission.[288] Linkage studies indicate that hemochromatosis gene is located in the vicinity of the HLA-A locus on the short arm of chromosome 6.[289] Because linkage is very tight, once the diagnosis of idiopathic (hereditary) hemochromatosis has been established in an index case, all other homozygotes in a pedigree may be identified with a high degree of confidence by demonstrating their identity in both HLA haplotypes. Haplotypes A3B7 and A3B14 are more frequent in hereditary hemochromatosis than in the whole population. However, it is not a particular haplotype but the genotypic identity of a sibling's HLA types with those of the index case that identifies additional homozygotes or heterozygotes in the same family. Approximately 10% of the population in the U.S., Sweden, Australia, and Scotland are heterozygotes for the hemochromatosis gene, and about 2 to 3 per 1000 are homozygotes.[287,290]

In transfusional iron overload, increased serum ferritin concentration is proportional to the amount of blood transfused and to the concentration of liver iron.[247] However, the rate of both liver iron accumulation and increase in serum ferritin tend to level off after the first 80 to 100 units of blood,[248] probably reflecting increased spontaneous excretion of iron. In thalassemic patients with advanced liver disease and very high serum ferritin, the proportion of glycosylated ferritin, probably derived from normal secretion from RE cells, is reduced, and an increased fraction of serum ferritin is derived from the cytosolic ferritin of disintegrating parenchymal cells. Such ferritin is nonglycosylated, and may be distinguished from the former by its inability to bind to concanavalin A.[212]

Malignant Disease

The first descriptions of ferritinemia in the literature were related to the high levels of serum ferritin encountered in Hodgkin's disease.[197,198] Since then, increased serum ferritin concentrations have been described in leukemia, non-Hodgkin's lymphoma, carcinoma of the pancreas, liver, breast, and other solid tumors.[210,212,213,249-251] There are three possible causes of increased serum ferritin levels in malignancy. First, as already noticed in the earliest reports on ferritinemia, hepatocellular damage caused by metastasis or drug toxicity may result in the release of ferritin stored in the liver. Second, the inflammatory response to tumor may produce increased serum ferritin, as outlined earlier. Finally, there may be increased ferritin production from the tumor cells themselves.

To correlate serum ferritin with disease activity, one may use ferritin assays that employ normal human liver or spleen isoferritins derived from the heart or various tumors. Figure 10 shows ferritin levels in various malignancies studied by Niitsu et al. employing antihuman-liver ferritin.[251] Some tumors, such as carcinoma of the pancreas, lung, and the acute leukemias are characterized by very high serum ferritin levels whereas others, such as most tumors of the GI tract and urogenital tumors, show normal values or a moderate increase only. Jacobs et al. measured serum ferritin concentrations in 229 women presenting with early breast cancer.[300] Ferritin levels were higher in cancer patients than in normal women, and patients with initial ferritin above 200 μg/ℓ had a higher tumor recurrence rate during the subsequent 4 years. Serum ferritin concentration greater than 120 μg/ℓ was found in only 5% of normal women, but 25% of patients with breast cancer. In patients with neuroblastoma, ferritin levels correlate closely with disease activity, and are useful in distinguishing patients with and without bone metastases.[301,302] Correlations between disease stage

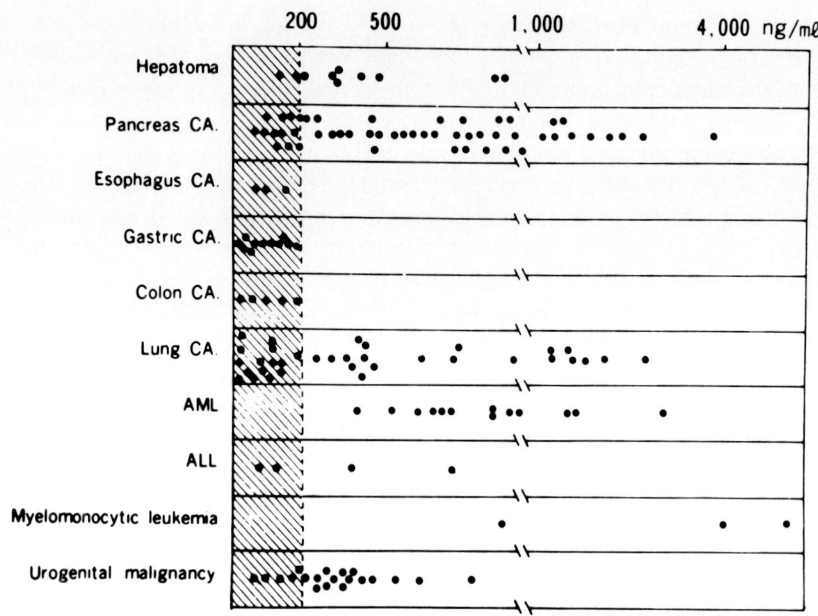

FIGURE 10. Serum ferritin in patients with malignant disease. (From Niitsu, Y., Goto, Y., Kohgo, Y., Adachi, C., Onodera, Y., and Urishicaki, I., *Radioimmunoassay of Hormones, Proteins and Enzymes,* Albertini, A., Ed., Excerpta Medica, Amsterdam, 1980, 256—266. With permission.)

and serum ferritin in Hodgkin's disease and diffuse histiocytic lymphoma show that patients in remission have striking reductions in their serum ferritin levels when compared to initial measurements made during the active phase of the disease[252,253] (Figure 11). Correlations between disease stage and serum ferritin concentration show that patients with Hodgkin's disease and diffuse histiocytic lymphoma have strikingly lower serum ferritin levels during remission than measurements during active phases of their disease.[252,253] In the acute leukemias, there is significant reduction in ferritin in patients with both ALL and ANLL when in prolonged remission, but whether this is related to the disappearance of tumor cells or to the discontinuation of aggressive therapy, and the resolution of severe infectious complications associated with therapy, is open to speculation.[252,254] Although these studies of disease activity and ferritin levels have disclosed some interesting correlations, their diagnostic significance is limited because of the nonspecific, multifactorial nature of the mechanisms responsible for increased serum ferritin concentration.

One of the ways to increase the specificity of serum ferritin measurements in malignancy is the development of selective assays for the measurement of acidic isoferritins. Many, although by no means all, tumors are characterized by the presence of isoferritins more acidic than normal liver or spleen ferritin. These "carcinofetal isoferritins" are not unique to malignant cells, as they correspond to acidic isoferritins normally found in adult heart.[255] They are believed to represent an increase in the relative proportion of H (heart-type) subunits of ferritin as against L (liver-type) subunits which are predominant in normal spleen and liver ferritin. Specific two-site IRMA assays are now available for the measurement of acidic isoferritins derived from human heart[250] or HeLa cells.[256]

Results obtained with isoferritin assays have produced conflicting data. Hazard and Drysdale found increased concentrations of acidic isoferritins using an assay based on HeLa cell ferritin, as compared to basic ferritins in the sera of the same patients with solid tumors.[249] Similarly, Niitsu et al.[251] found higher levels of acidic isoferritins using an assay based on heart ferritin. In contrast, Jones and Worwood[250] were unable to demonstrate acidic isofer-

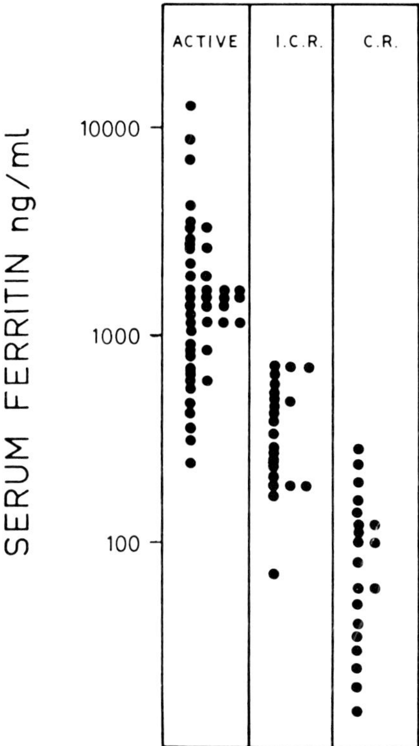

FIGURE 11. Serum ferritin concentration in patients with Stage III and Stage IV Hodgkin's lymphoma at presentation or relapse (active), incomplete remission (ICR), and in complete remission (CR). (From Matzner, Y., Konijn, A. M., and Hershko, C., *Am. J. Hematol.*, 9, 13, 1980. With permission.)

ritins in the sera of patients with various tumors using a two-site IRMA for acidic heart ferritin. It is possible that these seemingly conflicting data are the result of differences in methodology. In spite of the identity in pI of HeLa cell and heart ferritin, there are marked differences in their anion exchange affinity.[250] The immunological specificity of antibodies prepared against HeLa cell and heart ferritin may be different, and therefore tumor-derived ferritin may be recognized in the serum by one but not by the other assay system. The future development of monoclonal antibodies to various isoferritin species may resolve the present controversy over the existence of acidic isoferritins in the sera of patients with cancer, and could lead to the establishment of new and useful markers for clinical use.

Finally, it should be emphasized that more than one mechanism may be operative in the production of increased acidic isoferritins in cancer. According to the model proposed by Drysdale et al.,[257] isoferritins of various pI are produced by various combinations of H- and L-type ferritin subunits, with H-rich isoferritins having the most acidic pI. Tissue iron concentrations greatly influence isoferritin patterns, and the production of acidic isoferritins is increased under conditions of iron depletion. It is possible therefore that "carcinofetal isoferritins" merely reflect iron depletion in rapidly growing tumors. In addition, post-synthetic modification, such as glycosylation, may also contribute significantly to the heterogeneity of serum ferritin. Unlike tissue ferritin, a large proportion of serum ferritin is glycosylated. This is reflected in the fact that about 70% of normal serum ferritin binds to concanavalin A, a plant lectin which binds glycoproteins containing glucose and mannose residues. Glycosylated subunits of serum ferritin have an approximate molecular weight of

23,000 and they make up 32 to 47% of the ferritin binding to concanavalin A.[286] Binding to concanavalin A is a property of the more acidic isoferritins in serum. Incubation of serum ferritin with neuraminidase eliminates much of the microheterogeneity of ferritin on isoelectric focusing.[258] These observations suggest that acidic isoferritins, as are found in the sera of patients with cancer, may be the product of post-synthetic glycosylation without necessarily involving a difference in their protein subunit composition.

USE OF ISOTOPES IN THE STUDY OF IRON TURNOVER

Radioisotopes were first applied to the study of the physiology of iron in the circulation by Hahn et al.[259] in 1939. Within the next 10 years both ^{59}Fe and ^{55}Fe became established as useful radioiron tracers in the study of iron kinetics. It was shown that iron is not taken up directly by circulating erythrocytes[260] and that it is incorporated into hemoglobin by the erythroid precursor cells of the bone marrow. It was also recognized that the rate of radioiron uptake by the marrow was related to the number of erythroid precursors in that tissue.[261,262] The fundamentals of present-day ferrokinetic techniques were laid by Huff et al.,[263,264] who first used transferrin-bound radioiron to study the rate of red cell production. Red cell production rates were measured by calculating the rate of clearance from the plasma ($t_{1/2}$ ^{59}Fe), the fraction of radioiron incorporated into circulating erythrocytes at days 10 to 14, the plasma concentration, and the plasma volume.[214,265]

Plasma iron turnover (PIT) is calculated as follows:

$$\text{PIT} = \frac{\text{plasma iron (mg/d}\ell) \times 0.693 \times 1440}{t_{1/2}\ \text{(min)}} = \text{mg/d}\ell\ \text{plasma per day}$$

The above formula can be simplified to:

$$\frac{\text{Plasma iron } (\mu\text{g \%})}{t_{1/2}\ \text{min}}$$

or converted into milligrams per decaliter whole blood as a product of:

$$\frac{(100 - \text{Hct})}{100}$$

or converted into milligrams per kilogram per day as a product of:

$$\frac{\text{Plasma volume (m}\ell)}{\text{Weight (kg)} \times 100}$$

Red blood cell iron utilization (RBCU) expressed as activity of circulating RBC (percent of injected radioiron) is calculated by the formula:

$$\frac{\text{14 day activity/m}\ell\ \text{whole blood} \times 100}{\text{0 time activity/m}\ell\ \text{whole blood}}$$

Erythrocyte iron turnover (EIT) is the product of PIT × RBCU. The standard expression of milligrams per decaliter whole blood per day for PIT and EIT is preferred, since it does not require plasma volume measurement and permits comparison between different individuals. Ferrokinetic data published up to 1970 for various clinical conditions have been reviewed by Finch et al.[265] and are summarized in Table 6. The average normal PIT is 0.70

Table 6
FERROKINETIC DATA IN VARIOUS CLINICAL CONDITIONS[a]

Condition	PVC (%)	SI (μg/dℓ)	$t_{1/2}$ (min)	PIT (mg/dℓ/day)	Utilization (%)	EIT (mg/dℓ/day)
			Normal			
	45	105	86	0.70	80	0.56
			Anemia			
Disorders of proliferation						
Decreased erythropoietin						
Hypothyroidism	31	62	84	0.51	79	0.41
Renal failure						
I Transfused	24	220	221	0.84	34	0.29
II Nontransfused	27	76	79	0.81	81	0.66
Iron deficiency	26	21	20	0.80	94	0.75
Inflammation						
Infection	36	60	47	0.81	86	0.70
Rheumarthritis	37	68	48	0.89	78	0.70
Hodgkin's disease	31	55	42	0.90	76	0.68
Marrow damage						
Aplasia	21	182	351	0.45	0	0
Primary hypoplasia	25	199	310	0.48	26	0.12
Multiple myeloma	30	54	105	0.36	71	0.26
Acute leukemia	23	175	187	0.75	47	0.35
Disorders of maturation						
Nuclear abnormalities						
Pernicious anemia	19	153	51	2.43	28	0.68
Sprue	22	114	62	1.62	46	0.75
Impaired Hb synthesis						
Thalassemia major	24	169	24	5.36	18	0.96
Thalassemia trait	37	151	66	1.44	59	0.85
Refractory anemia with hypercellular marrow	23	152	55	2.13	31	0.66
Myelofibrosis	27	111	62	1.31	44	0.57
Hemolytic anemias						
Hereditary spherocytosis	35	118	27	2.84	61	1.73
Autoimmune hemolytic anemia	29	116	39	2.11	73	1.54
Sickle cell anemia	25	117	29	3.03	63	1.91
PNH	30	136	45	2.10	72	1.51
			Polycythemia			
Polycythemia vera	60	86	34	1.01	86	0.87
Secondary polycythemia	57	113	64	0.76	85	0.64
Hemochromatosis	44	213	121	0.98	74	0.73

[a] Average values of data. PCV = packed cell volume; SI = serum iron; PIT = plasma iron turnover; EIT = erythrocyte iron turnover.

From Finch, C. A., Deubelbeiss, K., Cook, J. D., Eschbacn, L. A., Harker, L. A., Funk, D. D., Marsaglia, G., Hillman, R. S., Slichter, S., Adamson, J. W., Ganzoni, A., and Giblett, E. R., *Medicine,* 49, 17, 1970. With permission of the Williams & Wilkins Co., Baltimore.

mg/dℓ whole blood per day and the EIT is 0.56. The standard deviation of the normal mean is ±24%.[266]

In terms of ferrokinetic measurements, anemias can be divided into three categories: (1) disorders of proliferation, (2) disorders of maturation, and (3) disorders of the mature erythrocyte.

Disorders of proliferation are seen in conditions with impaired erythropoietin production caused by a reduction in tissue metabolism, such as hypofunction of the thyroid, pituitary, or adrenal glands or testes, or in severe renal disease. These conditions are characterized by normal or increased serum iron and $t_{1/2}$ ^{59}Fe and reduced or normal PIT and EIT. In renal insufficiency, red cell lifespan is reduced,[267] and the survival of RBC is impaired.[269] Thus, in spite of an apparently normal rate of EIT, the circulating red cell mass cannot be sustained at normal levels in iron deficiency.

Inflammation caused by infection, connective tissue disorders, or malignancy is manifested in low-serum iron, a short $t_{1/2}$ ^{59}Fe, and normal PIT and EIT, in a fashion similar to that of iron deficiency. Iron supply is limited because of a block in iron release from tissues.[171] Red cell survival in inflammation is about half normal, and the normal rates of EIT are not sufficient to prevent a reduction in red cell mass. This relative bone marrow failure is caused by the limited supply of transferrin iron and an inadequate erythropoietin response to anemia.[270] Marrow damage ranging from leukemic infiltration of the marrow to complete aplasia is the most simple and straightforward manifestation of "disorders of proliferation". EIT is moderately or drastically reduced in this case; serum iron and $t_{1/2}$ ^{59}Fe are very high, and PIT reflects mostly nonerythroid iron turnover.

Disorders of maturation are conditions characterized by excessive death of nucleated red cells, or ineffective erythropoiesis. The mechanism responsible for this premature destruction of erythroid cells may be nuclear abnormality, an impairment of hemoglobin synthesis, a heterogenous group of anemias commonly referred to as refractory anemia with hypercellular marrow, and myelofibrosis.

Nuclear abnormality is responsible for ineffective erythropoiesis in the megaloblastic anemia of B12, and folate deficiency. PIT is twice to fourfold normal, but most of the iron turnover is wasted on early death of erythroid precursors, and EIT is only a small fraction of PIT. Following treatment, plasma iron becomes the limiting factor and PIT is often reduced to the range usually found in iron deficiency.[271]

Impaired hemoglobin synthesis is responsible for the extremely severe, ineffective erythropoiesis typical of thalassemia major. Expansion of the erythropoietic tissue throughout the medullary cavities is reflected in a nearly tenfold increase in PIT, with extensive breakdown of developing cells which, in turn, are rapidly catabolized with efficient recircuiting of hemoglobin iron. Because of the premature destruction of erythrocytes, EIT is reduced to about 20% of the PIT.[272] A similar, but less pronounced, discrepancy between PIT and EIT can be found in thalassemia minor and the sideroblastic anemias.[273]

In refractory anemia with hyperplastic marrow and in myelofibrosis ineffective erythropoiesis is the final common expression of a wide range of disorders characterized by abnormal erythroid maturation. The ferrokinetic pattern of these conditions is indistinguishable from that of the megaloblastic anemias or thalassemia.

Hemolytic anemias are characterized by increased serum iron, a very short $t_{1/2}$ ^{59}Fe, and increased PIT and EIT. Although EIT is about 30% less than PIT, this discrepancy does not necessarily represent ineffective erythropoiesis, but rather a dilution of the radioiron tracer in the labile iron pool, and, in addition, destruction of young erythrocytes within the 2-week observation period. Premature destruction of erythrocytes is also reflected in the accumulation of radioactivity in organs involved in red cell sequestration and destruction, such as the spleen.

Ferrokinetic studies are useful in defining differences between primary and secondary polycythemia. In both conditions a moderate increase in PIT and EIT may be found, but in polycythemia vera EIT is relatively higher than the rate required to maintain a constant level of circulating red cells, indicating a progressive expansion of the red cell mass. The $t_{1/2}$ ^{59}FE in polycythemia vera is often shorter than in secondary polycythemia, but this difference may be attributed to a coexistent iron deficiency, which is quite common in polycythemia vera.

Ferrokinetics are of limited value in the diagnosis and evaluation of idiopathic hemochromatosis. Although serum iron is usually very high, PIT and EIT are near normal, and nonerythroid iron turnover is not strikingly increased.

The above data, based on simple calculations of PIT and EIT, provide useful information for the clinical assessment of various pathologic conditions. However, the rate of radioiron disappearance from the plasma is a complex function and cannot be accurately expressed as a simple exponential curve. Normally, the slope of the radioiron disappearance curve changes from about 40% per hour initially to less than 1% on the second day because of a reflux of iron into the plasma from more peripheral compartments. Attempts have been made to formulate a reflux model by multicompartmental analysis of plasma radioactivity, but these models have not been validated by correlation with normal and pathologic states.[223-225,274-276]

An alternative approach has been the analysis of the radioiron disappearance curve in terms of a probability theory.[277] The distribution of sojourn times for returning particles was calculated from an integrodifferential equation by fitting the plasma iron disappearance curve with a linear combination of exponential functions. This method has been further extended to estimate total reflux based on the area underlying the disappearance curve.[3] Total reflux in turn was further subdivided into early and late components (Table 7). Total reflux amounts to about one third of total PIT in normal subjects, in iron overload, erythroid hypoplasia, and uremic patients without transfusion requirement. Reflux is over 50% in hemolytic anemia, iron deficiency, and ineffective erythropoiesis. Early reflux has a re-entry time of 7 to 10 hr. It is similar in all disease groups, amounting to 0.14 mg/dℓ/day of iron with an SD of +0.08. It is not affected by differences in erythropoietic activity, but is positively correlated to the level of plasma iron and plasmatocrit ($r = 0.711$, $p < 0.001$). Both the re-entry time and the amount of iron involved in early exchange are consistent with a lymphatic shunt of transferrin iron. Late reflux is usually larger than early reflux. It is not affected by the size of body iron stores or plasma iron levels, but is very sensitive to erythropoietic activity. Late reflux is very low in aplastic anemia and is greatly increased in hemolytic anemia. The $t_{1/2}$ of late reflux is 5 to 15 days as compared to $t_{1/2}$ of 7 to 10 hr in early reflux. The close correlation with erythropoietic activity and the time of return identify late reflux with wastage iron of erythropoiesis or iron taken up by the marrow but released without permanent incorporation into circulating erythrocytes.

Having defined the early and late reflux pathways, it is possible to construct a comprehensive model of iron exchange in the body (Figure 12). Fixed tissue turnover represents the amount of iron cleared from the plasma and not returned during the subsequent 2 weeks. It consists of fixed erythrocyte turnover, which indicates effective erythropoiesis, and fixed parenchymal turnover, represented by the hepatic parenchyma as the most important organ. In analogy with early reflux, fixed parenchymal turnover is closely related to the concentration of transferrin iron ($r = 0.085$, $p < 0.001$). Total plasma iron turnover is the sum of fixed tissue turnover and total reflux. Since both components of nonerythron turnover, namely early reflux and fixed parenchymal turnover, are proportional to plasma iron supply, they can be derived from the formula:

$$\text{Nonerythron turnover} + \text{SI } (\mu\text{g/d}\ell) \times \text{plasmatocrit} \times 0.0035$$

Table 7
IRON TURNOVER COMPARTMENTS

	Fixed (mg/dℓ whole blood/day)			Reflux (mg/dℓ whole blood/day)			
	Total	**RBC**	**Parenchymal**	**Total**	**Early**	**Late**	**Total erythron**
Normal subjects	0.50 ± 0.03[a]	0.41 ± 0.02	0.09 ± 0.01	0.25 ± 0.01	0.06 ± 0.01	0.19 ± 0.01	0.60 ± 0.02
Iron overload	0.85 ± 0.05	0.66 ± 0.05	0.18 ± 0.03	0.34 ± 0.03	0.12 ± 0.02	0.23 ± 0.02	0.89 ± 0.07
Iron deficiency	0.32 ± 0.10	0.32 ± 0.09	0.01 ± 0.01	0.37 ± 0.06	0.10 ± 0.03	0.27 ± 0.06	0.59 ± 0.15
Erythroid hypoplasia	0.31 ± 0.04	0.01 ± 0.01	0.30 ± 0.03	0.18 ± 0.02	0.16 ± 0.03	0.02 ± 0.002	0.03 ± 0.01
Renal patients							
I, Transfused	0.60 ± 0.09	0.15 ± 0.04	0.45 ± 0.05	0.38 ± 0.03	0.27 ± 0.02	0.11 ± 0.02	0.26 ± 0.06
II, Nontransfused	0.56 ± 0.08	0.45 ± 0.06	0.11 ± 0.02	0.36 ± 0.05	0.11 ± 0.02	0.24 ± 0.04	0.69 ± 0.10
Hemolytic anemia	1.56 ± 0.20	1.43[b] ± 0.12	0.13[b] ± 0.07	1.65 ± 0.27	0.15 ± 0.05	1.49 ± 0.25	2.92 ± 0.32
Ineffective erythropoiesis	1.07 ± 0.11	—	—	2.08 ± 0.32	—	—	2.67 ± 0.49

[a] Standard error of the mean.

[b] Values calculated indirectly by estimating the nonerythron iron turnover from plasma iron and plasmatocrit.

From Cook, J. D., Marsaglia, G., Eschbach, J. W., Funk, D. D., and Finch, C. A., *J. Clin. Invest.*, 49, 197, 1970. With permission.

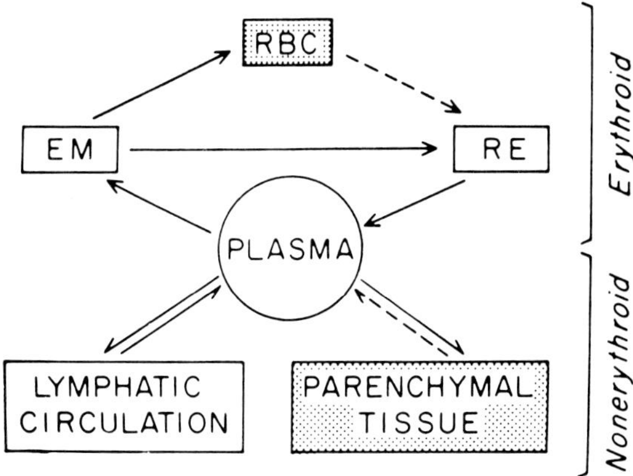

FIGURE 12. A biological model for plasma iron turnover. PIT is divided into iron which remains localized in tissue (shaded areas) and iron which will be returned to the plasma within 2 weeks. Total reflux consists of lymphatic circulation and the sojourn of nonviable erythrocyte precursors via the reticuloendothelial system. The intracellulary fixed tissue turnover is partitioned into an erythrocyte and parenchymal fraction. During a 2-week period of observation, there is no evidence for a return of iron from these sites (interrupted lines). Total erythron iron turnover, including both effective and ineffective erythropoiesis, is represented by the sum of the fixed erythrocyte and late reflux values. (From Cook, J. C., Marsaglia, G., Eschbach, J. W., Funk, D. D., and Finch, C. A., *J. Clin. Invest.*, 49, 197, 1970. With permission.)

Table 8
RETICULOENDOTHELIAL HANDLING OF ^{59}FE-LABELED ERYTHROCYTES

	Condition				
	Early release		Late release		$^{59}Fe/^{55}Fe^{a}$ at 15 days
	%	$t_{1/2}$ (min)	%	$t_{1/2}$ (min)	
Normal	64	33	36	5.6	92.5
Inflammation	44	42	56	12.0	64.0
Hemochromatosis					
Untreated	57	39	43	∞	69.5
Treated	92	29	8	<0.5	100
Iron deficiency	100	31	0	—	100

[a] Ratio of transferrin ^{55}Fe and DRBC ^{59}Fe in newly formed erythrocytes; used as an index of cumulative ^{59}Fe release from RE cells.

Erythron turnover can be obtained by subtracting nonerythron turnover from PIT. The relation between total erythron turnover and fixed erythrocyte turnover is determined by the efficiency of erythropoiesis.

The handling of iron by RE cells can be studied directly by the use of heat-denatured ^{59}Fe-labeled erythrocytes (^{59}Fe DRBC).[172,173,278] Following a short lag phase required for red cell phagocytosis and heme catabolism, ^{59}Fe derived from hemoglobin enters a labile pool from which it is either promptly returned to circulating transferrin (early release) or is retained (late release) in a more slowly exchanging iron pool (Table 8). The half-life of

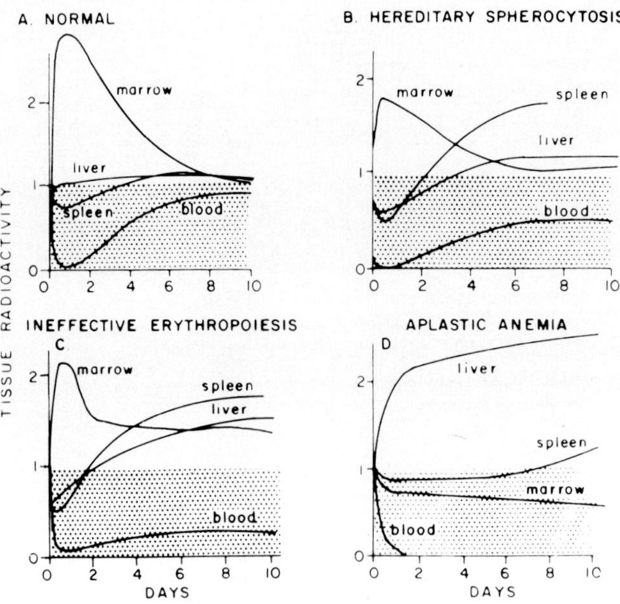

FIGURE 13. Blood and tissue ferrokinetic profiles. All measurements start at 1, representing radioactivity immediately after the injection of radioiron. In hereditary spherocytosis (B), the marrow produces cells which are trapped and subsequently destroyed in the spleen, indicated by the accumulation of radioactivity in the spleen and the reduced proportion of activity appearing in the circulating erythrocytes. In ineffective erythropoiesis (C), the marrow is active as shown by its initial uptake of radioiron, but radioactivity subsequently accumulates in the liver, spleen, and marrow, indicating that a large portion of the erythroid activity is wasted on the production of nonviable erythrocytes which are removed by the reticuloendothelial cells of these organs. In aplastic anemia (D), there is no marrow uptake of radioiron and none appears in circulating red cells. Instead, there is pathologic deposition of iron in the parenchymal cells of the liver. (From Finch, C. A., Deubelbeiss, K., Cook, J. D., Eschbach, L. A., Harker, L. A., Funk, D. D., Marsaglia, G., Hillman, R. S., Slichter, S., Adamson, J. W., Ganzoni, A., and Giblett, E. R., *Medicine*, 49, 17, 1970. With permission of the Williams & Wilkins Co., Baltimore.)

early and late release in normal man is 33 min and 5.6 days, respectively. Through a wide spectrum of clinical conditions, the half-life of early release was found to be constant, but the proportion of early release ranged from 100% in iron deficiency to as little as 10% in iron overload. The half-life of late release ranged from less than 1 day in iron deficiency or treated hemochromatosis to no measurable release in advanced untreated hemochromatosis. The cumulative release of radioiron within 2 weeks was 100% in patients with iron deficiency and treated hemochromatosis, 93% in normals, and less than 70% in patients with inflammation and untreated hemochromatosis.

Another approach to the study of iron exchange in the body is the in vivo measurement of transferrin ^{59}Fe uptake by the different tissues using surface counting (Figure 13). The distribution of ^{59}Fe radioactivity is measured within 12 days of injection and is expressed in relation to the radioactivity measured over the same organ immediately after injection of labeled transferrin. In normal subjects, ^{59}Fe is rapidly cleared from blood with a reciprocal increase in marrow radioactivity. Radioiron is subsequently released from the marrow in newly formed erythrocytes, with a corresponding increase in blood radioactivity. Because of its high vascularity, the spleen reflects blood radioactivity, and these is little change in hepatic radioactivity within the 12-day study period. In hemolytic anemia with a predominantly splenic destruction of erythrocytes, radioactivity accumulates over the spleen, with a reduced proportion of radioactivity in circulating erythrocytes. In ineffective erythropoiesis, radioactivity accumulates over the liver and marrow as well as over the spleen, indicating the production of nonviable erythrocytes which are removed by reticuloendothelial cells of those organs. Finally, in aplastic anemia, there is no marrow uptake of radioactivity and no production of labeled erythrocytes. Iron is accumulated mainly over the liver, reflecting the parenchymal uptake of transferrin ^{59}Fe.[228,279]

ACKNOWLEDGMENT

This work was supported in part by Grants No. 750 and No. 2851 of the United States-Israel Binational Science Foundation.

REFERENCES

1. **Harrison, P. M., Hoare, R. J., Hoy, T. Y., and Macara, I. G.,** Ferritin and haemosiderin: structure and function, in *Iron in Biochemistry and Medicine,* Jacobs, A. and Worwood, M., Eds., Academic Press, New York, 1974, 73.
2. **Crichton, R. R., Huebers, H., and Huebers, E.,** Comparative studies on ferritin, in *Proteins of Iron Storage and Transport in Biochemistry and Medicine,* Crichton, R. R., Eds., North-Holland, Amsterdam, 1975, 193.
3. **Cook, J. D., Marsaglia, G., Eschbach, J. W., Funk, D. D., and Finch, C. A.,** Ferrokinetics: a biologic model for plasma iro- exchange in man, *J. Clin. Invest.,* 49, 197, 1970.
4. **Callender, S. T., Mallett, B. J., and Smith, M. D.,** Absorption of haemoglobin iron, *Br. J. Haematol.,* 3, 186, 1957.
5. **Turnbull, A., Cleton, F., and Finch, C. A.,** Iron absorption. IV. The absorption of hemoglobin iron, *J. Clin. Invest.,* 41, 1897, 1962.
6. **Hwang, Y. F. and Brown, E. B.,** Effect of desferrioxamine in iron absorption, *Lancet,* 1, 135, 1965.
7. **Conrad, M. E., Weintraub, L. R., Sears, D. A., and Crosby, W. H.,** Absorption of hemoglobin iron, *Am. J. Physiol.,* 211, 1123, 1966.
8. **Hallberg, L. and Solvell, L.,** Absorption of hemoglobin iron in man, *Acta Med. Scand.,* 181, 335, 1967.
9. **Wheby, M. S., Suttle, G. E., and Ford, K. T.,** Intestinal absorption of hemoglobin iron, *Gastroenterology,* 58, 647, 1970.
10. **Callender, S. T., Marney, S. R., and Werner, G. T.,** Absorption of labelled iron from food, *Br. J. Radiol.,* 43, 284, 1970.
11. **Layrisse, M., Martinez-Torres, C., Cook, J. D., Walker, R., and Finch, C. A.,** Iron fortification of food: its measurement by the extrinsic tag method, *Blood,* 41, 333, 1973.
12. **Hallberg, L. and Solvell, L.,** Absorption of a single dose of iron in man, *Acta Med. Scand.,* 358(168), 19, 1960.
13. **Brown, E. B.,** The absorption of iron, *Am. J. Clin. Nutr.,* 12, 205, 1963.
14. **Wheby, M. S. and Crosby, W. H.,** The gastrointestinal tract and iron absorption, *Blood,* 22, 416, 1963.
15. **Dowdle, E. B., Schachter, D., and Schenker, H.,** Active transport of ^{59}Fe by everted segments of rat duodenum, *Am. J. Physiol.,* 198, 609, 1960.
16. **Jacobs, P., Bothwell, T. H., and Charlton, R. W.,** Intestinal iron transport: studies using a loop of gut with artificial circulation, *Am. J. Physiol.,* 210, 694, 1966.
17. **Greenberger, N. Y., Balcerzak, S. P., and Ackerman, G. A.,** Iron uptake by isolated intestinal brush borders: Changes induced by alterations in iron stores, *J. Lab. Clin. Med.,* 73, 711, 1969.
18. **Hübers, H., Hübers, E., Forth, W., Leopold, G., and Rummel, W.,** Binding of iron to non-ferritin protein in the mucosal cells of normal and iron deficient rats during absorption, *Acta Pharmacol. Toxicol.,* 29(4), 22, 1971.
19. **Richmond, V. S., Worwood, M., and Jacobs, A.,** The iron content of intestinal epithelial cells and its subcellular distribution: studies on normal, iron loaded and iron deficient rats, *Br. J. Haematol.,* 23, 605, 1972.

20. **Conrad, M. E. and Crosby, W. H.,** Intestinal mucosal mechanisms controlling iron absorption, *Blood,* 22, 406, 1963.
21. **Worwood, M. and Jacobs, A.,** The subcellular distribution of ^{59}Fe in small intestinal mucosa: studies with normal, iron deficient and iron loaded rats, *Br. J. Haematol.,* 22, 265, 1972.
22. **Brown, E. B. and Rother, M. L.,** Studies of the mechanism of iron absorption. II. Influence of iron deficiency and other conditions on iron uptake by rats, *J. Lab. Clin. Med.,* 62, 804, 1963.
23. **Worwood, M. and Jacobs, A.,** The subcellular distribution of ^{59}Fe during iron absorption in the rat, *Br. J. Haematol.,* 20, 587, 1971.
24. **Hubers, H., Hubers, E., Simon, J., and Forth, W.,** A method for preparing stable density gradients and their application for fractionation of intestinal mucosal cells, *Life Sci.,* 10, 377, 1971.
25. **Charlton, R. W., Jacobs, P., Torrance, J. D., and Bothwell, T. H.,** Regulation of the intestinal absorption of iron by the rate of erythropoiesis, *Br. J. Haematol.,* 2, 432, 1965.
26. **Sheehan, R. G. and Frenkel, E. P.,** The control of iron absorption in the gastrointestinal mucosal cell, *J. Clin. Invest.,* 51, 224, 1972.
27. **Blanc, B. and Isliker, H.,** Repartition du par dans diverses fractions tissulaires de la mugeuse intestinale au cours de l'absorption, *Helv. Physiol. Pharmacol. Acta,* 23, 145, 1965.
28. **Worwood, M. and Jacobs, A.,** Absorption of ^{59}Fe in the rat: iron binding substances in the soluble fraction of intestinal mucosa, *Life Sci.,* 10, 1363, 1971.
29. **Jacobs, A. and Worwood, M.,** Correlation between iron content and ferritin in hemochromatosis, *Br. J. Haematol.,* 27, 359, 1974.
30. **Pollack, S., Camparro, T., and Arcario, A.,** A search for mucosal iron carrier. Identification of mucosal fractions with rapid turnover of s;5^{9}Fe, *J. Lab. Clin. Med.,* 80, 322, 1972.
31. **Hübers, H., Hübers, E., Simon, J., and Forth, W.,** Binding of iron to a nonferritin protein in the mucosal cells of normal and iron deficient rats during absorption, *Life Sci.,* 10, 1141, 1971.
32. **Granick, S.,** Protein apoferritin and ferritin in iron feeding and absorption, *Science,* 103, 107, 1946.
33. **Boender, C. A., Mulder, E., Plaem, J. E., Wael, J., and Verloop, M. C.,** Iron absorption and retention in man, *Nature (London),* 213, 1236, 1967.
34. **Boender, C. A. and Verloop, M. C.,** Iron absorption, iron loss and iron retention in man: studies after oral iron administration of a tracer dose of $^{59}FeSO_4$ and $^{131}BaSO_4$, *Br. J. Haematol.,* 17, 45, 1969.
35. **Powell, L. W., Campbell, C. B., and Wilson, E.,** Intestinal mucosal uptake and iron retention in idiopathic hemochromatosis as evidence for a mucosal abnormality, *Gut,* 11, 727, 1970.
36. **Brittin, G. M. and Raval, D.,** Duodenal ferritin synthesis during iron absorption in the iron-deficient rat, *J. Lab. Clin. Med.,* 75, 811, 1970.
37. **Brittin, G. M. and Ravel, D.,** Duodenal ferritin synthesis during iron absorption in the iron-deficient rat, *J. Lab. Clin. Med.,* 77, 54, 1971.
38. **Schade, S. G., Felsher, B. F., Bernier, G. M., and Conrad, M. E.,** Effect of cobalt upon iron absorption, *J. Lab. Clin. Med.,* 75, 435, 1970.
39. **Bielig, H. J. and Bayer, E.,** Eisenkomplexe mit 3 ungepaarten Elektronen, *Naturwissenschaften,* 16, 466, 1955.
40. **Conrad, M. E., Benjamin, B. I., Williams, H. L., and Foy, A. L.,** Human absorption of hemoglobin iron, *Gastroenterology,* 53, 5, 1967.
41. **Brown, E. B., Hwang, Y. F., Nicol, S., and Turnberg, J.,** Absorption of radiation-labeled hemoglobin by days, *J. Lab. Clin. Med.,* 72, 58, 1968.
42. **Weintraub, L. R., Weinstein, M. B., Huser, H., and Rafal, S.,** Absorption of hemoglobin iron: the role of heme-splitting substance in the intestinal mucosa, *J. Clin. Invest.,* 47, 531, 1968.
43. **Dawson, R. B., Rafal, S., and Weintraub, L. R.,** Absorption of hemoglobin iron: the role of xantine oxidase in the intestinal heme-splitting reaction, *Blood,* 35, 94, 1970.
44. **Wynter, C. V. A. and Williams, R.,** Iron binding properties of gastric juice in idiopathic haemochromatosis, *Lancet,* 2, 534, 1968.
45. **Forth, W., Rummel, W., and Adres, H.,** Zur Frage der Regulation der Eisenresorption durch Gastroferrin, ein eisenbinden des Protein des Magensafts, *Klin. Wochenschr.,* 46, 1003, 1968.
46. **Jacobs, A.,** Availability and absorption of dietary iron, in *Progress in Gastroenterology,* Vol. 2, Glass, B. J., Ed., Grune & Stratton, New York, 1970, 221.
47. **Kavin, H., Charlton, R. W., Jacobs, P., Green, R., Torrance, J. D., and Bothwell, T. H.,** Effect of the exocrine pancreatic secretions on iron absorption, *Gut,* 8, 556, 1967.
48. **Murray, M. J. and Stein, N.,** Does pancreas influence iron absorption?, *Br. J. Haematol.,* 15, 87, 1968.
49. **Jacobs, A., Rhodes, J., and Eakins, J. D.,** Gastric factors influencing iron absorption in anaemic patients, *Scand. J. Haematol.,* 4, 105, 1967.
50. **Jacobs, A.,** Effect of gastric juice and pH in inorganic iron in solution, *Nature (London),* 216, 707, 1967.
51. **Smith, P. M., Studley, F., and Williams, R.,** Iron absorption in idiopathic haemochromatosis and its measurement using a whole body counter, *Clin. Sci.,* 37, 519, 1969.

52. **Crosby, W. H.,** The control of iron balance by the intestinal mucosa, *Blood,* 22, 441, 1963.
53. **Conrad, M. E., Weintraub, L. R., and Crosby, W. H.,** Role of intestine in iron kinetics, *J. Clin. Invest.,* 43, 963, 1964.
54. **Weintraub, L. R., Conrad, M. E., and Crosby, W. H.,** Regulation of the intestinal absorption of iron by rate of erythropoiesis, *Br. J. Haematol.,* 11, 432, 1965.
55. **Pirzio-Biroli, G., Bothwell, T. H., and Finch, B. A.,** Iron absorption. II. The absorption of radioiron administered with a standard meal in man, *J. Lab. Clin. Med.,* 51, 37, 1958.
56. **Weintraub, L. R., Conrad, M. E., and Crosby, W. H.,** The significance of iron turnover in the control of iron absorption, *Blood,* 24, 19, 1964.
57. **Chirashiri, L. and Izak, G.,** The effect of acute hemorrhages and acute hemolysis on the intestinal iron absorption in the rat, *Br. J. Haematol.,* 12, 611, 1966.
58. **Pearson, W. N., Reich, M., Frank, H., and Salamat, L.,** Effects of dietary iron level on gut iron levels and iron absorption in the rat, *J. Nutr.,* 92, 53, 1967.
59. **Kaufman, R. M., Pollack, S., and Crosby, W. H.,** Iron-deficient diet: effects in rats and humans, *Blood,* 28, 726, 1966.
60. **Balcerzak, S. P. and Greenberger, N. J.,** Iron content of isolated intestinal epithelial cells in relation to iron absorption, *Nature (London),* 20, 270, 1968.
61. **Pollack, S. and Campana, T.,** The relationship between mucosal iron and iron absorption in the guinea pig, *Scand. J. Haematol.,* 7, 208, 1970.
62. **Cook, J. D., Larysse, M., Martinez-Torres, C., Walker, R., Monsen, E., and Finch, C. A.,** Food iron absorption measured by an extrinsic tag, *J. Clin. Invest.,* 51, 805, 1972.
63. **Richmond, V. S., Worwood, M., and Jacobs, M.,** The iron content of intestinal epithelial cells and its subcellular distribution. Studies on normal, iron deficient and iron-overloaded animals, *Br. J. Haematol.,* 23, 605, 1972.
64. **Howard, J. and Jacobs, A.,** Iron transport by rat small intestine in vitro: effect of body iron status, *Br. J. Haematol.,* 23, 595, 1972.
65. **Worwood, M. and Jacobs, A.,** The subcellular distribution of ^{59}Fe in small intestinal mucosa, *Br. J. Haematol.,* 22, 265, 1972.
66. **Taylor, M. R. H. and Gatenby, P. B. B.,** Iron absorption in relation to transferrin saturation and other factors, *Br. J. Haematol.,* 16, 443, 1966.
67. **Pirzio-Biroli, G. and Finch, C. A.,** Iron absorption. III. The influence of iron stores on iron absorption in the normal subject, *J. Lab. Clin. Med.,* 55, 216, 1960.
68. **Heinrich, H. C.,** Iron deficiency without anaemia, *Lancet,* 2, 460, 1968.
69. **Hoglund, S. and Reizenstein, P.,** Studies on iron absorption. V. Effect of gastrointestinal factors on iron absorption, *Blood,* 34, 496, 1969.
70. **Hausmann, K., Kuse, R., Meinecke, K. H., Bartels, H., and Heinrich, H. C.,** Diagnostiche Kriterien des pralatenten, latenten und manifesten Eisenmangels, *Klin. Wochenschr.,* 49, 1971.
71. **Totze, C., Schmerlinska, E., and Heinrich, H. C.,** Cytochemide des Nichthämoglobineisens in Knochenmarkzellen und intestinale Eisenresorption bei verschiedenen Anämien des Kindersalters, *Monatsschr. Kinderheilkd.,* 119, 13, 1971.
72. **Bannerman, R. M., Callender, S. T., Hardistry, R. M., and Smith, R. S.,** Iron absorption in thalassemia, *Br. J. Haematol.,* 10, 490, 1964.
73. **Shahid, M. J. and Haydar, N. A.,** Absorption of inorganic iron in thalassemia, *Br. J. Haematol.,* 13, 713, 1967.
74. **Erlandson, M. E., Walden, B., Stern, G., Hilgartner, M. W., Wehman, J., and Smith, C. H.,** Studies on congenital hemolytic syndromes. IV. Gastrointestinal absorption of iron, *Blood,* 19, 359, 1962.
75. **Brain, M. C. and Herdan, A.,** Tissue iron stores in sideroblastic anaemia, *Br. J. Haematol.,* 11, 107, 1965.
76. **Fletcher, J. and Huens, E. R.,** Significance of the binding of iron by transferrin, *Nature (London),* 218, 1211, 1968.
77. **Lavie, R. S. and Finch, C. A.,** The in vivo plasma clearance of iron from transferrins of low and high iron saturation, *Clin. Sci.,* 38, 783, 1970.
78. **Krantz, S., Goldwasser, E., and Jacobson, L. O.,** Studies on erythropoiesis. XIV. The relationship of humoral stimulation to iron absorption, *Blood,* 14, 654, 1959.
79. **Beutler, E. and Buttenweiser, E.,** The regulation of iron absorption. A search for humoral factors, *J. Lab. Clin. Med.,* 55, 274, 1960.
80. **Mendel, G. A.,** Studies on iron absorption. I. The relationships between the rate of erythropoiesis, hypoxia, and iron absorption, *Blood,* 18, 727, 1961.
81. **Hathorn, M. K. S.,** The influence of hypoxia on iron absorption in the rat, *Gastroenterology,* 60, 76, 1971.
82. **Apte, S. V. and Brown, E. B.,** Effect of plasma from pregnant women on iron absorption by the rat, *J. Nutr.,* 101, 927, 1969.

83. **Larysse, M. and Martinez-Torres, C.,** Model for measuring the dietary absorption from heme iron. Measurement of the total iron absorption from a complete meal, *Am. J. Clin. Nutr.*, 25, 401, 1972.
84. **Larysse, M., Martinez-Torres, C., Cook, J. D., Walker, R., and Finch, C. A.,** Iron fortification of food: its measurement by the extrinsic tag method, *Blood,* 4, 333, 1973.
85. **Green, R., Charlton, R., Seftel, H., Bothwell, T., Mayet, F., Adams, B., and Finch, C. A.,** Body iron excretion in man, *Am. J. Med.*, 45, 336, 1968.
86. **Hallberg, L., Hagdahl, A. M., Nilsson, L., and Rylo, G.,** Menstrual blood loss in iron deficiency, *Acta Med. Scand.*, 180, 639, 1966.
87. **Kuhn, I. N., Mansen, E. R., Cook, J. D., and Finch, C. A.,** Iron absorption in man, *J. Lab. Clin. Med.*, 71, 715, 1968.
88. Committee on Iron Deficiency of the AMA Council on Foods and Nutrition. Iron deficiency in the United States, *JAMA,* 203, 407, 1968.
89. **Wheby, M. S. and Jones, L. G.,** Studies on iron absorption. Role of transferrin in iron absorption, *J. Clin. Invest.*, 42, 1007, 1963.
90. **Wheby, M. S. and Crosby, W. H.,** Studies on iron absorption. The gastrointestinal tract and iron absorption, *Blood,* 22, 416, 1963.
91. **Wheby, M. S.,** Studies on iron absorption, *N. Engl. J. Med.*, 271, 1391, 1964.
92. **Moore, C. V.,** The importance of nutritional factors in the pathogenesis of iron deficiency anemia, *Ser. Haematol.*, 6, 1, 1965.
93. **Peterson, R. E. and Manu, J. D.,** Transport of radioactive iron in the intestinal lymph, *Am. J. Physiol.*, 169, 763, 1952.
94. **Reizenstein, P. G., Cronkite, E. P., Meyer, L. M., and Usenik, A.,** Lymphatics in intestinal absorption of vitamin B_{12} and iron, *Proc. Soc. Exp. Biol. Med.*, 105, 233, 1960.
95. **Hyde, A. S.,** Absorption of radioiron perfused through the duodenum of the rat, *Am. J. Physiol.*, 191, 265, 1957.
96. **Solvell, L.,** Absorption of radioiron perfused through the duodenum of the rat, *Acta Med. Scand. Suppl.*, 358(168), 71, 1960.
97. **Charley, P. J., Sarkar, B., Stitt, C., and Saltman, P.,** Chelation of iron by sugars, *Biochim. Biophys. Acta,* 69, 313, 1963.
98. **Laurell, C. B. and Ingelman, B.,** The iron binding protein of swine serum, *Acta Chem. Scand.*, 1, 770, 1947.
99. **Aisen, P. and Brown, E. B.,** The iron-binding function of transferrin in iron metabolism, *Semin. Haematol.*, 14, 31, 1977.
100. **Roberts, R. C., Makey, D. G., and Seal, U. S.,** Human transferrin: molecular weight and sedimentation properties, *J. Biol. Chem.*, 84, 1907, 1966.
101. **Mann, K. G., Fish, W. W., Cox, A. C., and Tanford, C.,** Single chain nature of human serum transferrin, *Biochemistry,* 9, 1348, 1970.
102. **Leibman, A. and Aisen, P.,** Preparation of single crystals of transferrin, *Arch. Biochem. Biophys.*, 171, 717, 1967.
103. **Eriksson, S. and Sjognist, Y.,** Quantitative determination of N-terminal amino acids in some serum proteins, *Biochem. Biophys. Acta,* 45, 290, 1960.
104. **Ferney, R. E. and Komatsu, S. K.,** The role of tyrosyl groups in metal binding properties of transferrins, *Biochemistry,* 6, 1136, 1967.
105. **Jamieson, G. A., Jett, M., and de Barbados, S. L.,** The carbohydrate sequence of glycopeptide chains of human transferrin, *J. Biol. Chem.*, 246, 3686, 1971.
106. **Charlwood, P. A.,** Ultracentrifugal characteristics of human, monkey and rat transferrins, *Biochem. J.*, 88, 394, 1963.
107. **Roop, W. E. and Putnam, F. W.,** Purification and properties of human transferrin C and a slow moving genetic variant, *J. Biol. Chem.*, 242, 2507, 1967.
108. **Surgenor, D. M., Koechlin, B., and Strong, L. E.,** Chemical, clinical and immunological studies on products of human plasma fractionation, metal-combining globulin of human plasma, *J. Clin. Invest.*, 28, 73, 1949.
109. **Morgan, E. H.,** Transferrin and transferrin iron, in *Iron in Biochemistry and Medicine,* Jacobs, A. and Worwood, M., Eds., Academic Press, London, 1974, 29.
110. **MacGillivray, R. T. A. and Brew, K.,** Transferrin: internal homology in the amino acid sequence, *Science,* 190, 236, 1975.
111. **Warner, R. G. and Weber, I.,** Metal combining properties of conalbumin; cupric and ferric citrate complexes, *J. Am. Chem. Soc.*, 75, 5094, 1953.
112. **Lane, R. S.,** DEAE-cellulose chromatography of human transferrin: the effect of increasing iron saturation and copper (II) binding, *Biochim. Biophys. Acta,* 243, 193, 1971.
113. **Lane, R. S.,** Transferrin-reticulocyte binding: evidence for the functional importance of transferrin conformation, *Br. J. Haematol.*, 22, 309, 1972.

114. **Bezkorovainy, A., Rafelson, M. E., and Likhite, V.,** Isolation and partial characterization of transferrin from normal human plasma, *Arch. Biochem.*, 103, 371, 1963.
115. **Rosserieau-Motreff, M. Y., Soletewey, F., Lamote, R., and Peeters, H.,** Size and shape determination of apotransferrin and transferrin monomers, *Biopolymers,* 10, 1039, 1971.
116. **Azari, P. R. and Feeney, R. E.,** Resistance of metal complexes of conalbumin and transferrin to proteolysis and thermal denaturation, *J. Biol. Chem.*, 232, 293, 1958.
117. **Glazer, A. N. and McKenzie, H. A.,** The denaturation of proteins. IV. Conalbumin and iron. III. Conalbumin in urea solution, *Biochim. Biophys. Acta,* 71, 109, 1963.
118. **Clark, J. R., Osuga, D. T., and Feeney, R. E.,** A genetically varying minor protein constituent of chicken egg white, *J. Biol. Chem.*, 238, 3621, 1963.
119. **Bezkovainy, A.,** A comparative study of metal-free, iron-saturated and scialic acid-free transferrins, *Biochim. Biophys. Acta,* 127, 535, 1966.
120. **Bron, C., Blanc, C., and Isliker, H.,** Etude electrophoretique de la denaturation de transferrin humaine par l'uree, *Biochem. Biophys. Acta,* 154, 67, 1968.
121. **Faust, C. H. and Tengerdy, R. P.,** The role of antigenic conformation in antigen-antibody complex formation, *Immunochemistry,* 8, 211, 1971.
122. **Scuro, L. A., Dobrilla, G., Lo Carcio, V., Bosello, O., D'Andrea, F., and Innecco, A.,** Transferrin iron-binding capacity and total iron binding capacity. Discrepancy as an index of extra-transferrin iron transport, *Acta Hepato Gastroenterol.*, 19, 90, 1972.
123. **Ezekiel, E.,** The iron binding proteins in milk and the secretion of iron by the mammary gland in the rat, *Biochim. Biophys. Acta,* 107, 511, 1965.
124. **Jordan, S. M. and Morgan, E. H.,** Plasma protein synthesis by tissue slices from pregnant and lactating rats, *Biochim. Biophys. Acta,* 174, 373, 1969.
125. **Baker, E., Shaw, D. C., and Morgan, E. H.,** Isolation and characterization of rabbit serum and milk transferrins: evidence for difference in scialic acid content only, *Biochemistry,* 7, 1371, 1968.
126. **Jordan, S. M., Kaldor, I., and Morgan, E. H.,** Milk and serum iron-binding capacity in the rabbit, *Nature (London),* 215, 76, 1967.
127. **Jordan, S. M. and Morgan, E. H.,** Plasma protein metabolism during lactation in the rabbit, *Am. J. Physiol.*, 219, 1549, 1970.
128. **Morgan, E. H.,** Plasma protein turnover and transmission to the milk in the rat, *Biochim. Biophys. Acta,* 154, 478, 1968.
129. **Soltys, H. D. and Brody, J. I.,** Synthesis of transferrin by human peripheral blood lymphocytes, *J. Lab. Clin. Med.*, 75, 250, 1970.
130. **Gittin, D. and Pericelli, A.,** Synthesis of serum albumin, prealbumin, alpha-foetoprotein, alpha-1-antitrypsin and transferrin by the human yolk sac, *Nature (London),* 228, 995, 1970.
131. **Gitlin, D. and Boseman, M.,** Sites of serum alpha-fetoprotein synthesis in the human and in the rat, *J. Clin. Invest.*, 46, 1010, 1967.
132. **Masters, C. L., Bingold, L. P., and Morgan, E. H.,** Plasma protein metabolism and transfer to the fetus during pregnancy in the rat, *Am. J. Physiol.*, 216, 876, 1969.
133. **Morgan, E. H.,** A study of iron transfer from rabbit transferrin to reticulocytes using synthetic chelating agents, *Biochim. Biophys. Acta,* 244, 103, 1971.
134. **Morgan, E. H. and Peters, T.,** The biosynthesis of rat serum albumin. V. Effect of protein depletion and refeeding on albumin and transferrin synthesis, *J. Biol. Chem.*, 246, 3500, 1971.
135. **Antia, A. V., McFarlane, H., and Soothill, J. F.,** Serum siderophilin in kwashiorkor, *Arch. Dis. Child.*, 43, 459, 1967.
136. **McFarlane, H., Reddy, S., Adcock, K. J., Adeshina, H., Cooke, A. R., and Akere, J.,** Immunoglobulins, transferrin caeruloplasmin and heterophile antibodies in kwashiorkor, *Trop. Geogr. Med.*, 22, 61, 1970.
137. **Githri, D., Landing, B. H., and Whipple, A.,** Localization of homologous plasma proteins in tissues of young human beings as demonstrated with fluorescent antibodies, *J. Exp. Med.*, 97, 163, 1953.
138. **Von Ehrenstein, G.,** Iron transport through the lymph stream, *Acta Chem. Scand.*, 10, 703, 1956.
139. **Bogdanikowa, B. and Grabowski, R.,** Serum proteins present in edema fluid, *Clin. Chim. Acta,* 36, 351, 1972.
140. **Parker, W. C. and Bearn, A. G.,** Studies on the transferrins of adult serum, cord serum and cerebrospinal fluid. The effect of neuraminidase, *J. Exp. Med.*, 115, 83, 1962.
141. **Frick, E.,** Quantitative determination of transferrin in normal and pathological cerebrospinal fluid, *Klin. Wochenschr.*, 41, 75, 1963.
142. **Poortmens, J. and Jeanloz, R. W.,** Quantitative immunological determination of 12 plasma proteins excreted in human urine before and after exercise, *J. Clin. Invest.*, 47, 386, 1968.
143. **Morgan, E. H.,** Transferrin and albumin distribution and turnover in the rat, *Am. J. Physiol.*, 211, 1486, 1966.

144. **Morgan, E. H. and Peters, T.,** Intracellular aspects of transferrin synthesis and secretion in the rat, *J. Biol. Chem.*, 246, 3508, 1971.
145. **Morgan, E. H.,** Plasma iron binding capacity and iron stores in altered erythroid metabolism in the rat, *Q. J. Exp. Physiol.*, 48, 176, 1963.
146. **Wasserman, L. R., Sharney, L., Gevirtz, N. B., Schwartz, L., Weintraub, L. R., Tendler, D., Dumont, A. E., Dreiling, D., and Witte, M.,** Studies in iron kinetics. Interpretation of ferrokinetic data in man, *Proc. Soc. Exp. Biol. Med.*, 115, 817, 1964.
147. **Hampton, J. C.,** An electronmicroscope study of the source and distribution of ferritin in hepatic parenchymal cells of the newborn rabbit, *Blood,* 15, 480, 1960.
148. **Cheney, B. A., Lothe, K., Morgan, E. H., Sood, S. K., and Finch, C. A.,** Internal iron exchange in the rat, *Am. J. Physiol.*, 212, 376, 1967.
149. **Hoffenberg, R., Gordon, A. H., Black, E. G., and Louis, L. N.,** Plasma protein catabolism in the perfused rat liver. The effect of alteration of albumin concentration and dietary protein depletion, *Biochem. J.*, 118, 401, 1970.
150. **Waldmann, R. A., Wochner, R. D., and Strober, W.,** The role of the gastrointestinal tract in plasma protein metabolism, *Am. J. Med.*, 46, 275, 1969.
151. **Gardiner, M. E., Finlay-Jones, J. M., and Morgan, E. H.,** Catabolism and urinary excretion of albumin and transferrin before and after intravenous injection of albumin in the rat: with observations in the urinary excretion of IgG globulin, *Biochem. Med.*, 8, 287, 1973.
152. **Jarman, S. and Lassen, N. A.,** Albumin and transferrin metabolism in infectious and toxic diseases, *Scand. J. Clin. Lab. Invest.*, 13, 357, 1961.
153. **Awai, M. and Brown, E. B.,** Studies on the metabolism of I^{131} labeled human transferrin, *J. Lab. Clin. Med.*, 61, 363, 1963.
154. **Cromwell, S. M.,** The metabolism of transferrin, in *Protides of the Biological Fluids,* Peeters, H., Ed., Elsevier, Amsterdam, 1963, 484.
155. **Freeman, T. and Gordon, A. H.,** Albumin catabolism in hypoproteinemic states, studies with ^{131}I-albumin, *Bibl. Haematol.*, 23, 1108, 1966.
156. International Committee for Standardization in Hematology, Proposed recommendation for measurement of serum iron in human blood, *Br. J. Haematol.*, 20, 451, 1971.
157. International Committee for Standardization in Hematology, Studies on standardization of serum iron and iron binding capacity assays, in *Modern Concepts in Hematology,* Izak, G. and Lewis, S. M., Eds., Academic Press, New York, 197, 69.
158. International Committee for Standardization in Hematology, The measurement of total and unsaturated iron binding capacity in serum, *Br. J. Haematol.*, 1978.
159. **Dlott, D., Siegel, M. M., and Bersohn, R.,** A proposed flurometric determination of unsaturated iron-binding capacity, *Am. J. Clin. Pathol.*, 64, 217, 1975.
160. **Mazur, A., Green, S., Saha, A., and Carlton, A.,** Mechanism of release of ferritin iron in vivo by xanthine oxidase, *J. Clin. Invest.*, 37, 1809, 1958.
161. **Grace, N. D., Greenwald, M. A., and Greenberg, M. S.,** Effect of allopurinol on iron mobilization, *Gastroenterology,* 59, 103, 1970.
162. **Kozma, C., Salvador, R. A., and Elion, G. B.,** Allppurinol and iron storage, *Lancet,* 2, 1040, 1967.
163. **Freeden, E. and Osaki, S.,** Ferroxidases and ferrireductases; their role in iron metabolism, *Adv. Exp. Med. Biol.*, 48, 235, 1974.
164. **Bryce, C. F. A. and Crichton, R. R.,** The catalytic activity of horse spleen apoferritin. Preliminary kinetic studies and the effect of chemical modification, *Biochem. J.*, 133, 301, 1973.
165. **Drysdale, J. W. and Munro, H. N.,** Regulation of synthesis and turnover of ferritin in rat liver, *J. Biol. Chem.*, 241, 3630, 1966.
166. **Drysdale, J. W. and Shafritz, D. A.,** In vitro stimulation of apoferritin synthesis by iron, *Biochim. Biophys. Acta,* 383, 97, 1975.
167. **Zahringer, J., Baliga, B. S., and Munro, H. N.,** Novel mechanism for translational control in regulation of ferritin synthesis by iron, *Proc. Natl. Acad. Sci. U.S.A.*, 73, 857, 1976.
168. **Osaki, S., Johnson, D. A., and Frieden, E.,** The mobilization of iron from the perfused mammalian liver by a serum copper enzyme, ferroxidase. I, *J. Biol. Chem.*, 246, 3018, 1971.
169. **Lipschitz, D. A., Bothwell, T. H., Seftel, H. C., Wapnick, A. A., and Charlton, R. W.,** The role of ascorbic acid in the metabolism of storage iron, *Br. J. Haematol.*, 20, 155, 1971.
170. **Wapnick, A. A., Bothwell, T. H., and Seftel, H.,** The relationship between serum iron levels and ascorbic acid stores in siderotic Bantu, *Br. J. Haematol.*, 19, 271, 1970.
171. **Hershko, C., Cook, J. D., and Finch, C. A.,** Storage iron kinetics. VI. The effect of inflammation on iron exchange in the rat, *Br. J. Haematol.*, 28, 67, 1974.
172. **Fillet, G., Cook, J. D., and Finch, C. A.,** Storage iron kinetics. VII. A biologic model for reticuloendothelial iron transport, *J. Clin. Invest.*, 53, 1527, 1974.

173. **Noyes, W. D., Bothwell, T. H., and Finch, C. A.,** The role of the reticuloendothelial cell in iron metabolism, *Br. J. Haematol.*, 6, 43, 1960.
174. **Unger, A. and Hershko, C.,** Hepatocellular uptake of ferritin in the rat, *Br. J. Haematol.*, 28, 169, 1974.
175. **Schade, S. G. and Fried, W.,** The utilization of senescent red cell and hemolysate iron for erythropoiesis, *Proc. Soc. Exp. Biol. Med.*, 151, 78, 1976.
176. **Cook, J. D., Hershko, C., and Finch, C. A.,** Storage iron kinetics. IV. Cellular distribution of ferritin iron stores in rat liver, *Proc. Soc. Exp. Biol. Med.*, 145, 1378, 1974.
177. **Van Wyk, C. P., Linder-Horowitz, M., and Munro, H. N.,** Effect of iron loading on non heme iron compounds in different liver cell populations, *J. Biol. Chem.*, 246, 1025, 1971.
178. **Hershko, C., Cook, J. D., and Finch, C. A.,** Storage iron kinetics. II. The uptake of hemoglobin iron by hepatic parenchymal cells, *J. Lab. Clin. Med.*, 80, 624, 1972.
179. **Hershko, C.,** The fate of circulating haemoglobin, *Br. J. Haematol.*, 29, 199, 1975.
180. **Muller-Eberhard, U., Bosman, C., and Liem, H. H.,** Tissue localization of the heme-hemopexin complex in the rabbit and the rat as studied by light microscopy with the use of radioisotopes, *J. Lab. Clin. Med.*, 76, 426, 1970.
181. **Bissell, D. M., Hammaker, L., and Schmid, R.,** Hemoglobin and erythrocyte catabolism in rat liver. The separate roles of parenchymal and sinusoidal cells, *Blood*, 40, 812, 1972.
182. **Bothwell, T. H. and Finch, C. A.,** *Iron Metabolism*, Little, Brown, Boston, 1962, 286.
183. **Douglas, A. S. and Dacie, J. V.,** The incidence and significance of iron-containing granules in human erythrocytes and their precursors, *J. Clin. Pathol.*, 6, 307, 1953.
184. **Henderson, P. A. and Hillman, R. S.,** Characteristics of iron dextran utilization in man, *Blood*, 34, 357, 1969.
185. **Balcerzak, S. P., Westerman, M. P., Heinle, E. W., and Taylor, R. H.,** Measurement of iron stores using deferoxamine, *Ann. Intern. Med.*, 68, 518, 1968.
186. **Ploem, J. E., de Wael, J., Verloop, M. C., and Punt, H.,** Sideruria following a single dose of desferrioxamine-B as a diagnostic test in iron overload, *Br. J. Haematol.*, 12, 396, 1966.
187. **Barry, M., Cartei, G., and Sherlock, S.,** Quantitative measurement of iron stores with diethylenetriamine penta-acetic acid, *Gut*, 11, 291, 1970.
188. **Waxman, H. S. and Brown, E. B.,** Clinical usefulness of iron chelating agents, *Progr. Hematol.*, 6, 338, 1969.
189. **Hallberg, L., Hedenberg, L., and Weinfeld, A.,** Liver iron and desferrioxamine-induced urinary iron excretion, *Scand. J. Haematol.*, 3, 85, 1966.
190. **Harker, L. A., Funk, D. D., and Finch, C. A.,** Evaluation of storage iron by chelates, *Am. J. Med.*, 45, 105, 1968.
191. **Hershko, C., Cook, J. C., and Finch, C. A.,** Storage iron kinetics. III. Study of desferrioxamine action by selective radioiron labels of R.E. and parenchymal cells, *J. Lab. Clin. Med.*, 81, 876, 1973.
192. **Wapnick, A. A., Lynch, S. R., Charlton, R. W., Seftel, H. C., and Bothwell, T. H.,** The effect of ascorbic acid deficiency on desferrioxamine-induced urinary iron excretion, *Br. J. Haematol.*, 17, 563, 1969.
193. **Hershko, C. and Rachmilewitz, E. A.,** The inhibitory effect of vitamin E on desferrioxamine-induced iron excretion in rats, *Pro. Soc. Exp. Biol. Med.*, 152, 249, 1976.
194. **Haskins, D., Stevens, A. R., Finch, S., and Finch, C. A.,** Iron metabolism. Iron stores in man as measured by phlebotomy, *J. Clin. Invest.*, 31, 543, 1952.
195. **Walters, G. O., Miller, F. M., and Worwood, M.,** Serum ferritin concentration and iron stores in normal subjects, *J. Clin. Pathol.*, 26, 770, 1973.
196. **Charlton, R. W., Hawkins, D. M., Mavor, W. O., and Bothwell, T. H.,** Hepatic storage iron concentrations in different population groups, *Am. J. Clin. Nutr.*, 23, 358, 1970.
197. **Reissmann, K. R. and Dietrich, M. R.,** On the presence of ferritin in the peripheral blood of patients with hepatocellular disease, *J. Clin. Invest.*, 35, 588, 1956.
198. **Aungst, C. W.,** A specific and sensitive method for the detection of ferritin in body fluids, *J. Lab. Clin. Med.*, 67, 307, 1966.
199. **Addison, G. M., Beamish, M. B., Hales, C. N., Hodgkins, M., Jacobs, A., and Llewellin, P.,** An immunoradioactive assay for ferritin in the serum of normal subjects and patients with iron deficiency and iron overload, *J. Clin. Pathol.*, 25, 326, 1972.
200. **Miles, L. E. M., Lipschitz, D. A., Bieber, C. P., and Cook, J. D.,** Measurement of serum ferritin by a 2-site immunoradiometric assay, *Anal. Biochem.*, 61, 209, 1974.
201. **Worwood, M.,** Serum ferritin, in *Meth. Hematol.*, 1, 59—89, 1980.
202. **Luxton, A. W., Walker, W. H. C., Gauldie, J., Ali, M. A. M., and Pelletier, C.,** A radioimmunoassay for serum ferritin, *Clin. Chem.*, 23, 683, 1977.
203. **Barnett, M. D., Gordon, Y. B., Amess, J. A. L., and Mollin, D. L.,** The measurement of ferritin in serum by radioimmunoassay, *J. Clin. Pathol.*, 31, 742, 1978.

204. **Deppe, W. M., Joubert, S. M., and Naidoo, P.,** Radioimmunoassay of serum ferritin, *J. Clin. Pathol.,* 31, 872, 1978.
205. **Wide, L. and Birgegard, G. A.,** A solid phase radioimmunoassay for serum ferritin using ^{125}I-labelled ferritin, *Uppsala J. Med. Sci.,* 82, 15, 1977.
206. **Halliday, J. W., Gera, K. L., and Powell, L. W.,** Solid phase radioimmunoassay for serum ferritin, *Clin. Chim. Acta,* 58, 207, 1975.
207. **Theriault, L. and Page, M.,** A solid phase enzyme immunoassay for serum ferritin, *Clin. Chem.,* 23, 2142, 1977.
208. **Zuyderhoudt, F. M. J., Boers, W., Linthorst, C., Jörning, G. G. A., and Hengeveld, P.,** An enzyme-linked immunoassay for ferritin in human serum and rat plasma and the influence of the iron in serum ferritin on serum iron measurement, during acute hepatitis, *Clin. Chim. Acta,* 88, 37, 1978.
209. **Watanabe, N., Niitsu, Y., Ohtsuka, S., Koseki, J., Kohgo, Y., Urushizaki, I., Mato, K., and Ishikawa, E.,** Enzyme immunoassay for human ferritin, *Clin. Chem.,* 25, 80, 1979.
210. **Marcus, D. M. and Zinberg, N.,** Measurement of serum ferritin by radioimmunoassay: results in normal individuals and patients with breast cancer, *J. Natl. Cancer Inst.,* 55, 791, 1975.
211. **Konijn, A. M., Levy, R., Link, G., and Hershko, C.,** A rapid and sensitive ELISA for serum ferritin employing a fluorogenic substrate, *J. Immunol. Meth.,* 54, 297, 1982.
212. **Worwood, M.,** Serum ferritin, *CRC Crit. Rev. Clin. Lab. Sci.,* 10, 171, 1979.
213. **Halliday, J. W. and Powell, L. W.,** Serum ferritin and isoferritins in clinical medicine, *Progr. Hematol.,* 11, 229—266, 1979.
214. **Bezwoda, W. R., Bothwell, T. H., Torrance, J. D., MacPhail, A. P., and Charlton, R. W.,** The relationship between marrow iron stores, plasma ferritin concentrations and iron absorption, *Scand. J. Haemat.,* 22, 113, 1979.
215. **Heinrich, H. C., Bruggemann, J., Gabbe, E. E., and Glazer, M.,** Correlation between diagnostic FE^{59} (2+) absorption and serum ferritin concentration in man, *Z. Naturforsch.,* 32C, 1023, 1977.
216. **Cook, J. D., Lipschitz, D. A., Miles, L. E. M., and Finch, C. A.,** Serum ferritin as a measure of iron stores in normal subjects, *Am J. Clin. Nutr.,* 27, 681, 1974.
217. **Walters, G. O., Jacobs, A., Worwood, M., Trevett, D., and Thomson, W.,** Iron absorption in normal subjects and patients with idiopathic haemochromatosis: relationship with serum ferritin concentration, *Gut,* 16, 188, 1975.
218. **Cook, J. D., Skikne, B. S., and Lynch, S. R.,** Serum ferritin in the evaluation of anemia, in *Radioimmunoassay of Hormones, Proteins and Enzymes,* Albertini, A., Ed., Excerpta Medica, Amsterdam, 1980, 239—248.
219. **Valberg, L. S., Sorbie, J., Ludwig, J., and Pelletiev, O.,** Serum ferritin and the iron status of Canadians, *Can. Med. J.,* 114, 417, 1976.
220. **Lundström, U., Siimes, M. A., and Dallman, P. R.,** At what age does iron supplementation become necessary in low-birth weight infants?, *J. Pediatr.,* 91, 878, 1977.
221. **Fenton, V., Cavill, I., and Fisher, J.,** Iron stores in pregnancy, *Br. J. Haematol.,* 37, 145, 1977.
222. **Finch, C. A., Cook, J. D., Labbe, R. F., and Culala, M.,** Effect of blood donation on iron stores as evaluated by serum ferritin, *Blood,* 50.
223. **Bentley, D. P. and Jacobs, A.,** Accumulation of storage iron in patients treated for iron deficiency anaemia, *Br. Med. J.,* 2, 64, 1975.
224. **Hershko, C., Bar-Or, D., Gaziel, E., Naparstek, E., Konijn, A. M., Grossowicz, N., Kaufman, N., and Izak, G.,** Diagnosis of iron deficiency anemia in a rural population of children. Relative usefulness of serum ferritin, red cell protoporphyrin, red cell indices, and transferrin saturation determinations, *Am. J. Clin. Nutr.,* 39, 1600, 1981.
225. **Dallman, P. R.,** Serum ferritin in the diagnosis of iron deficiency, in *Radioimmunoassay of Hormones, Proteins, and Enzymes,* Albertini, A., Ed., Excerpta Medica, Amsterdam, 1980, 230—238.
226. **Cartwright, G. E. and Lee, G. R.,** The anaemia of chronic disorders, *Br. J. Haematol.,* 21, 147, 1971.
227. **Hershko, C., Cook, J. D., and Finch, C. A.,** Storage iron kinetics. VI. The effect of inflammation on iron exchange in the rat, *Br. J. Haematol.,* 28, 67, 1974.
228. **Lipschitz, D. A., Cook, J. D., and Finch, C. A.,** A clinical evaluation of serum ferritin as an index of iron stores, *N. Engl. J. Med.,* 290, 1213, 1974.
229. **Bentley, D. P. and Williams, P.,** Serum ferritin concentration as an index of storage iron in rheumatoid arthritis, *J. Clin. Pathol.,* 27, 786, 1974.
230. **Smith, R. J., Davis, P., Thomson, A. B. R., Wadsworth, L. D., and Fackre, P.,** Serum ferritin levels in anemia of rheumatoid arthritis, *J. Rheum.,* 4, 389, 1977.
231. **Koerper, M. A., Stempel, D. A., and Dallman, P. R.,** Anemia in patients with juvenile rheumatoid arthritis, *J. Pediatr.,* 92, 930, 1978.
232. **Hussein, S., Prieto, J., O'Shea, M., Hoffbrand, A. V., Baillod, R. A., and Moorhead, J. F.,** Serum ferritin assay and iron status in chronic renal failure and haemodialysis, *Br. Med. J.,* 1, 546, 1975.

233. **Mirahmadi, K. S., Wellington, L. P., Winer, R. L., Dabir-Vaziri, N., Byer, B., Gorman, J. T., and Rosen, S. M.**, Serum ferritin level. Determinant of iron requirement in hemodialysis patients, *JAMA*, 238, 601, 1977.
234. **Aljama, P., Ward, M. K., Pierides, A. M., Eastham, E. J., Ellis, H. A., Feest, T. G., Conceirao, S., and Kerr, D. N. S.**, Serum ferritin concentration; a reliable guide to iron overload in uremic and hemodialyzed patients, *Clin. Nephrol.*, 10, 101, 1978.
235. **Ellis, D.**, Serum ferritin compared with other indices of iron status in children and teenagers undergoing maintenance hemodialysis, *Clin. Chem.*, 25, 741, 1979.
236. **Cotterill, A. M., Flather, J. N., Cattell, W. R., Barnett, M. D., and Baker, L. R. I.**, Serum ferritin concentration and oral iron treatment in patients on regular haemodialysis, *Br. Med. J.*, 1, 790, 1979.
237. **Lynn, K. L., Mitchell, T. R., and Sheppard, J.**, Serum ferritin concentration in patients receiving maintenance hemodialysis, *Clin. Nephrol.*, 14, 124, 1980.
238. **Bell, J. D., Kincaid, W. R., Morgan, R. Y., Bunce, H., Alperin, J. B., Sarles, H. E., and Remmers, A. R.**, Serum ferritin assay and bone-marrow iron stores in patients on maintenance hemodialysis, *Kidney Int.*, 17, 237, 1980.
239. **Birgegard, G., Nilsson, P., and Wide, L.**, Regulation of iron therapy by serum ferritin estimations in patients on chronic hemodialysis, *Scand. J. Urol. Nephrol.*, 15, 69, 1981.
240. **Moreb, J., Popovtzer, M. M., Friedlaender, M. M., Konijn, A. M., and Hershko, C.**, Evaluation of iron status in patients on chronic hemodialysis: relative usefulness of bone marrow hemosiderin serum ferritin, transferrin saturation, mean corpuscular volume and red cell protoporphyrin, *Nephron*, in press, 1985.
241. **Halliday, J. W., Russo, A. M., Cowlishaw, J. L., and Powell, L. W.**, Serum ferritin in diagnosis of hemochromatosis, *Lancet*, 2, 621, 1977.
242. **Prieto, J., Barry, M., and Sherlock, S.**, Serum ferritin in patients with iron overload and with acute and chronic liver diseases, *Gastroenterology*, 68, 525, 1975.
243. **Edwards, C. O., Carroll, M., Bray, P., and Cartwright, G. E.**, Hereditary hemochromatosis. Diagnosis in siblings and children, *N. Engl. J. Med.*, 297, 7, 1977.
244. **Wands, J. R., Rowe, J. A., and Mezey, S. E.**, Normal serum ferritin concentrations in precirrhotic hemochromatosis, *N. Engl. J. Med.*, 294, 302, 1976.
245. **Powell, L. W. and Halliday, J. W.**, Serum ferritin in hemochromatosis, *N. Engl. J. Med.*, 294, 1185, 1976.
246. **Crosby, W. H.**, Normal serum ferritin in precirrhotic hemochromatosis, *N. Engl. J. Med.*, 296, 1116, 1977.
247. **Letsky, E. A., Miller, F., Worwood, M., and Flynn, D. M.**, Serum ferritin in children with thalassemia regularly transfused, *J. Clin. Pathol.*, 27, 652, 1974.
248. **Hershko, C., Konijn, A. M., and Loria, A.**, Serum ferritin in beta thalassemia, in *Radioimmunoassay of Hormones, Proteins and Enzymes*, Albertini, A., Ed., Excerpta Medica, Amsterdam, 1980, 249—255.
249. **Hazard, J. T. and Drysdale, J. W.**, Ferritinaemia in cancer, *Nature (London)*, 265, 755, 1977.
250. **Jones, B. M. and Worwood, M.**, An immunoradiometric assay for the acidic ferritin of human heart; application to human tissues, cells and serum, *Clin. Chim. Acta*, 85, 81, 1978.
251. **Niitsu, Y., Goto, Y., Kohgo, Y., Adachi, C., Onodera, Y., and Urushizaki, I.**, Evaluation of heart isoferritin assay for diagnosis of cancer, in *Radioimmunoassay of Hormones, Proteins and Enzymes*, Albertini, A., Ed., Excerpta Medica, Amsterdam, 1980, 256—266.
252. **Matzner, Y., Konijn, A. M., and Hershko, C.**, Serum ferritin in hematologic malignancies, *Am. J. Hematol.*, 9, 13, 1980.
253. **Jacobs, A., Slater, A., Whittaker, J. A., Canellos, G., and Wiernik, P. H.**, Serum ferritin concentration in untreated Hodgkin's disease, *Br. J. Cancer*, 34, 162, 1976.
254. **Parry, D. H., Ricketts, C., and Jacobs, A.**, Serum ferritin in unmaintained remission in acute lymphoblastic leukaemia, *Br. Med. J.*, 2, 1341, 1978.
255. **Arosio, P., Yokota, M., and Drysdale, J. W.**, Structural and immunological relationships of isoferritins in normal and malignant cells, *Cancer Res.*, 36, 1735, 1976.
256. **Hazard, J. T., Yokota, M., Srosio, P., and Drysdale, J. W.**, Immunologic differences in human isoferritins; implications for immunologic quantitation of serum ferritin, *Blood*, 49, 139, 1977.
257. **Drysdale, J., Kohgo, Y., and Watanabe, N.**, Ferritin phenotypes, in *Radioimmunoassay of Hormones, Proteins and Enzymes*, Albertini, A., Ed., Excerpta Medica, Amsterdam, 1980, 213—220.
258. **Worwood, M.**, Structure and metabolism of serum ferritin, in *Radioimmunoassay of Hormones, Proteins and Enzymes*, Albertini, A., Ed., Excerpta Medica, Amsterdam, 1980, 213—220.
259. **Hahn, P. F., Bale, W. F., Laurence, E. O., and Whipple, G. H.**, Radioactive iron and its metabolism in anemia. Its absorption, transportation and utilization, *J. Exp. Med.*, 69, 739, 1939.
260. **Hahn, P. F., Baie, W. F., Ross, J. F., Hettig, R. A., and Whipple, G. H.**, Radioiron in plasma does not exchange with hemoglobin iron in red cells, *Science*, 92, 131, 1940.

261. **Huff, R. L. and Judd, O. J.,** Kinetics of iron metabolism, in *Advances in Biology and Medical Physics,* Vol. 4, Lawrence, J. H. and Tobias, C. A., Eds., Academic Press, New York, 1956, 223.
262. **Finch, C. A., Gibson, J. G., Peacock, W. C., and Fluharty, R. G.,** Iron metabolism. Utilization of intravenous radioactive iron, *Blood,* 4, 905, 1949.
263. **Huff, R. L., Hennessy, T. G., Austin, R. E., Garcia, J. F., Roberts, B. M., and Lawrence, J. H.,** Plasma and red cell iron turnover in normal subjects and in patients having various hematopoietic disorders, *J. Clin. Invest.,* 29, 1041, 1950.
264. **Huff, R. L., Elmlinger, P. J., Garcia, J. F., Oda, J. M., Cockrell, M. C., and Lawrence, J. H.,** Ferrokinetics in normal persons and in patients having various erythropoietic disorders, *J. Clin. Invest.,* 30, 1512, 1951.
265. **Finch, C. A., Deubelbeiss, K., Cook, J. D., Eschbach, L. A., Funk, D. D., Marsaglia, G., Hillman, R. A., Schlichter, S., Adamson, J. W., Ganzoni, A., and Giblett, E. R.,** Ferrokinetics in man, *Medicine,* 49, 17, 1970.
266. **Funk, D. D.,** Plasma iron turnover in normal subjects, *J. Nucl. Med.,* 11, 107, 1970.
267. **Adamson, J. W., Eschbach, J., and Finch, C. A.,** The kidney and erythropoiesis, *Am. J. Med.,* 44, 725, 1968.
268. **Pollycove, M.,** Iron metabolism and kinetics, *Semin. Hematol.,* 3, 235, 1966.
269. **Layrisse, M., Linares, J., and Roche, M.,** Excess hemolysis in subjects with severe iron deficiency anemia associated and nonassociated with hookworm infection, *Blood,* 25, 73, 1965.
270. **Cartwright, G. E. and Lee, G. R.,** The anemia of chronic disorders, *Br. J. Haematol.,* 21, 147, 1971.
271. **Finch, C. A., Coleman, D. H., Motulsky, A. G., Donohue, D. M., and Reiff, R. H.,** Erythrokinetics in pernicious anemia, *Blood,* 11, 807, 1956.
272. **Sturgeon, P. and Finch, C. A.,** Erythrokinetics in Cooley's anemia, *Blood,* 12, 64, 1957.
273. **Roath, S., Bourne, M. S., and Israels, M. C. G.,** Ferrokinetics in pyridoxine-responsive anemia, *Acta Haematol.,* 32, 1, 1964.
274. **Pollycove, M. and Mortimer, R.,** A quantitative determination of iron kinetics and hemoglobin synthesis in human subjects, *J. Clin. Invest.,* 40, 753, 1961.
275. **Garby, L., Schneider, W., Sundquist, O., and Vuille, J. C.,** A ferro-erythrokinetic model and its properties, *Acta Physiol. Scand.,* 59(216), 1, 1963.
276. **Cavill, I. and Ricketts, C.,** The kinetics of iron metabolism, in *Iron in Biochemistry and Medicine,* Jacobs, A. and Worwood, M., Eds., Academic Press, London, 1974, 614.
277. **Hosain, F., Marsaglia, G., and Finch, C. A.,** Blood ferrokinetics in normal man, *J. Clin. Invest.,* 46, 1, 1967.
278. **Fillet, G.,** Etuderadioisotopique de la reutilisation du fer chez l'animal et chez l'homme, These du grade d'Agrege de l'Enseignement Superieur, Universite de Liege, 1977.
279. **Hillman, R. S. and Finch, C. A.,** Erythropoiesis: normal and abnormal, *Semin. Hematol.,* 4, 327, 1967.
280. **Olsson, K. S.,** Iron stores in normal men and male blood donors, *Acta Med. Scand.,* 192, 401, 1972.
281. **Pritchard, J. and Mason, R. A.,** Iron stores of normal adults and replenishment with oral iron therapy, *JAMA,* 190, 897, 1964.
282. **Konijn, A. M., Levy, R., and Tal, R.,** Isolation of basic and acid isoferritins from human term placenta for use as antigens in serum ferritin immunoassays. Abstracts Iron Club Meeting, September 2—5, 1982, Os, Bergen, Norway.
283. **Marechal, J. C., Dublet, B., Wustefeld, C., Charlier, G., and Crichton, R. R.,** Immunological characteristics of human ferritins: consequences for human serum ferritin determination, *Clin. Chim. Acta,* 111, 99, 1981.
284. **Imagawa, M., Yoshitake, S., Ishikawa, E., Niitsu, Y., Urushizaki, Y., Kanazawa, R., Tachibana, S., Nakazawa, N., and Ogawa, H.,** Development of a highly sensitive sandwich enzyme immunoassay for human ferritin using affinity-purified anti-ferritin labelled with β-D-galactodidase from *Escherichia coli, Clin. Chim. Acta,* 121, 277, 1982.
285. **Ghielmi, S., Pizzoccolo, G., Jacobello, C., Albertini, A., and Arosio, P.,** Methodological effects on the quantitation of serum ferritin by radio- and enzymeimmunoassays, *Clin. Chim. Acta,* 120, 285, 1982.
286. **Cragg, S. J., Wagstaff, M., and Worwood, M.,** Detection of glycosylated subunit in human serum ferritin, *Biochem. J.,* 199, 565, 1981.
287. **Cartwright, G. E., Edwards, C. O., Krevits, K., Skolnick, M., Amos, D. B., Johnson, A., and Buskjaer, L.,** Hereditary hemochromatosis: phenotype expression of the disease, *N. Engl. J. Med.,* 301, 175, 1979.
288. **Simon, M., Bourel, M., Genetet, B., and Fauchet, R.,** Idiopathic hemochromatosis. Demonstration of recessive transmission and early detection by family HLA typing, *N. Engl. J. Med.,* 297, 1017, 1977.
289. **Edwards, C. O., Skolnick, M. H., and Kushner, J. P.,** Hereditary hemochromatosis: contribution of genetic analyses, *Progr. Hematol.,* 12, 43, 1981.
290. **MacSween, R. N. M. and Scott, A. R.,** Hepatic cirrhosis: a clinicopathological review of 520 cases, *J. Clin. Pathol.,* 26, 936, 1973.

291. **Crichton, R. R., Heuterspreute, M., Mathijs, M. M., Wustefeld, C., Charlier, G., and Chen, M.,** Structural studies on ferritins, in *The Biochemistry and Physiology of Iron,* Saltman, P. and Begenauer, J., Eds., Elsevier/North-Holland, Amsterdam, 1982, 353—358.
292. **Heuterspreute, M. and Crichton, R. R.,** Amino acid sequence of horse spleen ferritin, *FEBS Lett.,* 129, 322, 1981.
293. **Bourne, P. E., Harrison, P. M., Lewis, W. G., Rice, D. W., Smith, J. M. A., and Stansfield, R. F. D.,** The structure and function of ferritin. Past progress and future promise, in *The Biochemistry and Physiology of Iron,* Saltman, P. and Hegenauer, J., Eds., Elsevier/North-Holland, Amsterdam, 1982, 345—351.
294. **Banyard, S. H., Stammers, D. K., and Harrison, P. M.,** Electron density map of apoferriton at 2.8 Å resolution, *Nature (London),* 271, 282, 1978.
295. **Jandl, J. H. and Katz, J. H.,** The plasma-to-cell cycle of transferrin, *J. Clin. Invest.,* 42, 314, 1963.
296. **Kornfeld, S.,** The effect of metal attachment to human apotransferrin on its binding to reticulocytes, *Biochem. Biophys. Acta,* 194, 25, 1969.
297. **Morgan, E. H. and Appleton, T. C.,** Autoradiographic localization of ^{125}I-labelled transferrin in rabbit reticulocytes, *Nature (London),* 223, 1371, 1979.
298. **Armstrong, N. J. and Morgan, E. H.,** The effect of intracellular pH on the uptake of transferrin-bound iron by immature erythroid cells, in *Biochemistry and Physiology of Iron,* Saltman, P. and Hegenauer, J., Eds., Elsevier/North-Holland, Amsterdam, 1982, 149—157.
299. **Hemmaplardh, D. and Morgan, E. H.,** The role of endocytosis in transferrin uptake by reticulocytes and bone marrow cells, *Br. J. Haematol.,* 36, 85, 1977.
300. **Jacobs, A., Jones, B., Ricketts, C., Hayward, J. C., Bulbrook, R. D., and Wang, D. Y.,** Serum ferritin concentration in early breast cancer, *Br. J. Cancer,* 34, 286, 1976.
301. **Hann, H. L., Levy, H. M., and Evans, A. E.,** Serum ferritin as a guide to therapy in neuroblastoma, *Cancer Res.,* 40, 1411, 1980.
302. **Hann, H. L., Evans, A. E., Cohen, I. J., and Leitmeyer, B. A.,** Biologic differences between neuroblastoma stages IV-S and IV. Measurement of serum ferritin and E-rosette inhibition in 30 children, *N. Engl. J. Med.,* 305, 425, 1981.
303. **Romslo, I.,** Intracellular transport of iron, in *Iron in Biochemistry and Medicine,* Vol. 2, Jacobs, A. and Worwood, M., Eds., Academic Press, New York, 1980, 325.
304. **Pollack, S. and Lasky, F. D.,** Guinea pig intestinal iron binding protein, *Biochem. Biophys. Res. Commun.,* 70, 533, 1976.
305. **Huebers, H., Huebers, E., Rummel, W., and Crichton, R. R.,** Isolation and characterization of iron-binding proteins from rat intestinal mucosa, *Eur. J. Biochem.,* 66, 447, 1976.
306. **El-Shobaki, F. A. and Rummel, W.,** The role of mucosal iron binding proteins in adaptation of iron absorption during protein deficiency and rehabilitation, *Res. Exp. Med. (Berl.),* 173, 119, 1978.
307. **Harrison, P. M., Clegg, G. A., and May, K.,** Ferritin structure and function, in *Iron in Biochemistry and Medicine,* Vol. 2, Jacobs, A. and Worwood, M., Eds., Academic Press, New York, 1980, 131—171.

RED CELL ENZYMES

Hisaichi Fujii and Shiro Miwa

INTRODUCTION

Since there are no nucleus, mitochondria, or microsomes in mature red cells, the red cell supports itself through the most primitive and universal pathway of metabolism. Glucose, the main metabolic substrate of red cells, is metabolized via two major pathways: (1) the Embden-Meyerhof or glycolytic pathway and (2) the hexose monophosphate pathway (Figure 1). Under normal circumstances, about 90% of glucose entering the red cell is metabolized by the glycolytic pathway and 10% by the hexose monophosphate pathway. The glycolytic pathway is the only pathway of ATP synthesis in the mature red cell, 2 mol of ATP being generated per mole of glucose consumed. Important functions of red cell ATP include active transport of sodium and potassium, maintenance of low intracellular calcium levels, phosphorylation of membrane protein, and sustenance of glycolysis itself. Glycolysis is also the major source of red cell reduced nicotinamide adenine dinucleotide (NADH), an essential cofactor for methemoglobin reductase, which catalyzes the conversion of methemoglobin to functional hemoglobin. At the step of phosphoglycerate kinase (PGK), energy generation is by-passed by the Rapoport-Leubering cycle, as a result of which 2,3-diphosphoglycerate (2,3-DPG) is formed. The 2,3-DPG has an important role in regulating the oxygen-dissociation curve of hemoglobin and also provides a reservoir of triose.

Of the 11 glycolytic enzymes, at least 7 enzyme anomalies associated with congenital nonspherocytic hemolytic anemia have been reported (Table 1). Under such circumstances, the viability of the red cell is reduced, and hemolytic anemia results.

The most important product of the hexose monophosphate pathway is reduced nicotinamide adenine dinucleotide phosphate (NADPH). Another important function is to provide ribose for nucleotide and nucleic acid synthesis. NADPH, by serving as a cofactor in the reduction of oxidized glutathione (GSSG), is a major reducing agent in the red cell and the ultimate source of protection against oxidative attack. In the syndromes associated with dysfunction of the hexose monophosphate pathway and glutathione metabolism, oxidative denaturation of hemoglobin is the major contributor to the hemolytic process.

Deficiency of glycolytic enzymes, of enzymes of the hexose monophosphate pathway and closely related GSH metabolism, and of enzymes of nucleotide metabolism have emerged as causes of hereditary nonspherocytic hemolytic anemia as shown in Table 1. The purpose of this chapter is to review congenital nonspherocytic hemolytic anemia associated with red cell enzyme deficiency, hereditary methemoglobinemia, and the significance of the determination of red cell enzyme activities for nonhematologic disorders.

HEREDITARY HEMOLYTIC ANEMIA ASSOCIATED WITH RED CELL ENZYME DEFICIENCY

Defects in the Embden-Meyerhof Pathway and Rapoport-Leubering Cycle

Hexokinase Deficiency

The initial step in glycolysis, whereby glucose is catalytically phosphorylated to glucose 6-phosphate by hexokinase (Hx), is especially critical to human red cell metabolism. Of all the glycolytic enzymes of the red cell, Hx is the lowest in activity, and is the most influenced by red cell age. It has been estimated that the mature red cell may have no more than 2 to 3% of the Hx activity originally presented in the reticulocyte.[1] Hx is monomer with a molecular weight of 100,000, and exists as four isozymes (Hx I, II, III, and IV) with distinct

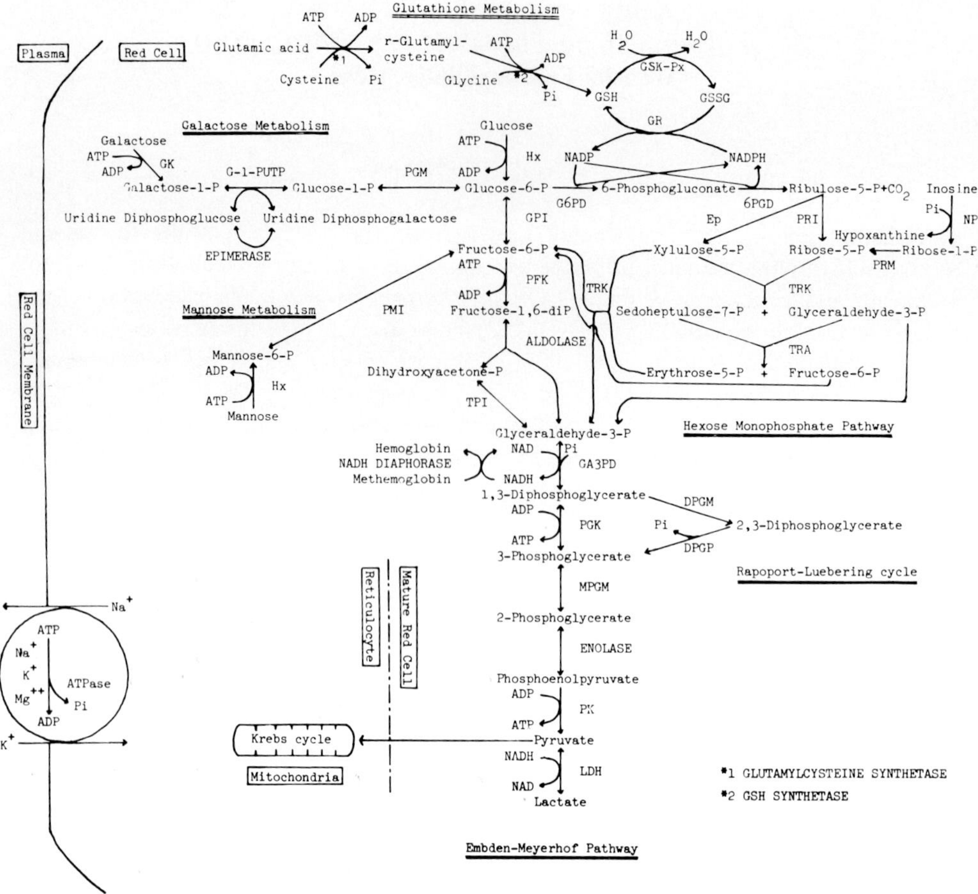

FIGURE 1. Major pathways of energy metabolism in human red cells. Abbreviations: GK, galactokinase; G-1-PUTP, galactose-1-P uridyl transferase; PGM, phosphoglucomutase; PMI, phosphomannose isomerase; Hx, hexokinase; GPI, phosphoglucose isomerase; PFK, phosphofructokinase; TPI, triosephosphate isomerase; GA3PD, glyceraldehyde 3-phosphate dehydrogenase; PGK, phosphoglycerate kinase; DPGM, diphosphoglyceromutase; DPGP, diphosphoglycerophosphatase; MPGM, monophosphoglyceromutase; PK, pyruvate kinase; LDH, lactate dehydrogenase; GR, glutathione reductase; GSH-Px, glutathione peroxidase; G6PD, glucose 6-phosphate dehydrogenase; 6-PGD, 6-phosphogluconate dehydrogenase; EP, epimerase; PRI, phosphoribose isomerase; TRK, transketolase; TRA, transaldolase; NP, nucleoside phosphorylase; PRM, phosphoribomutase.

kinetic properties and tissue distribution. Red cell Hx is mainly of type I, which is separated into three major forms, designated Hx Ia, Ib, and Ic. In young red cells, Hx Ib is predominant. The mature red cell contains Hx III, which is not found in the fetal cell, and lower levels of Hx Ib.[2]

Congenital nonspherocytic hemolytic anemia with Hx deficiency was first reported by Valentine et al.[3] in 1967. Following this article, there have been 12 further reports as shown in Table 2.[4-15] Family studies are most consistent with an autosomal recessive mode of inheritance, but a dominant mode of inheritance was suggested in the case reported by Newman et al.[13] Red cell morphology is unremarkable except for one patient who showed striking morphological abnormalities, such as spherocytes, target cells, ''sickle'' cells, and ''pincered'' cells.[13] In general, anemia and hyperbilirubinemia are prominent in the newborn period or the first decade of life. Goebel et al.[7] reported a woman who revealed hemolytic anemia, multiple malformations, and a latent diabetes mellitus. The diagnosis of Hx deficiency is not always simple. Because Hx is one of the most age-dependent enzymes, a

Table 1
RED CELL ENZYME ANOMALIES ASSOCIATED WITH HEMOLYTIC ANEMIA

Red cell enzyme anomalies	Mode of inheritance
Embden-Meyerhof pathway	
Hexokinase deficiency	Autosomal recessive
Glucosephosphate isomerase deficiency	Autosomal recessive
Phosphofructokinase deficiency	Autosomal recessive
Aldolase deficiency	Autosomal recessive
Triosephosphate isomerase deficiency	Autosomal recessive
Phosphoglycerate kinase deficiency	Sex-linked
Pyruvate kinase deficiency	Autosomal recessive
Rapoport-Luebering cycle	
Diphosphoglyceromutase deficiency	Autosomal recessive
Hexose monophosphate pathway and glutathione metabolism	
Glucose 6-phosphate dehydrogenase deficiency	Sex-linked
Glutathione reductase deficiency	Autosomal recessive
Glutathione peroxidase deficiency	Autosomal
Glutathione synthetase deficiency	Autosomal recessive
γ-Glutamyl-cysteine synthetase deficiency	Autosomal recessive
Nucleotide metabolism	
Adenylate kinase deficiency	Unknown
Pyrimidine 5′-nucleotidase deficiency	Autosomal recessive
Overproduction of adenosine deaminase	Autosomal dominant

Table 2
HEXOKINASE DEFICIENCY

Kindred	Age (years)	Sex	Hemoglobin (g/dℓ)	Reticulocyte (%)	Red cell hexokinase activity (% of normal)	Ref.
1	5 months	F	9.4	13.4	63	3
2	38	F	(Ht:36%)	7—13	79	4
3	22	M	—	1.7—6.3	49	5
4	2	M	6.5	5	75	6
5	28	F	8.5—9.6	2.4	39	7
6	30	F	11.3	39	53	8
7	33 months	M	8.6—9.4	6.7—8.5	53	9
8	11	F	11.6	5.1	83	10
9	9	F	8.7	11.6	68	11
10	1	F	7.0—9.2	3.1—8.1	48	12
11	19	M	13.8	33	180	13
12	7	M	9.7	3.6	70	14
13	19	F	9.8	50	25	15

deficiency of the enzyme may easily be masked by reticulocytosis. Valentine et al.[3] used the ratio of Hx to two other age-dependent enzymes, i.e., pyruvate kinase (PK) and glucose 6-phosphate dehydrogenase (G6PD) for detecting the true Hx-deficient patient. Measurement of the enzyme activity in old red cells is also valuable after red cell fractionation.

In most cases of Hx deficiency a decreased affinity of the residual enzyme for glucose and ATP has been observed,[4-7,12,15] and heat instability has been observed in two cases.[4,13] In other cases, kinetic studies did not reveal any differences between patient red cell Hx and normal enzyme. In most cases the results of electrophoresis have not been reported. In two patients, however, the electrophoretic pattern of the mutant enzyme showed a decrement or absence of Hx type I and a relatively increased Hx activity in the type III band.[8,15]

Glucosephosphate Isomerase Deficiency

Glucosephosphate isomerase (GPI) catalyzes the reversible interconversion of glucose 6-phosphate and fructose 6-phosphate. The structural gene for GPI is located on chromosome 19.[16] GPI from a variety of human tissues have been studied by electrophoretic techniques. A single genetic form of GPI is synthesized in all the cells of the body.[17,18] GPI is a dimer with a molecular weight of 134,000,[19] or 132,000.[20]

The congenital defect in GPI activity is the third most common erythroenzymopathy in the red cell after G6PD and PK deficiency. After the first report on GPI deficiency by Baughan et al.[21] in 1968, at least 41 patients from 35 families have been described (Table 3).[22-52] The GPI-deficient patients show a typical chronic nonspherocytic hemolytic anemia from the neonatal period or early childhood. The severity of the hemolytic anemia is quite variable as shown in Table 3. In most cases of GPI deficiency, other organ dysfunction was not observed. Only two cases showed mental retardation,[24,41] and one patient showed excessive glycogen storage in the enlarged liver.[41] The defect is inherited as an autosomal recessive.

About half of the cases in Table 3 are true homozygotes and the remaining cases are either heterozygotes or heterozygous for two different mutant GPI genes (double heterozygotes). Red cell GPI activities of homozygous or doubly heterozygous patients were decreased to about 25% of normal. Obligate heterozygotes for mutant alleles are hematologically normal, but have reduced red cell GPI activity. The characteristic feature of GPI deficiency is thermal instability of the enzyme and normal affinity for glucose 6-phosphate except for GPI Cowen.[30] This disorder may be caused by a structural gene mutation resulting in the synthesis of an abnormal molecule, as disclosed in G6PD and PGK deficiency. In fact, single amino acid substitution of genetic variants, i.e., Singh variant[20] and PHI 5-1,[53] have been considered.

The precise mechanism of hemolysis of GPI deficiency is still unknown. GPI-deficient red cells had a markedly increased rigidity and an abnormally strong attachment of hemoglobin to the inner surface of membranes. It is suggested that the metabolic environment of the spleen impairs the deformability of GPI-deficient red cells and predisposes them to splenic sequestration.[54,55]

Phosphofructokinase Deficiency

Phosphofructokinase (PFK), the key regulatory enzyme of glycolysis, catalyzes the conversion of fructose 6-phosphate to fructose 1,6-diphosphate (F-1,6-DP). PFK is a tetrameric enzyme, and three types of subunits, i.e., muscle type subunit (PFK-M), liver type subunit (PFK-L), and fibroblast or platelet type subunit (PFK-F or P), exist in human tissues.[56] Molecular weights of PFK-M, PFK-L, and PFK-F subunits are 85,000, 80,000, and 85,000, respectively.[57,58] Structural genes for PFK-M, PFK-L, and PFK-F are located on chromosomes 1, 21, and 10, respectively.[59,60] Human muscle and liver enzymes consist of distinct homotetramers (M_4 and L_4). Red cell PFK consists of a heterozygous mixture of five tetramers

Table 3
GLUCOSEPHOSPHATE ISOMERASE DEFICIENCY

Kindred	Variant	Age (years)	Sex	Hemoglobin (g/dℓ)	Reticulocyte (%)	Red cell GPI activity (% of normal)	Electro-phoretic mobility	Ref.
1	Seattle	15	M	9.8	28	19	Fast	21
2	Whitley-Country	13	F	8.0	72	16	Slow	22
		12	M	7.6	42	14		
		2	M	6.0	71	30		
3		5				40	Normal	23
4	Espeln	24	M	12.3	11	25	Fast	24
		21	M			23		
5		10	F				50	25
6	Valle Hermoso	14	F	9—10	15—20	25	Normal	26
7	Paderborn	20	M	8—20	8—20	22	Fast	27, 28
8		12	M			10		29
9	Cowen					45	Fast	30
10	Hay					45	Fast	
11	Los Angeles	1	M	7.4	34	14	Slow	31
12	Winnipeg	26	F	11.1	33	29	Slow	
13	Narita	2	M	8.0	24	40	Fast	32
14	Matsumoto	24	F	8.6	7	38	Normal	33
15		23	M	13.8	2.6	21	Normal	34
		20	F	10.9	3.1	20	Normal	
16		34	M	11.2	5.1	20	Normal	
17		40	F	9.4	8.4	16	Normal	
18		5	M	10	5	15	Normal	35
19	Recklinghausen	9	F	7—9	16	15	Slow	36
20	Elyria	13	F		0.2—51.6	15	Slow	37
21	Nordhorn	1	M	5.1—10.4	22	22	Fast	38
22	Kentucky	19	F	11	35		Normal	39
		10	M	10	20			

Table 3 (continued)
GLUCOSEPHOSPHATE ISOMERASE DEFICIENCY

Kindred	Variant	Age (years)	Sex	Hemoglobin (g/dℓ)	Reticulocyte (%)	Red cell GPI activity (% of normal)	Electro-phoretic mobility	Ref.
23		4	F	10	20			40
24	Utrecht	8	F	5.4—13	28	20—25	Normal	41
25	Nijmegen	14	F	4.1—8.9	48	20	Slow	42
26	Barcelona	12	F			15	Fast	43
27	Kortrijk					25—30	Fast	44
28		8	F	2.2—10.7	15—83	24	Normal	45
29	Liége	3	F	7.5	10.4	18	Slow	46
30		17	M	12.4	4.7	15	Normal	47
31	Roma	5	F	4—15.8	13.8—28.2	41	Fast	48
32	Augsburg	1	M	5.1—7.0	13.4—38.8	50	Fast	49
33		3	F	11.1	1.3	23	Fast	50
		1	F	10.2	1.4	19	Fast	
34	Tokyo	9	M	10.3	1.7	59	Normal	51
35	Kinki	13	F	10.7	10.2	10	Normal	52

Table 4
PHOSPHOFRUCTOKINASE DEFICIENCY

Kindred	Age (years)	Sex	Myopathy	Hemolytic anemia	Muscle PFK activity[a]	Red cell PFK activity[a]	Ref.
1	20	F	+	+	1	30	63
	23	M	+	+	2	48	
	27	M	+	+	2.6	42	
2	18	M	+	+	1	51	64
3	38	F	−	+	ND[b]	8	65
4	23	M	−	+	ND	59	66
5	37	M	+	?	0	17	67
6	20	M	+	?	6	ND	68
7		M	−	−	ND	28	69
8	18	F	−	+	100	61	70
9	53	M	−	+	ND	Decreased	71
10	23	M	+	+	5	32	72
	21	F	+	+	ND	58	
11	31	M	+	+	0	50	73
12	6 months	M	+	−	ND	ND	74
	14 months	F	+	−	6	75	
13	23	M	+	+	0	64	75
14	39	M	+	−	0	ND	
15	61	F	+	+	1	43	76
16	4	F	+	−	1.5	ND	77
17	61	M	+	+	1	40	78
18	19	M	+	+	80	58	79
	15	F	+	+	ND	48	
19	35	M	+	+	Decreased	59	

[a] Percent of normal.
[b] Not determined.

(M_4, M_3L, M_2L_2, ML_3, and L_4) with the two subunits being present in approximately equal proportion.[61] Vora et al.[62] also suggest that as many as 15 kinds of tetramers which consist of combinations of the 3 subunits (PFK-M, PFK-L, and PFK-F) could exist in some normal red cell PFK.

Since PFK deficiency associated with myopathy and congenital hemolytic anemia was first described by Tarui et al.[63] 24 cases of congenital PFK deficiency occurring in 19 unrelated families have been reported (Table 4).[64-79] In these cases, 11 cases had the typical features of glycogen storage disease, type VII (Tarui's disease), i.e., hemolytic anemia and myopathy, such as exercise intolerance, muscle cramps, and occasionally myoglobinuria.[63,64,72,73,75,76,78,79] The other cases exhibited myopathy alone,[67,68,74,77] hemolytic anemia alone,[65,66,70,71] or no clinical symptoms at all.[69] Red cell PFK deficiency may be due to a defect of either PFK-L or PFK-M subunit. The complete absence of PFK-M subunit activity leads to both hematological and muscular symptoms, and it may arise from a defect of synthesis[64] or from a mutant PFK-M subunit.[75,78] Recently, we discovered two families of PFK deficiency with hemolytic anemia and mild myopathy.[79] Starch gel electrophoresis and DEAE-Sephadex chromatography could not determine the PFK-M subunit in the patient's red cell PFK (Figures 2 and 3). Enzyme activity of the patient's PFK-M was decreased to about half of normal. Furthermore, the patient's enzyme was quite thermolabile. The patient's clinical symptoms, i.e., hemolytic anemia and myopathy, was considered to be due to unstable mutant PFK-M subunit in the red cells and muscle.

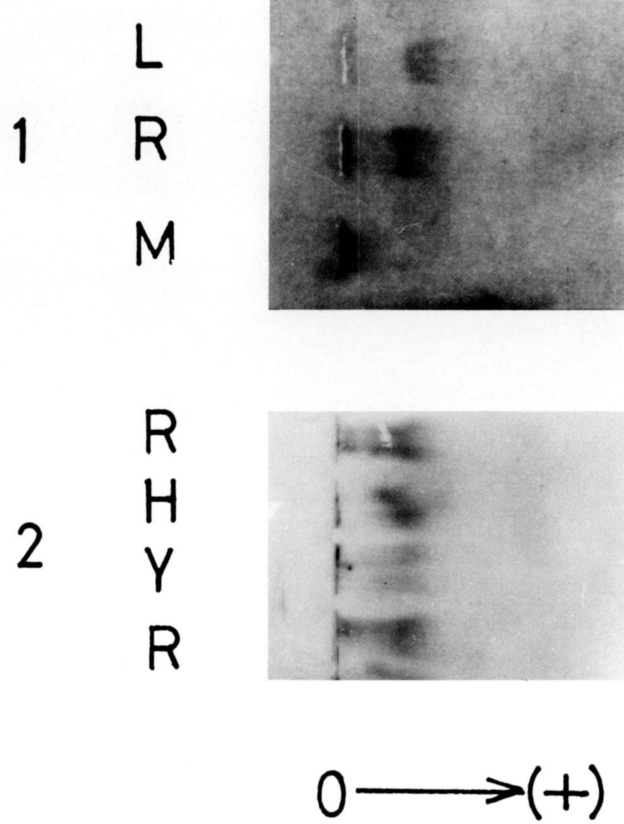

FIGURE 2. Starch-gel electrophoresis of liver PFK (L), muscle PFK (M), normal red cell PFK (R), and probands' red cell PFKs (Case 1 (Y), Case 2 (H)).[79]

Aldolase Deficiency

The hexose phosphate, F-1,6-DP, is split by aldolase into two triose phosphates: glyceraldehyde 3-phosphate and dihydroxyacetone phosphate. Aldolase has a molecular weight of 158,000 and consists of four subunits.[80] It has been said that three types of aldolase isozyme are found in human tissues.[81,82] Aldolase A is the type found in muscle and in red cells; aldolase B is found in the liver; aldolase C occurs in the brain along with aldolase A. Recently, messenger RNA for aldolase B was isolated from adult and fetal human liver. Messenger RNA specifying synthesis of aldolase B exhibited a sedimentation coefficient of 16S both in adult and fetal liver.[83]

Red cell aldolase deficiency is very rare, and only two kindreds are reported. Beutler et al.[84] reported the first case of this enzyme deficiency associated with hereditary nonspherocytic hemolytic anemia of mild to moderate degree. The patient was the offspring of first cousins. The patient showed many dysmorphic features, and mental and growth retardation. Red cell aldolase activity of the patient was 16% of normal, but Beutler et al.[84] were unable to detect any structural abnormality either by electrophoresis or kinetic studies. The decreased aldolase activity with normal enzymatic characteristics led Beutler et al. to consider that the depression of aldolase activity represented a disorder in regulation of aldolase levels rather than in the structural gene for aldolase itself.

The proband reported by us[85] was a 14-year-old Japanese boy. Consanguineous marriage was not proven (Figure 4). The proband had moderate to mild anemia aggravated by upper

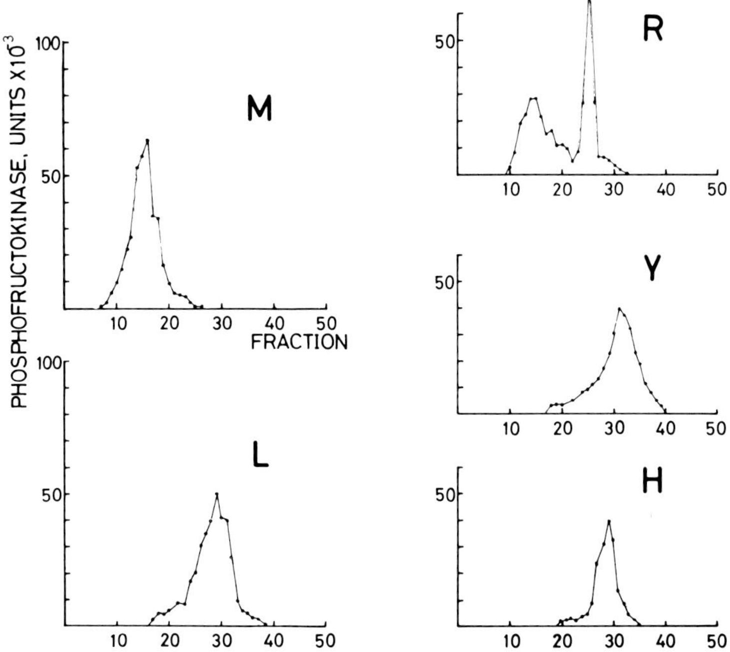

FIGURE 3. Chromatographic separation of muscle PFK (M), liver PFK (L), normal red cell PFK (R), and red cell PFKs of probands (Case 1 (Y), Case 2 (H)).[79]

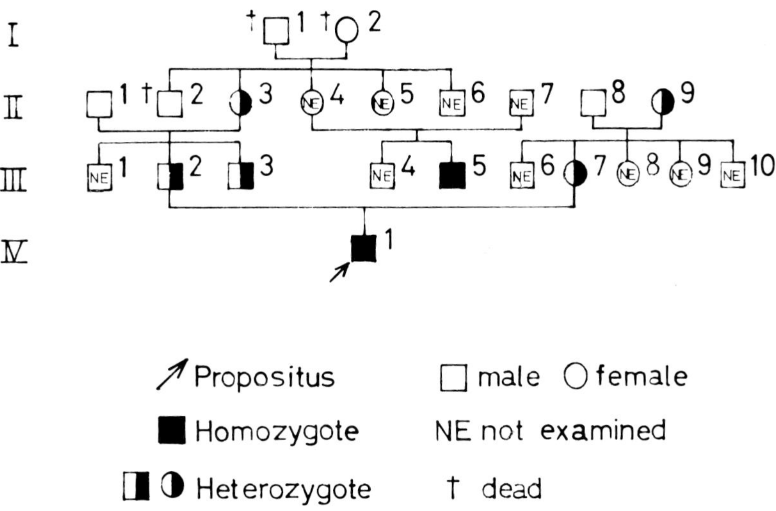

FIGURE 4. Pedigree of the Japanese family with red cell aldolase deficiency.[85]

respiratory infections and hepatosplenomegaly, but he did not show any dysmorphic feature or mental and growth retardation. The red cell aldolase activity was 6% of the normal mean. Red cell F-1,6-DP was remarkably increased (Figure 5). The patient's enzyme was unstable to heat, and showed an increased Michaelis constant for F-1,6-DP. Family studies disclosed that a nephew of the proband's paternal grandmother also had homozygous aldolase deficiency (Figure 4). In this case, red cell aldolase deficiency was considered to be due to a structural gene mutation.

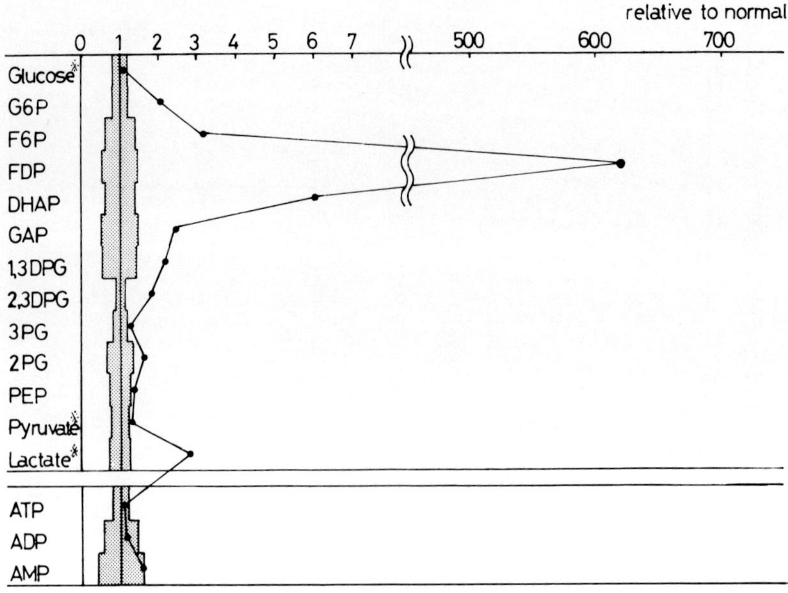

FIGURE 5. Red cell glycolytic intermediates and adenine nucleotides of the patient with red cell aldolase deficiency.[85]

Triosephosphate Isomerase Deficiency

Triosephosphate isomerase (TPI) catalyzes the interconversion of glyceraldehyde 3-phosphate and dihydroxyacetone phosphate. TPI is a dimeric enzyme, and its subunit size is 26,500.[86] Human TPI exists as multiple electrophoretic forms, i.e., three major forms: A, B, and C. The A and C forms are homodimers, $\alpha\alpha$ and $\beta\beta$, and the form B is heterodimer, $\alpha\beta$. The two polypeptide chains (α and β) appear to be identical (amino acid composition, molecular weight, and antigenicity), and since the electrophoretic banding pattern changes with cell aging, it is considered that the multiple forms of TPI are the consequence of minor post-synthetic alteration of form A.[87] TPI A and TPI B isozymes are products of the same structural locus,[88] which is located on chromosome 12.[89]

TPI deficiency is a rare inherited disease characterized by chronic hemolytic anemia, progressive neurological impairment, and in some instances, frequently recurring bacterial infections. Since the first description of TPI deficiency by Schneider et al.,[90] 15 cases from 7 unrelated families have been reported.[91-96] The mode of inheritance of this disease is autosomal recessive. Cases of decreased TPI activities associated with cat cry syndrome[97] and pancytopenia[98] were reported, whereas the correlation between TPI deficiency and these disorders was not clear. Although the degree of anemia is variable, most patients require blood transfusions. Neurologic involvement, such as paraparesis, weakness, and hypotonia, is progressive in most cases. Early death, usually in childhood, is observed.

A rapid screening method reported by Kaplan et al.[99] could prove useful for the presumptive detection of TPI deficiency.

Phosphoglycerate Kinase Deficiency

Phosphoglycerate kinase (PGK) is a key enzyme for ATP generation in the glycolytic pathway, and catalyzes the conversion of 1,3-diphosphoglycerate to 3-phosphoglycerate. The PGK reaction is by-passed by the Rapoport-Leubering cycle. The structural locus for PGK is on the long arm of X chromosome, and human PGK in red cells and other tissues, except for sperm, is controlled by a single structural gene.[100,101] Human PGK is a single-chain polypeptide with a molecular weight of about 49,000.[102] Recently, the complete amino

```
                                   10                                              20
N-Acetyl-Ser-Leu-Ser-Asn-Lys-Leu-Thr-Leu-Asp-Lys-Leu-Asp-Val-Lys-Gly-Lys-Arg-Val-Val-Met-
                              30                                              40
     Arg-Val-Asp-Phe-Asn-Val-Pro-Met-Lys-Asn-Asn-Gln-Ile-Thr-Asn-Asn-Gln-Arg-Lys-Ile-
                              50                                              60
     Lys-Ala-Ala-Val-Pro-Ser-Ile-Lys-Phe-Cys-Leu-Asp-Asp-Gly-Ala-Lys-Ser-Val-Val-Leu-
                              70                                              80
     Met-Ser-His-Leu-Gly-Arg-Pro-Asp-Gly-Val-Pro-Met-Pro-Asp-Lys-Tyr-Ser-Leu-Glu-Pro-
                              90                                              100
     Val-Ala-Val-Glu-Leu-Lys-Ser-Leu-Leu-Gly-Lys-Asp-Val-Leu-Phe-Leu-Lys-Asp-Cys-Val-
                              110                                             120
     Gly-Pro-Glu-Val-Glu-Lys-Ala-Cys-Ala-Asp-Pro-Ala-Ala-Gly-Ser-Val-Ile-Leu-Leu-Glu-
                              130                                             140
     Asn-Leu-Arg-Phe-His-Val-Glu-Glu-Glu-Gly-Lys-Gly-Lys-Asp-Ala-Ser-Gly-Asn-Lys-Val-
                              150                                             160
     Lys-Ala-Glu-Pro-Ala-Lys-Ile-Glu-Ala-Phe-Arg-Ala-Ser-Leu-Ser-Lys-Leu-Gly-Asp-Val-
                              170                                             180
     Tyr-Val-Asn-Asp-Ala-Phe-Gly-Thr-Ala-His-Arg-Ala-His-Ser-Ser-Met-Val-Gly-Val-Asn-
                              190                                             200
     Leu-Pro-Gln-Lys-Ala-Gly-Gly-Phe-Leu-Met-Lys-Lys-Glu-Leu-Asn-Tyr-Phe-Ala-Lys-Ala-
                              210                                             220
     Leu-Glu-Ser-Pro-Glu-Arg-Pro-Phe-Leu-Ala-Ile-Leu-Gly-Gly-Ala-Lys-Val-Ala-Asp-Lys-
                      ●(Pro)  230                                             240
     Ile-Gln-Leu-Ile-Asn-Asn-Met-Leu-Asp-Lys-Val-Asn-Glu-Met-Ile-Ile-Gly-Gly-Gly-Met-
                              250                                             260
     Ala-Phe-Thr-Phe-Leu-Lys-Val-Leu-Asn-Asn-Met-Glu-Ile-Gly-Thr-Ser-Leu-Phe-Asp-Glu-
                              270                                             280
     Glu-Gly-Ala-Lys-Ile-Val-Lys-Asp-Leu-Met-Ser-Lys-Ala-Glu-Lys-Asp-Gly-Val-Lys-Ile-
                        ✱(Met) ■(Asn) 290                                     300
     Thr-Leu-Pro-Val-Asp-Phe-Val-Thr-Ala-Asp-Lys-Phe-Asp-Glu-Asn-Ala-Lys-Thr-Gly-Glu-
                              310                                             320
     Ala-Thr-Val-Ala-Ser-Gly-Ile-Pro-Ala-Gly-Trp-Met-Gly-Leu-Asp-Cys-Gly-Pro-Glu-Ser-
                              330                                             340
     Ser-Lys-Lys-Tyr-Ala-Glu-Ala-Val-Thr-Arg-Ala-Lys-Gln-Ile-Val-Trp-Asp-Gly-Pro-Val-
                              350                                             360
     Gly-Val-Phe-Glu-Trp-Glu-Ala-Phe-Ala-Arg-Gly-Thr-Lys-Ala-Leu-Met-Asp-Glu-Val-Val-
                              370     ▲(Asn)                                  380
     Lys-Ala-Thr-Ser-Arg-Gly-Cys-Ile-Thr-Ile-Ile-Gly-Gly-Gly-Asp-Thr-Ala-Thr-Cys-Cys-
                              390                                             400
     Ala-Lys-Trp-Asn-Thr-Gln-Asp-Lys-Val-Ser-His-Val-Ser-Thr-Gly-Gly-Gly-Ala-Ser-Leu-
                              410                         417
     Glu-Leu-Leu-Glu-Gly-Lys-Val-Leu-Pro-Gly-Val-Asp-Ala-Leu-Ser-Asn-Ile-OH
```

FIGURE 6. Complete amino acid sequence of normal human phosphoglycerate kinase (PGK). Specific amino acid substitutions of four PGK variants, i.e., PGK II (Thy→Asn at 352), PGK München (Asp→Asn at 268), PGK Uppsala (Arg→Pro at 206), and PGK Tokyo (Val→Met at 266) are also shown.

acid sequence of normal human PGK was determined. The enzyme consists of 417 amino acid residues with acetylserine at the NH_2-terminal and isoleucine at the COOH-terminal (Figure 6).[103,104]

Inherited deficiency of PGK is associated with nonspherocytic hemolytic anemia and often with mental disorders in man. At the present time, 11 unrelated families have been reported (Table 5).[105-115] The first case reported by Kraus et al.[105] is a heterozygous female, and the results are not very clear. The second family reported by Valentine et al.[106] is a large Chinese family, and pedigree study indicates that the expression of PGK deficiency is compatible with X-linked inheritance. Besides these deficient variants, several other electrophoretic variants, which are not associated with enzyme deficiency, also have been reported.[100] Red cell PGK deficiency is severe in red cells of affected males. A significant accumulation of several glycolytic intermediates, i.e., glyceraldehyde 3-phosphate, dihydroxyacetone phosphate, and F-1,6-DP, was observed in red blood cells of these hemolytic subjects. Exacerbation of hemolytic anemia may occur during periods of crisis, often brought by intercurrent infections. Mild mental retardation, behavioral aberrations, and neurological symptoms are often associated with the severe enzyme deficiency.

The electrophoretic mobility and enzymatic properties of the residual enzymes from three unrelated subjects, i.e., PGK Matsue,[116] PGK München,[117] and PGK variant found in France,[118] have been reported. These studies suggest that the enzyme deficiency is a result of structural gene mutation. Recently, single amino acid substitutions of PGK II,[119] PGK München,[120]

Table 5
PHOSPHOGLYCERATE KINASE DEFICIENCY

Kindred	Variant	Red cell PGK activity (% of normal)	Hemolytic anemia	Mental disorder	Electro-phoretic mobility (% of normal)	Ref.
1		75	±	−		105
2		5	+	+		106
3	Uppsala	10	+	+	Fast	107
4		20	+	−		108
5	Matsue	5	+	+	Slow	109
6		42	±	−		110
7		10	+	+		111
8	Tokyo	15	+	+	Slow	112
9		10	+	±	Normal	113
10	München	21	−	−	Slow	114
11	Creteil	3	−	+	Slow	115

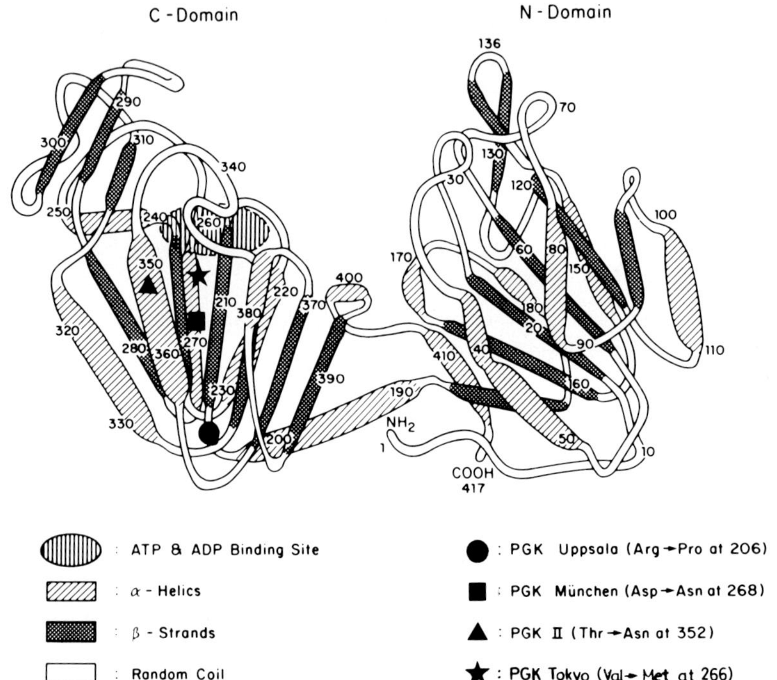

FIGURE 7. Three-dimensional model of human phosphoglycerate kinase (PGK). This figure is based on the three-dimensional model of horse PGK published by Banks et al.[123] Positions of the amino acid substitutions of four variant enzymes are also shown.

PGK Uppsala,[121] and PGK Tokyo[122] were reported, and the correlation between the functional and structural abnormalities of these variants was clarified (Figures 6 and 7 and Table 6). PGK II is an electrophoretic variant found in New Guinea populations. Red cell enzyme activity, specific activity, and the kinetic properties of PGK II are normal. However, PGK II strongly binds with citrate and moves towards the anode much faster than the normal enzyme using the citrate buffer system. The structural abnormality of PGK II is a single amino acid substitution from threonine to asparagine at the 352nd position. PGK München is associated with red cell enzyme deficiency, but not with hemolytic anemia or clinical

Table 6
ENZYMATIC PROPERTIES OF PHOSPHOGLYCERATE KINASE VARIANTS

PGK Variant	Specific activity (% of normal)	K_m (μM) ADP	1,3-DPG	ATP	3-PG	pH Optimum	Heat stability
Normal	100	106 ± 16	2.4 ± 0.5	343 ± 14	540 ± 80	7—10	Stable
PGK II	100	—	—	Normal	Normal	Normal	Stable
PGK München	38	85	2.0	340	440	Acidic	Unstable
PGK Uppsala	29	556	4.9	930	2800	Normal	Unstable
PGK Tokyo	31	143	2.0	667	870	Acidic	Unstable

symptoms. The variant has normal Michaelis constants for the substrates, decreased specific activity, and slower than normal anodal electrophoretic mobility. However, the heat stability in vitro of PGK München is substantially decreased from that of the normal. The amino acid substitution of PGK München is asparagine for aspartic acid at the 258th position of the normal enzyme. PGK Uppsala is associated with severe red cell enzyme deficiency, chronic nonspherocytic hemolytic anemia, and mental disorders. The variant enzyme has lower specific activity, thermal instability, and higher than normal Michaelis constants for the substrates. The structural abnormality of PGK Uppsala is a single amino acid substitution from arginine to proline at the 206th position. PGK Tokyo is associated with enzyme deficiency, nonspherocytic hemolytic anemia, and neurological disturbances. The variant enzyme was purified from the cultured lymphoblastoid cells. PGK Tokyo has a lower specific activity, higher than normal Michaelis constants for the substrates, acidic shift in pH optimum, and thermal instability. The structural abnormality of PGK Tokyo is found to be a single amino acid substitution from valine to methionine at the 266th position.

In PGK II, the substitution of one neutral amino acid for another occurs on the protein surface and does not affect enzyme catalysis. Consequently, PGK II shows no abnormalities except for the unusual interaction with citrate. PGK München has quite similar catalytic properties to that of normal subjects, but shows marked thermal instability. It is conceivable that the aspartyl residue at the 268th position forms a hydrogen bond with a basic residue in a neighboring strand, stabilizing the molecule against heat denaturation. Substitution of PGK Uppsala and PGK Tokyo are proximal to the substrate binding site of the enzyme. The substitutions at these positions are expected to induce a dislocation of the ATP and ADP binding site, resulting in markedly disadvantageous enzyme properties and severe clinical symptoms.

Splenectomy had a favorable outcome in three out of four patients.[105,106,108,115]

Pyruvate Kinase Deficiency

Pyruvate kinase (PK) is one of the three postulated rate-controlling enzymes of glycolysis. The high-energy phosphate of phosphoenolpyruvate is transfered to ADP by this enzyme to generate 2 mol of ATP per mole of glucose oxidized. Enolpyruvate formed in this reaction is converted spontaneously to the keto form of pyruvate. In mammalian tissues at least three different isozymes of PK exist.[124,125] Type M_1 is found in skeletal muscle, heart, and brain. Type L is the major isozyme in liver and the minor one in renal cortex and also occurs in the small intestine. The main PK isozyme in the kidney is type M_2 which is also found in most other tissues (Figure 8). The red cell enzyme (type R or L′) is kinetically and immunologically identical with the major isozyme found in the liver. The M_1 and M_2 isozymes display Michaelis-Menten kinetics with respect to phosphoenolpyruvate. The M_1 isozyme is not affected by F-1,6-DP and the M_2 is allosterically activated by this compound. Type L and R exhibit cooperativity in their kinetics towards phosphoenolpyruvate, and both are allosterically activated by F-1,6-DP. It has been established that both L- and R- type PK differ from M_1- and M_2-type PK by kinetic, electrophoretic, and immunological properties,

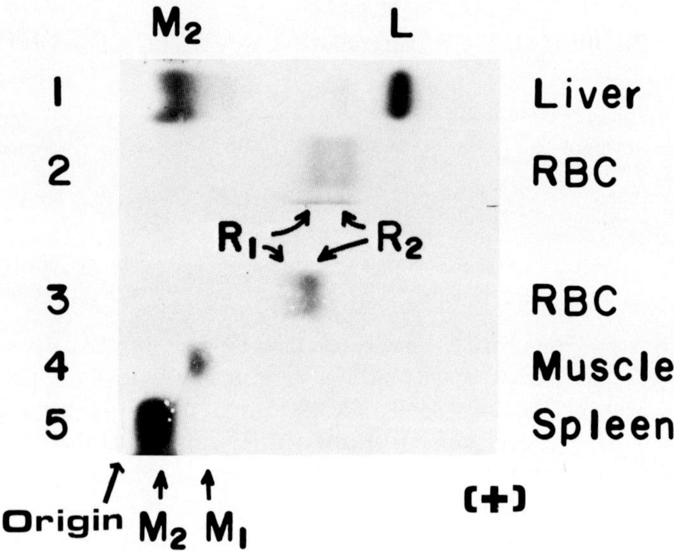

FIGURE 8. Pyruvate kinase zymogram of liver, red cell, muscle, and spleen. Supporting medium: 3.34% acrylamide gel, 1 mm in thickness. Buffer: 10 m*M* Tris-Cl, 5 m*M* $MgCl_2$, 0.5 m*M* F-1, 6-DP, pH 8.3.

and that they are probably under control of different genes.[126-128] Recent work suggests that the M_1 and M_2 isozymes of PK are the products of the same gene,[129,130] and that the L- and L′-type isozymes are encoded by the same structural gene[131-135] and are translated from different messenger RNAs.[136] The structural studies of the rat PK were performed extensively by Saheki et al.[128] Their apparent subunit molecular weights were 59,000 (type M_1), 60,000 (type M_2), 58,500 (type L), and 62,000 (type R). Human red cell PK is a tetramer having an estimated molecular weight of 225,400.[137,138] From the hypothesis reported by Kahn et al.,[133,139,140] L-type PK is synthesized as L'_4 form (molecular weight, 62,000) in the erythroblast. Red cell maturation and aging are accompanied by a partial proteolysis of two subunits, such that L'_4 is transformed into the heterotetramer $L_2L'_2$; the molecular weight of the L subunit is about 58,000. Kahn et al. proposed that erythrocyte-type PK (L'_4) may be considered as a ''precursor form'' of L-type enzyme (L_4), the former being transformed into the latter by partial proteolysis. In mature blood cells, there is a distinct distribution pattern of PK isozymes, i.e., M_2-type PK in leukocytes and platelets, and L-type PK in red cells. Recently, we examined the PK isozymes during the erythroid cell maturation using a immunofluorescent method.[141] M_2-type PK was seen in erythroid precursor cells and L-type PK production occurred after the reduction of M_2-type PK. Different genes seem to code for M_2- and L-type PK and regulation of PK isozyme switch during erythroid cell maturation might occur just like the switch from fetal to adult hemoglobin.

Deficiency of red cell PK is the most common enzymatic cause of hereditary hemolytic anemia.[142] More than 300 cases with red cell PK deficiency have been reported since the first report by Valentine et al.[143] Although this disorder has been reported from around the world, most cases of PK deficiency have been found in persons of Northern European origin.[144,145] An autosomal recessive mode of inheritance has been observed in most family studies. Clinical symptoms are observed in the homozygous or doubly heterozygous state. The clinical expression of PK deficiency is highly variable, ranging from pronounced neonatal jaundice requiring multiple exchange transfusions to a fully compensated hemolytic anemia. As a rule, hemolytic anemia and jaundice are observed in infancy or childhood, and splenomegaly of slight to moderate degree is also seen. The chronic hemolytic process may be exacerbated by infections.[142,143,146] After the first decade of life, gallstones are detected with

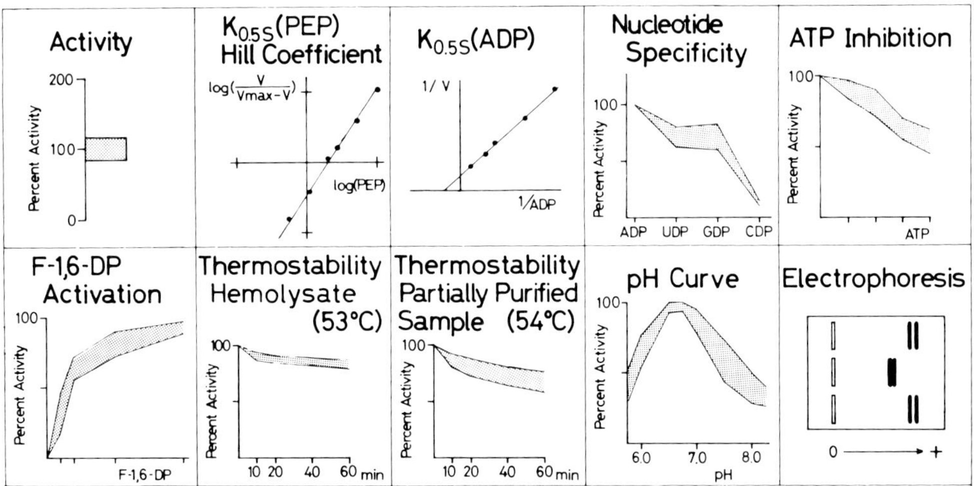

FIGURE 9. The biochemical properties of pyruvate kinase variant.

high frequency. The clinical polymorphism may be due to the characteristics of mutant enzymes.

The degree of anemia varies widely among patients. The hemoglobin value is usually in the range of 6 to 12 g/dℓ. Red cell morphologic abnormalities are not a prominent feature of PK deficiency. The red cell is normochromic with a slight anisocytosis and poikilocytosis. Echinocytes may be seen occasionally before splenectomy, but they increase in number and may become conspicuous after splenectomy. Serum indirect bilirubin is moderately increased, and haptoglobin is decreased or absent.

The diagnosis of PK deficiency depends on the demonstration of quantitatively decreased enzyme activity or qualitative abnormalities of the enzyme. Spectrophotometric assay method of the red cell PK activity is proposed by a working group of the International Committee for Standardization in Haematology.[147,148] Red cells and leukocytes are under separate genetic control. Furthermore, leukocytes are a rich source of PK, and the activity of this enzyme is not diminished in leukocytes in red cell PK deficiency. It is therefore important that leukocytes be removed completely for the determination of red cell PK activity. Most deficient individuals show 5 to 25% of the normal mean activity. Heterozygous carriers of PK variant have approximately one half normal activity. In general, no relationship between measurable activity and severity of hemolysis can be demonstrated in PK deficiency.[149-156] Mutations which result in the formation of an enzyme with normal or high PK activity at high substrate concentration are known to occur. Most of these variants show low substrate affinity for phosphoenolpyruvate. These variants can be detected under the assay condition of low substrate concentration (low S system).[147,148] In addition to this, determination of glycolytic intermediates by enzymatic method[157] is another useful tool for the detection of these PK variants. Phosphoenolpyruvate, 2-phosphoglycerate, 3-phosphoglycerate, and 2,3-DPG are high in PK-deficient red cells. It has been increasingly apparent that most, if not all, cases of PK deficiency are caused by the production of mutant enzymes due to structural gene alterations.[131,152,158-161] The standard method for the analysis of PK variant has been recently established by a working group of the International Committee for Standardization in Haematology Expert Panel on Red Cell Enzymes (Figure 9.)[162] Table 7 shows seven new PK variants characterized by this method.[163] These cases were all true homozygotes as evidenced by consanguineous marriages of the parents. All patients showed moderate chronic hemolytic anemia. Out of 7 variants, 4 showed normal or high PK activity. From these results, low substrate affinity (high $K_{0.5s}$ for phosphoenolpyruvate) and thermal instability

Table 7
CHARACTERISTICS OF PYRUVATE KINASE VARIANTS[162]

Kindred	1	2	3	4	5	6	7
Activity (%)	156	136	147	39	51	92	63
$K_{0.5S}$(PEP)	H	H	H	H	H	H	H
Hill coefficient	L	N	N	N	L	Slightly H	N
$K_{0.5S}$(ADP)	N	L	L	N	N	N	N
Nucleotide specificity	Slightly Abn	N	Abn	N	Abn	Abn	Abn
ATP inhibition	N	N	More	N	More	More	More
F-1,6-DP activation	N	N	N	Less	N	Less	Less
Thermostability	Lab	Lab	N	Lab	Lab	Lab	Lab
pH curve	Acid	Acid	N	Narrow	Narrow	N	N
Electrophoretic mobility	Slow	Slow	Fast	N	Slow	Slow	N

Note: N, normal; H, high; L, low; Abn, abnormal; More, more inhibition than the normal; Less, less activation (more F-1,6-DP required than the normal required for 50% activation); Lab, labile; Acid, acidic shift.

appear to play major roles in causing defective enzyme function, resulting in hemolytic anemia. Product inhibition of PK by ATP may also play an additional role in causing hemolysis.

The mechanism of hemolysis in PK-deficient red cells is still unknown. PK deficiency results in impaired glycolysis and diminished capacity to generate ATP. Impaired ATP synthesis seems to be the most severe metabolic consequence of PK deficiency. However, some patients with marked reticulocytosis have a normal or elevated ATP level. PK-deficient reticulocytes depend upon mitochondrial oxidative phosphorylation rather than on glycolysis to maintain an adequate ATP level. If oxidative phosphorylation is possibly compromised in the splenic environment, the ATP level declines rapidly, producing a decreased red cell deformability mainly due to marked loss of potassium and water, and finally leading to recognition, sequestration, and destruction of the red cells in the reticuloendothelial system.[164-168] Recently, Zanella et al.[169] reported that PK-deficient red cells display a membrane abnormality responsible for the abnormal membrane autolysis (glycoprotein self-digestion) and the increased susceptibility of red cells to macrophage.

2,3-Diphosphoglyceromutase Deficiency

2,3-Diphosphoglyceromutase (2,3-DPGM) catalyzes the formation of 2,3-DPG, an important effector of the dissociation of oxygen from hemoglobin. 2,3-DPG is the most abundant glycolytic intermediates in red cells and combines with deoxyhemoglobin, reducing the affinity of hemoglobin for oxygen and thereby shifting the oxygen-hemoglobin dissociation curve to the right. 2,3-DPG is converted to 3-phosphoglycerate by diphosphoglycerate phosphatase (DPGP). Rosa et al.[170] and Sasaki et al.[171] demonstrated that 2,3-DPGM and DPGP are displayed by the same enzyme protein which has phosphoglyceromutase activity.

Schröter[172] reported about 50% of normal 2,3-DPGM activity in the asymptomatic parents, sister, and paternal grandmother of a child with severe transfusion-dependent hemolysis. 2,3-DPGM activity could not be measured in the child due to the presence of a large amount of transfused blood, but the child was considered to represent homozygosity for 2,3-DPGM deficiency. More recently, several partial deficiencies of this enzyme were reported.[173-177] Rosa et al.[178] reported a case of the complete deficiency of 2,3-DPGM. The patient was a 42-year-old man of French origin whose blood hemoglobin concentration was 19.0 g/dℓ. He was normal on physical examination except for a ruddy cyanosis. There was no evidence of hemolysis. The red cell 2,3-DPG level was below 3% of normal and, as a consequence, the affinity of the red cell for oxygen was increased. Both DPGM and DPGP activities were undetectable in the red cell.

Hexose Monophoshate Pathway and Glutathione Metabolism

Glucose 6-Phosphate Dehydrogenase

Glucose 6-phosphate dehydrogenase (G6PD), an NADP-dependent enzyme, catalyzes the dehydrogenation of glucose 6-phosphate to 6-phosphogluconate. The next oxidative step is catalyzed by 6-phosphogluconate dehydrogenase (6-PGD), which also requires $NADP^+$ as hydrogen acceptor, to give the pentose, ribulose 5-phosphate. Ribulose 5-phosphate is converted back to the main stream of glycolysis by transketolase and transaldolase. NADPH, provided from the hexose monophosphate pathway, reduces oxidized glutathione (GSSG) to reduced glutathione (GSH), catalyzed by glutathione reductase (GR). In turn, GSH removes oxidants, such as superoxide anion (O_2^-) and hydrogen peroxide (H_2O_2) from the red cell in a reaction catalyzed by glutathione peroxidase (GSH-Px). This reaction is important since the accumulation of oxidants may decrease the lifespan of the red cell by increasing the rate of oxidation of protein, i.e., hemoglobin, red cell membrane, and enzyme protein.

Human G6PD has been purified and characterized.[179] The G6PD molecule appears to consist of several identical subunits, each with a molecular weight of 55,000. Under the optimal assay conditions in vitro, and presumably also in red cells, the enzyme is predominantly dimeric. The enzyme has tightly bound NADP which cannot be easily removed by dialysis.[180,181] G6PD is a peptide chain, consisting of about 500 amino acid residues, with pyroglutamic acid at the NH_2-terminal and glycine at the COOH-terminal. All tryptic peptides and cyanogen bromide peptides of G6PD have been isolated and analyzed,[182] and most of the amino acid sequence has been determined.[183] Recently, human G6PD complementary DNA has been cloned from human messenger RNA.[184]

It has been recognized that certain oxidant drugs, such as primaquine, produced an acute hemolytic anemia in some susceptible individuals since the 19th century. Beginning in 1952, systematic studies were done in the U.S. to determine the cause of this type of drug sensitivity. Cross-transfusion studies with ^{51}Cr-labeled red cells indicated that primaquine sensitivity was due to an intrinsic abnormality of the red cell.[185] Thereafter, the content of GSH was found to be lower in primaquine-sensitive red cells than in normal cells.[186] Finally, deficiency of the enzyme G6PD was identified by Carson et al.[187] in 1956.

Deficiency of G6PD is the most common metabolic disorder of the red blood cell. It is estimated that 100 million people are affected in the world. The incidence of this disorder is approximately 20% among African Bantu males, 12% in American black males, and 8% in Brazilian blacks. A high prevalence of G6PD deficiency is also seen in the people of the Mediterranean basin, East Indians, Orientals, and Filipinos.[145,188] Northern European people and Japanese rarely have G6PD deficiency. The incidence in Japanese is considered to be 0.1 to 0.5%.[189,190] Because of its high prevalence in populations where malaria is endemic, the geographic distribution of G6PD deficiency led to the suggestion that this gene may confer some degree of resistance to *Plasmodium falciparum* malaria.[191,192] From studies on the distribution of *Plasmodium falciparum* rings in red cells with normal and deficient activity of G6PD, the parasite-rate was 2 to 80 times higher in normal than in the deficient red cells. These results were interpreted by Luzzatto et al.[193] that the gene for G6PD deficiency confers a selective advantage aganist malaria. On the other hand, more recent studies report that evidence for the possible role of malaria in selecting for G6PD-deficient genes solely consists of the geographic association of high frequencies of G6PD deficiency with endemic malaria.[194] The precise reason for the geographic distribution of G6PD deficiency is still unknown.

The genes controlling G6PD structure and synthesis are located on the X-chromosome.[195,196] Thus, the inheritance is sex-linked. G6PD in all tissues seems to be under the same genetic control. Enzyme deficiency finds full expression in males carrying a G6PD-

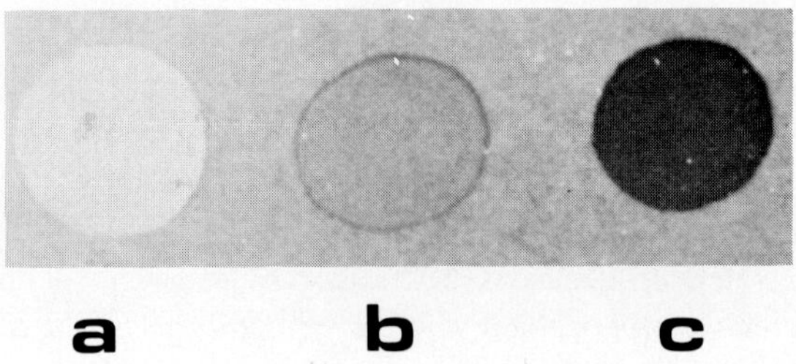

FIGURE 10. The fluorescent spot test for glucose 6-phosphate dehydrogenase (G6PD) deficiency. a, Normal G6PD; b, G6PD Ube[303]; c, G6PD Fukushima.[243]

deficient gene. Mean enzyme activity in females who carry a gene for G6PD deficiency may be normal, moderately reduced, or grossly deficient. This can be explained according to the Lyon hypothesis.[197] Only one X-chromosome is active in any somatic cell; the other X-chromosome is randomly inactivated early in embryonic life.[198] Therefore, individual red cells of heterozygous females are either normal or deficient.

Clinical manifestations of G6PD deficiency are divided into three types; acute hemolysis, chronic nonspherocytic hemolytic anemia, and favism. Acute severe hemolysis occurs after the exposure of certain drugs, such as antimalarials, sulfonamides, nitrofurans, analgesics, and sulfones. Infection and diabetic acidosis also induce hemolysis, and infection is thought to be a more common inciting factor than drug exposure in hemolytic events. In some G6PD variants, chronic hemolysis occurs. Anemia and jaundice are often noted in the newborn period, and some patients show marked neonatal hyperbilirubinemia. The anemia is clinically and hematologically indistinguishable from that due to glycolytic enzyme deficiency. Favism produces one of the most severe hemolytic episodes following exposure to fava beans and is the more frequent manifestation in Mediterranean countries. It is considered that some factors, e.g., allergy, in addition to G6PD deficiency is required for the development of favism.

Diagnosis of G6PD deficiency can be done by a quantitative enzyme assay with the ICSH procedure.[148] Several screening methods for the detection of G6PD deficiency have been reported. The fluorescent spot test recommended by the ICSH Expert Panel of Red Cell Enzymes seems to be the most generally useful and reliable;[199] 50% of enzyme-deficient subjects can be easily detected by this method (Figure 10).

Electrophoretic and kinetic studies of G6PD-deficient subjects' enzymes were performed extensively within a few years of the discovery of G6PD deficiency. Most genetic variants of G6PD presumably have arisen through single amino acid substitutions. A direct chemical proof has been obtained in two G6PD variants, i.e., G6PD A (a replacement of asparagine to aspartic acid)[200] and G6PD Hektoen (a replacement of histidine to tyrosine).[201] Due to the difficulty of obtaining sufficient amounts of blood from variant subjects, such kinds of studies could not be performed. In 1967, international agreement was reached regarding standardization of methods for characterization of G6PD variants (Figure 11).[188] It consists of the following parameters: (1) red cell enzyme activity; (2) electrophoretic mobility; (3) the Michaelis constants for its substrates, glucose 6-phosphate, and NADP; (4) capacity to utilize 2-deoxy-glucose 6-phosphate, galactose 6-phosphate, and deamino-NADP; (5) heat stability; (6) pH optimum; (7) inhibition constant by NADPH (Figure 11). Up to now, over 200 variants of G6PD have been distinguished on the basis of their physicochemical properties (Table 8).[202-342] Some are sporadic variants, others occur with high frequency in certain populations, such as the A^- variant in Africa or the Mediterranean variant. It is now clear that clinical polymorphism of G6PD deficiency is the results of characteristics of mutant enzymes which differ from one another with respect to stability, kinetics, and other physicochemical properties. Concerning correlations between molecular changes in G6PD and

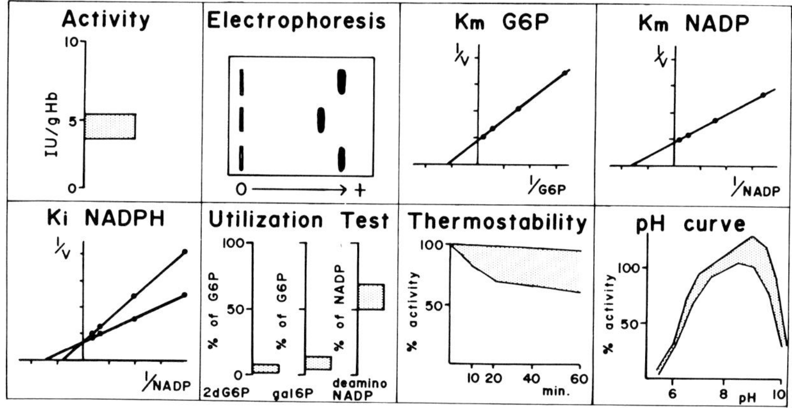

FIGURE 11. The biochemical properties of glucose 6-phosphate dehydrogenase variant.

Table 8
G6PD VARIANTS

Class 1 Variants (Associated With Nonspherocytic Hemolytic Anemia)

	Ref.
Electrophoretically fast variants	
St. Louis[c,h,j,q,r,]	202
Baudelocque[b,h,j,q,r]	203
Ohio[c,f,g,q]	204
Lincoln Park[b,f,h,j,p,u]	205
Heian[c,f,h,k,s]	206
Charleston[b,f,h,k,q,s]	207
Lawndale[c,f,q,r]	208
Torrance[a,e,q,u]	209
Jackson[b,f,g,k,o,r]	210
San Diego[b,g,o,r]	211
East Harlem[c,f,g,j,p]	212
Linda Vista[b,f,h,k,m,q,t]	213
Hotel Dieu[b,f,h,k,n,p,t]	214
Quadalajara[b,f,h,k,l,o,r]	215
Barcelona[b,f,h,i,o,r]	216
Pea Ridge[a,f,g,j,n,q,r]	217
Electrophoretically normal variants	
Chinese[a,g,i,o,r]	218
Bat-Yam[b,h,q,t]	219
Albuquerque[c,f,g,q,u]	220
Bangkok[a,f,h,q,u]	221
Oklahoma[c,f,g,p,u]	222
Duarte[a,f,h,q,u]	220
Hong Kong[b,d,h,o,r]	223
Chicago[a,d,g,q,r]	224
Boston[b,e,h,k,p,u]	225
Englewood[a,e,h,p,t]	226
New York[a,d,h,p,u]	226
Hawaii[b,f,g,j,q,t]	227
Cornell[a,f,g,j,q,u]	228
Tokushima[a,f,g,i,l,q,r]	229
Hayem[b,h,k,p,r]	202
Missoula[b,d,g,j,q,u]	230
Aarau[b,f,h,k,q,t]	231
Helsinki[c,e,g,i,o,r]	232
Kaluga[b,e,o,t]	233
Ogikubo[a,d,h,i,l,q,r]	234
Yokohama[a,d,g,i,m,p,r]	234
Akita[a,d,g,i,l,p,r]	234
Dublin[a,d,h,p,r]	235
Kremenchug[b,e,h,k,p,t]	236
Dothan[a,f,g,j,m,q,r]	237
Sapporo[a,d,h,k,n,o,r]	238
Electrophoretically slow variants	
Arlington Heights[c,f,g,j,q,u]	205
Long Prairie[b,d,h,k,q,r]	239
Panama[b,e,h,k,n,p,t]	240
Tripler[b,g,k,m,q,s]	241
Alhambra[a,e,g,p,u]	242
Kurume[a,d,h,i,m,q,t]	243
Rotterdam[b,d,h,o,t]	226
Atlanta[a,f,g,j,q,r]	244
Milwaukee[c,g,u]	245
Hong Kong Pokfulan[a,g,k,o,r]	218
Ramat-Gan[b,h,q,t]	219
Ashdod[c,h,p,t]	219
Tokyo[a,d,g,i,l,q,r]	229
Manchester[a,f,g,k,m,p,s]	246
Wakayama[a,d,g,i,m,q,r]	243
Freiburg[c,d,t]	247
Worcester[b,f,g,j,q,u]	248
Fukushima[a,d,g,j,m,p,r]	243
Yamaguchi[a,f,g,k,l,q,u]	243
Johannesburg[c,e,h,j,p,r]	249
Minneapolis[c,f,h,j,q,u]	250
Santa Barbara[a,f,g,j,n,q,u]	251
West Town[a,f,h,k,q,r]	205
San Francisco[c,f,g,k,m,q,r]	252
Kobe[c,d,g,k,l,q,u]	239

Table 8 (continued)
G6PD VARIANTS

Class 2 Variants (Severely Deficient, Less Than 10% Residual Activity)

Variant	Ref.
Electrophoretically fast variants	
San Jose[a,d,h,j,n,o]	253
Hualien-Chi[b,h,o,t]	254
San Juan[b,h,k,q,t]	255
Ankara[a,f,g,k,p,t]	256
Markham[b,h,p,t]	257
Taiwan-Hakka[b,h,k,p,t]	258
Union[b,d,h,k,p,t]	259
Ferrara[b,d,h,k,q,r]	260
Lublin[b,f,g,o]	261
Teheran[b,g,o,t]	254
Hualien[b,h,q,t]	254
Betica[a,g,j,o,r]	262
N-Sawan[b,e,h,k,q,t]	263
Baku[b,e,h,o,u]	264
Padrew[b,f,h,k,p,t]	263
Muret[b,e,h,k,o,u]	265
Laghouat[b,h,j,o,r]	266
Haad Yai[c,h,k,p,r]	263
Fukuoka[c,d,g,i,l,p,t]	267
Long Xuyen[b,h,k,p,t]	263
Castilla-like[b,f,h,k,p,r]	268
Dhon[b,g,k,p,r]	263
Amboin[b,f,h,k,p,r]	268
Birmingham[b,f,g,k,m,o,t]	269
Bukitu[c,f,h,k,p,r]	270
Goodenough[b,f,h,k,p,t]	268
Electrophoretically normal variants	
Indonesia[b,f,p,s]	271
Campbellpore[b,h,q,t]	272
Mediterranean[b,e,h,k,p,t]	273
Corinth[b,e,h,i,p,t]	274
'Mali'[b,d,h,p,u]	275
Siriraj[b,h,k,p,t]	276
El-Fayoum[b,h,k,q,t]	277
El-Morro[b,h,k,p,t]	255
Matam[b,e,h,k,p,t]	278
Abrami[b,f,h,k,p,t]	279
Hamm[b,d,h,k,q,u]	280
Tarsus[b,f,h,k,p,u]	280
Bagdad[c,f,h,t]	281
Blida[b,h,j,p,u]	266
Bnei Brak[a,f,h,o,t]	282
Petrich[b,f,h,k,p,s]	283
Ogori[a,d,g,i,o,r]	284
Gotze Delchev[b,f,h,k,s,v]	283
Gifu[a,d,g,k,l,p,r]	267
Bielefeld[b,f,h,k,n,o]	285
Nucus[c,e,h,j,o,u]	286
Selim[b,d,h,p,t]	264
Tashkent[b,e,h,k,p,t]	286
Moscow[b,e,h,k,p,u]	287
Electrophoretically slow variants	
Kirovograd[b,d,p,u]	288
Jammu[a,f,g,i,o,r]	289
Toulouse[a,e,h,k,q,s]	290
Panay[b,f,g,p,t]	291
Orchomenos[b,e,h,k,t]	292
Zhitomir[b,e,h,k,p,t]	288
Poznan[b,e,h,p,t]	293
Aachen[a,f,h,j,q,r]	294
Lifta[b,h,q,u]	219
Carswell[b,f,g,o,u]	295
Onoda[b,d,h,k,p,t]	296
Swit[b,e,h,k,p,t]	268
Kaluan[c,f,h,j,p,r]	297
Bogia[a,f,h,k,o,r]	297
Chainat[a,f,h,k,q,r]	263
Manus[b,e,h,k,p,t]	268
Madang[b,d,h,k,p,r]	268
Mainoki[b,d,h,k,p,r]	268
Colomiers[b,e,h,k,o,u]	265
Palakau[a,f,h,j,p,r]	268
Wewak[b,e,h,k,p,r]	268
Popondetta[b,e,h,k,p,t]	268
Zakataly[b,d,h,k,p,t]	298
Okhut I[b,d,h,k,p,t]	298
Shirin-Bulakh[b,e,h,k,p,u]	298
Titteri[b,h,j,o,u]	266
Salata[c,f,h,i,o,r]	297
Bideiz[b,d,h,k,p,t]	298
Ciudad de la Habana[b,d,h,k,n,p,t]	299
Angoram[b,d,h,k,o,r]	268
Shekii[b,e,h,k,p,t]	298
Alger[b,h,j,q,t]	266

Class 3 Variants (Moderately Deficient, 10—60% Residual Activity)

Variant	Ref.
Electrophoretically fast variants	
Barbieri[c,f,o]	300
Puerto Rico[b,g,p,r]	255
A-[a,d,g,i,o,r]	301
Debrousse[b,e,h,o,r]	302
Ube[a,d,g,i,n,o,r]	303
Castilla[a,f,h,k,m,p,r]	304
Toronto[b,f,h,i,p,r]	305
Taipei-Hakka[b,d,p,r]	258
Kabyle[a,g,o,r]	306
Chibuto[b,f,g,p,r]	307
Melissa[b,d,g,k,u]	308
Canton[b,h,p,t]	309
Velletri[c,d,h,k,m,q,t]	310

Table 8 (continued)
G6PD VARIANTS

	Ref.
Tahta[b,h,k,p,t]	277
Kan[h,k,q]	311
Gallura[b,f,g,k,n,p,r]	302
Chiapas[b,e,g,i,l,p,u]	312
Lozere[b,f,h,i,p,s]	313
Konan[a,d,g,i,l,o,r]	314
Electrophoretically normal variants	
Columbus[a,d,g]	204
Anant[b,h,k,o,r]	311
El-Kharga[a,h,j,p,u]	277
Hofu[b,d,g,k,o,r]	284
Mahidol[b,h,i,o,r]	263
Kamiube[a,d,g,i,l,o,r]	314
Electrophoretically slow variants	
Siwa[b,h,k,q,t]	277
Agrigento[b,d,g,k,p,r]	315
Athens[b,d,h,k,p,s]	316
Intanon[a,e,g,j,o,s]	317
Los Angeles[b,f,h,j,o,t]	318

	Ref.
Washington[a,g,o,r]	254
Benevento[b,h,p,t]	255
Trinacria[b,e,h,k,p,t]	319
Camperdown[b,e,h,k,o,s]	274
Kuanyama[b,e,h,k,o,r]	249
West Bengal[b,f,h,o,r]	320
Mexico[b,e,h,k,u]	321
Seattle[b,e,h,o,s]	322
Kerala[b,e,h,o,t]	320
Porbandar[b,e,h,k,o,r]	323
Port-Royal[b,h,j,p]	324
Vientiane[b,f,h,k,n,u,v]	325
Ferrara II[b,e,h,k,o,t]	326
Okhut II[b,f,h,k,p,r]	298
Yangoru[b,f,h,k,p,w]	268
Napoli[b,e,h,k,o,t]	326
Tenganan[b,f,h,k,p,r]	327
Thenia[a,g,j,o,s]	266

Class 4 Variants (Very Mild or Normal Activity, 60—150%)

	Ref.
Electrophoretically fast variants	
Inhambane[b,f,g,o,s]	307
LuzSaint Sauveur[b,e,h,k,o,r]	328
Steilacom[a,d,g,o,r]	329
A+[a,d,g,i,o,r]	330
Levadia[b,d,g,i,r]	331
Laurenzo Marques[a,d,g,o,r]	307
King County[a,d,h,r]	274
Thessaly[b,f,h,k,r]	332
Chao Phya[a,f,g,j,o,r]	333
S-Sakorn[c,f,g,j,o,r]	333
Bali[a,f,g,j,p,r]	327
Kiwa[a,d,g,i,l,o,r]	314
Electrophoretically normal variants	
B[a,d,g,i,l,o,r]	334
Martinique-like[b,f,h,i,p,r]	298

	Ref.
Electrophoretically slow variants	
Kardista[b,f,h,j,r]	308
Western[b,e,g,j,r]	335
Alexandra[b,d,g,j,o,r]	274
Manjacase[c,d,g,o,r]	307
Baltimore Austin[a,d,g,o,r]	336
Ijebu-Ode[a,f,p,t]	337
Minas Gerais[b,d,h,r]	338
Tacoma[a,d,g,k,r]	335
Madrona[b,d,g,r]	339
Ibadan-Austin[a,d,g,o,r]	336
Ita-Bale[c,f,p,r]	336
Ayutthaya[b,e,h,k,o,t]	333
Pinar Del Rio[b,d,g,n,p,t]	340
Porbandar[b,e,h,k,o,r]	341

Class 5 Variants (Increased Activity)

	Ref.
Electrophoretically fast variant	
Hektoen[a,d,g,j,o,r]	342

a Normal K_m G6P (50—70 μM).
b Low K_m G6P.
c High K_m G6P.
d Normal K_m NADP (2.9—4.4 μM.)
e Low K_m NADP.
f High K_m NADP.
g Normal 2-deoxy G6P utilization (4% of G6P).
h High 2-deoxy G6P utilization.
i Normal deamino NADP utilization (55—60% of NADP).
j Low deamino NADP utilization.
k High deamino NADP utilization.
l Normal K_i NADPH (19.22 ± 5.82).
m Low K_i NADPH.
n High K_i NADPH.
o Heat-stable.
p Labile.
q Very labile.
r Normal pH optimum.
s Slightly biphasic pH optimum.
t Biphasic.
u pH activity curve, monobasic, abnormal.
v Thermal stability; abnormal, activity increased with heating.
w No clear pH optimum.

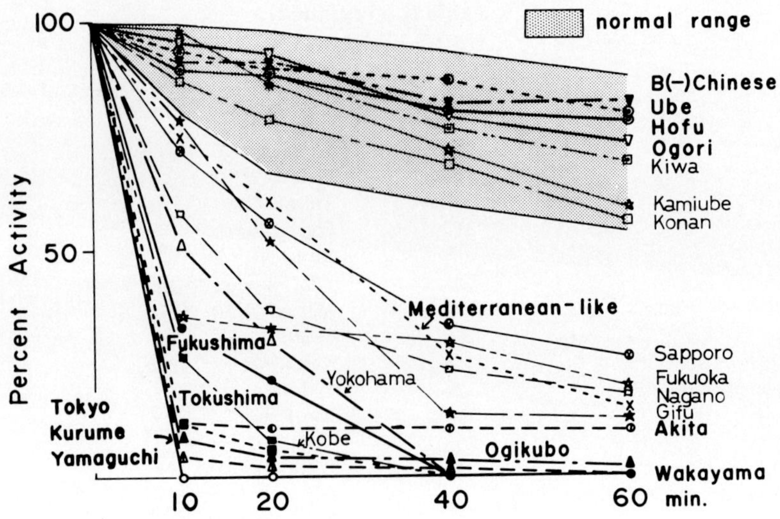

FIGURE 12. Thermostability test of glucose 6-phosphate dehydrogenase performed by WHO recommended method.[188]

clinical expression, Yoshida[182] emphasized particularly the role of the affinities of each variant for NADP and NADPH in determining whether it is associated with congenital hemolytic anemia or not. The hemolytic variants associated with relatively mild enzyme deficiency were very strongly inhibited by physiological concentration of NADPH, while nonhemolytic variants associated with severe enzyme deficiency were resistant to inhibition by NADPH. Figure 12 shows the results of a thermostability test of G6PD variants discovered by us. So-called Class 1 variants in the WHO classification[188] showed marked thermolability. Among Class 2 variants, G6PD Mediterranean-like, thermolabile variant, was associated with drug-induced hemolysis, whereas G6PD Ogori, a thermostable variant, showed no clinical symptoms at all. Thermostability was normal in all Class 3 variants which showed mild to moderate enzyme deficiency without clinical symptoms. Thus, thermostability and product inhibition by NADPH seem to be the most important kinetic properties determining whether a G6PD-deficient will be associated with acute or chronic hemolysis.

The direct cause of hemolysis of the G6PD-deficient red cells seems to be the decrease of the NADPH production by the hexose monophosphate pathway. When the G6PD-deficient red cells are unable to provide NADPH at a sufficient rate, the recycling of GSSG to GSH is limited. GSH depletion induces an oxidation of protein, especially globin, due to the reduction of oxidant removal in the red cells. Denatured globin forms insoluble masses that are attached by disulfide bridge to membrane sulfhydryl group (Heinz bodies). Presumably, the rigid Heinz bodies are removed from the cell by reticuloendothelial cells, ultimately resulting in extravascular hemolysis.[343] Recently, red cell membrane polypeptide and lipid profiles in G6PD-deficient subjects has been studied. High membrane spectrin and lipid content were demonstrated in the red cells of drug-sensitive G6PD-deficient individuals, while it was normal in nonsensitive G6PD-deficient subjects.[344]

Glutathione Reductase Deficiency

Glutathione reductase (GR) catalyzes the reduction of GSSG to GSH using NADPH provided from the hexose monophosphate pathway. GR, a ubiquitous flavoenzyme, maintains a high value for the ratio 2 GSH:GSSG in the red cell. GR is composed of two identical subunits, and the molecular weight of each subunit is 50,000.[345]

Since the first report of decreased GR activity by Löhr and Waller[346] in 1962, several cases of GR deficiency were reported. GR deficiency is a relatively common feature of disorders that are compounded by suboptimal nutrition and are associated with a variety of hematological disorders. The poorly defined clinical effects of the putative deficiency and the unconvincing nature of the family studies led to the suggestion that GR deficiency was a secondary manifestation of a poorly understood basic disorder. In fact, GR activity in the hemolysates of riboflavin-deficient humans was activated by a small amount of flavine adenine nucleotide (FAD). Furthermore, the administration of riboflavin restored the GR level of the red cells of secondary deficient individuals to normal within a few days.[347] Genetically determined GR deficiency has been reported in three cases by Loos et al.[348] They were offsprings of a consanguineous marriage. Complete GR deficiency was not affected by FAD in vitro and riboflavin in vivo. Clinically, this deficiency was manifested by hemolytic crisis after eating fava beans. The amount of GSH in the red cells was normal, but severely diminished glutathione stability during incubation with acetylphenylhydrazine was observed.

Glutathione Peroxidase Deficiency

Glutathione peroxidase (GSH-Px) catalyzes the destruction of H_2O_2 by GSH, protecting membrane lipids and hemoglobin against oxidation by H_2O_2. Necheles et al.[349,350] first reported a genetically determined partial and homozygous GSH-Px deficiency associated with neonatal jaundice and mild hemolysis. Spontaneous recovery from hemolysis was noted 3 months after birth. Thereafter, several cases with GSH-Px deficiency have been reported. Newborn infants exhibited significantly lower red cell GSH-Px activity and serum selenium concentrations than adult controls, and a significantly positive correlation between serum selenium concentration and GSH-Px activity has been observed.[351] Furthermore, the addition of selenium stimulates, both in vivo and in vitro, the GSH-Px activity.[352] Perona et al.[353] reported recently that the neonatal red cell GSH-Px deficiency may be partially due to insufficient availability of selenium during pregnancy. Therefore, the diagnosis of GSH-Px deficiency in newborn infants must be made carefully.

Defects in Glutathione Synthesis

Glutathione, a simple tripeptide, is synthesized in two steps, catalyzed by γ-glutamylcysteine synthetase (GC-S) and glutathione synthetase (GSH-S), respectively, from L-glutamate, L-leucine, and glycine. One molecule of ATP is broken down to ADP and phosphate for each peptide bond generated. Several families with GC-S deficiency[354,355] and GSH-S deficiency[356-362] have been reported. GC-S deficiency and GSH-S deficiency both appear to be inherited as an autosomal recessive and have been clearly associated with a moderate hemolytic anemia and a marked decrement of red cell GSH. Spinocerebellar degeneration and aminoaciduria were present in homozygous sibs of both families with GC-S deficiency.[354,355] Reduced levels of GSH were found in red cells, leukocytes, and muscle. In GSH-S deficiency, two clinically distinct syndromes are recognized. One shows only hemolysis,[356-358] and the other shows variable hemolysis with marked pyroglutamic aciduria.[359-362]

Nucleotide Metabolism

Adenylate Kinase Deficiency

Adenylate kinase (AK) is a ubiquitous enzyme which catalyzes the interconversion of AMP, ADP, and ATP. This interconversion of the adenine nucleotides seems to be of particular importance in regulating the equilibrium of adenine nucleotides in tissues, especially in red cells. Genetic polymorphism of this enzyme has been studied extensively.[363] Three common (AK 1, AK 2-1, and AK 2) and two rare phenotypes (AK 4-1 and AK 5-1) of AK are known, and phenotypes in Caucasians are mostly AK 1 (90%) or AK 2-1 (10%) with rare occurrence of AK 2.[364,365] The AK_2 allele is completely absent in Japanese.[366] The AK_1 has been assigned to a gene locus on chromosome 9 and AK_2 to a locus on the

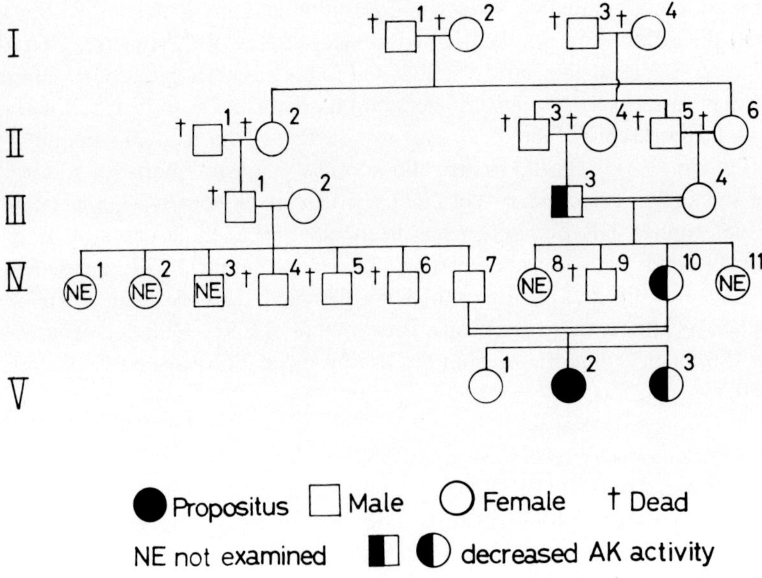

FIGURE 13. Pedigree of the Japanese family with red cell adenylate kinase deficiency.[371]

short arm of chromosome 1. The primary structure of human AK from skeletal muscle was determined to be a single polypeptide chain of 194 amino acid residues with an acetylmethionine at the NH_2-terminal and lysine at the COOH-terminal.[367]

Hereditary hemolytic anemia with red cell AK deficiency has been reported in an Israeli Arab boy,[368,369] a French child,[370] and a Japanese.[371] The proband reported by Szeinberg et al.[368,369] had chronic anemia due to a deficiency of AK and a deficiency of G6PD since the neonatal period. A sister also showed mild anemia. Both were found to have decreased AK activity, being less than 5 to 10% of the normal mean. All three adenine nucleotides were observed in increased concentrations in the proband and his AK-deficient sister. Starch-gel electrophoresis showed near absence of AK activity. Kinetic studies of the patient's AK had not yet been performed. The parents had intermediate red cell AK activity but no clinical symptoms. As the genes for AK deficiency and G6PD deficiency segregated independently in this family, the investigators proposed that the AK deficiency was transmitted most probably by an autosomal gene.

Subsequently, Boivin et al.[370] reported a second family with this enzyme deficiency. The proband had psychomotor retardation and moderate congenital hemolytic anemia with marked diminution of red cell AK activity. No AK activity band was found on starch-gel electrophoresis. The parents had half-normal AK activity with a phenotype of AK 1. Genetic inheritance was thought to be an autosomal recessive trait. In both families, the role of the enzyme deficiency in the observed anemia was not defined.

Quite recently, we found the third family of this disorder (Figure 13).[371] The proband is a 10-year-old Japanese girl. Her physical and mental development was normal. She showed moderate to mild hemolytic anemia since the neonatal period, and hepatosplenomegaly. The red cell AK activity was 44% of normal. Enzymatic characterization was performed using hemolysate in this case. The patient's AK had an increased Michaelis constant for ADP and slight thermal instability. The patient's enzyme migrated approximately halfway between the AK 1 and AK 2 position on starch-gel electrophoresis (Figure 14). The mechanism of hemolysis was considered to be due to a structural gene mutation which caused altered electrophoretic and kinetic properties. The proband's mother, younger sister, and maternal grandfather showed a half-normal enzyme activity but no clinical symptoms. Electrophorogram of these AK-deficient family members as well as that of the father was a phenotype

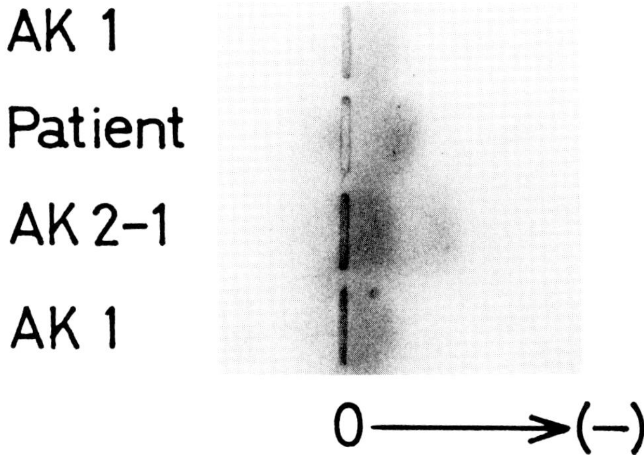

FIGURE 14. Starch-gel electrophoresis of the patient's adenylate kinase in the Japanese family.[371]

Table 9
ADENINE NUCLEOTIDES IN RED CELLS OF DIFFERENT AGE GROUPS

	Normal (retics, 0.8%)		Patient (retics, 4.8%)	
	Younger	**Older**	**Younger**	**Older**
Retics (%)	1.6	0.2	7.7	1.6
ATP[a]	1000	930	802	793
ADP[a]	282	311	326	311
AMP[a]	34.6	28.1	52.5	62.2

[a] Nanomoles per milliliter RBC.

of AK 1 while the proband showed a different electrophoretic pattern. An autosomal dominant mode of inheritance appears unlikely from the electrophoretic studies. The genetic pattern of these disorders remains to be proven.

The nature of the metabolic impairment imposed by the AK deficiency has not yet been elucidated. The physiological function of AK is to maintain the equilibrium of adenine nucleotides by the interconversion of ATP and AMP on the one hand and ADP on the other. Paglia and Valentine[372] speculated that AK is critical to the nucleotide salvage pathway mediated by adenosine kinase, and this salvage pathway is of great relative importance as glycolysis diminished. In the third family, adenine nucleotides were measured after red cell fractionation to elucidate this point. There was no significant difference in the contents of adenine nucleotides between the younger and older cells (Table 9). The causative relationship between AK deficiency and hemolysis is not clear.

Pyrimidine 5′-Nucleotidase Deficiency

Pyrimidine 5′-nucleotidase (P5N) has been identified in the soluble fraction of normal human red cells. The enzyme catalyzes the hydrolytic dephosphorylation of pyrimidine 5′-nucleotides but not purine nucleotides.[373] This enzyme was partially purified from human red cells, and had a molecular weight of 28,000.[374] Although the precise role of this enzyme in overall red cell metabolism is not clear, it is well established that hereditary deficiency

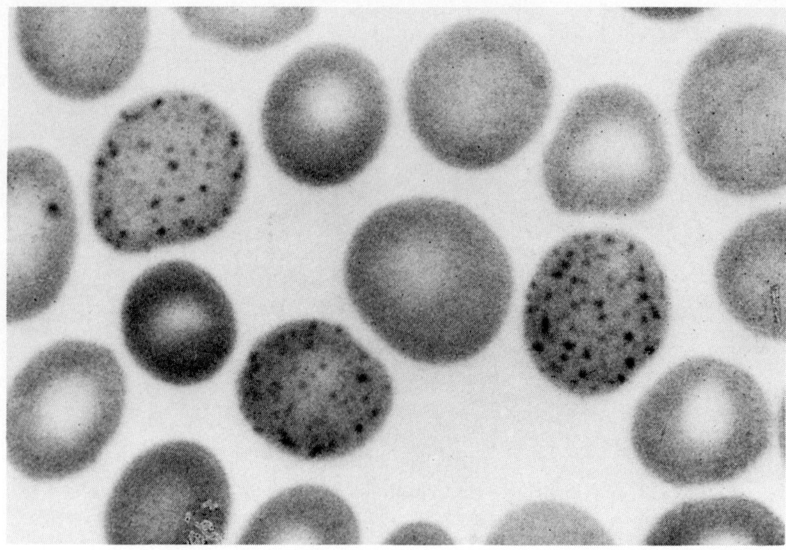

FIGURE 15. Basophilic stippling in peripheral blood smear of a patient with pyrimidine 5′-nucleotidase deficiency.

of this enzyme results in nonspherocytic hemolytic anemia since the first report by Valentine et al.[373] Up to now, 36 cases from 25 different families have been described from Israel,[375] Spain,[376] the U.S.,[377-379] France,[380,381] South Africa,[382] Turkey,[383] and Japan.[384-386] P5N deficiency is inherited as an autosomal recessive. It appears that P5N deficiency is one of the more common causes of hereditary nonspherocytic hemolytic anemia.

This syndrome is characterized by hemolytic anemia, pronounced basophilic stippling of red cells (Figure 15), and marked increase in both red cell GSH and pyrimidine-containing nucleotides. In normal red cells, adenine nucleotides form 96% of the nucleotide pool,[387] but more than 50% of the nucleotide pool consist of pyrimidine nucleotides in P5N-deficient cells. Spectroscopic examination of the perchloric-acid extract of red cells shows that the position of the absorption maximum is shifted from 260 nm in normal to 270 nm in the deficient cells (Figure 16). The maximum at 260 nm corresponds to that of adenine nucleotides. The shift to 270 nm indicates the presence of abnormal nucleotides and suggests that a major part of the abnormal nucleotide pool consists of cytidine nucleotides which have a maximum at 280 nm. Basophilic stippling of the red cells is the hallmark of this enzyme deficiency; it has been noted in most of all reported cases. It may be a reflection of retarded degradation of ribosomal RNA, secondary to feedback inhibition resulting from the high concentration of pyrimidine nucleotides.[373] A similar observation has been made in the case of lead poisoning.[388]

Electrophoretic and kinetic studies of the patient's enzyme have been reported in several of them (Table 10).[380,386,389-391] They showed an increased Michaelis constant for substrate in all cases and abnormal electrophoretic mobility in all but one case. Presumably, P5N deficiency is a consequence of structural alteration of the enzyme protein caused by a structural gene mutation. Recently, Vives-Corrons et al.[392] found that normal P5N consists of two isozymes and P5N deficiency is caused by a defect of major isozyme. The precise nature is still unknown.

Although the precise mechanism of hemolysis in P5N deficiency is not clear, Valentine et al.[373] have suggested that pyrimidine nucleotides can act as competitive cofactors capable of occupying the binding sites of enzymes, such as Hx, PGK, and PK, where ADP and ATP are much more efficient cofactors. Torrance and Whittaker,[387] on the other hand,

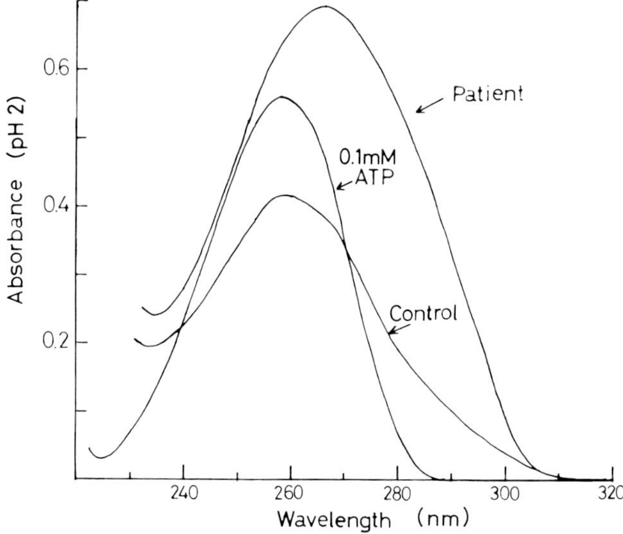

FIGURE 16. Absorption spectra of perchloric acid extracts of whole blood from normal subjects and a patient with pyrimidine 5′-nucleotidase (P5N) deficiency. Absorption peak shift occurs in P5N deficiency, reflecting intracellular accumulation of pyrimidine nucleotides.

Table 10
CHARACTERISTICS OF PYRIMIDINE 5′-NUCLEOTIDASE VARIANTS

Kindred	1[380]	2[391]	3[389]	4[390]	5[386]	6[386]	7[386]
P5N activity (% of normal)	10—14	19	5	9	24	11	48
K_m for CMP or UMP	High	High	High	High	High	High	High
Thermostability	Stable	Stable	Stable	Stable	Stable	Labile	Stable
pH optimum	Acidic	Acidic	Acidic	Acidic	Basic	Normal	Basic
Electrophoretic mobility	Slow	Slow	Normal	Slow	Slow	Slow	Slightly slow

suggested that both CTP and UTP may replace ATP as substrate for enzymes such as ATPase, resulting in the upset of the ionic balance of the red cells. Electron microscopic observation of the spleen revealed that in red cell P5N deficiency both intravascular hemolysis and erythrophagocytosis occur in the red pulp of the spleen.[393]

Hyperactivity of Adenosine Deaminase

Adenosine deaminase (ADA) is an amino hydrolase which catalyzes the deamination of the purine riboside, adenosine, to produce inosine and ammonia. It is widely distributed in human tissues,[394] and reduced or absent ADA is associated with one form of severe combined immunodeficiency disease.[396] Several isozymes of red cell ADA can be detected by starch-gel electrophoresis, and phenotypes in European populations are ADA 1 (90%) and ADA 2-1 (10%) with rare occurrence of ADA 2.[396,397] ADA has been shown to exist in different molecular and electrophoretic forms. Two forms have been well characterized. A small form (molecular weight, 38,000) of the enzyme predominates in the spleen, stomach, and red cells, while the large form (molecular weight, 298,000) predominates in the kidney, liver, and skin fibroblasts. The small form can be converted to the large form by complexing with a 200,000-dalton protein known as the adenosine deaminase binding protein of conversion factor.[398-402] Adenosine deaminase binding protein is on human chromosome 6; the structural

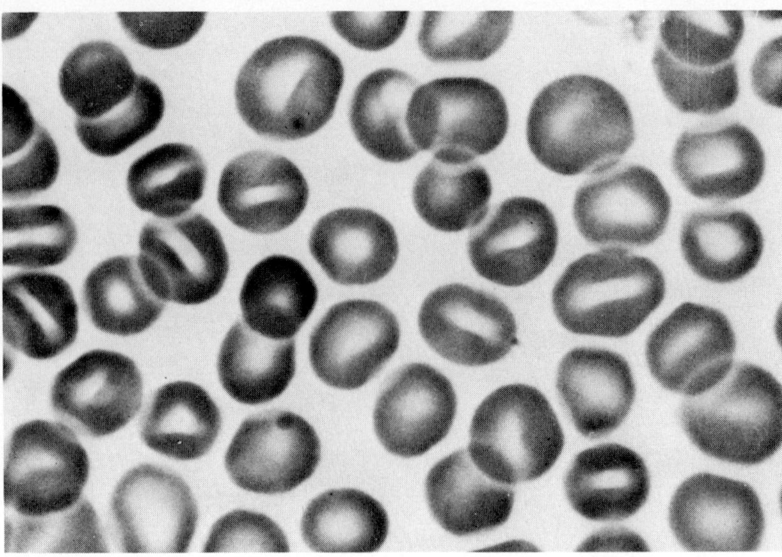

FIGURE 17. Stomatocytosis in peripheral blood smear of a patient with overproduction of adenosine deaminase.

gene for ADA 1 is on chromosome 20.[403] The human ADA locus is under manipulable genetic regulation.[404]

Hereditary hemolytic anemia with increased red cell ADA activity and decreased ATP was first reported by Valentine et al.[405] in 12 members from 3 generations of a single kindred. The disease was transmitted by an autosomal dominant trait. The enzyme activities were 45- to 70-fold of the normal whereas the concentration of ATP in the red cells was about half that of comparably reticulocyte-rich control.

Subsequently, we reported the additional family of the same disorder,[406] and quite recently, a third case was reported in an Algerian child.[407] In general, anemia was mild or fully compensated. Reticulocytosis, hyperbilirubinemia, and shortened red cell half-life were seen in all cases. Red cell morphology in our case revealed stomatocytosis as shown in Figure 17. A splenectomy was performed in a third case and rapid improvement was noted.

Red cell ADA from normal subjects and from a patient were purified using antibody affinity chromatography in the second kindred.[408] There were no differences in the molecular weight, specific activity, polyacrylamide gel electrophoresis (Figure 18), Michaelis constant for substrate, thermal stability, optimum pH, immunological reactivity, amino acid composition, and tryptic peptide mapping. These studies strongly suggest that increased red cell ADA activity is caused by an overproduction of a structurally normal enzyme. Moreover, the mechanism of red cell ADA accumulation in this disorder was investigated.[409] The rate of ADA synthesis in erythroid colony cells cultured from the patient's bone marrow cells was 11-fold greater than that from the normal (Figure 19). The accumulation of ADA in the patient seems to be due to the increased synthesis in precursors of red cells. The precise mechanism of this abnormality remains unknown, but it may be a defect in which mutation at a control gene results in increased rate of synthesis of ADA of normal structure. The defect appears to be confined to red cells, since lymphocyte and skin fibroblast ADA activity were normal.[405-407] This is consistent with evidence that tissue-specific isozymes of ADA share a common protein.

Increased ADA activity interferes with nucleotide generation via adenosine kinase, since ADA and adenosine kinase compete for a common substrate, adenosine. Hemolytic anemia

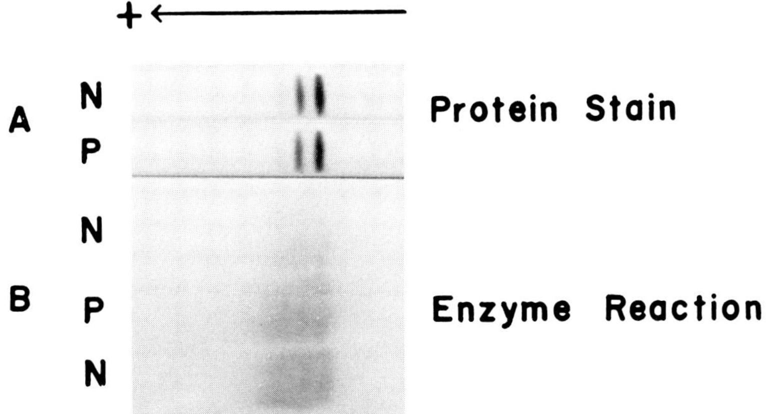

FIGURE 18. Polyacrylamide gel electrophoresis of purified adenosine deaminase. N, normal enzyme; P, patient's enzyme.

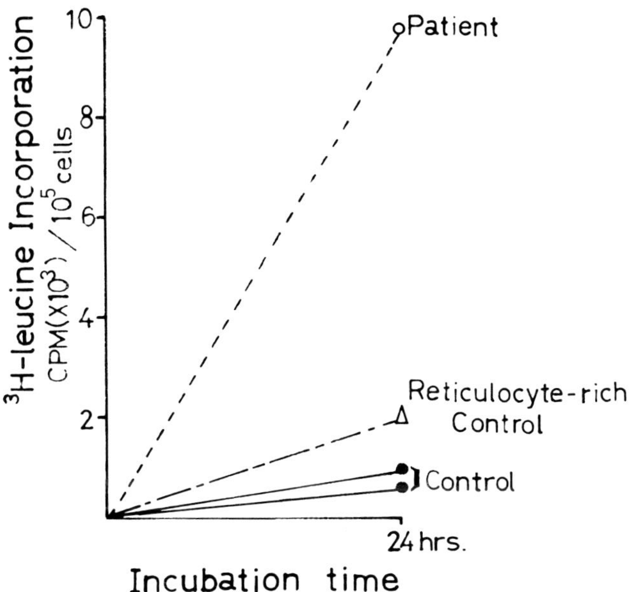

FIGURE 19. Rate of adenosine deaminase synthesis in erythroid colony cells cultured from normal, reticulocyte-rich control, and the patient's bone marrow cells.

may result from an inability to salvage sufficient adenine nucleotides to maintain red cell integrity.

HEREDITARY METHEMOGLOBINEMIA WITH DEFICIENCY OF NADH CYTOCHROME b_5 REDUCTASE

The NADH-dependent methemoglobin reductase system (NADH methemoglobin ferrocyanide reductase, NADH diaphorase, or NADH cytochrome b_5 reductase) is the most important one for the conversion of methemoglobin to functional, oxygen-binding hemoglobin. Methemoglobin reduction needs a hemoprotein, cytochrome b_5, and the electron flow of the NADH-methemoglobin reductase system is NADH cytochrome b_5 reductase-

Table 11
HEREDITARY NONHEMATOLOGIC DISORDERS WHICH CAN BE DIAGNOSED BY DETERMINATION OF RED CELL ENZYME ACTIVITY

Disorder	Deficient enzyme	Mode of inheritance
Acatalasemia	Catalase	Autosomal recessive
Lesch-Nyhan syndrome	Hypoxanthine guanine phosphoribosyltransferase	Sex-linked
Galactosemia	Galactose 1-phosphate uridyltransferase or galactokinase	Autosomal recessive
Severe combined immunodeficiency	Adenosine deaminase	Autosomal recessive
Immunodeficiency (defective T-cell immunity)	Purine nucleoside phosphorylase	Autosomal recessive
Renal tubular acidosis	Carbonic anhydrase-I	Autosomal recessive

cytochrome b_5-methemoglobin. Most patients with hereditary methemoglobinemia have been found to have red cells deficient in NADH cytochrome b_5 reductase activity. The great majority of these patients show only the diffuse, persistent, slate-gray cyanosis not associated with cardiac or pulmonary disease. A minority of patients have a severe neurological disorder with mental retardation that predisposes them to early death.[410] Kaplan et al.[411] disclosed that the molecular basis for uncomplicated hereditary methemoglobinemia without neurological involvement arises from a defect limited to the soluble cytochrome b_5 reductase, and that a combined deficiency of both the cytosolic and the microsomal cytochrome b_5 reductase occurs in subjects with mental retardation. Diagnosis of hereditary methemoglobinemia can be done by direct assay of NADH methemoglobin ferrocyanide reductase activity (Hegesh assay),[412] NADH diaphorase (Scott assay),[413] or NADH cytochrome b_5 reductase activity (Strittmatter assay).[414]

RED CELL ENZYMES FOR THE DIAGNOSIS OF CONGENITAL NONHEMATOLOGIC DISORDERS

It is possible to diagnose nonhematologic heritable disorders by measuring red cell enzyme activities, if the enzyme of the red cell and the target organ(s) demonstrating abnormality is under the same genetic control. Such disease and the defective enzymes involved are listed in Table 11.

Acatalasemia is a rare hereditary deficiency of tissue catalase. The patient shows an ulcerating gangrenous lesion of the oral cavity.

The Lesch-Nyhan syndrome is an inherited disorder associated with a virtually complete deficiency of hypoxanthine guanine phosphoribosyltransferase, and is characterized clinically by the excessive production of uric acid and certain characteristic neurologic features, such as self-mutilation, choreoathetosis, spasticity, and mental retardation.

Galactosemia is an inherited disorder associated with a cellular deficiency of galactokinase or galactose 1-phosphate uridyltransferase. The clinical manifestation in galactokinase deficiency is only cataracts. In transferase deficiency, galactose ingestion is characterized by inanition, failure to thrive, vomiting, liver disease, cataracts, and mental retardation.

Hereditary deficiency of adenosine deaminase (ADA) is associated with a severe immunodeficiency disease characterized by lymphopenia, thymic involution, and defective T- and B-cell function. A similar deficiency in purine nucleoside phosphorylase (PNP) engenders a selective cellular immune deficit with normal B-cell immunity. The causes of clinical symptoms may be that deoxyadenosine and deoxyguanosine accumulate in ADA and PNP deficiency, respectively, and are selectively phosphorylated by lymphoid cells to the corresponding deoxynucleoside triphosphate, resulting in inhibition of DNA synthesis.

A certain type of carbonic anhydrase (carbonic anhydrase 1) deficiency is known to cause renal tubular acidosis and nerve deafness.

REFERENCES

1. **Rogers, P. A., Fisher, R. A., and Harris, H.,** An examination of the age related patterns of decay of the hexokinase of human red cells, *Clin. Chim. Acta,* 65, 291, 1975.
2. **Stocchi, V., Magnani, M., Canestrari, F., Dachã, M., and Fornaini, G.,** Multiple forms of human red blood cell hexokinase, *J. Biol. Chem.,* 257, 2357, 1982.
3. **Valentine, W. N., Oski, F. A., Paglia, D. E., Baughan, M. A., Schneider, A. S., and Naiman, J. L.,** Hereditary hemolytic anemia with hexokinase deficiency. Role of hexokinase in erythrocyte aging, *N. Engl. J. Med.,* 276, 1, 1967.
4. **Keitt, A. S.,** Hemolytic anemia with impaired hexokinase activity, *J. Clin. Invest.,* 48, 1997, 1969.
5. **Moser, K., Ciresa, M., and Schwarzmeier, J.,** Hexokinasemangel bei hämolytischer Anämie, *Med. Welt.,* 46, 1977, 1970.
6. **Necheles, T. F., Rai, U. S., and Cameron, D.,** Congenital nonspherocytic hemolytic anemia associated with an unusual erythrocyte hexokinase abnormality, *J. Lab. Clin. Med.,* 76, 593, 1970.
7. **Goebel, K. M., Gassel, W. D., Goebel, F. D., and Kaffarnik, H.,** Hemolytic anemia and hexokinase deficiency associated with malformations, *Klin. Wochenschr.,* 50, 349, 1972.
8. **Rijksen, G. and Staal, G. E. J.,** Human erythrocyte hexokinase deficiency. Characterization of a mutant enzyme with abnormal regulatory properties, *J. Clin. Invest.,* 62, 294, 1978.
9. **Board, P. G., Trueworthy, R., Smith, J. E., and Moore, K.,** Congenital nonspherocytic hemolytic anemia with an unstable hexokinase variant, *Blood,* 51, 111, 1978.
10. **Beutler, E., Dyment, P. G., and Matsumoto, F.,** Hereditary nonspherocytic hemolytic anemia and hexokinase deficiency, *Blood,* 51, 935, 1978.
11. **Gilsanz, F., Meyer, E., Paglia, D. E., and Valentine, W. N.,** Congenital hemolytic anemia due to hexokinase deficiency, *Am. J. Dis. Child.,* 132, 636, 1978.
12. **Siimes, M. A., Rahiala, E.-L., and Leisti, J.,** Hexokinase deficiency in erythrocytes: a new variant in 5 members of a Finnish family, *Scand. J. Haematol.,* 22, 214, 1979.
13. **Newman, P., Muir, A., and Parker, A. C.,** Non-spherocytic haemolytic anaemia in mother and son associated with hexokinase deficiency, *Br. J. Haematol.,* 46, 537, 1980.
14. **Paglia, D. E., Shende, A., Lanzkowsky, P., and Valentine, W. N.,** Hexokinase "New Hyde Park": a low activity erythrocyte isozyme in a Chinese kindred, *Am. J. Hematol.,* 10, 107, 1981.
15. **Staal, G. E. J., Akkerman, J. W. N., Hofstede, D. P., van de Wall Bake, A. W. L., and Rijksen, G.,** Hexokinase deficiency in non-spherocytic hemolytic anemia, in *Proc. 19th Cong. Int. Soc. Hematol.,* Budapest, Hungary, 1982, 226.
16. **McMorris, F. S., Chen, T. R., Ricciuti, F., Tischfield, J., Greagan, R., and Ruddle, F.,** Chromosome assignments in man of the genes for two hexose phosphate isomerase, *Science,* 179, 1129, 1973.
17. **Nakashima, K., Miwa, S., Oda, S., Oda, E., Matsumoto, N., Fukumoto, Y., and Yamada, T.,** Electrophoretic and kinetic studies of glucosephosphate isomerase (GPI) in two different Japanese families with GPI deficiency, *Am. J. Hum. Genet.,* 25, 294, 1972.
18. **Payne, D. M., Porter, D. W., and Gracy, R. W.,** Evidence against the occurrence of tissue specific variants and isoenzymes of phosphoglucose isomerase, *Arch. Biochem. Biophys.,* 151, 122, 1972.
19. **Carter, N. D. and Yoshida, A.,** Purification and characterization of human phosphoglucose isomerase, *Biochim. Biophys. Acta,* 181, 12, 1969.
20. **Tilley, B. E., Gracy, R. W., and Welch, S. G.,** A point mutation increasing the stability of human phosphoglucose isomerase, *J. Biol. Chem.,* 249, 4571, 1974.
21. **Baughan, M. A., Valentine, W. N., Paglia, D. E., Ways, P. O., Simon, E. R., and DeMarsh, Q. B.,** Hereditary hemolytic anemia associated with glucose-phosphate isomerase (GPI) deficiency — a new enzyme defect of human erythrocytes, *Blood,* 32, 236, 1968.
22. **Paglia, D. E., Holland, P., Baughan, M. A., and Valentine, W. N.,** Occurrence of defective hexosephosphate isomerization in human erythrocytes and leukocytes, *N. Engl. J. Med.,* 280, 66, 1969.
23. **Cartier, P., Temkine, H., and Griscelli, C.,** Etude biochimique d' une anemie hemolytique avecdedicit familial en phosphohexisomerase, *Enzymol. Biol. Clin.,* 10, 439, 1969.

24. **Arnold, H., Blume, K. G., Busch, D., Lenkeit, U., Löhr, G. W., and Lübs, E.,** Klinische und biochemische Untersuchungen zur Glucosephosphatisomerase normaler menschlicher Erythrozyten une bei Glucosephosphatisomerase-Mangel, *Klin. Wochenschr.*, 48, 1299, 1970.
25. **Leger, J., Bost, M., Kolodie, L., Schaerer, R., and Hollard, D.,** Anemie hemolytique congenitale et familia avec deficit en phospho-hexoseisomerase (PHI) et elliptocytose, in *Proc. 13th Cong. Int. Soc. Hematol.*, München, West Germany, 1970, 293.
26. **Paglia, D. E., Paredes, R., Valentine, W. N., Dorantes, S., and Konrad, P. N.,** Unique phenotypic expression of glucosephosphate isomerase deficiency, *Am. J. Hum. Genet.*, 27, 62, 1970.
27. **Schröter, W., Brittinger, G., Zimmerschitt, E., König, E., and Schrader, D.,** Combined glucose-phosphate isomerase and glucose-6-phosphate dehydrogenase deficiency of the erythrocytes: a new hemolytic syndrome, *Br. J. Haematol.*, 20, 249, 1971.
28. **Schröter, W. and Tillmann, W.,** Congenital nonspherocytic hemolytic anemia associated with glucose-phosphate isomerase deficiency: Variant Paderborn, *Klin. Wochenschr.*, 55, 393, 1977.
29. **Oski, F. and Fuller, E.,** Glucose-phosphate isomerase (GPI) associated with abnormal osmotic fragility and spherocytes, *Clin. Res.*, 19, 427, 1971.
30. **Welch, S. G.,** Qualitative and quantitative variants of human phosphoglucose isomerase, *Hum. Hered.*, 21, 467, 1971.
31. **Blume, K. G., Hryniuk, W., Powars, D., Trinidad, F., West, C., and Beutler, E.,** Characterization of new variant of glucosephosphate isomerase deficiency with hereditary nonspherocytic hemolytic anemia, *J. Lab. Clin. Med.*, 97, 942, 1972.
32. **Miwa, S., Nakashima, K., Oda, S., Oda, E., Matsumoto, N., Ogawa, H., and Fukumoto, Y.,** Glucosephosphate isomerase (GPI) deficiency hereditary nonspherocytic hemolytic anemia. Report of the first case found in Japan, *Acta Haematol. Jpn.*, 36, 65, 1973.
33. **Miwa, S., Nakashima, K., Oda, S., Matsumoto, N., Ogawa, H., Kobayashi, R., Kotani, M., Harata, A., Onaya, T., and Yamada, Y.,** Glucosephosphate isomerase (GPI) deficiency hereditary nonspherocytic hemolytic anemia. Report of the second case found in Japanese, *Acta Haematol. Jpn.*, 36, 70, 1973.
34. **Miwa, S., Nakashima, K., Tajiri, M., Ono, J., Abe, S., Oda, E., Nonaka, H., Matsumoto, I., Shimoyama, S., Hirata, Y., Amaki, I., Horiuchi, A., Yamguchi, H., and Nishina, Y.,** Three cases in two families with congenital nonspherocytic hemolytic anemia due to defective glucosephosphate isomerase: GPI Matsumoto, *Acta Haematol. Jpn.*, 38, 238, 1975.
35. **Arakawa, M.,** personal communication, 1976.
36. **Arnold, H., Engelhardt, R., Löhr, G. W., Jacobi, H., and Liebold, I.,** Glucosephosphate-Isomerase Typ Recklinghausen: eine neue Defektvariante mit hämolytischer Anämie, *Klin. Wochenschr.*, 51, 1198, 1973.
37. **Beutler, E., Sigalove, W. H., Angusmuir, W., Matsumoto, F., and West, C.,** Glucosephosphate isomerase (GPI) deficiency: GPI Elyria, *Ann. Intern. Med.*, 80, 730, 1974.
38. **Arnold, H., Blume, K. G., Löhr, G. W., Schröter, W., Koch, H. H., and Wonneberger, B.,** Glucose phosphate isomerase deficiency with congenital nonspherocytic hemolytic anemia: a new variant (Type Nordhorn). II. Purification and biochemical properties of the defective enzyme, *Pediatr. Res.*, 8, 26, 1974.
39. **Hutton, J. J. and Chilcote, R. R.,** Glucose phosphate isomerase deficiency with hereditary nonspherocytic hemolytic anemia, *J. Pediatr.*, 85, 494, 1974.
40. **Müller, E., Marti, H. R., Bach, J., Micheli, J. L., and Gasser, C.,** Hereditäre nicht-sphärozytäre hämolytische Anämie durch Glukosephosphatisomerase-Mangel: Der erste in der Schweiz beobachtete Fall, *Schweiz. Med. Wochenschr.*, 104, 1379, 1974.
41. **Van Biervliet, J. P. G. M., Van Milligen-Boersma, L., and Staal, G. E. J.,** A new variant of glucosephosphate isomerase deficiency (GPI Utrecht), *Clin. Chim. Acta*, 65, 157, 1975.
42. **Rotteveel, J. J., de Vaan, G. A. M., Staal, G. E. J., Van Biervliet, J. P. G. M., and Schretlen, E. D. A. M.,** Glucosephosphate isomerase deficiency, a new variant in a Dutch family. Case report, *Eur. J. Pediatr.*, 125, 21, 1977.
43. **Kahn, A., Vives-Corron, J. L., Bertrand, O., Cottreau, D., Marie, J., and Boivin, P.,** Glucose-phosphate isomerase deficiency due to a new variant (GPI Barcelona) and to a silent gene. Biochemical, immunological and genetic studies, *Clin. Chim. Acta*, 66, 145, 1976.
44. **Staal, G. E. J., Akkerman, J. W. N., Eggermont, E., and Van Biervliet, J. P. G. M.,** A new variant of glucosephosphate isomerase deficiency: GPI-Kortrijk, *Clin. Chim. Acta*, 78, 121, 1977.
45. **Cayanis, E., Penfold, G. K., Freiman, I., and MacDougall, L. G.,** Haemolytic anaemia associated wtih glucosephosphate isomerase (GPI) deficiency in black South African child, *Br. J. Haematol.*, 37, 363, 1977.
46. **Arnold, H., Dodinval-Versie, J., Lambotte, C., Löhr, G. W., and van der Hofstadt, J.,** Glucose-phosphate isomerase deficiency type Liège: a new variant with congenital nonspherocytic hemolytic anemia, *Blut*, 35, 187, 1977.

47. **Zanella, A., Rebulla, P., Izzo, C., Zanuso, F., Kahane, I., Molinari, E., and Sirchia, G.,** A new mutant erythrocyte glucosephosphate isomerase (GPI) associated with GSH abnormality, *Am. J. Hematol.*, 5, 11, 1978.
48. **Isacchi, G., Cottreau, D., Mandelli, F., Papa, G., Ciccone, F., and Kahn, A.,** 'GPI Roma', a new glucose phosphate isomerase deficient variant, *Hum. Genet.*, 46, 219, 1979.
49. **Arnold, H., Löhr, G. W., Hasslinger, K., and Podgajny, T. H.,** Augsburg type glucosephosphate isomerase deficiency — a new variant causing congenital nonspherocytic hemolytic anemia in a German family, *Blut*, 40, 107, 1980.
50. **Uga, N., Nishina, T., Ohyama, K., Kitamura, M., Tsuchida, M., Rin, K., Yanagawa, Y., Fukushima, O., and Yoshihara, S.,** Two cases in a family with new variants of glucose phosphate isomerase deficiency, *Jpn. J. Clin. Hematol.*, 21, 633, 1980 (in Japanese).
51. **Soeda, A., Yokoi, S., Chiba, H., Kitani, N., Akatsuka, J., and Nishina, T.,** A case of congenital nonspherocytic hemolytic anemia associated with defective glucose phosphate isomerase, *Jpn. J. Clin. Hematol.*, 23, 1228, 1982 (in Japanese).
52. **Takegawa, S., Fujii, H., Miwa, S., Ohba, Y., Yamauchi, H., and Miyata, H.,** A case of congenital nonspherocytic hemolytic anemia associated wtih glucosephosphate isomerase (GPI) deficiency — GPI 'Kinki', *Acta Haematol. Jpn.*, 46, 11, 1983.
53. **Hopkinson, D. A.,** The investigation of reactive sulfhydryls in enzymes and their variants by starch-gel electrophoresis: studies on the human phosphohexose isomerase variant PHI 5-1, *Ann. Hum. Genet.*, 34, 79, 1970.
54. **Schröter, W. and Tillmann, W.,** Decreased deformability of erythrocytes in haemolytic anaemia associated with glucosephosphate isomerase deficiency, *Br. J. Haematol.*, 36, 475, 1977.
55. **Matsumoto, N., Ishihara, T., Oda, E., Miwa, S., Nakashima, K., Uchino, F., and Fukumoto, Y.,** Fine structure of the spleen and liver in glucosephosphate isomerase (GPI) deficiency hereditary nonspherocytic hemolytic anemia — selective reticulocyte destruction as a mechanism of hemolysis, *Acta Haematol. Jpn.*, 36, 46, 1973.
56. **Kahn, A., Meienhofer, M.-C., Cottreau, D., Lagrange, J.-L., and Dreyfrus, J.-C.,** Phosphofructokinase (PFK) isozymes in man. I. Studies of adult human tissues, *Hum. Genet.*, 48, 93, 1979.
57. **Karadsheh, N. S., Uyeda, K., and Oliver, R. M.,** Studies on structure of human erythrocyte phosphofructokinase, *J. Biol. Chem.*, 252, 3515, 1977.
58. **Cottreau, D., Levin, M. J., and Kahn, A.,** Purification and partial characterization of different forms of phosphofructokinase in man, *Biochim. Biophys. Acta*, 568, 183, 1979.
59. **Vora, S. and Francke, U.,** Assignment of the human gene for liver-type 6-phosphofructokinase isozyme (PFKL) to chromosome 21 by using somatic cell hybrids and monoclonal anti-L antibody, *Proc. Natl. Acad. Sci. U.S.A.*, 78, 3738, 1981.
60. **Vora, S., Durham, S., de Martinville, B., George, D. L., and Francke, U.,** Assignment of the human gene for muscle-type phosphofructokinase (PFKM) to chromosome 1 (Region cen → q 32) using somatic cell hybrides and monoclonal anti-M antibody, *Somat. Cell Genet.*, 8, 95, 1982.
61. **Vora, S., Seaman, C., Durham, S., and Piomelli, S.,** Isozymes of human phosphofructokinase: identification and subunit structural characterization of a new system, *Proc. Natl. Acad. Sci. U.S.A.*, 77, 62, 1980.
62. **Vora, S.,** Isozymes of human phosphofructokinase in blood cells and cultured cell lines: molecular and genetic evidence for a trigenic system, *Blood*, 57, 724, 1981.
63. **Tarui, S., Okuno, G., Ikuno, Y., Tanaka, T., Suda, M., and Nishikawa, M.,** Phosphofructokinase deficiency in skeletal muscle. A new type of glycogenosis, *Biochem. Biophys. Res. Commun.*, 19, 517, 1965.
64. **Layzer, R. B., Rowland, L. P., and Ranney, H. M.,** Muscle phosphofructokinase deficiency, *Arch. Neurol.*, 17, 512, 1967.
65. **Miwa, S., Sato, T., Murano, H., Kozuru, M., and Ibayashi, H.,** A new type of phosphofructokinase deficiency hereditary nonspherocytic hemolytic anemia, *Acta Haematol. Jpn.*, 35, 113, 1972.
66. **Waterbury, L. and Frenkel. E. P.,** Hereditary nonspherocytic hemolysis with erythrocyte phosphofructokinase deficiency, *Blood*, 39, 415, 1972.
67. **Serratrice, G., Monges, A., Roux, H., Aquaron, R., and Gambarelli, D.,** Forme myopathique du dèficit en phosphofructokinase, *Rev. Neurol. (Paris)*, 120, 271, 1969.
68. **Tobin, W. E., Huijing, F., Porro, R. S., and Salzman, R. T.,** Muscle phosphofructokinase deficiency, *Arch. Neurol.*, 28, 128, 1973.
69. **Boulard, M. R., Meienhofer, M. C., Bois, M., Reviron, M., and Najean, Y.,** Red cell phosphofructokinase deficiency, *N. Engl. J. Med.*, 291, 978, 1974.
70. **Kahn, A., Etiemble, J., Meienhofer, M., and Boivin, P.,** Erythrocyte phosphofructokinase deficiency associated with an unstable variant of muscle phosphofructokinase, *Clin. Chim. Acta*, 61, 415, 1975.
71. **Oda, S., Oda, E., and Tanaka, K. R.,** Erythrocyte phosphofructokinase (PFK) deficiency. Characterization and metabolic studies, *Clin. Res.*, 25, 344, 1977.

72. **Dupond, J. L., Carbillet, J. P., and Leconte des Floris, R.,** Glycogénose musculaire et anèmie hémolytique par déficit enzymatique chez deux germains. Forme familiale de maladie de Tarui, par déficit en phosphofructokinase musculaire et érythrocytaire, *Nouv. Presse Med.*, 6, 2665, 1977.
73. **Vora, S., Corash, L., and Piomelli, S.,** The molecular mechanism of inherited red cell phosphofructokinase deficiency associated with hemolysis and myopathy (Tarui's disease), *Blood,* 52(Suppl. 1), 105, 1978.
74. **Guibaud, P., Carrier, H., Mathieu, M., Dorche, C. L., Parchoux, B., Béthenod, M., and Larbre, F.,** Observation familiale de dystrophie musculaire congenitale par déficit en phosphofructokinase, *Arch. Fr. Pediatr.*, 35, 1105, 1978.
75. **Agamanolis, D. P., Askari, A. D., Mauro, S. D., Hays, A., Kumar, D., Lipton, M., and Raynor, A.,** Muscle phosphofructokinase deficiency: two cases with unusual polysaccharide accumulation and immunologically active enzyme protein, *Muscle Nerve,* 3, 456, 1980.
76. **Hays, A. P., Hallet, M., Delfs, J., Morris, J., Sotrel, A., Shevchuk, M. M., and DiMauro, S.,** Muscle phosphofructokinase deficiency: Abnormal polysaccharide in a case of late-onset myopathy, *Neurology (Ny),* 31, 1077, 1981.
77. **Danon, M. J., Carpenter, S., Manaligod, J. R., and Schliselfeld, L. H.,** Fetal infantile glycogen storage disease: deficiency of phosphofructokinase and phosphofructokinase b kinase, *Neurology (Ny),* 31, 1303, 1981.
78. **Zanella, A., Mariani, M., Meola, G., Fagnani, G., and Sirchia, G.,** Phosphofructokinase (PFK) deficiency due to a catalytically inactive mutant M-type subunit, *Am. J. Hematol.*, 12, 215, 1982.
79. **Tani, K., Fujii, H., Miwa, S., Koyama, W., Kanayama, M., Imanaka, F., and Kuramoto, A.,** Two cases of phosphofructokinase deficiency associated with congenital hemolytic anemia found in Japan, *Am. J. Hematol.*, 14, 165, 1983.
80. **Eagles, P. A. M. and Iqbal, M.,** A comparative study of aldolase from human muscle and liver, *Biochem. J.*, 133, 429, 1973.
81. **Penhoet, E., Rajkumar, T., and Rutter, W. J.,** Multiple forms of fructose diphosphate aldolase in mammalian tissues, *Proc. Natl. Acad. Sci. U.S.A.*, 56, 1275, 1966.
82. **Lebherz, H. G. and Rutter, W. J.,** Distribution of fructose diphosphate aldolase variants in biological systems, *Biochemistry,* 8, 109, 1969.
83. **Grégori, C., Besmond, C., Kahn, A., and Dreyfus, J.-C.,** Characterization of messenger RNA for aldolase B in adult and fetal human liver, *Biochem. Biophys. Res. Commun.*, 104, 369, 1982.
84. **Beutler, E., Scott, S., Bishop, A., Margolis, N., Matsumoto, F., and Kuhl, W.,** Red cell aldolase deficiency and hemolytic anemia: a new syndrome, *Trans. Assoc. Am. Physicians,* 76, 154, 1973.
85. **Miwa, S., Fujii, H., Tani, K., Takahashi, K., Takegawa, S., Fujinami, N., Sakurai, M., Kubo, M., Tanimoto, Y., Kato, T., and Matsumoto, N.,** Two cases of red cell aldolase deficiency associated with hereditary hemolytic anemia in a Japanese family, *Am. J. Hematol.*, 11, 425, 1981.
86. **Yuan, P. M., Dewan, R. N., Zaun, M., Thompson, R. E., and Gracy, R. W.,** Isolation and characterization of triosephosphate isomerase isozymes from human placenta, *Arch. Biochem. Biophys.*, 198, 42, 1979.
87. **Eber, S. W. and Krietsch, W. K. G.,** The isolation and characterization of the multiple forms of human skeletal muscle triosephosphate isomerase, *Biochim. Biophys. Acta,* 614, 173, 1980.
88. **Decker, R. S. and Mohrenweiser, H. W.,** Origin of the triosephosphate isomerase isozymes in humans: genetic evidence for the expression of a single structural locus, *Am. J. Hum. Genet.*, 33, 683, 1981.
89. **Jongsma, A. P. M., Hagmeijer, J., and Meeralhan, P.,** Regional mapping of TPI, LDH-B and Pep-B on chromosome 12 of man, *2nd Int. Workshop on Human Gene Mapping,* Basel, Switzerland, 1975, 189.
90. **Schneider, A. S., Valentine, W. N., Hattori, M., and Heins, H. L.,** Hereditary hemolytic anemia with triosephosphate isomerase deficiency, *N. Engl. J. Med.*, 272, 229, 1965.
91. **Valentine, W. N., Schneider, A. S., Baughan, M. A., Paglia, D. E., and Heins, H. L.,** Hereditary hemolytic anemia with triosephosphate isomerase deficiency, *Am. J. Med.*, 41, 27, 1966.
92. **Harris, S. R., Paglia, D. E., Jaffé, E. R., Valentine, W. N., and Klein, A. L.,** Triose phosphate isomerase deficiency in adult, *Clin. Res.*, 18, 529, 1970.
93. **Angelman, H., Brain, M. C., and Iver, M.,** A case of triosephosphate isomerase deficiency with sudden death, in *Proc. 13th Cong. Int. Soc. Hematol.*, Munich, West Germany, 1970, 122.
94. **Skala, H., Dreyfus, J. C., Vives-Corrons, J. L., Matsumoto, F., and Beutler, E.,** Triose phosphate isomerase deficiency, *Biochem. Med.*, 18, 226, 1977.
95. **Vives-Corrons, J. L., Rubinson-Skala, H., Mateo, M., Estella, J., Feliu, E., and Dreyfus, J.-C.,** Triosephosphate isomerase deficiency with hemolytic anemia and severe neuromuscular disease. Familial and biochemical studies of a case found in Spain, *Hum. Genet.*, 42, 171, 1978.
96. **Eber, S. W., Dünnwald, M., Belohradsky, B. H., Bidlingmaier, F., Schievelbein, H., Weinmann, H. M., and Krietsch, W. K. G.,** Hereditary deficiency of triosephosphate isomerase in four unrelated families, *Eur. J. Clin. Invest.*, 9, 195, 1979.
97. **Sparkes, R. S., Carrel, R. E., and Paglia, D. E.,** Probable localization of a triosephosphate isomerase gene to the short arm of the number 5 human chromosome, *Nature (London),* 224, 367, 1969.

98. **Moser, K., Fischer, M., Krepler, P., and Lechner, K.,** Glutathionreductase-und Triosephosphatisomerase-mangel in Erythrocyten und Thrombocyten bei Pancytopenie (Typ Estren-Damashek), *Klin. Wochenschr.,* 46, 995, 1968.
99. **Kaplan, J. C., Shore, N., and Beutler, E.,** The rapid detection of triose phosphate isomerase deficiency, *Am. J. Clin. Pathol.,* 50, 656, 1968.
100. **Chen. S.-H., Malcolm, L. A., Yoshida, A., and Giblett, E. R.,** Phosphoglycerate kinase: an X-linked polymorphism in man, *Am. J. Hum. Genet.,* 23, 87, 1971.
101. **Deys, B. F., Grzeschick, K. H., Grzeschick, A., Jaffe, E. R., and Siniscalco, M.,** Human phosphoglycerate kinase and inactivation of the X chromosome, *Science,* 175, 1002, 1972.
102. **Yoshida, A. and Watanabe, S.,** Human phosphoglycerate kinase. I. Crystalization and characterization of normal enzyme, *J. Biol. Chem.,* 247, 440, 1972.
103. **Huang, I.-Y., Rubinfien, E., and Yoshida, A.,** Complete amino acid sequence of human phosphoglycerate kinase. Isolation and amino acid sequence of tryptic peptides, *J. Biol. Chem.,* 255, 6408, 1980.
104. **Huang, I.-Y., Welch, C. D., and Yoshida, A.,** Complete amino acid sequence of human phosphoglycerate kinase. Cyanogen bromide peptides and complete amino acid sequence, *J. Biol. Chem.,* 255, 6412, 1980.
105. **Kraus, A. P., Langston, M. F., Jr., and Lynch, B. L.,** Red cell phosphoglycerate kinase deficiency. A new cause of non-spherocytic hemolytic anemia, *Biochem. Biophys. Res. Commun.,* 30, 173, 1968.
106. **Valentine, W. N., Hsieh, H., Paglia, D. E., Anderson, H. M., Baughan, M. A., Jaffé, E. R., and Garson, D. M.,** Hereditary hemolytic anemia associated with phosphoglycerate kinase deficiency in erythrocytes and leukocytes, *N. Engl. J. Med.,* 280, 528, 1969.
107. **Hjelm, M. and Wadman, B.,** Nonspherocytic hemolytic anemia with phosphoglycerate kinase deficiency, in *Proc. 13th Int. Cong. Haemat.,* Munich, Germany, 1970, 121.
108. **Cartier, P., Habibi, B., Leroux, J.-P., and Marchand, J.-C.,** Anémie hémolytique congénitale associée a un déficit en phosphoglycérate-kinase dans les globules rouges, les polynucléaires et les lymphocytes, *Nouv. Rev. Fr. Hématol.,* 11, 565, 1971.
109. **Miwa, S., Nakashima, K., Oda, S., Ogawa, H., Nagafuji, H., Arima, M., Okuna, T., and Nakashima, T.,** Phosphoglycerate kinase (PGK) deficiency hereditary nonspherocytic hemolytic anemia: report of a case found in Japanese family, *Acta Haematol. Jpn.,* 35, 571, 1972.
110. **Arese, P., Bosia, A., Gallo, E., Mazza, U., and Pescarmona, G. P.,** Red cell glycolysis in a case of 3-phosphoglycerate kinase deficiency, *Eur. J. Clin. Invest.,* 3, 86, 1973.
111. **Konrad, P. N., McCarthy, D. J., Mauer, A. M., Valentine, W. N., and Paglia, D. E.,** Erythrocyte and leukocyte phosphoglycerate kinase deficiency with neurologic disease, *J. Pediatr.,* 82, 456, 1973.
112. **Akatsuka, J., Saito, F., Okabe, N., Maekawa, K., Kitani, N., Nishina, T., and Hashimoto, F.,** Studies on erythrocyte and leukocyte phosphoglycerate kinase deficiency with neurologic disease, *Jpn. J. Clin. Hematol.,* 14, 1189, 1973 (in Japanese).
113. **Boivin, P., Hakim, J., Mandereau, J., Galand, C., Degos, F., and Schaison, G.,** Erythrocyte and leukocyte 3-phosphoglycerate kinase deficiency. Studies of properties of the enzyme, phagocytic activity of the polymorphonuclear leukocytes and a review of the literature, *Nouv. Rev. Fr. Hématol.,* 14, 496, 1974.
114. **Krietsch, W. K. G., Krietsch, H., Kaiser, W., Dünnwald, M., Kuntz, G. W. K., Duhm, J., and Bücher, T.,** Hereditary deficiency of phosphoglycerate kinase: a new variant in erythrocytes and leucocytes, not associated with haemolytic anaemia, *Eur. J. Clin. Invest.,* 7, 427, 1977.
115. **Rosa, R., George, C., Fardeau, M., Calvin, M.-C., Rapin, M., and Rosa, J.,** A new case of phosphoglycerate kinase deficiency: PGK Creteil associated with rhabdomyolysis and lacking hemolytic anemia, *Blood,* 60, 84, 1982.
116. **Yoshida, A. and Miwa, S.,** Characterization of a phosphoglycerate kinase variant associated with hemolytic anemia, *Am. J. Hum. Genet.,* 26, 378, 1974.
117. **Krietsch, W. K. G., Eber, S. W., Haas, B., Ruppelt, W., and Kuntz, G. W. K.,** Characterization of a phosphoglycerate kinase deficiency variants not associated with hemolytic anemia, *Am. J. Hum. Genet.,* 32, 364, 1980.
118. **Kahn, A., Cottreau, D., Galand, C., and Boivin, P.,** Human erythrocyte phosphoglycerate kinase deficiency: presence in a deficient patient of a stable variant with lowered catalytic activity, *Clin. Chim. Acta,* 69, 21, 1976.
119. **Yoshida, A., Watanabe, S., Chen, S.-H., Giblett, E. R., and Malcolm, L. A.,** Human phosphoglycerate kinase. II. Structure of a variant enzyme, *J. Biol. Chem.,* 247, 446, 1972.
120. **Fujii, H., Krietsch, W. K. G., and Yoshida, A.,** A single amino acid substitution (Asp $\rightarrow$ Asn) in a phosphoglycerate kinase variant (PGK München) associated with enzyme deficiency, *J. Biol. Chem.,* 255, 6421, 1980.
121. **Fujii, H. and Yoshida, A.,** Molecular abnormality of phosphoglycerate kinase-Uppsala associated with chronic nonspherocytic hemolytic anemia, *Proc. Natl. Acad. Sci. U.S.A.,* 77, 5461, 1980.

122. **Fujii, H., Chen, S.-H., Akatsuka, J., Miwa, S., and Yoshida, A.,** Use of cultured lymphoblastoid cells for the study of abnormal enzymes: molecular abnormality of a phosphoglycerate kinase variant associated with hemolytic anemia, *Proc. Natl. Acad. Sci. U.S.A.*, 78, 2587, 1981.
123. **Banks, R. D., Blake, C. C. F., Evans, P. R., Haser, R., Rice, D. W., Hardy, G. W., Merrett, M., and Phillips, A. W.,** Sequence, structure and activity of phosphoglycerate kinase: a possible hinge-bending enzyme, *Nature (London)*, 279, 773, 1979.
124. **Imamura, K. and Tanaka, T.,** Multimolecular forms of pyruvate kinase from rat and other mammalian tissues. I. Electrophoretic studies, *J. Biochem.*, 71, 1043, 1972.
125. **Ibsen, K. H.,** Interrelationships and function of the pyruvate kinase isozymes and their variant forms: a review, *Cancer Res.*, 37, 341, 1977.
126. **Tanaka, T., Harano, Y., Sue, F., and Morimura, H.,** Crystallization, characterization and metabolic regulation of two types of pyruvate kinase isolated from rat tissues, *J. Biochem.*, 62, 71, 1967.
127. **Harada, K., Saheki, S., Wada, K., and Tanaka, T.,** Purification of four pyruvate kinase isozymes of rats by affinity elution chromatography, *Biochim. Biophys. Acta*, 524, 327, 1978.
128. **Saheki, S., Saheki, K., and Tanaka, T.,** Peptide structures of pyruvate kinase isozymes. I. Comparison of the four pyruvate kinase isozymes of the rat, *Biochim. Biophys. Acta*, 704, 484, 1982.
129. **Noguchi, T. and Tanaka, T.,** The M_1 and M_2 subunits of rat pyruvate kinase are encoded by different messenger RNAs, *J. Biol. Chem.*, 257, 1110, 1982.
130. **Hance, A. J., Lee, J., and Feitelson, M.,** The M_1 and M_2 isozymes of pyruvate kinase are the products of the same gene, *Biochem. Biophys. Res. Commun.*, 106, 492, 1982.
131. **Bigley, R. H. and Koler, R. D.,** Liver pyruvate kinase (PK) isozymes in a PK-deficient patient, *Ann. Hum. Genet.*, 31, 383, 1968.
132. **Nakashima, K., Miwa, S., Oda, S., Tanaka, T., Imamura, K., and Nishina, T.,** Electrophoretic and kinetic studies of mutant erythrocyte pyruvate kinases, *Blood*, 43, 537, 1974.
133. **Kahn, A., Marie, J., Galand, C., and Boivin, P.,** Chronic haemolytic anaemia in two patients heterozygous for erythrocyte pyruvate kinase deficiency. Electrofocusing and immunological studies of erythrocyte and liver pyruvate kinase, *Scand. J. Haematol.*, 16, 250, 1976.
134. **Kahn, A., Marie, J., Garreau, H., and Sprengers, E. D.,** The genetic system of the L-type pyruvate kinase forms in man, *Biochim. Biophys. Acta*, 523, 59, 1978.
135. **Nakashima, K., Miwa, S., Fujii, H., Shinohara, K., Yamauchi, K., Tsuji, Y., and Yanai, M.,** Characterization of pyruvate kinase from the liver of a patient with aberrant erythrocyte pyruvate kinase, PK Nagasaki, *J. Lab. Clin. Med.*, 90, 1012, 1977.
136. **Marie, J., Simon, M.-P., and Kahn, A.,** Cotranslation of L and L′ pyruvate kinase messenger RNAs from human fetal liver, *Biochim. Biophys. Acta*, 696, 340, 1982.
137. **Chern, C. J., Rittenberg, M. B., and Black, J. A.,** Purification of human erythrocyte pyruvate kinase, *J. Biol. Chem.*, 247, 7173, 1972.
138. **Marie, J., Kahn, A., and Boivin, P.,** Human erythrocyte pyruvate kinase. Total purification and evidence for its antigenic identity with L-type enzyme, *Biochim. Biophys. Acta*, 481, 96, 1977.
139. **Marie, J., Garreau, H., and Kahn, A.,** Evidence for a postsynthetic proteolytic transformation of human erythrocyte pyruvate kinase into L-type enzyme, *FEBS Lett.*, 78, 91, 1977.
140. **Marie, J. and Kahn, A.,** Proteolytic processing of human erythrocyte pyruvate kinase: study of normal and deficient enzyme, *Biochem. Biophys. Res. Commun.*, 91, 123, 1979.
141. **Takegawa, S., Fujii, H., and Miwa, S.,** Conversion of pyruvate kinase isozymes from M_2- to L-type during development of the red cell, *Br. J. Haematol.*, 54, 467, 1983.
142. **Miwa, S.,** Pyruvate kinase deficiency and other enzymopathies of the Embden-Meyerhof pathway, *Clin. Haematol.*, 10, 57, 1981.
143. **Valentine, W. N., Tanaka, K. R., and Miwa, S.,** A specific erythrocyte glycolytic enzyme defect (pyruvate kinase) in three subjects with congenital non-spherocytic hemolytic anemia, *Trans. Assoc. Am. Physicians*, 74, 100, 1961.
144. **Tanaka, K. R., Valentine, W. N., and Miwa, S.,** Pyruvate kinase (PK) deficiency hereditary nonspherocytic hemolytic anemia, *Blood*, 19, 267, 1962.
145. **Beutler, E.,** *Hemolytic Anemia in Disorders of Red Cell Metabolism*, Plenum Press, New York, 1978.
146. **Tanaka, K. R. and Paglia, D. E.,** Pyruvate kinase deficiency, *Semin. Hematol.*, 8, 367, 1971.
147. **Beutler, E.,** *Red Cell Metabolism. A Manual of Biochemical Methods*, 2nd ed., Grune & Stratton, New York, 1975.
148. **Beutler, E., Blume, K. G., Kaplan, J. C., Löhr, G. W., Ramot, B., and Valentine, W. N.,** International committee for standardization in haematology: recommended methods for red-cell enzyme analysis, *Br. J. Haematol.*, 35, 331, 1977.
149. **Boivin, P., Galand, C., Mallarme, J., and Perrot, T.,** Mise en évidence d'une enzyme à cinétique anormale dans deux nouveaux cas de déficit en pyruvate kinase érythrocytaire, *Pathol. Biol.*, 17, 597, 1969.

150. **Staal, G. E. J., Koster, J. F., and Van Milligen-Boersma, L.,** Some properties of abnormal red blood cell pyruvate kinase, *Biochim. Biophys. Acta,* 220, 613, 1970.
151. **Blume, K. G., Arnold, H., Löhr, G. W., and Scholz, G.,** On the molecular basis of pyruvate kinase deficiency, *Biochim. Biophys. Acta,* 370, 601, 1974.
152. **Miwa, S., Nakashima, K., Ariyoshi, K., Shinohara, K., Oda, E., and Tanaka, T.,** Four new pyruvate kinase (PK) variants and a classical PK deficiency, *Br. J. Haematol.,* 29, 157, 1975.
153. **Kahn, A., Marie, J., Galand, C., and Boivin, P.,** Molecular mechanism of erythrocyte pyruvate-kinase deficiency, *Hum. Genet.,* 29, 271, 1975.
154. **Paglia, D. E., Gray, G. R., Growe, G. H., and Valentine, W. N.,** Simultaneous inheritance of mutant isoenzymes of erythrocyte pyruvate kinase associated with chronic haemolytic anaemia, *Br. J. Haematol.,* 34, 61, 1976.
155. **Paglia, D. E., Konrad, P. N., Wolff, J. A., and Valentine, W. N.,** Biphasic reaction kinetics in an anomalous isozyme of erythrocyte pyruvate kinase, *Clin. Chim. Acta,* 73, 395, 1976.
156. **Garreau, H., Buc. H., Columelli, S., and Najman, A.,** Molecular alterations in congenital erythrocyte pyruvate-kinase deficiency, *Clin. Chim. Acta,* 68, 245, 1976.
157. **Minakami, S., Suzuki, C., Saito, T., and Yoshikawa, H.,** Studies on erythrocyte glycolysis. I. Determination of the glycolytic intermediates in human erythrocytes, *J. Biochem.,* 58, 543, 1965.
158. **Waller, H. D. and Löhr, G. W.,** Hereditary nonspherocytic enzymopenic hemolytic anemia with pyruvate kinase deficiency, in *Proc. 9th Congr. Int. Soc. Hematol.,* Mexico City, Mexico, 1964, 257.
159. **Paglia, D. E., Valentine, W. N., Baughan, M. A., Miller, D. R., Reed, C. F., and McIntyre, O. R.,** An inherited molecular lesion of erythrocyte pyruvate kinase. Identification of a kinetically aberrant isozyme associated with premature hemolysis, *J. Clin. Invest.,* 47, 1929, 1968.
160. **Ohyama, H., Kumatori, T., Nishina, T., and Miwa, S.,** Functionally abnormal pyruvate kinase in congenital hemolytic anemia, *Acta Haematol. Jpn.,* 32, 330, 1969.
161. **Imamura, K., Tanaka, T., Nishina, T., Nakashima, K., and Miwa, S.,** Studies on pyruvate kinase (PK) deficiency. II. Electrophoretic, kinetic and immunological studies on pyruvate kinase of erythrocyte and other tissues, *J. Biochem.,* 74, 1165, 1973.
162. **Miwa, S., Boivin, P., Blume, K. G., Arnold, H., Black, J. A., Kahn, A., Staal, G. E. J., Nakashima, K., Tanaka, K. R., Paglia, D. E., Valentine, W. N., Yoshida, A., and Beutler, E.,** International committee for standardization in haematology: recommended methods for the characterization of red cell pyruvate kinase variants, *Br. J. Haematol.,* 43, 275, 1979.
163. **Miwa, S., Fujii, H., Takegawa, S., Nakatsuji, T., Yamato, K., Ishida, Y., and Ninomiya, N.,** Seven pyruvate kinase variants characterized by the ICSH recommended methods, *Br. J. Haematol.,* 45, 575, 1980.
164. **Shohet, S. B. and Ness, P. M.,** Hemolytic anemias. Failure of the red cell membrane, *Med. Clin. N. Am.,* 60, 913, 1976.
165. **Bernard, J. F.,** Anomalies des transferts cationiques transmembranaires au cours des anémies hémolitiques congénitals, *Nouv. Rev. Fr. Hematol.,* 18, 117, 1977.
166. **Mentzer, W. C., Jr., Baehner, R. L., Schmidt-Schönbein, H., Robinson, S. H., and Nathan, D. G.,** Selective reticulocyte destruction in erythrocyte pyruvate kinase deficiency, *J. Clin. Invest.,* 50, 688, 1971.
167. **Matsumoto, N., Ishihara, T., Nakashima, K., Miwa, S., Uchino, F., and Kondo, M.,** Sequestration and destruction of reticulocyte in the spleen in pyruvate kinase deficiency hereditary nonspherocytic hemolytic anemia, *Acta Haematol. Jpn.,* 35, 525, 1972.
168. **Matsumoto, N., Ishihara, T., Miwa, S., and Uchino, F.,** The mechanism of mitochondrial extrusion from reticulocytes in the spleen from patients with erythrocyte pyruvate kinase (PK) deficiency, *Acta Haematol. Jpn.,* 37, 25, 1974.
169. **Zanella, A., Brovelli, A., Mantovani, A., Izzo, C., Rebulla, P., and Balduini, C.,** Membrane abnormalities of pyruvate kinase deficient red cells, *Br. J. Haematol.,* 42, 101, 1979.
170. **Rosa, R., Gaillardon, J., and Rosa, J.,** Diphosphoglycerate mutase and 2,3-diphosphoglycerate phosphatase activities of red cells: comparative electrophoretic study, *Biochem. Biophys. Res. Commun.,* 51, 536, 1973.
171. **Sasaki, R., Ikura, K., Sugimoto, E., and Chiba, H.,** Purification of bisphosphoglyceromutase, 2,3-bisphosphoglycerate phosphatase and phosphoglycerate mutase from human erythrocytes, *Eur. J. Biochem.,* 50, 581, 1975.
172. **Schröter, W.,** Kongenitale nichtsphärocytäre hämolytische Anämie bei 2,3-Diphosphoglyceratmutase-Mangel der Erythrocyten im frühen Säuglingalter, *Klin. Wochenschr.,* 43, 1147, 1965.
173. **Labie, D., Leroux, J.-P., Najman, A., and Reyrolle, C.,** Familial diphosphoglyceratemutase deficiency. Influence on the oxygen affinity curves of hemoglobin, *FEBS Lett.,* 9, 37, 1970.
174. **Cartier, P. P., Labie, D., Leroux, J.-P., Najman, A., and Demaugre, F.,** Déficit familial en diphosphoglycératemutase: Étude hématologique et biochimique, *Nouv. Rev. Fr. Hematol.,* 12, 269, 1972.

175. **Rosa, R., Galacteros, F., Calvin, M. C., and Rosa, J.,** New cases of partial diphosphoglycerate mutase (DPGM) deficiency associated with erythrocytosis, in *Proc. 19th Congr. Int. Soc. Hematol.*, Budapest, Hungary, 1982, 227.
176. **Nishina, T.,** personal communication, 1973.
177. **Travis, S. F., Martinez, J., Garvin, J., Jr., Atwater, J., and Gillmer, P.,** Study of a kindred with partial deficiency of red cell 2,3-diphosphoglycerate mutase (2,3-DPGM) and compensated hemolysis, *Blood,* 51, 1107, 1978.
178. **Rosa, R., Prehu, M.-U., Beuzard, Y., and Rosa, J.,** The first case of a complete deficiency of diphosphoglyceromutase in human erythrocytes, *J. Clin. Invest.*, 62, 907, 1978.
179. **Yoshida, A.,** Glucose 6-phosphate dehydrogenase of human erythrocytes. I. Purification and characterization of normal (B+) enzyme, *J. Biol. Chem.*, 241, 4966, 1966.
180. **Yoshida, A.,** Subunit structure of human glucose 6-phosphate dehydrogenase and its genetic implication, *Biochem. Genet.*, 2, 237, 1968.
181. **Yoshida, A. and Hoagland, V. D., Jr.,** Active molecular unit and NADP content of human glucose 6-phosphate dehydrogenase, *Biochem. Biophys. Res. Commun.*, 40, 1167, 1970.
182. **Yoshida, A.,** Glucose-6-phosphate dehydrogenase abnormality and hemolysis, *Acta Biol. Med. Germ.*, 36, 689, 1977.
183. **Yoshida, A.,** personal communication, 1982.
184. **Persico, M. G., Toniolo, D., Nobile, C., D'Urso, M., and Luzzato, L.,** cDNA sequence of human glucose 6-phosphate dehydrogenase cloned in pBR 322, *Nature (London),* 294, 778, 1981.
185. **Dern, R. J., Weinstein, I. M., Le Roy, G. V., Talmage, D. W., and Alving, A. S.,** The hemolytic effect of primaquine. I. The localization of the drug-induced hemolytic defect in primaquine-sensitive individuals, *J. Lab. Clin. Med.*, 43, 303, 1954.
186. **Beutler, E., Dern, R. J., Flanagan, C. L., and Alving, A. S.,** The hemolytic effect of primaquine. VII. Biochemical studies of drug-sensitive erythrocytes, *J. Lab. Clin. Med.*, 45, 286, 1955.
187. **Carson, P. E., Flanagan, C. L., Ickes, C. E., and Alving, A. S.,** Enzymatic deficiency in primaquine-sensitive erythrocytes, *Science,* 124, 484, 1956.
188. WHO Scientific Group: Standardization of procedures for the study of glucose-6-phosphate dehydrogenase, *WHO Tech. Rep. Ser.*, 366, 1, 1967.
189. **Fujii, H., Nakashima, K., and Miwa, S.,** Incidence and characteristics of G6PD deficiency in Japan, *Jpn. J. Hum. Genet.*, 23, 271, 1978.
190. **Nakatsuji, T. and Miwa, S.,** Studies on the incidence of G6PD deficiency in Japan using both Beutler's spot test and starch gel electrophoresis, *Jpn. J. Hum. Genet.*, 24, 215, 1979.
191. **Allison, A. C.,** Genetic factors in resistance to malaria, *Ann. N.Y. Acad. Sci.*, 91, 710, 1961.
192. **Motulsky, A. C.,** Glucose-6-phosphate dehydrogenase deficiency haemolytic disease of the new born, and malaria, *Lancet,* i, 1168, 1961.
193. **Luzzatto, L., Usanga, E. A., and Reddy, S.,** Glucose 6-phosphate dehydrogenase deficient red cells: resistance to infection by malarial parasites, *Science,* 164, 839, 1969.
194. **Kartin, S. K., Miller, L. H., Alling, D., Okoye, V. C., Esan, G. J. F., Osunkoya, B. O., and Deane, M.,** Severe malaria and glucose-6-phosphate dehydrogenase deficiency: a reappraisal of the malaria/G-6-P.D. hypothesis, *Lancet,* i, 524, 1979.
195. **Childs, B., Zinkham, W., Browne, E. A., Kimbro, E. L., and Torbert, J. V.,** A genetic study of a defect in glutathione metabolism of the erythrocyte, *Johns Hopkins Med. J.*, 102, 21, 1958.
196. **Kirkman, H. N. and Hendrickson, E. M.,** Sex-linked electrophoretic difference in glucose-6-phosphate dehydrogenase, *Am. J. Hum. Genet.*, 15, 241, 1963.
197. **Lyon, M.,** Gene action in the X-chromosome of the mouse (*Mus musculus* L.), *Nature (London),* 190, 372, 1961.
198. **Beutler, E., Yeh, M., and Fairbanks, V. F.,** The normal human female as a mosaic of X-chromosome activity: studies using the gene for G-6-PD deficiency as a marker, *Proc. Natl. Acad. Sci. U.S.A.*, 48, 9, 1962.
199. **Beutler, E., Blume, K. G., Kaplan, J. C., Löhr, G. W., Ramot, B., and Valentine, W. N.,** International committee for standardization in haematology: recommended screening test for glucose-6-phosphate dehydrogenase (G-6-PD) deficiency, *Br. J. Haematol.*, 43, 469, 1979.
200. **Yoshida, A.,** A single amino acid substitution — asparagine to aspartic acid — between normal (B+) and the common Negro variant (A+) of human glucose-6-phosphate dehydrogenase, *Proc. Natl. Acad. Sci. U.S.A.*, 57, 835, 1967.
201. **Yoshida, A.,** Amino acid substitution (histidine to tyrosine) in a glucose-6-phosphate dehydrogenase variant (G6PD Hektoen) associated with overproduction, *J. Mol. Biol.*, 52, 483, 1970.
202. **Kahn, A., Boulard, M., Hakim, J., Schaison, G., Boivin, P., and Bernard, J.,** Anemie hemolytique congenitale non spherocytaire par deficit en glucose 6-phosphate dehydrogenase erythrocytaire. Description de deux nouvelles variants: Gd(−)Saint Louis (Paris) et Gd(−)Hayem, *Nouv. Rev. Fr. Hematol.*, 14, 587, 1974.

203. **Junien, C., Kaplan, J.-C., Meienhofer, M. C., Maigret, P., and Sender, A.,** G6PD Baudelocque: a new unstable variant characterized in cultured fibroblasts, *Enzyme,* 18, 48, 1974.
204. **Pinto, P. V. C., Newton, W. A., Jr., and Richardson, K. E.,** Evidence for four types of erythrocyte glucose-6-phosphate dehydrogenase from G-6-PD deficient human subjects, *J. Clin. Invest.,* 45, 823, 1966.
205. **Honig, G. R., Habacon, E., Vida, L. N., Matsumoto, F., and Beutler, E.,** Three new variants of glucose-6-phosphate dehydrogenase associated with chronic nonspherocytic hemolytic anemia: G-6-PD Lincoln Park, G-6-PD Arlington Heights, and G-6-PD West Town, *Am. J. Hematol.,* 6, 353, 1979.
206. **Nakai, T. and Yoshida, A.,** G6PD Heian, a glucose-6-phosphate dehydrogenase variant associated with hemolytic anemia found in Japan, *Clin. Chim. Acta,* 51, 199, 1974.
207. **Beutler, E., Grooms, A. M., Morgan, S. K., and Trinidad, F.,** Chronic severe hemolytic anemia due to G-6-PD Charleston: a new deficient variant, *J. Pediatr.,* 80, 1005, 1972.
208. **Grossman, A., Ramanathan, K., Justice, P., Gordon, J., Shahidi, N. T., and Hsia, D.,** Congenital nonspherocytic hemolytic anemia associated with erythrocyte G-6-PD deficiency in a Negro family, *Pediatrics,* 37, 624, 1966.
209. **Tanaka, K. R. and Beutler, E.,** Hereditary hemolytic anemia due to glucose-6-phosphate dehydrogenase Torrance: a new variant, *J. Lab. Clin. Med.,* 73, 657, 1969.
210. **Thigpen, J. T., Steinberg, M. H., Beutler, E., Gillespie, G. T., Jr., Dreiling, B. J., and Morrison, F. S.,** Glucose-6-phosphate dehydrogenase Jackson. A new variant associated with hemolytic anemia, *Acta Haematol.,* 51, 310, 1974.
211. **Howell, E. B., Nelson, A. J., and Jones, O. W.,** A new G-6-PD variant associated with chronic nonspherocytic haemolytic anaemia in a Negro family, *J. Med. Genet.,* 9, 160, 1972.
212. **Feldman, R., Gromisch, D. S., Luhby, A. L., and Beutler, E.,** Congenital nonspherocytic hemolytic anemia due to glucose-6-phosphate dehydrogenase East Harlem: a new deficient variant, *J. Pediatr.,* 90, 89, 1977.
213. **Smith, J. W. and Beutler, E.,** personal communication, 1982.
214. **Kahn, A., Pao, C., Cottreau, D., and Bilski-Pasquier, G.,** Gd(−)Hotel Dieu: a new G-6PD variant with chronic hemolysis in a Negro patient from Senegal, *Hum. Genet.,* 39, 353, 1977.
215. **Vaca, G., Ibarra, B., Romero, F., and Olivares, N.,** G-6-PD Quadalajara: a new mutant associated with chronic non-spherocytic hemolytic anemia, personal communication, 1982.
216. **Vives, Corrons, J. L., Feliu, E., Pujades, M. A., Rozman, C., Carreras, A., and Vallespi, M. T.,** Severe glucose-6-phosphate dehydrogenase (G6PD) deficiency associated with chronic hemolytic anemia, granulocyte dysfunction and increased susceptibility to infections. Description of a new molecular variant (G6PD Barcelona), *Blood,* 59, 428, 1982.
217. **Fairbanks, V. F., Nepo, A. G., Beutler, E., Dickson, E. R., and Honig, G.,** Glucose-6-phosphate dehydrogenase variants: re-evaluation of G6PD Chicago and Cornell and a new variant (G6PD Pea Ridge) resembling G6PD Chicago, *Blood,* 55, 216, 1980.
218. **Chan, T. K. and Lai, M. C. S.,** Glucose 6-phosphate dehydrogenase: Identity of erythrocyte and leukocyte enzyme with report of a new variant in Chinese, *Biochem. Genet.,* 6, 119, 1972.
219. **Ramot, B., Ben-Bassat, I., and Shchory, M.,** New glucose-6-phosphate dehydrogenase variants observed in Israel and their association with congenital nonspherocytic hemolytic disease, *J. Lab. Clin. Med.,* 74, 895, 1969.
220. **Beutler, E., Mathai, C. K., and Smith, J. E.,** Biochemical variants of glucose-6-phosphate dehydrogenase giving rise to congenital nonspherocytic hemolytic disease, *Blood,* 31, 131, 1968.
221. **Talalak, P. and Beutler, E.,** G-6-PD Bangkok: a new variant found in congenital nonspherocytic hemolytic disease (CNHD), *Blood,* 33, 772, 1969.
222. **Kirkman, H. N. and Riley, H. D., Jr.,** Congenital nonspherocytic hemolytic anemia, *Am. J. Dis. Child.,* 102, 313,, 1961.
223. **Wong, P. W. K., Shih, L.-Y., and Hsia, D. Y. Y.,** Characterization of glucose-6-phosphate dehydrogenase among Chinese, *Nature (London),* 208, 1323, 1965.
224. **Kirkman, H. N., Rosenthal, I. M., Simon, E. R., Carson, P. E., and Brinson, A. G.,** "Chicago I" variant of glucose-6-phosphate dehydrogenase in congenital hemolytic disease, *J. Lab. Clin. Med.,* 63, 715, 1964.
225. **Necheles, T. F., Snyder, L. M., and Strauss, W.,** Glucose-6-phosphate dehydrogenase Boston. A new variant associated with congenital nonspherocytic hemolytic disease, *Humangenetik,* 13, 218, 1971.
226. **Rattazzi, M. C., Corash, L. M., Van Zanen, G. E., Jaffe, E. R., and Piomelli, S.,** G6PD deficiency and chronic hemolysis: Four new mutants — relationships between clinical syndrome and enzyme kinetics, *Blood,* 38, 205, 1971.
227. **Beutler, E.,** unpublished data, 1975.
228. **Miller, D. R. and Wollman, M. R.,** A new variant of glucose-6-phosphate dehydrogenase deficiency hereditary hemolytic anemia, G6PD Cornell: erythrocyte, leukocyte, and platelet studies, *Blood,* 44, 323, 1974.

229. **Miwa, S., Ono, J., Nakashima, K., Abe, S., Kageoka, T., Shinohara, K., Isobe, J., and Yamaguchi, H.,** Two new glucose 6-phosphate dehydrogenase variants associated with congenital nonspherocytic hemolytic anemia found in Japan: Gd(−)Tokushima and Gd(−)Tokyo, *Am. J. Hematol.*, 1, 443, 1976.
230. **Wilson, W. W.,** Congenital hemolytic anemia due to deficiency of glucose-6-phosphate dehydrogenase, *Rocky Mt. Med. J.*, 73, 160, 1976.
231. **Gahr, M., Schroeter, W., Sturzenegger, M., Bornhalm, D., and Marti, H. R.,** Glucose-6-phosphate dehydrogenase (G-6-PD) deficiency in Switzerland, *Helv. Paediatr. Acta*, 31, 159, 1976.
232. **Vuopio, P., Harkonen, R., Johnsson, R., and Nuutinen, M.,** Red cell glucose-6-phosphate dehydrogenase deficiency in Finland, *Ann. Clin. Res.*, 5, 168, 1973.
233. **Shatskaya, T. L., Krasnopolskaya, K. D., and Idelson, L. I.,** The new form of glucose-6-phosphate dehydrogenase (G6PD "Kaluga") from erythrocytes of a patient with chronic nonspherocytic hemolytic anemia, *Vopr. Med. Khim.*, 22, 764, 1976.
234. **Miwa, S., Fujii, H., Nakashima, K., Miura, Y., Yamada, K., Hagiwara, T., and Fukuda, M.,** Three new electrophoretically normal glucose-6-phosphate dehydrogenase variants associated with congenital nonspherocytic hemolytic anemia found in Japan: G6PD Ogikubo, Yokohama, and Akita, *Hum. Genet.*, 45, 11, 1978.
235. **McCann, S. R., Smithwick, A. M., Temperley, I. J., and Tipton, K.,** Chronic nonspherocytic hemolytic anemia resulting from glucose-6-phosphate dehydrogenase deficiency in an Irish kindred, *J. Med. Genet.*, 17, 191, 1980.
236. **Tokarev, Y. N., Chernyak, N. B., Batishchev, A. I., Lanzina, N. V., and Alexeyev, G. A.,** Étude des proprietés électrophorétiques et cinétiques de la glucose-6-phosphate déshydrogénase (Gd) d'érythrocytes dans les déficits héréditaires de l'enzyme: Description d'une nouvelle variante de glucose-6-phosphate déshydrogénase: La Gd Kremenchug, *Nouv. Rev. F. Hematol.*, 20, 557, 1978.
237. **Prchal, J., Moreno, H., Conrad, M., and Vitek, A.,** G-6-PD Dothan: a new variant associated with chronic hemolytic anemia, *I.R.C.S.*, 7, 348, 1979.
238. **Fujii, H., Miwa, S., Tani, K., Takagawa, S., Fujinami, N., Takahashi, K. Nakayama, S., Konno, M. and Sato, T.,** Glucose-6-phosphate dehydrogenase variants: a unique variant (G6PD Kobe) showed an extremely increased affinity for galactose-6-phosphate and a new variant (G6PD Sapporo) resembling G6PD Pea Ridge, *Hum. Genet.*, 58, 405, 1981.
239. **Johnson, G. J., Kaplan, M. E., and Beutler, E.,** G-6-PD Long Prairie: a new mutant exhibiting normal sensitivity to inhibition by NADPH and accompanied by nonspherocytic hemolytic anemia, *Blood*, 49, 247, 1977.
240. **Beutler, E., Matsumoto, F., and Daiber, A.,** Nonspherocytic hemolytic anemia due to G-6-PD Panama, *I.R.C.S.*, 2, 1389, 1974.
241. **Engstrom, P. F. and Beutler, E.,** G-6-PD Tripler: a unique variant associated with chronic hemolytic disease, *Blood*, 36, 10, 1970.
242. **Beutler, E. and Rosen, R.,** Nonspherocytic congenital hemolytic anemia due to a new G-6-PD variant: G-6-PD Alhambra, *Pediatrics*, 45, 230, 1970.
243. **Miwa, S., Fujii, H., Nakatsuji, T., Ishida, Y., Oda, E., Kaneto, A., Motokawa, M., Ariga, Y., Fukuchi, S., Sasai, S., Hiraoka, K., Kashii, H., Kodama, T., and Miwa, Y.,** Four new electrophoretically slow-moving glucose-6-phosphate dehydrogenase variants associated with congenital nonspherocytic hemolytic anemia found in Japan. Gd(−)Kurume, Gd(−)Fukushima, Gd(−)Yamaguchi, and Gd(−)Wakayama, *Am. J. Hematol.*, 5, 131, 1978.
244. **Beutler, E., Keller, J. W., and Matsumoto, F.,** A new glucose-6-phosphate dehydrogenase (G-6-PD) variant associated with nonspherocytic hemolytic anemia: G-6-PD Atlanta, *I.R.C.S.*, 4, 579, 1976.
245. **Westring, D. W. and Pisciotta, A. V.,** Anemia, cataracts, and seizures in patient with glucose-6-phosphate dehydrogenase deficiency, *Arch. Intern. Med.*, 118, 385, 1966.
246. **Milner, G., Delamore, I. W., and Yoshida, A.,** G-6-PD Manchester: a new variant associated with chronic nonspherocytic hemolytic anemia, *Blood*, 43, 271, 1974.
247. **Weinreich, J., Busch, D., Gottstein, U., Schaefer, J., and Rohr, J.,** Ueber zwei neue faelle von hereditaerer nichtsphaerocytaerer haemolytischner Anaemie bei Glucose-6-Phosphat-Dehydrogenase-Defekt in einer nord Deutschen Familie, *Klin. Wochenschr.*, 46, 146, 1968.
248. **Snyder, L. M., Necheles, T. F., and Reddy, W. J.,** G-6-PD Worcester: a new variant, associated with X-linked optic atrophy, *Am. J. Med.*, 49, 125, 1970.
249. **Balinsky, D., Gomperts, E., Cayanis, E., Jenkins, T., Bryer, D., Bersohn, I., and Metz, J.,** Glucose-6-phosphate dehydrogenase Johannesburg: a new variant with reduced activity in a patient with congenital nonspherocytic haemolytic anaemia, *Br. J. Haematol.*, 25, 385, 1973.
250. **Johnson, G. J. and Beutler, E.,** personal communication, 1980.
251. **Kidder, W. R. and Beutler, E.,** personal communication, 1979.
252. **Mentzer, W. C., Warner, R., Addiego, J., Smith, B., and Walter, T.,** G6PD San Francisco: a new variant of glucose-6-phosphate dehydrogenase associated with congenital nonspherocytic hemolytic anemia, *Blood*, 55, 195, 1980.

253. **Castro, A. M. and Snyder, L. M.,** G6PD San Jose: a new variant characterized by NADPH inhibition studies, *Humangenetik,* 21, 361, 1974.
254. **McCurdy, P. R.,** unpublished data, 1975.
255. **McCurdy, P. R., Maldonado, N., Dillon, D. E., and Conrad, M. E.,** Variants of glucose-6-phosphate dehydrogenase (G-6-PD) associated with G-6-PD deficiency in Puerto Ricans, *J. Lab. Clin. Med.,* 82, 432, 1973.
256. **Kahn, A., North, M. L., Messer, J., and Boivin, P.,** G-6-PD Ankara, a new G-6PD variant with deficiency found in a Turkish family, *Humangenetik,* 27, 247, 1975.
257. **Kirkman, H. N., Kidson, C., and Kennedy, M.,** Variants of human glucose-6-phosphate dehydrogenase. Studies of samples from New Guinea. Hereditary disorders of erythrocyte metabolism, in *City of Hope Symp. Series,* Vol. 1, Beutler, E., Ed., Grune & Stratton, New York, 1968, 126.
258. **McCurdy, P. R., Blackwell, P. Q., Todd, D., Tso, S. C., and Tuchinda, S.,** Further studies on glucose-6-phosphate dehydrogenase deficiency in Chinese subjects, *J. Lab. Clin. Med.,* 75, 788, 1970.
259. **Yoshida, A., Baur, E. W., and Motulsky, A. G.,** A Philippino glucose-6-phosphate dehydrogenase variant (G6PD Union) with enzyme deficiency and altered substrate specificity, *Blood,* 35, 506, 1970.
260. **Carandina, G., Moretto, E., Zecchi, G., and Conighi, C.,** Glucose 6-phosphate dehydrogenase Ferrara. A new variant of G6PD identified in Northern Italy, *Acta Haematol.,* 56, 116, 1976.
261. **Pawlak, A. L., Zagorski, Z., Rozynkowa, D., and Horst, A.,** Polish variant of glucose-6-phosphate dehydrogenase (G-6-PD Lublin), *Humangenetik,* 10, 340, 1970.
262. **Vives Corrons, J. L., Pujades, A., and Curia, M. D.,** Caracterización molecular de la glucose-6-fosfato deshidrogenase (G6PD) en 24 casos de déficit enzimático y descripción de una nreva variante (G6PD-Bética), *Sangre,* 25, 1049, 1980.
263. **Panich, V. and Na-Nakorn, S.,** G6PD variants in Thailand, *J. Med. Assoc. Thai,* 63, 537, 1980.
264. **Shatskaya, T. L., Krasnopolskaya, K. D., and Annenkov, G. A.,** A description of new mutant forms of erythrocyte glucose-6-dehydrogenase isolated at the territory of the Soviet Union, *Genetika,* 11(12), 116, 1975.
265. **Vergnes, H., Ribet, A., Bommelaer, G., Amadieu, J., and Brun, H.,** Gd(−)Muret and Gd(−)Colomiers, two new variants of glucose-6-phosphate dehydrogenase associated with favism, *Hum. Genet.,* 57, 332, 1981.
266. **Benabadji, M., Merad, F., Benmoussa, M., Trabuchet, G., Junien, C., Dreyfus, J. C., and Kapaln, J. C.,** Heterogeneity of glucose-6-phosphate dehydrogenase-deficiency in Algeria, *Hum. Genet.,* 40, 177, 1978.
267. **Miwa, S.,** personal communication, 1982.
268. **Chockkalingam, K., Board, P. G., and Nurse, G. T.,** Glucose-6-phosphate dehydrogenase deficiency in Papua New Guinea: the description of 13 new variants, *Hum. Genet.,* 60, 189, 1982.
269. **Prchal, J. T., Crist, W. M., Malluah, A., Vitek, A., Tauxe, W. N., and Carroll, A. J.,** A new glucose-6-phosphate dehydrogenase deficient variant in a patient with Chediak-Higasi syndrome, *Blood,* 56, 476, 1980.
270. **Chockkalingam, K. and Board, P. G.,** Further evidence for heterogeneity of glucose-6-phosphate dehydrogenase deficiency in Papua New Gunea, *Hum. Genet.,* 56, 209, 1980.
271. **Kirkman, H. N. and Luan Eng, L.-I.,** Variants of glucose-6-phosphate dehydrogenase in Indonesia, *Nature (London),* 221, 959, 1969.
272. **McCurdy, P. R. and Mahmood, L.,** Red cell glucose-6-phosphate dehydrogenase deficiency in Pakistan, *J. Lab. Clin. Med.,* 76, 943, 1970.
273. **Kirkman, H. N., Schettini, F., and Pickard, B. M.,** Mediterranean variant of glucose-6-phosphate dehydrogenase, *J. Lab. Clin. Med.,* 63, 726, 1964.
274. **Yoshida, A.,** unpublished data, 1975.
275. **Kahn, A., Boivin, P., Hakim, J., and Lagneau, J.,** Hétérogénéité des glucose-6-phosphate déshydrogénase erythrocytaire deficitaires dans la race noire Etude cinétique et description de deux nouvelles variantes Gd(−)Dakar et Gd(−)Mali, *Nouv. Rev. Fr. Hematol.,* 11, 741, 1971.
276. **Panich, V., Sungnate, T., and NaNakorn, S.,** Acute intravascular hemolysis and renal failure in a new glucose 6-phosphate dehydrogenase variant: G6PD Siriraj, *J. Med. Assoc. Thai,* 55, 726, 1972.
277. **McCurdy, P. R., Kamel, K., and Selim, O.,** Heterogeneity of red cell glucose 6-phosphate dehydrogenase (G6PD) deficiency in Egypt, *J. Lab. Clin. Med.,* 84, 673, 1974.
278. **Kahn, A., Hakim, J., Cottreau, D., and Boivin, P.,** Gd(−)Matam, an African glucose-6-phosphate dehydrogenase variant with enzyme deficiency. Biochemical and immunological properties in various hemopoietic tissues, *Clin. Chim. Acta,* 59, 183, 1975.
279. **Kahn, A., Bernard, J.-F., Cottreau, D., Marie, J., and Boivin, P.,** Gd(−)Abrami. A deficient G6PD variant with hemizygous expression in blood cells of a woman with primary myelofibrosis, *Humangenetik,* 30, 41, 1975.

280. **Gahr, M., Bornhalm, D., and Schroeter, W.,** Haemolytic anemia due to glucose 6-phosphate dehydrogenase (G6PD) deficiency: demonstration of two new biochemical variants, G6PD Hamm and G6PD Tarsus, *Br. J. Haematol.*, 33, 363, 1976.
281. **Geerdink, R. A., Horst, R., and Staal, G. E. J.,** An Iraqi Jewish family with a new red cell glucose-6-phosphate dehydrogenase variant (Gd-Bagdad) and kernicterus, *Isr. J. Med. Sci.*, 9, 1040, 1973.
282. **Sidi, Y., Aderka, D., Brok-Simoni, F., Benjamin, D., Ramot, B., and Pinkhas, J.,** Viral hepatitis with extreme hyperbilirubinemia, massive hemolysis and encephalopathy in a patient with a new G6PD variant, *Isr. J. Med. Sci.*, 16, 130, 1980.
283. **Shatskaya, T. L., Krasnopolskaya, K. D., and Zakharova, T. V.,** Regularities of distribution of Gd-alleles in Azerbaijan. II. Identification of G6PD munant forms, *Genetika,* 16(12), 2217, 1980.
284. **Miwa, S., Nakashima, K., Ono, J., Fujii, H., and Suzuki, E.,** Three glucose-6-phosphate dehydrogenase variants found in Japan, *Hum. Genet.*, 36, 327, 1977.
285. **Gahr, M., Bornhalm, D., and Schroeter, W.,** Biochemishe Eigenschaften einer neuen Variante des Glucose-6-phosphate Dehydrogenase (G6PD)-Mangels mit Favismus: G-6-PD Bielafeld, *Klin. Woch.*, 55, 379, 1977.
286. **Yermakov, N., Tokarev, F., Chernjak, N., Schoenian, G., Griger, M., Guckler, G., Jacobasch, G., Mahmudova, M., and Bahramov, S.,** New stable mutant Gd(−) variants: G5PD Tashkent and G6PD Nucus. Molecular basis of hereditary enzyme deficiency, *Acta Biol. Med. Germ.*, 40, 559, 1981.
287. **Batischev, A. I., Chernyak, N. B., and Tokarev, Y. N.,** Detection of a new abnormal variant of glucose-6-phosphate dehydrogenase in human red cells, *Byull. Exsp. Biol. Med.*, 84(12), 728, 1977.
288. **Shatskaya, T. L., Krasnopolskaya, K. D., and Idelson, L. J.,** Mutant forms of erythrocyte glucose 6-phosphate dehydrogenase in Ashkenazi. Description of two new variants: G6PD Kirovograd and G6PD Zhitomir, *Humangenetik,* 33, 175, 1976.
289. **Beutler, E.,** Glucose 6-phosphate dehydrogenase deficiency. A new Indian variant G6PD Jammu., in *Trneds in Haematology,* Sen, N. N. and Basu, A. K., Eds., Calcutta, India, 1975, 279.
290. **Vergnes, H., Yoshida, A., Gourdin, D., Gherardi, M., Bierme, R., and Ruffie, J.,** Glucose 6-phosphate dehydrogenase Toulouse. A new variant with marked instability and severe deficiency discovered in a family of Mediterranean ancestry, *Acta Haematol.*, 51, 240, 1974.
291. **Fernandez, M., and Fairbanks, V. F.,** Glucose-6-phosphate dehydrogenase deficiency in the Phillipines: report of a new variant G-6-PD Panay, *Mayo Clin. Proc.*, 43, 645, 1968.
292. **Stamatoyannopoulos, G., Voigtlander, V., Kotsakis, P., and Akrivakis, A.,** Genetic diversity of the "Mediterranean" glucose-6-phosphate dehydrogenase deficiency phenotype, *J. Clin. Invest.*, 50 1253, 1971.
293. **Pawlak, A. L., Mazurkiewicz, C. A., Ordynski, J., Ruzynkowa, D., and Horst, A.,** G6PD Poznan. Variant with severe enzyme deficiency, *Humangenetik,* 28, 163, 1975.
294. **Kahn, A., Esters, A., and Habedank, M.,** Gd(−)Aachen. A new variant of deficient glucose 6-phosphate dehydrogenase, *Humangenetik,* 32, 171, 1976.
295. **Siegel, N. H., and Beutler, E.,** Hemolytic anemia caused by G-6-PD Carswell, a new variant, *Ann. Intern. Med.*, 75, 437, 1971.
296. **Miwa, S.,** unpublished data, 1976.
297. **Chockkalingam, K. and Board, P. G.,** Further evidence for heterogeneity of glucose-6-phosphate dehydrogenase deficiency in Papua New Guinea, *Hum. Genet.*, 56, 209, 1980.
298. **Krasnopolskaya, K. D., Shatskaya, T. L., Filippov, I. K., Annenkov, G. A., Aakharova, T. V., Mekhtiev, N. K., and Movsum-Zade, K. M.,** Genetic heterogeneity of G6PD deficiency: Study of mutant G6PD alleles in Shekii district of Azerbaijan, *Acad. Sci. Genet. U.S.S.R.*, 13(8), 1455, 1977.
299. **Gonzalez R., Estrada, M., Garcia, M., and Guiteirrez, A.,** G6PD Ciudad de la Habana: a new slow variant with deficiency found in a Cuban family, *Hum. Genet* 55, 133, 1980.
300. **Marks, P. A., Banks, J., and Gross, R.,** Genetic heterogeneity of glucose-6-phosphate dehydrogenase deficiency, *Nature (London),* 194, 454, 1962.
301. **Yoshida, A., Stamatoyannopoulos, G., and Motulsky, A.,** Negro variant of glucose-6-phosphate dehydrogenase deficiency (A−) in man, *Science* 155, 97, 1967.
302. **Kissin, C. and Cotte, J.,** Etude d'un variant de glucose-6-phosphate deshydrogenase: le type constantine, *Enzyme,* 11, 277, 1970.
303. **Nakashima, K., Ono, J., Abe, S., Miwa, S., and Yoshida, A.,** G6PD Ube. A glucose-6-phosphate dehydrogenase variant found in four unrelated Japanese families, *Am. J. Hum Genet.*, 29, 24, 1977.
304. **Lisker, R., Briceno, R. P., Zavala, C., Navarrete, J. I., Wessels, M., and Yoshida, A.,** A glucose 6-phosphate dehydrogenase Gd(−)Castilla variant characterized by mild deficiency associated with drug induced hemolytic anemaia, *J. Lab. Clin. Med.*, 90, 754, 1977.
305. **Crookston, J. H., Yoshida, A., Lin, M., and Booser, D. J.,** G-6-PD Toronto, *Biochem. J.*, 8, 259, 1973.
306. **Kaplan, J. C., Rosa, R., Seringe, P., and Hoeffel, J. C.,** La polyorphisme genetique de la glucose-6-phosphate deshydrogenase erythrocytaire chez l'homme. *Enzyme,* 8, 332, 1967.

307. **Reys, L., Manso, C., and Stamatoyannopoulos, G.,** Genetic studies on Southeastern Bantu of Mozambique. I. Variants of glucose-6-phosphate dehydrogenase, *Am J. Hum. Genet.*, 22, 203, 1970.
308. **Stamatoyannopoulos, G.,** unpublished data, 1975.
309. **McCurdy, P. R., Kirkman, H. N., Naiman, J. L., Jim, r. T. S., and Pickard, B. M.,** A Chinese variant of glucose-6-phosphate dehydrogenase, *J. Lab. Clin. Med.*, 67, 374, 1966.
310. **Mandelli, F., Amadori, S., De Laurenzi, A., Kahn, A., Isacchi, G., and Papa, G.,** Glucose-6-phosphate dehydrogenase Velletri, *Acta Haematol.*, 57, 121, 1977.
311. **Panich, V. and Sungate, T.,** Characterization of glucose-6-phosphate dehydrogenase in Thailand, *Humangenetik*, 18, 39, 1973.
312. **Lisker, R., Briceno, R. P., Agrilar, L., and Yoshida,** Avariant glucose-6-phosphate dehydrogenase Gd(−)Chiapas associated with moderate enzyme deficiency and occasional hemolytic anemia, *Hum. Genet.*, 43, 81, 1978.
313. **Vergnes, H., Gherardi, M., and Yoshida, A.,** G6PD Lozere and Trinacria-like: segregation of two nonhemolytic variants in a French family, *Hum. Genet.*, 34, 293, 1976.
314. **Nakatsuji, T. and Miwa, S.,** Incidence and characteristics of Glucose-6-phosphate dehydrogenase variant in Japan, *Hum. Genet.*, 51, 297, 1979.
315. **Sansone, G., Perroni, L., and Yoshida, A.,** Glucose-6-phosphate dehydrogenase variants from Italian subjects associated with severe neonatal jaundice, *Br. J. Haematol.*, 31, 159, 1975.
316. **Stamatoyannopoulos, G., Yoshida, A., Bacopoulos, C., and Motulsky, A.,** Athens variant of glucose-6-phosphate dehydrogenase, *Science*, 157, 831, 1967.
317. **Panich, V.,** G6PD Intanon. A new glucose 6-phosphate dehydrogenase variant, *Humangenetik*, 21, 203, 1974.
318. **Beutler, E. and Matsumoto, F.,** A new glucose 6-phosphate dehydrogenase variant: G6PD (−) Los Angeles, *I.R.C.S.*, 5, 89, 1977.
319. **Sansone, G., Perroni, L., Yoshida, A., and Dave, V.,** A new glucose 6-phosphate dehydrogenase variant (Gd Trinacria) in two unrelated families of Sicilian ancestry. *Ital. J. Biochem.*, 26, 44, 1977.
320. **Azevedo, E., Kirkman, H. N., Morrow, A. C., and Motulsky, A. G.,** Variants of red cell glucose-6-phosphate dehydrogenase among Asiatic Indians, *Ann. Hum. Genet.*, 31, 373, 1968.
321. **Lisker, R., Linares, C., and Motulsky, A, G.,** Glucose-6-phosphate dehydrogenase Mexico. A new variant with enzyme deficiency, abnormal mobility and absence of hemolysis, *J. Lab. Clin. Med.*, 79, 788, 1972.
322. **Kirkman, H. N., Simon, E. R., and Pickard, B. M.,** Seattle variant of glucose-6-phosphate dehydrogenase, *J. Lab. Clin. Med.*, 66, 834, 1965.
323. **Nurse, G. T. and Balinsky, D.,** unpublished data, 1975.
324. **Kaplan, J. C., Hanzlickova Leroux, A., Nicholas, A. M., Rosa, R., Weiler, C., and Lepercq, G,** A new glucose-6-phosphate dehydrogenase variant (G6PD Port-Royal), *Enzyme*, 12, 25, 1970.
325. **Kahn, A., North, M. L., Cottreau, D., Giron, G., and Lang, J. M.,** G6PD Vientiane: a new glucose-6-phosphate dehydrogenase variant with increased stability, *Hum. Genet.*, 43, 85, 1978.
326. **DeFlora, A., Morelli, A., Benatti, U., Ciuntini, P.., Ferraris, A. M., Galiano, S., Ravazzalo, R., and Gaetani, G. F.,** Two new glucose-6-phosphate dehydrogenase variants having similar characteristics but different intracellular lability and specific activity, *Br. J. Haematol.*, 48, 417, 1981.
327. **Chockkalingam, K., Board, P. G., and Breguet, G.,** Glucose-6-phosphate dehydrogenase variants of Bali Islands (Indonesia), *Hum. Genet.*, 60, 60, 1982.
328. **Vergnes, H., Gherardi, M., Quilici, J. C., Yoshida, A., and Giacardy, R.,** G-6-PD Luz-Saint-Sauveur: a new variant with abnormal electrophoretic mobility mild enzyme deficiency and absence of haematological disorders, *I.R.C.S.*, (73-7)3-1-14 (Abstr.), 1973.
329. **Yoshida, A., Baur, E., and Voigtlander, B.,** unpublished data, 1975.
330. **Yoshida, A.,** Human glucose-6-phosphate dehydrogenase: purification and characterization of Negro type variant (A+) and comparison with normal enzyme (B+), *Biochem. Genet.*, 1, 81, 1967.
331. **Stamatoyannopoulos, G., Kotsakis, P., Voigtlander, V., and Motulsky, A. G.,** Electrophoretic diversity of glucose-6-phosphate dehydrogenase among Greeks, *Am. J. Hum. Genet.*, 22, 587, 1970.
332. **Stamatoyannopoulos, G, Voigtlaender, V., and Akrivakis, A.,** Thessaly variant of glucose-6-phosphate dehydrogenase, *Humangenetik*, 9, 23, 1970.
333. **Panich, V.,** Glucose-6-phosphate dehydrogenase in Thailand. The occurrence of three electrophoretic variants among 1115 non-deficient males, *Hum. Genet.*, 53, 227, 1980.
334. **Yoshida, A.,** Glucose-6-phosphate dehydrogenase of human erythrocytes. I. Purification and characterization of normal (B+) enzyme, *J. Biol. Chem.*, 241, 4966, 1966.
335. **Yoshida, A. and Baur, E.,** unpublished data, 1975.
336. **Long, W. K., Kirkman, H. N., and Sutton, H. E.,** Electrophoretically slow variants of glucose-6-phosphate dehydrogenase from red cells of Negroes, *J. Lab. Clin. Med.*, 65, 81, 1965.
337. **Luzzatto, L. and Afolayan, A.,** Different types of human erythrocyte glucose-6-phosphate dehydrogenase, with characterization of two new genetic variants, *J. Clin. Invest.*, 47, 1833, 1968.

338. **Azevedo, E. S. and Yoshida, A.,** Brazilian variant of glucose-6-phosphate dehydrogenase (Gd Minas Gerais), *Nature (London),* 222, 380, 1969.
339. **Hook, E. B., Stamatoyannopoulos, G., Yoshida, A., and Motulsky, A. G.,** Glucose-6-phosphate dehydrogenase Madrona: a slow electrophoretic glucose-6-phosphate dehydrogenase variant with kinetic characteristics similar to those of normal type, *J. Lab. Clin. Med.,* 72, 404, 1968.
340. **González, R., Wude, M., Estrada, M., Svarch, E., and Colombo, B.,** G6PD Pinar Del Rio: a new variant discovered in a Cuban family, *Biochem. Genet.,* 15, 909, 1977.
341. **Cayanis, E., Lane, A. B., Jenkins, T., Nurse, G. T., and Balinsky, D.,** Glucose-6-phosphate dehydrogenase Porbandar: a new slow variant with slightly reduced activity in a South African family of Indian descent, *Biochem. Genet.,* 15, 765, 1977.
342. **Dern, R. J., McCurdy, P. R., and Yoshida, A.,** A new structural variant of glucose-6-phosphate dehydrogenase with a high production rate (G6PD), *J. Lab. Clin. Med.,* 73, 283, 1969.
343. **Beutler, E.,** Abnormalities of the hexose monophosphate shunt, *Semin. Hematol.,* 8, 311, 1971.
344. **Bapat, J. P. and Baxi, A. J.,** Mechanism of hemolysis of G-6-PD deficient red cells: changes in membrane lipids and polypeptides, *Blut,* 44, 355, 1982.
345. **Krohne-Ehrich, G., Schirmer, R. H., and Untucht-Grau, R.,** Glutathione rductase from human erythrocytes: isolation of the enzyme of sequence analysis of the redox-active peptide, *Eur. J. Biochem.,* 80, 65, 1971.
346. **Löhr, G. W. and Waller, H. D.,** Eine neue enzymopenische hämolytische Anämie mit Glutathionreduktase-Mangel, *Med. Klin.,* 57, 1521, 1962.
347. **Beutler, E.,** Effect of flavin compounds on glutathione reductase activity: in vivo and in vitro studies, *J. Clin. Invest.,* 48, 1957, 1969.
348. **Loos, H., Roos, D., Weening, R., and Houwerziji, J.,** Familial deficiency of glutathione reductase in human blood cells, *Blood,* 48, 53, 1976.
349. **Necheles, T. F., Boles, T. A., and Allen, D. M.,** Erythrocyte glutathione-peroxidase deficiency and hemolytic disease in the newborn infant, *J. Pediatr.,* 72, 319, 1968.
350. **Necheles, T. F., Steinberg, M. H., and Cameron, D.,** Erythrocyte glutathione-peroxidase deficiency, *Br. J. Haematol.,* 19, 605, 1970.
351. **Flohé, L., Günzler, W. A., and Schock, H. H.,** Glutathione peroxidase: a selenoenzyme, *FEBS Lett.,* 32, 132, 1973.
352. **Perona, G., Guidi, G. C., Piga, A., Cellerino, R., Menna, R., and Zatti, M.,** In vivo and in vitro variations of human erythrocyte glutathione peroxidase activity as result of cell aging, selenium availability and peroxide activation, *Br. J. Haematol.,* 39, 399, 1978.
353. **Perona, G., Guidi, G. C., Piga, A., Cellerino, R., Milani, G., Colautti, P., Moschini, G., and Stievano, B. M.,** Neonatal erythrocyte glutathione peroxidase deficiency as a consequence of selenium imbalance during pregnancy, *Br. J. Haematol.,* 42, 567, 1979.
354. **Konrad, P. N., Richards, F., Valentine, W. N., and Paglia, D. E.,** Gamma-glutamyl-cysteine synthetase deficiency, *N. Engl. J. Med.,* 286, 557, 1972.
355. **Richards, F., Cooper, M. R., Pearce, L. A., Cowan, R. J., and Spurr, C. L.,** Familial spinocerebullar degeneration, hemolytic anemia, and glutathione deficiency, *Arch. Intern. Med.,* 134, 534, 1974.
356. **Oort, M., Loos, J. A., and Prins, H. K.,** Hereditary absence of reduced glutathione in the erythrocyte, a new clinical and biochemical entity?, *Vox Sang.,* 6, 370, 1961.
357. **Boivin, P. and Galand, C.,** La synthése du glutathion au cours de l'anémie hémolytique congénitale avec déficit en glutathion-synthétase érythrocytaire?, *Nouv. Rev. Fr. Hématol.,* 5, 707, 1965.
358. **Mohler, D. N., Majerus, P. W., Minnich, V., Hess, C. H., and Garrick, M. D.,** Glutathione synthetase deficiency as a cause of hereditary hemolytic disease, *N. Engl. J. Med.,* 283, 1253, 1970.
359. **Larsson, A. and Zetterstroem, R.,** Pyroglutamic aciduria (5-oxoprolinuria), an inborn error in glutathione metabolism, *Pediatr. Res.,* 8, 852, 1974.
360. **Wellner, V. P., Sekura, R., Meister, A., and Larsson, A.,** Glutathione synthetase deficiency, an inborn error of metabolism involving the gamma-glutamyl cycle in patients with 5-oxoprolinuria (pyroglutamic aciduria), *Proc. Natl. Acad. Sci. U.S.A.,* 71, 2505, 1974.
361. **Marstein, S., Jellum, E., Halpern, B., Eldjarn, L., and Perry, T. L.,** Biochemical study of erythrocytes in a patient with pyroglutamic acidemia (5-oxoprolinemia), *N. Engl. J. Med.,* 295, 406, 1976.
362. **Spielberg, S. P., Garrick, M. D., Corash, L. M., Butler, J. D., Tietze, F., Rogers, L., and Schulman, J. D.,** Biochemical heterogeneity in glutathione synthetase deficiency, *J. Clin. Invest.,* 61, 1417, 1978.
363. **Fildes, R. A. and Harris, H.,** Genetically determined variation of adenylate kinase in man, *Nature (London),* 209, 261, 1966.
364. **Bowman, J. E., Frischer, H., Ajmar, F., Carson, P. E., and Gower, M. K.,** Population, family and biochemical investigation of human adenylate kinase polymorphism, *Nature (London),* 214, 1156, 1967.
365. **Russell, P. J., Jr., Hornstein, J. M., Goins, L., Jones, D., and Laver, M.,** Adenylate kinase in human tissues. I. Organ specificity of adenylate kinase isoenzymes, *J. Biol. Chem.,* 249, 1874, 1974.

366. **Ishimoto, G.,** Red cell enzymes, in *Anthropological and Genetic Studies on the Japanese,* Watanabe, S., Kondo, S., and Matsunaga, E., Eds., University of Tokyo Press, Tokyo, 1975, 109.
367. **Von Zabern, I., Wittmann-Liebold, B., Untucht-Grau, R., Schirmer, R. H., and Pai, E. F.,** Primary and tertiary structure of the principal human adenylate kinase, *Eur. J. Biochem.,* 68, 281, 1976.
368. **Szeinberg, A., Gavendo, S., and Cahana, D.,** Erythrocyte adenylate-kinase deficiency, *Lancet,* i, 315, 1969.
369. **Szeinberg, A., Kahana, D., Gavendo, S., Zaidman, J., and Ben-Ezzer, J.,** Hereditary deficiency of adenylate kinase in red blood cells, *Acta Haematol.,* 42, 111, 1969.
370. **Boivin, P., Galand, C., Hakim, J., Simony, D., and Seligman, M.,** Une nouvelle érythroenzymopathie: Anémie hémolytique congénitale non sphérocytaire et déficit héréditaire en adénylate-kinase erythrocytaire, *Presse Med.,* 79, 215, 1971.
371. **Miwa, S., Fujii, H., Tani, K., Takahashi, K., Takizawa, T., and Igarashi, T.,** Red cell adenylate kinase deficiency associated with hereditary nonspherocytic hemolytic anemia: clinical and biochemical studies, *Am. J. Hematol.,* 14, 325, 1983.
372. **Paglia, D. E. and Valentine, W. N.,** Haemolytic anaemia associated with disorders of the purine and pyrimidine salvage pathways, *Clin. Haematol.,* 10, 81, 1981.
373. **Valentine, W. N., Fink, K., Paglia, D. E., Harris, S. R., and Adams, W. S.,** Hereditary hemolytic anemia with human erythrocyte pyrimidine 5′-nucleotidase deficiency, *J. Clin. Invest.,* 54, 866, 1974.
374. **Torrance, J. D., Whittaker, D., and Beutler, E.,** Purification and properties of human erythrocyte pyrimidine 5′-nucleotidase, *Proc. Natl. Acad. Sci. U.S.A.,* 74, 3701, 1977.
375. **Ben-Bassat, I., Brok-Simon, F., Kende, G., Holtzmann, F., and Ramot, B.,** A family with red cell pyrimidine 5′-nucleotidase deficiency, *Blood,* 47, 919, 1976.
376. **Vives-Corrons, J. L., Montserrat-Costa, E., and Rozman, C.,** Hereditary hemolytic anemia with erythrocyte pyrimidine 5′-nucleotidase deficiency in Spain, *Hum. Genet.,* 34, 285, 1976.
377. **Oda, S. and Tanaka, K. R.,** Metabolic studies in erythrocyte pyrimidine 5′-nucleotidase deficiency, *Clin. Res.,* 24, 149, 1976.
378. **Paglia, D. E., Fink, K., and Valentine, W. N.,** Additional data from two kindreds with genetically induced deficiencies of erythrocyte pyrimidine nucleotidase, *Acta Haematol.,* 63, 262, 1980.
379. **Beutler, E., Baranko, P. V., Feagler, J., Matsumoto, F., Miro-Quesdada, M., Selby, G., and Singh, P.,** Hemolytic anemia due to pyrimidine-5′-nucleotidase deficiency: report of eight cases in six families, *Blood,* 56, 251, 1980.
380. **Rosa, R., Rochant, H., Dreyfus, B., Valentin, C., and Rosa, J.,** Electrophoretic and kinetic studies of human erythrocyte deficient in pyrimidine 5′-nucleotidase, *Hum. Genet.,* 38, 209, 1977.
381. **Buc, H.-A., Kaplan, J.-C., and Najman, A.,** Study of a case with severe red-cell pyrimidine 5′-nucleotidase deficiency, *Clin. Chim. Acta,* 95, 83, 1979.
382. **Torrance, J. D., Karabus, C. D., Shnier, M., Meltzer, M., Katz, J., and Jenkins, T.,** Haemolytic anaemia due to erythrocyte pyrimidine 5′-nucleotidase deficiency. Report of the first South African family, *S. Afr. Med. J.,* 52, 671, 1977.
383. **Ozsoylu, S. and Gurgey, A.,** A case of hemolytic anemia due to erythrocyte pyrimidine 5′-nucleotidase deficiency, *Acta Haematol.,* 66, 56, 1981.
384. **Miwa, S., Nakashima, K., Fujii, H., Matsumoto, M., and Nomura, K.,** Three cases of hereditary hemolytic anemia with pyrimidine 5′-nucleotidase deficiency in a Japanese family, *Hum. Genet.,* 37, 361, 1977.
385. **Miwa, S., Ishida, Y., Kibe, A., Uekihara, S., and Kishimoto, S.,** Two cases of hereditary hemolytic anemia with pyrimidine 5′-nucleotidase deficiency, *Acta Haematol. Jpn.,* 44, 187, 1981.
386. **Hirono, A., Fujii, H., Miyajima, H., Kawakatsu, T., Hiyoshi, Y., and Miwa, S.,** Three families of hereditary hemolytic anemia with pyrimidine 5′-nucleotidase deficiency: electrophoretic and kinetic studies, *Clin. Chim. Acta,* 130, 189, 1983.
387. **Torrance, J. D. and Whittaker, D.,** Distribution of erythrocyte nucleotides in pyrimidine 5′-nucleotidase deficiency, *Br. J. Haematol.,* 43, 423, 1979.
388. **White, J. M. and Selhi, H. S.,** Lead and the red cell, *Br. J. Haematol.,* 30, 133, 1975.
389. **Fujii, H., Nakashima, K., Miwa, S., and Nomura, K.,** Electrophoretic and kinetic studies of a mutant red cell pyrimidine 5′-nucleotidase, *Clin. Chim. Acta,* 95, 89, 1979.
390. **Ishida, Y., Miwa, S., Miura, Y., and Kibe, A.,** Electrophoretic and kinetic studies of human erythrocyte deficient in pyrimidine 5′-nucleotidase, *Clin. Chim. Acta,* 108, 285, 1980.
391. **Shinohara, K. and Tanaka, K. R.,** Kinetic and electrophoretic studies of human erythrocyte deficient in pyrimidine 5′-nucleotidase, *Hum. Genet.,* 51, 107, 1979.
392. **Vives-Corrons, J. L.,** personal communication, 1982.
393. **Matsumoto, N., Adachi, H., Miwa, S., Takahashi, M., Kamei, T., Ishida, Y., and Kibe, A.,** Electron microscopic observation of the red pulp of the spleen in hereditary hemolytic anemia with erythrocyte pyrimidine 5′-nucleotidase deficiency: evidence for intravascular hemolysis, *Acta Haematol. Jpn.,* 45, 17, 1982.

394. **Edwards, Y. H., Hopkinson, D. A., and Harris, H.,** Adenosine deaminase isozymes in human tissues, *Ann. Hum. Genet. Lond.*, 35, 207, 1971.
395. **Giblett, E. R., Anderson, J. E., Cohen, F., Pollara, B., and Meuwissen, H. J.,** Adenosine deaminase deficiency in two patients with severely impaired cellular immunity, *Lancet*, ii, 1067, 1972.
396. **Spencer, N., Hopkinson, D. A., and Harris, H.,** Adenosine deaminase polymorphism in man, *Ann. Hum. Genet. London*, 32, 9, 1968.
397. **Hopkinson, D. A., Cook, P. J. L., and Harris, H.,** Further data on the adenosine deaminase (ADA) polymorphism and a report of a new phenotype, *Ann. Hum. Genet. London*, 32, 361, 1969.
398. **Schrader, W. P., Stacy, A. R., and Pollara, B.,** Purification of human erythrocyte adenosine deaminase by affinity column chromatography, *J. Biol. Chem.*, 251, 4026, 1976.
399. **Daddona, P. E. and Kelley, W. N.,** Human adenosine deaminase. Purification and subunit structure, *J. Biol. Chem.*, 252, 110, 1977.
400. **Schrader, W. P. and Stacy, A. R.,** Purification and subunit structure of adenosine deaminase from human kidney, *J. Biol. Chem.*, 252, 6409, 1977.
401. **Daddona, P. E. and Kelley, W. N.,** Human adenosine deaminase binding protein. Assay, purification and properties, *J. Biol. Chem.*, 253, 4617, 1978.
402. **Schrader, W. P., Woodward, F. J., and Pollara, B.,** Purification of an adenosine deaminase complexing protein from human plasma, *J. Biol. Chem.*, 254, 11964, 1979.
403. **Koch, G. and Shows, T. B.,** A gene of human chromosome 6 functions in assembly of tissue-specific adenosine deaminase isozymes, *Proc. Natl. Acad. Sci. U.S.A.*, 75, 3876, 1978.
404. **Siciliano, M. J., Bordelon, M. R., and Kohler, P. O.,** Expression of human adenosine deaminase after fusion of adenosine deaminase-deficient cells with mouse fibroblasts, *Proc. Natl. Acad. Sci. U.S.A.*, 75, 936, 1978.
405. **Valentine, W. N., Paglia, D. E., Tartaglia, A. P., and Gilsantz, F.,** Hereditary hemolytic anemia with increased red cell adenosine deaminase (45- to 70-fold) and decreased adenosine triphosphate, *Science*, 195, 783, 1977.
406. **Miwa, S., Fujii, H., Matsumoto, N., Nakatsuji, T., Oda, S., Asano, H., Asano, S., and Miura, Y.,** A case of red-cell adenosine deaminase overproduction associated with hereditary hemolytic anemia found in Japan, *Am. J. Hematol.*, 5, 107, 1978.
407. **Pérignon, J.-L., Hamet, M., Buc, H. A., Cartier, P. H., and Derycke, M.,** Biochemical study of a case of hemolytic anemia with increased (85-fold) red cell adenosine deaminase, *Clin. Chim. Acta*, 124, 205, 1982.
408. **Fujii, H., Miwa, S., and Suzuki, K.,** Purification and properties of adenosine deaminase in normal and hereditary hemolytic anemia with increased red cell activity, *Hemoglobin*, 4, 693, 1980.
409. **Fujii, H., Miwa, S., Tani, K., Fujinami, N., and Asano, Y.,** Overproduction of structurally normal enzyme in man: hereditary haemolytic anaemia with increased red cell adenosine deaminase activity, *Br. J. Haematol.*, 51, 427, 1982.
410. **Jaffé, E. R.,** Hereditary methemoglobinemia associated with abnormalities in the metabolism of erythrocytes, *Am. J. Med.*, 41, 786, 1966.
411. **Kaplan, J.-C., Leroux, A., and Beauvais, P.,** Formes cliniques et biologiques du déficit en cytochrome b_5 réductase, *C. R. Seances Soc. Biol.*, 173, 368, 1979.
412. **Hegesh, E., Calmanovici, N., and Avron, M.,** New method for determining ferrihemoglobin reductase (NADH-methemoglobin reductase) in erythrocytes, *J. Lab. Clin. Med.*, 72, 339, 1968.
413. **Scott, E. M.,** The relation of diaphorase of human erythrocytes to inheritance of methemoglobinemia, *J. Clin. Invest.*, 39, 1176, 1960.
414. **Passon, P. G. and Hultquist, D. E.,** Soluble cytochrome b_5 reductase from human erythrocytes, *Biochim. Biophys. Acta*, 275, 62, 1972.

THE RED CELL MEMBRANE: BIOCHEMICAL COMPOSITION AND "ANATOMY" IN HEALTH AND DISEASE

Joel Anne Chasis and Stephen B. Shohet

INTRODUCTION

In the past decade, major strides have been made in our understanding of the composition of the red cell. Technical advances in both lipid and protein analysis have enabled us to determine the detailed composition of the membrane and to begin to probe some of the interactions between components. Previous advances in chromatographic and spectrographic methods for separating and analyzing the membrane lipids have now been supplemented with highly sensitive electrophoretic methods for solubilizing and separating membrane proteins. In addition, the use of affinity chromatography purification techniques and immunologic blotting methods have extended the sensitivity and specificity of the basic electrophoretic procedures such that proteins present in trace amounts can be prepared in highly purified form. This, in turn, is beginning to allow us to conduct structural analyses of membrane proteins using newly developed tryptic mapping and sequencing procedures which were previously beyond the reach of students of the red cell membrane. Further, elegant electron micrographic methods for the topographic localization of specific membrane protein associations have enabled us to begin to visualize the biochemically active structures of membrane elements. Finally, the application of newer physical techniques utilizing fluorescence probes and advanced spectrographic techniques involving magnetic or spin resonance have enabled us to begin to study the interactions of some of the membrane components under in vivo conditions.

Although the fruits of these later developments are still to be gathered, sufficient new information on the basic composition and disposition of the red cell membrane components has now accumulated to warrant the present review. We will concentrate mostly on the new knowledge of the membrane proteins which has accumulated in the past several years. The lipids which, of course, are a major component of the membrane as well, will also be discussed, although recent developments in this area have been less active. Finally, although this review is designed primarily to describe the composition and disposition of membrane components, some comments on the normal functional role and the clinical importance of abnormalities in these components will be introduced when relevant. The organization of this review will be as follows. The first section will discuss the composition and character of membrane proteins, some of their important interactions, and, when known, their role in normal physiology and abnormal pathology. The second section will consist of a similar treatment of the membrane lipids.

RED CELL MEMBRANE PROTEINS

When considering membrane proteins, it is convenient to divide them into integral membrane proteins, which in the red cell often span the bilayer, and peripheral, skeletal proteins which form a supporting lattice, attached to, and underneath the inner leaflet of the lipid bilayer. We will first discuss the integral red cell membrane proteins band 3, and the glycophorins. A current conception of the structural anatomy of the red cell membrane is presented in Figure 1.

Structure and Function of Integral Proteins

Band 3

Band 3, also known as the anion transport protein, is the major transmembrane glycoprotein

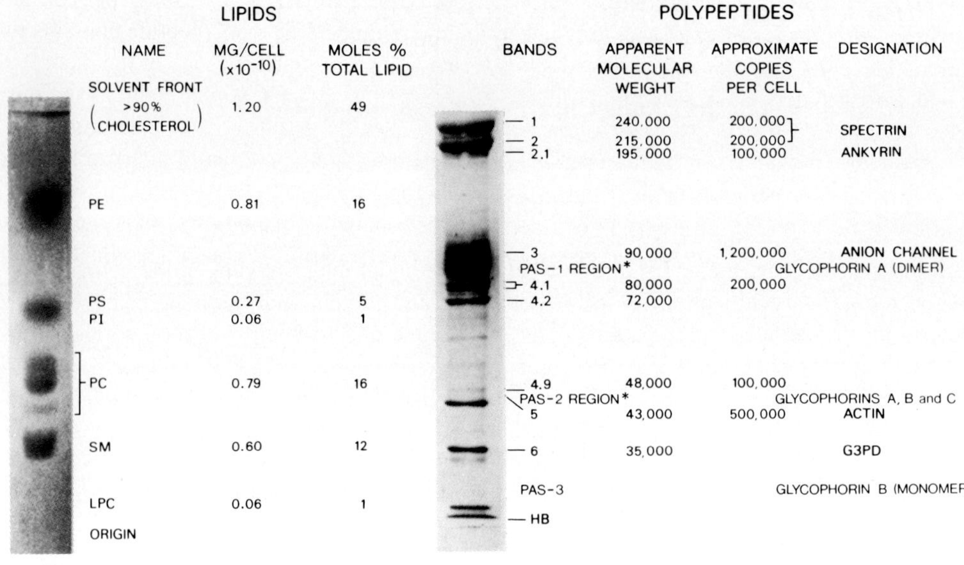

A

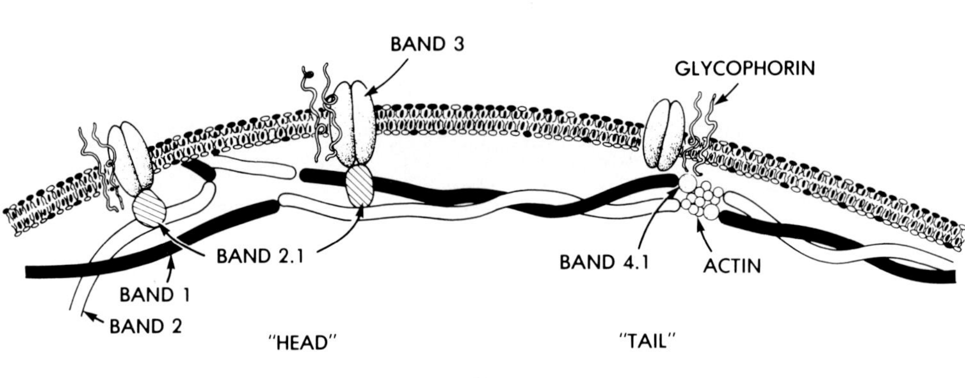

B

FIGURE 1. Current concepts of red cell membrane composition and organization. (a) Thin-layer chromatogram of red cell membrane lipids (left) and Coomassie blue-stained SDS polyacrylamide gel electrophoretogram of red cell membrane proteins (right). (b) Diagrammatic cross-section of membrane bilayer and supporting "skeleton". The predominant protein of the membrane, spectrin, occurs as a heterodimer (bands 1 and 2) linked together into a fibrous network. The linkage between the "tail", or amino ends of the dimers appears to be mediated by actin (band 5) and band 4.1. Linkage between the "head", or carboxy, ends of the dimers occurs by direct contact between complimentary strands of the heterodimer. Attachment of the skeleton to the membrane is produced by a specific association between band 2 of spectrin and band 3 in the lipid bilayer via the spectrin-binding protein, band 2.1 (ankyrin), near the head end of the spectrin dimer. An additional association of the skeletal complex with the lipid bilayer may be provided by a connection between spectrin and another bilayer protein, PAS2 via band 4.1. Bands 2, 2.1, 3, and 4.1 can be phosphorylated, and some of that phosphorylation is cAMP-dependent. The phosphorylation sites of spectrin band 2, which are not shown in this diagram, appear to be close to the end of the dimer. The outer leaflet of the bilayer is composed predominantly of choline-containing phospholipids (indicated by black head groups), and the inner leaflet is predominantly composed of acidic phospholipids, such as phosphatidylethanolamine and phosphatidylserine (indicated by white head groups). Cholesterol (indicated by black ovals) is shown embedded symmetrically in each leaflet among the fatty acid side groups of the phospholipid, although this has not yet been experimentally verified. The PAS1 and PAS2 bands have been better defined by additional biochemical studies, including gel electrophoresis techniques with improved resolution. It is now known that the PAS1 region contains the dimer of the sialoglycopeptide glycophorin A and that the PAS2 region resolves into three bands: the dimer of glycophorin B (47,000 daltons), the monomer of glycophorin A (38,000 daltons), and glycophorin C, also called glyconnectin (35,000 daltons). Unfortunately, there is not, as of yet, a universally accepted nomenclature for these PAS-staining sialoglycopeptides. (From Williams, W. J., et al., Eds., *Hematology*, McGraw-Hill, New York, 1983. With permission.)

with a molecular weight of approximately 95,000. There are 1.2×10^6 copies per cell[2] and the protein appears to exist as a tetramer in the membrane.[3,4] This polypeptide contains two domains, a 40,000-mol wt portion which is located on the cytoplasmic side of the membrane and which includes the N-terminus, and a 55,000-mol wt domain which includes the intramembranous and cell surface portions of the polypeptide ending in the C-terminus. The carbohydrate residues are linked to this C-terminal domain and consist of a single N-linked oligosaccharide made up of a variable number of repeating N-acetyllactosamine disaccharide units. It is partially because of this heterogeneity in number of units that band 3 migrates as a diffuse band on polyacrylamide gels. In the adult erythrocyte, the N-acetyllactosamine disaccharide units are branched and substituted into the N-linked oligosaccharide core.[5] This structure terminates in galactose residues and carries the I as well as ABH blood group antigenic determinants.[6] In the fetal cell, the oligosaccharide is not branched, thereby creating a different blood group antigen, the i antigen. There appears to be a further heterogeneity in the carbohydrate structure of band 3 since some of the polypeptides have mannose residues with GlcNAc and Gal-GlcNAc substitutions but no chains of *N*-acetyllactosamine units.[7]

The intramembranous portion of band 3 passes through the lipid bilayer several times[8] and comprises the major component of the intramembranous particles described by freeze etching.[9,10] In addition, protein diffusion measurements suggest that an association exists between the intramembranous components of band 3 and those of a second membrane-spanning protein glycophorin A.[11]

The cytoplasmic portion of band 3 is known to have binding sites for several cytoplasmic proteins although the biological significance of some of these associations is not yet understood. Close to the N-terminus is an acidic segment of the polypeptide where electrostatic binding of glyceraldehyde-3-phosphate dehydrogenase (band 6) and aldolase occurs. The metabolites bound to these glycolytic enzymes, in turn, influence the binding of the enzymes to band 3.[12,13] Some experiments strongly suggest that hemoglobin also binds to this segment of band 3.[14,15] However, these is some controversy about this binding since, under certain experimental conditions, this anionic portion of band 3 can be very sticky.[16]

In addition to binding to these cytoplasmic proteins, the N-terminal domain of band 3 is known to bind to band 2.1 (ankyrin)[17,18] and, thus, links the bilayer to its supporting skeletal infrastructure. Binding studies have shown about 100,000 to 125,000 ankyrin binding sites per cell.[17,19,20] Since there are 1.2×10^6 copies of band 3 per cell, there would be one binding site for every two tetramers if indeed band 3 exists in the membrane as a tetramer. However, no difference between band 3 molecules that are bound to 2.1 in the membrane, and those that are not has been found by peptide mapping.[21] In addition, if purified band 3 is incorporated into liposomes, most of the molecules can bind ankyrin.[20] Thus, more needs to be learned about band 3 and its association with ankyrin.

The band 3 molecule has at least two very important but very different functions. The cytoplasmic domain through ankyrin serves as a bilayer attachment site for the spectrin, actin, protein 4.1 skeleton. These skeletal proteins play an important role in determining cellular shape, deformability, and membrane stability.[22-24] In addition, recent evidence suggests that the assembly of the skeletal proteins into a lattice may occur at the bilayer and be controlled by the binding affinities of band 3 for ankyrin and ankyrin for spectrin.[25]

The surface and intramembranous domain of band 3 is the anion transport system which exchanges HCO_3^- and Cl^- thereby increasing the capacity of the blood to carry CO_2 from the tissues to the lungs.[26,27] There is also some evidence that part of this domain may play a role in recognition of senescent red cells and their removal from the circulation by macrophages. The mechanism of removal of senescent cells has not yet been elucidated but it has been shown that when whole blood is separated on a density gradient, the most dense cells have an antibody on their surface that the less dense cells do not have.[28,29] Since there is some evidence suggesting that the most dense cells correspond to the oldest cells, this antibody may provide an immunologic marker of aged cells. The antigenic determinants for this antibody have been shown by Kay on proteolytic cleavage products of band 3.[30]

The Glycophorins

There are three main PAS-positive sialoglycoproteins in the red cell membrane. Several nomenclatures for the glycophorins exist (see Anstee[31] for comparison) and in this review we will use that of Furthmayr. Glycophorin A, with a molecular weight of about 31,000 comprises approximately 70% of the sialoglycopeptides; glycophorin B with a molecular weight of about 24,000 comprises approximately 15%, and glycophorin C comprises approximately 6%. Extensive structural analyses have been done on glycophorins A and B. Glycophorin A is a bilayer-spanning protein with its carboxy terminus and about 40 amino acids on the cytoplasmic side of the membrane, 23 amino acids in a hydrophobic segment traversing the bilayer as an apolar α-helix, and about 70 amino acids on the cell surface.[32-34] Some 60% of this glycoprotein is carbohydrate and these sugar residues are exclusively located on the extracellular domain. There are 15 O-linked sialotetrasaccharides[35,36] and one N-linked oligosaccharide.[37] Glycophorin A carries the blood group M, N antigenic determinants. Polypeptide sequencing and carbohydrate analysis reveal that the only differences between the antigenic portions of M and N are different amino acids at positions 1 and 5.[38]

Two variants of glyphorin A, M^g and M^c, have been described which contain several amino acid substitutions; however, these changes appear to be clinically insignificant.[39] In addition, several families have been described who, by PAS stain, radiolabeling, and immunologic studies, appear to lack at least the extracellular and cytoplasmic portions of glycophorin A in their circulating cells.[40-42] This condition has been termed En(a−) and whether the glycophorin A molecule is completely absent has not yet been determined. Clinically En(a−) individuals seem well although careful erythrocyte survival studies would be helpful in a more complete evaluation.

Although glycophorin A is known to carry the MN antigen determinants and receptors for influenza and Sendai viruses,[9] any additional biological roles have not been determined. Experiments from several laboratories show that when erythrocytes bind either a lectin or antibody with specificity for glycophorin A, membrane deformability decreases and the cell shape change induced by echinocytic agents is inhibited.[43,44] The loss in deformability appears to occur because glycophorin A has become associated with the skeletal proteins, which are known to play an important role in determining membrane deformability.[44] Binding studies demonstrate that band 4.1 associates with glycophorin A[45] and that this association may be dependent on the extent of phosphorylation of phosphoinositides.[46] Thus, protein 4.1 may be the protein link between glycophorin A and the skeletal proteins.

Structural studies of glycophorin B show that it possesses appreciable peptide and carbohydrate homology with glycophorin A.[38] In fact, the first 26 residues in from the N-terminus are identical to those of the N phenotype of glycophorin A, and glycophorin B does indeed carry N blood group activity. The carbohydrate residues of this region are also similar except that glycophorin B does not have the N-linked oligosaccharide. In addition to N activity, this glycophorin possesses blood group antigen S, or s activity, which is associated with the presence at residue 29 of a methionine or threonine, respectively.[47] Miltenberger classes III and IV and S-s are variants which involve structural changes in glycophorin B.[48] None of these variants, however, seem to cause clinically significant disease. If glycophorin B possesses a function in addition to carrying blood group antigens, that function remains to be elucidated.

Glycophorin C, which only contributes about 6% of the sialoglycopeptide content of the cell, has an amino acid sequence which is very different from glycophorins A and B. However, the carbohydrate content and lectin binding properties taken together suggest similarities with glycophorin A. There appear to be mannose and N-acetylglucosamine residues, possibly in an N-glycosidically linked oligosaccharide. In addition, the presence of N-acetylgalactosamine, sialic acid, and galactose, and certain lectin binding specificities suggest the presence of O-glycosidically linked oligosaccharides.[31,38,48] One group of investigators believes glycophorin C is associated with band 4.1 and they therefore call it ''glycoconnectin''.[49]

Band 4.5 Region

The protein constituents which migrate in the band 4.5 region on gel electrophoresis have not been as extensively characterized as other membrane proteins. There is preliminary evidence from immunologic studies and peptide mapping that at least some 4.5 components may be proteolytic pieces of band 3. However, this region is mentioned here because of its probable functional importance: one of the components of the 4.5 region has been shown by cytochalasin B and reconstitution studies to play a role in glucose transport as reviewed by Baldwin and Llenhard.[50]

Structure and Function of Skeletal Proteins

Underlying the bilayer and associated with it through several protein-protein and protein-lipid linkages is a lattice of proteins known as the membrane skeleton.[51-53] This lattice includes spectrin, actin, protein 4.1, and protein 2.1 and plays an important role in supporting the bilayer and determining the membrane properties of deformability and stability.[23] In describing the membrane skeleton, we will first discuss the structure and intermolecular associations of each of the component proteins, and then discuss the diseases associated with abnormalities of these proteins.

Spectrin

Spectrin is the central protein of the membrane skeleton and is composed of two subunits: α, with a molecular weight of 240,000, and β, with a molecular weight of 225,000. The α- and β-chains are known to self-associate into dimer (αβ spectrin), tetramer, and in concentrated solutions, higher-order oligomers.[54,55] It is felt by many that spectrin is present as oligomers in its native state on the membrane since concentrations similar to those which produce oligomers in vitro (>5 mg/mℓ) must be present near the inner surface of the membrane. The configuration of the dimer, when examined under the electron microscope after rotary shadowing with platinum, is that of a flexible, rod-shaped molecule. The α- and β-subunit are associated head-to-head and parallel to form a dimer. Two dimers associate in the same head region to form a tetramer and when a concentrated solution of spectrin (>5 mg/mℓ) is examined, higher oligomers can be seen.[54,55]

With the use of peptide mapping of trypsin and nitrothiocyanobenzoic acid-generated peptides and with monoclonal antibody probes, the alignment of peptides in both the α- and β-chain has been elegantly determined.[56] The amino acid compositions of the α- and β-chains are similar and their sequencing is now in progress. Data available reveal that the α- and β-subunits contain many areas of homology.[57] The sequence of the amino terminal domain of the α-subunit has been completely determined and this 595 amino acid region contains a repeating unit of 106 amino acids which suggests that in the evoluation of spectrin, multiple gene duplications occurred. This repeating unit is not present in the 17 residues next to the N-terminus, and it is this segment which is felt to contain the oligomer binding site.[58,59]

Not only does spectrin self-associate, but it also has been shown to form noncovalent associations with actin, protein 4.1, and protein 2.1. Protein 2.1, also known as ankyrin, is one of the molecules which anchors the membrane skeleton to the bilayer through an association both with spectrin and with the cytoplasmic portion of the transmembrane protein band 3. By biochemical and electron microscopic studies, protein 2.1 has been shown to bind about 20 nm from the head (site of dimer formation) of the spectrin molecule.[60,61] Further studies have placed the binding site within the first two peptide domains of the β-subunit.[62] Since there are only 100,000 copies of ankyrin per cell[63] and 200,000 spectrin dimers, that would mean there would be one binding site per tetramer. Less is known about the binding of protein 4.1 and actin to spectrin, but morphological data suggest that they bind to the opposite terminal end from that of 2.1.[61]

In addition to binding sites for these structural proteins, spectrin also has binding sites for several other kinds of cytoplasmic molecules. The polyphosphate, 2,3-DPG binds to spectrin at possibly seven sites.[64] In addition, several groups of investigators agree that calmodulin binds to spectrin although some believe it binds to the α-subunit[65,66] while others find it binds to the β-subunit.[57] Both calmodulin and polyphosphate binding may well play roles in membrane stability and cell shape.

Protein 4.1

Protein 4.1 is an approximately 80,000-dalton protein which is present at 200,000 copies per erythrocyte. Initially, it was felt to be a single polypeptide since it migrated as a single band in continuous buffer systems.[67] However, with the use of the discontinuous buffer system, it is now apparent that there is a doublet in the 4.1 region, the components of which have been termed 4.1a and 4.1b.[68] The relationship of these two polypeptides to one another is not yet fully understood. It is, however, known through peptide mapping that 4.1a and 4.1b contain closely related sequences.[68] Additional studies which compare the proportion of 4.1a and 4.1b in mouse cells of varying ages show that young cells have proportionally more 4.1b while older cells have more 4.1a.[69] It appears, therefore, that there may be some post-translational modification responsible for the differences between these two bands.

Ultrastructural studies of protein 4.1 show it to be globular in form. When examined by rotary shadowing in solution with spectrin, protein 4.1 binds to the tail ends of the spectrin tetramer.[60,61] Binding studies of spectrin and protein 4.1, done in solution, confirm such an association.[60,61] It appears that spectrin-protein 4.1 binding facilities the interaction of spectrin with actin which is discussed below.

Recent evidence from studies of inside-out vesicles and protein 4.1 suggests that protein 4.1 may bind to glycophorin A and hence provide another means for spectrin to associate with the membrane.[45] Preliminary studies suggest that the extent of binding of protein 4.1 and glycophorin A is influenced by the state of phosphorylation of the phosphoinositides[46] and so may have interesting functional significance.

One group has, in addition, suggested an association between protein 4.1 and glycophorin C based on the behavior of glycophorin A and protein 4.1 during Triton extraction of the membrane.[49] However, this association remains controversial in part because of the vast difference between the number of copies of protein 4.1 (200,000) and of glycophorin C (35,000).

Actin

Actin, as a monomer, has a molecular weight of 42,000 and appears as band 5 when red cell membranes are subjected to polyacrylamide gel electrophoresis. Traditionally employed extraction procedures yield a depolymerized form of actin but it has been felt that the polymerized, filamentous form, F-actin, is present in the membrane. Recently, biochemical and ultrastructural studies seem to confirm the presence of F-actin. For example, it has been shown by several investigators that an oligomeric complex of spectrin-actin-protein 4.1 can stimulate actin polymerization[70-72] and that this polymerization is inhibited by cytochalsin B which is known to inhibit F-actin-induced actin polymerization.[73] In addition, phalloidin can be used to stabilize actin filaments in the membrane and a subsequent actin extraction yielded oligomers made up of 30 monomers.[74]

Using binding studies, sedimentation analysis, and viscometry, different investigators have shown that F-actin forms weak bonds with spectrin and that this association is enhanced by protein 4.1.[71,75-79] Electron microscopic studies have shown that F-actin binds to the tail region of spectrin,[80,81] the same region as that which binds protein 4.1. At this time, it is not known whether or not protein 4.1 forms a link between F-actin and spectrin.

Ankyrin

Ankyrin, otherwise known as band 2.1,[2] is present in the membrane skeleton along with a series of its proteolytic products. Taken together, these polypeptides have been called "syndeins", from the Greek "to connect", because of their role in associating spectrin with band 3 and thus to the bilayer.[82] Ankyrin has a globular form and about 100,000 copies are present per cell.[63] As discussed in detail above, ankyrin is responsible for the high-affinity binding of spectrin to the membrane. Its binding site on spectrin has been localized microscopically to within the first two domains of the head region of the β-chain. Binding studies show that saturation occurs at a molar ratio of one ankyrin per spectrin dimer.[61] This stoichiometry is supported by a rotary shadowing experiment in which two ankyrin molecules can be seen binding symmetrically to a spectrin tetramer.[60,61] As previously noted, ankyrin also binds with high affinity to the cytoplasmic end of band 3 and thus links the skeletal protein lattice to the bilayer.

Band 4.9

Band 4.9 is a 48,000-dalton polypeptide about which little was known until very recently when it was shown that band 4.9 can associate with actin and reduces the rate of actin polymerization.[83] Its concentration is equimolar with spectrin tetramers[83] and it may serve the important function of stabilizing short actin oligomers.

Membrane Protein Defects in Hemolytic Anemias

Armed with an increased understanding of the normal protein structure of the erythrocyte membrane, it has been possible to begin to define the molecular basis for some of the congenital and hereditary hemolytic anemias. The abnormalities thus far appear to fall into two main categories: either a quantitative or a qualitative change in a membrane protein. In almost all cases, only circulating erythrocytes have been studied, so whether the defined abnormalities exist in maturing cells is unknown. This becomes particularly pertinent when discussing quantitative defects since an observed protein deficiency in mature cells may result, for example, from a qualitatively altered protein which was rendered more susceptible to proteolysis. However, until we can examine erythroid precursors in the bone marrow, and, in the more distant future, define the pertinent gene structure, these ambiguities will persist.

It is now known that within the phenotypic categories of hereditary spherocytosis and hereditary elliptocytosis, individuals with different skeletal protein abnormalities can be found. Thus, different molecular characteristics can result in the same cell shape but produce different severities of anemia. In the near future, it will be important to develop a new terminology for these anemias based on their molecular defects.

Hereditary Spherocytosis

Hereditary spherocytosis (HS) is the most common of the group of hereditary and congenital hemolytic anemias which involve membrane dysfunction. The majority of patients with this disorder have red cells which range from discocytic to stomatocytic but have only a small number of truly spherocytic cells.[84] These individuals have a compensated or mild anemia and, despite intense effort in several laboratories, no biochemical defect has been documented.

In contrast, a small number of individuals have marked spherocytosis and fragmented cells in their peripheral blood and have severe hemolysis.[85,86] Biochemical studies reveal that within this group there are at least two different molecular defects found. Agre has documented a 50% reduction in α- and β-spectrin content of red cells in one family with a severe form of HS.[85] When cellular deformability is measured using the ektacytometer, these cells have markedly decreased deformability which is due to a reduced surface area to volume ratio.[23] Membrane stability, as assayed in the ektacytometer, is decreased[23] and it thus appears that a deficiency in spectrin results in an unstable membrane which undergoes fragmentation leading to cells with a reduced surface area.

A second defect has been reported in several kindreds with marked spherocytosis.[86,87] This defect appears to involve the region of the spectrin molecule that binds to protein 4.1 and it results in a defective association between spectrin and protein 4.1. These cells also have decreased cellular deformability and decreased membrane stability when examined in the ektacytometer.[23]

It therefore appears that either a quantitative or qualitative defect in the spectrin molecule can give rise to membrane instability and subsequent fragmentation.

Hereditary Pyropoikilocytosis

Hereditary pyropoikilocytosis (HPP) is a second form of hemolytic anemia in which the molecular defect involves the spectrin molecule.[57,88-91] Individuals with this disorder have dramatic pyropoikilocytosis in their peripheral blood with microspherocytes, fragments, and budding forms and experience moderate to severe hemolysis improved by splenectomy.[92] When the cellular deformability and membrane stability are measured by ektacytometry, the membranes are extremely unstable and cellular deformability is reduced as a result of fragmentation-induced loss of membrane surface area.[57,93]

Because the red cell morphology resembled that induced by heat injury, patients' cells were heated and their morphology studied. Normal red cells fragment at 49°C, but these patients' cells were observed to fragment at 45 to 46°C.[92] Subsequently, spectrin purified from HPP cells was shown to undergo similar thermal denaturation[94] and the molecular defect has been localized to the domain on the α-chain involved in oligomer formation.[57,90]

Hereditary Elliptocytosis

Hereditary elliptocytosis (HE), like hereditary spherocytosis, is now known to be a group of diseases all resulting in some degree of elliptocytes but with different clinical severities and different molecular defects. At present, three skeletal protein abnormalities resulting in elliptocytosis have been defined.

The first of these protein abnormalities is a decreased spectrin dimer-dimer association. This abnormality results in a mild anemia with fragmented forms in the peripheral blood. When membrane stability was measured by ektacytometry, an intermediate degree of reduction was found.[95] In low ionic strength extracts prepared at 4°C, there is an increase in the proportion of spectrin in the dimer state.[96,97] As with HPP, the molecular defect appears to involve the 80,000-dalton peptide of the α-chain, which is the site of spectrin oligomerization.[98]

A second protein defect which is associated with elliptocytosis is characterized by a decreased binding of normal protein 2.1 (ankyrin) to patients' inside-out red cell membrane vesicles which have been depleted of their own ankyrin.[99] Individuals with this defect have moderate to severe hemolysis with marked microcytosis, poikilocytosis, and membrane fragmentation in vivo. The defect appears to involve the site of ankyrin binding on the cytoplasmic domain of band 3 since the patients' ankyrin and ankyrin-spectrin interactions are normal.

The third molecular defect that has been identified in association with elliptocytosis is a deficiency in protein 4.1.[100,101] The North African family identified with this disorder has elliptocytes. There is no in vivo fragmentation in heterozygous family members with partial deficiency of protein 4.1 (50% decrease) while elliptocytes and dramatic in vivo fragmentation occur in the homozygous individuals with >95% decrease in protein 4.1. When membrane stability is measured by ektacytometry, it is markedly reduced in the homozygous state and intermediately reduced in the heterozygous state.[95] The basis for this protein deficiency is not yet known.

RED CELL MEMBRANE LIPIDS

Structure and Function

Cholesterol and phospholipids in a molar ratio of 6:5 comprise more than 95% of the lipid content of the erythrocyte membrane. The remainder is made up of small amounts of free fatty acids, polyglycerol-phosphatides, glycerides, and phosphatidic acid.[102-106] A thin-layer chromatogram of the red cell membrane lipids is depicted in Figure 1.

The phospholipids which are present include phosphatidylcholine at a concentration of about 30%, phosphatidylethanolamine and sphingomyelin, both about 25%, and phosphatidylserine and phosphatidylinositol, both about 15%.[102,103,106-108] The structure of these phospholipids, other than sphingomyelin, is characterized by a glycerol backbone, with either fatty acids in ester linkage to the first and second carbons, or vinyl and saturated ether linkages. A base (i.e., choline, serine) is linked by a phosphodiester bond to the third carbon atom. Between 1 and 2% of phospholipids exist with only one fatty acid and are known as lysophosphatides.[109] In contrast to the molecules with two fatty acids which are lipophilic, these compounds are both lipophilic and hydrophilic. Because of these solubility characteristics, they have detergent-like qualities and an increase in their rate of exchange with the plasma.[110]

The phospholipids are amphipathic molecules having a hydrophilic (polar) head group and two hydrocarbon hydrophobic (nonpolar) tails. In an aqueous environment, these molecules form a bilayer with the head groups exposed and the tails buried.[111,112] This lipid bilayer is the fluid matrix of the erythrocyte membrane, as it is in other biological membranes. Within this bilayer, the distribution of phospholipids is nonrandom and asymmetric.[109,113,114] Using nonpenetrating chemical reagents, phospholipases, and exchange onto transfer proteins, their topology has been defined. The neutral phospholipids, phosphatidylcholine and sphingomyelin, are predominantly in the outer monolayer, while the charged molecules, phosphatidylserine and phosphatidylethanolamine, are predominantly in the inner monolayer.[110,115,116] Phospholipids with saturated fatty acids esterified to their head group are more easily "ordered" and form more stable arrays than those containing unsaturated fatty acids. In the erythrocyte bilayer, the inner monolayer is composed of phospholipids with unsaturated fatty acids and is more fluid, while the outer monolayer, being composed of phospholipids with saturated fatty acids, is more gel-like.[117,118]

Phospholipid asymmetry may be maintained, at least in part, by the membrane skeletal proteins. In intact cells exposed to SH-oxidizing agents, cross-linking of spectrin and hydrolysis of PS and PE by phospholipase A_2 occur.[119] Since PS and PE are not susceptible to this phospholipase in fresh cells, it is possible that in SH-oxidized cells these phospholipids have moved to the outer monolayer as a result of the release of constraints normally imposed on them by spectrin or by the membrane skeletal network.

Data obtained from recombination experiments of spectrin-actin with PS and PS/PC vesicles using NMR, freeze-etching, and scanning calorimetry suggest that spectrin interacts with anionic phospholipids.[120,121] Further studies supporting the role of spectrin in maintaining lipid asymmetry were done with a fluorescent probe, merocyanine 540, which binds to lipids in a fluid state and does not stain the plasma membrane of normal intact erythrocytes, presumably because the outer monolayer is in a gel-like state. In cells pretreated with an oxidizing agent, tetrathionate, and in mouse cells deficient in spectrin, the bilayer stained with merocyanin, suggesting that with a qualitative or quantitative change in spectrin, the outer monolayer became more disordered, or "fluid".[118]

Further support for the requirement of a normal skeleton in maintaining lipid bilayer asymmetry comes from additional studies with sickle cells. In deoxygenated, reversibly sickled cells, all of the PC present in the membrane is available for exchange, as determined by studies with a PC-specific exchange protein.[122] Thus, in these membranes, PC must undergo rapid transbilayer movement since a substantial amount of it is in the inner leaflet in these cells. Studies of the equilibrium time for radiolabeled PC introduced into the outer membrane revealed four times lower levels for deoxygenated vs. oxygenated cells. Reoxygenation restored the equilibrium time.

Lipid asymmetry is lost if discoid cells from patients with sickle cell anemia are deoxygenated to the sickle form. Upon oxygenation and resultant unsickling, the asymmetry is regained.[123,124] This loss of asymmetry upon sickling most likely results from a disruption of the membrane skeleton, which is thought to occur in sickle cell disease.[125]

Transmembrane movement of lipids, also called translocation, has been documented in biological membranes and model membranes by NMR, chemical labeling, exchange techniques, and phospholipases. Lipid translocation can be seen as essential in establishing the bilayer and renewing the phospholipids within it, most noticeably phosphatidylcholine.[109] Although no *de novo* lipid synthesis occurs, there are mechanisms for lipid turnover and renewal because of the existence of (1) exchange between plasma lipids and RBC lipids and (2) enzymatic pathways for acylation and methylation. Unesterified plasma cholesterol is in equilbrium with RBC cholesterol. Since the plasma enzyme lecithin-cholesterol acyl transferase (LCAT) partially regulates the level of plasma-free cholesterol, it also influences RBC cholesterol. Plasma phosphatidylcholine, lysophosphatidylcholine, and free fatty acid are also involved in passive exchange equilibria with the membrane.[105,126-128]

Translocation, from the outer to the inner surfaces of the membrane, is probably essential for one major phospholipid renewal process, PC synthesis by acylation of lsyo PC. The site for PC acylation is the inner monolayer and, therefore, the lysophosphatidylcholine must move from the plasma to reach the enzymes on the inner leaflet through the outer monolayer. Once in the inner monolayer, PC is synthesized through the acylation of LPC with free fatty acid. The resultant molecules can then move back to the outer monolayer.[109,129]

Factors influencing translocation in intact human erythrocytes were studied using the differential extraction of lysophosphatidylcholine from membranes by saline and albumin.[130] At 37°C, the rate of translocation across the bilayer was 1.87% per hour, equilibrium approximately 27 hr. The rate was found to be strongly influenced by temperature and cholesterol content but not by ATP depletion. In addition, oxidative cross-linking with diamide resulted in increased translocation rates. These studies support the importance to translocation of lipid and protein organization within the membrane.

A second enzymatic pathway involving translocation has been identified in red cell and other cell membranes which may participate in transmembrane signaling.[131] By studies with labeled methyl donors and inside-out and right-side-out ghosts, it has been shown that methyltransferase I is localized on the cytoplasmic side of the bilayer where it converts phosphatidylethanolamine to phosphatidyl-*N*-monomethylethanolamine. Methyltransferase II then catalyzes the stepwise methylation of this compound to phosphatidylcholine. During the methylation process, lipids are translocated across the membrane since methyltransferase II faces the outside of the bilayer.[132,133] During these processes, a decrease in the microviscosity of the membrane can be observed.[134] Reticulocytes have β-adrenergic receptors which can be coupled to adenylate cyclase to generate cyclic AMP.[135] Increasing phospholipid methlylation or directly increasing membrane fluidity facilitated receptor and adenylate cyclase coupling thereby increasing response to β-adrenergic stimulation.[136] In addition, increased phospholipid methylation has been shown to lead to increased Ca^{2+}-ATPase activity.[137] Therefore, this methylation process appears to play a role in certain receptor-mediated events and may be important in regulating erythrocyte calcium.

In the erythrocyte membrane lipids determine passive cation permeability and influence cell shape. The more saturated and less branched the fatty acids, the greater the ion permeability barrier.[138] In addition, increased cholesterol tends to increase the "order" of the membrane and its barrier function. Lysophosphatides and amphipathic agents have been shown to have a profound influence on cell shape in vitro. These effects may be related to the distribution of the agent between the inner and outer leaflets of the bilayer. An elegant hypothesis advanced by Sheetz and Singer[139] suggests that the lipid membrane acts as a "bilayer couple" in which a slight expansion of the outer leaflet due to preferential insertion of the amipath induces a bending moment which results in the echinocytic cell shape. Conversely, expansion of the inner leaflet produces an opposite bending moment which results in the stomatocytic cell shape. A detailed discussion of the role of lipids in cell shape is beyond the scope of this article, but has been thoroughly reviewed by Deutike.[24,140]

Diseases Associated with Lipid Abnormalities

Abetalipoproteinemia

In abetalipoproteinemia, an autosomally recessively inherited disease, the red cell has an abnormal spiny or acanthocytic shape. Its lipids reflect some of the abnormalities seen in the plasma lipids. In the plasma and red cell phospholipids, the proportion of sphingomyelin is increased and the proportion of lecithin is decreased in comparison to normal cells.[103,105] This abnormality is accentuated in the red cells as they age.[141] The change in lipid composition may well cause the observed decrease in the fluidity of acanthocyte membranes[108] since liposome studies have shown that sphingomyelin is more rigid in bilayer lipid arrays than lecithin.[129] Individuals with this disease have a slightly shortened red cell survival.[103]

Liver Disease

In individuals with severe hepatocellular disease, usually alcoholic cirrhosis, there is an abnormal plasma low-density lipoprotein and an increased molar ratio of unesterified cholesterol to phospholipid.[136] Because of the passive exchange between plasma and RBC lipids, this plasma abnormality influences the red cell and the RBC membrane contains 50 to 70% more cholesterol than normal.[136] Although the total phospholipid content is normal, the relative amount of lecithin is increased and that of sphingomyelin decreased. These cells have an abnormal shape with spiny projections and are called either spur cells or, again, acanthocytes. The fluidity of lipids within the bilayer appears to be decreased as a result of the increase in cholesterol and the red cell deformability is decreased.[119,125,135] In this disorder, red cell survival is appreciably shortened and severe hemolytic anemia is common. Moreover, this development is often a bad prognostic sign for the underlying liver disease.

Perioxidative Damage

α-Tocopherol (vitamin E) plays a role in protecting against oxidative damage in human cells, including erythrocytes. Deficiencies in this vitamin are seen primarily in individuals with chronic fat malabsorption and in low birth weight infants. In these instances, a hemolytic anemia with morphologic abnormalities can be seen which is reversible with vitamin E.[142-144] Individuals with erythrocytes less able to cope with oxidant damage because of hereditary deficiencies in glucose-6-phosphate dehydrogenase or glutathione synthetase have had increases in their red cell survivals when treated with vitamin E in some studies.[145,146] Relative vitamin E deficiency has also been found in the red cells of patients with other chronic hemolytic anemias such as thalassemia and sickle cell disease. Treatment of these disorders with supplemental vitamin E has had only equivocal results; however, Rachmilewitz has shown responses in some patients.[147]

High Phosphatidylcholine Hemolytic Anemia

Finally, a rare, congenital hemolytic disorder has been described in patients with excess phosphatidylcholine in their RBC membrane.[148] The red cells in this condition have increased cation permeability, decreased whole cell deformability, and decreased in vivo survival. Interestingly, membrane fluidity, as determined by spin resonance studies, is nearly normal — perhaps because of a ''compensatory'' associated increase in membrane cholesterol.[149] The biochemical basis for the excess phosphatidylcholine appears to be a defect in a fatty acid transfer reaction which normally converts a fraction of newly acylated PC into PE.[150] Patients with this autosomal dominant disorder have mild to moderate chronic hemolysis which is clinically ameliorated by splenectomy.

CONCLUSION

In this review, we have tried to describe much of the progress which has enabled us to define most of the protein and lipid constituents of the red cell membrane, and to begin to develop a concept of their structural and functional interrelationships. We have also discussed some selected hemolytic conditions in which abnormalities in red cell membrane constituents and their interrelationships have been defined. Although this characterization of molecular defects in hemolytic disorders is just beginning, appreciable progress has already been made and some understanding of the membrane has been advanced through the examples of clinical hemolytic anemia which have been studied. With the advent of the newer techniques — including, especially, the powerful tools of molecular genetics — we anticipate that there will be a further major increase in the understanding of the pathophysiology of these disorders and, in turn, our understanding of fundamental membrane function.

NOTE ADDED IN PROOF

Since submission of this manuscript, Agre and colleagues have reported partial deficiency of spectrin in patients with the common form of hereditary spherocytosis (*Nature (London)*, 314, 380, 1985).

REFERENCES

1. **Shohet, S. B. and Beutler, E.,** The red cell membrane, in *Hematology,* Williams, W. J., Beutler, E., Erslev, A. J., and Lichtman, M. A., Eds., McGraw Hill, New York, 1983, 345—353.
2. **Steck, T.,** The organization of proteins in the human red cell, *J. Cell Biol.,* 62, 1—19, 1974.
3. **Nigg, E. and Cherry, R.,** Influence of temperature and cholesterol on the rotational diffusion of band 3 in the human erythrocyte membrane, *Biochemistry,* 18, 3457—3465, 1979.
4. **Weinstein, R., Kitodadad, J., and Steck, T.,** The band 3 protein in transmembrane particle of the human red blood cell, in *Membrane Transport in Erythrocytes,* Lassen, U., Ussing, H., and Wieth, J., Eds., Rinnksgaarad, Copenhagen, 1980, 33—50.
5. **Fukuda, M. and Fukuda, M. N.,** Changes in cell surface glycoproteins and carbohydrate structures during the development and differentiation of human erythroid cells, *J. Supramol. Struct.,* 17, 313—324, 1981.
6. **Finne, J.,** Identification of the blood group ABH active glycoprotein components of human erythrocyte membrane, *Eur. J. Biochem.,* 104, 181—189, 1980.
7. **Tsuji, T., Irimura, T., and Osawa, T.,** The carbohydrate moiety of band 3 glycoprotein of human erythrocyte membranes, *J. Biol. Chem.,* 256, 10497—10502, 1981.
8. **Tanner, M. J. A., Williams, D. G., and Jenkins, R. E.,** Structure of the erythrocyte anion transport protein, *Ann. N.Y. Acad. Sci.,* 341, 455—464, 1980.

9. **Tillack, T. W., Scott, R. E., and Marchesi, V. T.,** The structure of erythrocyte membranes studied by freeze-etching. II. Localization of receptors for phytohemagglutinin and influenza virus to the intramembranous particles, *J. Exp. Med.*, 135, 1209—1227, 1972.
10. **Pinto da Silva, P. and Nicolson, G. L.,** Freeze-etch localization of concanavalin A receptors to the membrane intercalated particles of human erythrocyte ghost membranes, *Biochim. Biophys. Acta*, 363, 311—319, 1974.
11. **Nigg, E. A., Bron, C., Girardet, M., and Cherry, R. J.,** Band 3-glycophorin A association in erythrocyte membranes demonstrated by combining protein diffusion measurements with antibody-induced cross-linking, *Biochemistry*, 19, 1887—1893, 1980.
12. **Murthy, S. N. P., Lie, T., Kaul, R. J., et al.,** The aldolase binding site of the human erythrocyte membrane is at the NH_2-terminus of band 3, *J. Biol. Chem.*, 256, 11203—11208, 1981.
13. **Gillies, R. J.,** The binding site for aldolase and G3PDH in erythrocyte membranes, *Trends Biochem. Sci.*, 37, 45—46, 1982.
14. **Shaklai, N., Ranney, H. M., and Sharma, V.,** Interactions of hemoglobin S with erythrocyte membranes, in *The Function of Red Blood Cells: Erythrocyte Pathobiology*, Wallach, D. F. M., Ed., Alan R. Liss, New York, 1981, 1—16.
15. **Eisinger, J., Flores, J., and Salhany, J. M.,** Association of erythrocyte membranes with cytosol hemoglobin, *Proc. Natl. Acad. Sci. U.S.A.*, 79, 408—412, 1982.
16. **Tanner, M. J. A.,** Erythrocyte membrane structure and function, *Malaria and the Red Cell*, Ciba Pharmaceuticals, Summit, N.J., Evered, D. and Whelan, J., Eds., Ciba Foundation Symposium, 1983, 3—23.
17. **Bennett, V. and Stenbuck, P.,** Association between ankyrin and the cytoplasmic domain of band 3 isolated from the human erythrocyte membrane, *J. Biol. Chem.*, 255, 6424—6432, 1980.
18. **Bennett, V.,** The molecular basis for membrane-cytoskeleton association in human erythrocytes, *J. Cell. Biochem.*, 18, 49—65, 1982.
19. **Bennett, V. and Stenbuck, P.,** The membrane attachment protein for spectrin is associated with band 3 in human erythrocyte membranes, *Nature (London)*, 280, 468—473, 1979.
20. **Hargreaves, W., Giedd, K., Verkleij, A., et al.,** Reassociation of ankyrin with band 3 in erythrocyte membranes and in lipid vesicles, *J. Biol. Chem.*, 255, 11965—11972, 1980.
21. **Bennett, V.,** Isolation of an ankyrin-band 3 oligomer from human erythrocyte membranes, *Biochim. Biophys. Acta*, 689, 475—484, 1982.
22. **Evans, E. A. and Hochmuth, R. M.,** A solid-liquid composite model of the red cell membrane, *J. Membr. Biol.*, 30, 351—362, 1977.
23. **Mohandas, N., Chasis, J. A., and Shohet, S. B.,** The influence of membrane skeleton on red cell deformability, membrane material properties, and shape, *Semin. Hematol.*, 20, 225—242, 1983.
24. **Sheetz, M. P.,** Membrane skeletal dynamics: role in modulation of red cell deformability, mobility of transmembrane proteins, and shape, *Semin. Hematol.*, 20, 175—188, 1983.
25. **Lazarides, E. and Moon, R. T.,** Assembly and topogenesis of the spectrin-based membrane skeleton in erythroid development, *Cell*, 37, 354—356, 1984.
26. **Cabantchik, Z. I. and Rothstein, A.,** Membrane proteins related to anion permeability of human red blood cells, *J. Membr. Biol.*, 15, 207—226, 1974.
27. **Lepke, S., Fasold, H., Pring, M., and Passaow, H. J.,** A study of the relationship between inhibition of anion exchange and binding to the red blood cell membrane of 4.4′-diisothiocyano stilbene-2,2′-disulfonic acid (DIDS) and its dihydroderivative (H_2DIDS), *J. Membr. Biol.*, 29, 147—177, 1976.
28. **Alderman, E. M., Fudenberg, H. H., and Lovins, B. E.,** Isolation and characterization of an age-related antigen present on senescent human red blood cells, *Blood*, 58, 341—349, 1981.
29. **Kay, M. M. B.,** Isolation of the phagocytosis-inducing IgG-binding antigen on senescent somatic cells, *Nature (London)*, 289, 491—494, 1981.
30. **Kay, M. M. B.,** Glucose transport protein is structurally and immunologically related to band 3 and senescent cell antigen, *Proc. Natl. Acad. Sci. U.S.A.*, 82, 1731, 1985.
31. **Anstee, D. J.,** The blood group MN Ss-active sialoglycoproteins, *Semin. Hematol.*, 18, 13—31, 1981.
32. **Marchesi, V. T., Tillack, T. W., Jackson, R. L., et al.,** Chemical characterization and surface orientation of the major glycoprotein of the human erythrocyte membrane, *Proc. Natl. Acad. Sci. U.S.A.*, 69, 1445—1449, 1972.
33. **Schulte, T. H. and Marchesi, V. T.,** Conformation of human erythrocyte glycophorin A and its constituent peptides, *Biochemistry*, 18, 275—280, 1979.
34. **Ross, A. H., Radhakrishnan, R., Robson, R. J., and Khurana, H. G.,** The transmembrane domain of glycophorin A as studied by cross-linking using photo-activatable phospholipids, *J. Biol. Chem.*, 257, 4152—4161, 1982.
35. **Thomas, D. B. and Winzler, R. J.,** Structural studies on human erythrocyte glycoproteins: alkali-labile oligosaccharides, *J. Biol. Chem.*, 244, 5943—5946, 1969.
36. **Lisowska, E., Dur, M., and Dahr, W.,** Comparison of alkali-labile oligosaccharide chains of M and N blood group glycopeptides from human erythrocyte membrane, *Carbohyd. Res.*, 79, 103—113, 1980.

37. **Yoshima, H., Furthmayr, H., and Kobata, A.,** Structures of the asparagine-linked sugar chains of glycophorin A, *J. Biol. Chem.,* 255, 9713—9718, 1980.
38. **Furthmayr, H.,** Structural comparison of glycophorins and immuochemical analysis of genetic variants, *Nature (London),* 271, 519—524, 1978.
39. **Anstee, D. J., Mawby, W. J., and Tanner, M. J. A.,** Structural variation in human erythrocyte sialoglycoproteins, in *Membranes and Transport,* Vol. 2, Martonosi, A., Ed., Plenum Press, New York, 1982, 429—432.
40. **Dahr, W., Uhlenbruck, G., Leikola, J., et al.,** Studies on membrane glycoprotein defect of En(a−) erythrocytes, *J. Immunogenet.,* 31, 329—346, 1976.
41. **Tanner, J. A. and Anstee, D. J.,** The membrane change in En(a−) human erythrocytes, *Biochem. J.,* 153, 271—277, 1976.
42. **Cotmore, S. F., Furthmayr, H., and Marchesi, V. T.,** Immunochemical evidence for the transmembrane orientation of glycophorin A: location of ferritin-antibody conjugates in intact cells, *J. Mol. Biol.,* 113, 539—553, 1977.
43. **Lovrien, R. E. and Anderson, R. A.,** Stoichiometry of wheat germ agglutinin as a morphology controlling agent and as a morphology protective agent for the human erythrocyte, *J. Cell. Biol.,* 85, 534—548, 1980.
44. **Chasis, J. A., Mohandas, N., and Shohet, S. B.,** Erythrocyte membrane rigidity induced by glycophorin A-ligand interaction, *J. Clin. Invest.,* 75, 1919, 1985.
45. **Anderson, R. A. and Lovrien, R. E.,** Glycophorin is linked by band 4.1 protein to the human erythrocyte membrane skeleton, *Nature (London),* 307, 655—658, 1984.
46. **Anderson, R. A. and Marchesi, V. T.,** Polyphosphoinositide modulation of glycophorin-protein 4.1 interactions: a possible mechanism for regulation of the red cell membrane skeleton, *J. Cell. Biol.,* 97, 297a, 1983.
47. **Dahr, W., Beyreuther, K., Steinbach, H., Gielan, W., and Krüger, J.,** Structure of the Ss blood group antigens. II. A methionine/threonine polymorphism within the N-terminal sequence of the Ss glycoprotein, *Hoppe-Seyler's Z. Physiol. Chem.,* 361, 895—906, 1980.
48. **Tanner, M. J. A. and Anstee, D. J.,** A method for the direct demonstration of lectin-binding components of the human erythrocyte membrane, *Biochem. J.,* 153, 265—270, 1976.
49. **Mueller, T. and Morrison, M.,** Glycoconnectin (PAS 2), a membrane attachment site for the human erythrocyte cytoskeleton, in *Erythrocyte Membranes 2: Recent Clinical and Experimental Advances,* Kruckeberg, W., Eaton, J., and Brewer, J., Eds., Alan R. Liss, New York, 1981, 95—112.
50. **Baldwin, S. A. and Lienhard, G. E.,** Glucose transport across plasma membranes: facilitated diffusion systems, *Trends Biochem. Sci.,* 6, 208—211, 1981.
51. **Lux, S.,** Dissecting the red cell membrane skeleton, *Nature (London),* 281, 426—429, 1979.
52. **Branton, D., Cohen, C. M., and Tyler, J.,** Interaction of cytoskeletal proteins on the human erythrocyte membrane, *Cell,* 24, 24—32, 1981.
53. **Marchesi, V. T.,** The red cell membrane skeleton: recent progress, *Blood,* 61, 1—11, 1983.
54. **Morrow, J., Haigh, W., and Marchesi, V. T.,** Spectrin oligomers: a structural feature of the erythrocyte cytoskeleton, *J. Supramol. Struct.,* 17, 275—287, 1981.
55. **Morrow, J. and Marchesi, V. T.,** Self-assembly of spectrin oligomers in vitro: a basis for a dynamic cytoskeleton, *J. Cell. Biol.,* 88, 463—468, 1981.
56. **Speicher, D., Morrow, J., and Knowles, W.,** A structural model of human erythrocyte spectrin: alignment of chemical and functional domains, *J. Biol. Chem.,* 257, 9093—9101, 1982.
57. **Knowles, W. J., Morrow, J. S., Speicher, D. W., et al.,** Molecular and functional changes in spectrin from patients with hereditary pyropoikilocytosis, *J. Clin. Invest.,* 71, 1867—1877, 1983.
58. **Speicher, D. W., Davis, G., Yurchenco, P. D., and Marchesi, V. T.,** Structure of human erythrocyte spectrin. I. Isolation of the α-I domain and its cyanogen bromide peptides, *J. Biol. Chem.,* 258, 14931—14937, 1983.
59. **Speicher, D. W., Davis, G., and Marchesi, V. T.,** Structure of human erythrocyte spectrin. II. The sequence of the α-I domain, *J. Biol. Chem.,* 258, 14938—14947, 1983.
60. **Tyler, J., Hargreaves, W., and Branton, D.,** Purification of two spectrin binding proteins. Biochemical and electron microscopic evidence for site-specific reassociation between spectrin and bands 2.1 and 4.1, *Proc. Natl. Acad. Sci. U.S.A.,* 76, 5192—5196, 1979.
61. **Tyler, J., Reinhardt, B., and Branton, D.,** Associations of erythrocyte membrane proteins. Binding of purified bands 2.1 and 4.1 to spectrin, *J. Biol. Chem.,* 255, 7034—7039, 1980.
62. **Morrow, J., Speicher, D., and Knowles, W.,** Identification of functional domains of human erythrocyte spectrin, *Proc. Natl. Acad. Sci. U.S.A.,* 77, 6592—6596, 1980.
63. **Bennett, V.,** Immunoreactive forms of human erythrocyte ankyrin are present in diverse cells and tissues, *Nature (London),* 281, 597—599, 1979.
64. **Shaklai, N., Benitz, L., and Ranney, H. M.,** Binding of 2,3-diphosphoglycerate by spectrin and its effect on oxygen affinity of hemoglobin, *Am. J. Physiol.,* 234, 36—40, 1978.

65. **Glenney, J., Glenney, P., and Weber, K.,** Erythroid spectrin, brain fodrin, and intestinal brush border proteins (TW-260/240) are related molecules containing a common calmodulin-binding subunit bound to a variant cell type-specific subunit, *Proc. Natl. Acad. Sci. U.S.A.*, 79, 4002—4005, 1982.
66. **Sobue, K., Muramoto, Y., and Fujita, M.,** Calmodulin-binding protein of erythrocyte cytoskeleton, *Biochem. Biophys. Res. Commun.*, 100, 1063—1070, 1981.
67. **Fairbanks, G., Steck, T., and Wallach, D.,** Electrophoretic analysis of the major polypeptides of the human erythrocyte membrane, *Biochemistry*, 10, 2606—2617, 1971.
68. **Goodman, S. R., Yu, J., Whitfield, C. F., Culp, E. N., and Posnak, E. J.,** Erythrocyte membrane skeleton protein bands 4.1a and b are sequence-related phosphoproteins, *J. Biol. Chem.*, 257, 4564—4569, 1982.
69. **Jackson, C. W., Mueller, T. J., Dockter, M. E., and Morrison, M.,** Cytoskeletal alterations during red cell aging, *Blood*, 58, 29a, 1981.
70. **Cohen, C. and Branton, D.,** The role of spectrin in erythrocyte membrane-stimulated actin polymerization, *Nature (London)*, 279, 163—165, 1979.
71. **Pinder, J., Ungewickell, E., Calvert, R., et al.,** Polymerization of G-actin by spectrin preparations: identification of the active constituent, *FEBS Lett.*, 104, 396—400, 1979.
72. **Brenner, S. L. and Korn, E. D.,** Spectrin/actin complex isolated from sheep erythrocytes accelerates actin polymerization by simple nucleation, *J. Biol. Chem.*, 255, 1670—1676, 1980.
73. **Lin, D.,** Spectrin-4.1-actin complex of the human erythrocyte: Molecular basis of its ability to bind cytochalasins with high affinity and to accelerate actin polymerization in vitro, *J. Supramol. Struct.*, 15, 129—138, 1981.
74. **Atkinson, M., Morrow, J., and Marchesi, V.,** The polymeric state of actin in the human erythrocyte cytoskeleton, *J. Cell. Biochem.*, 18, 493—505, 1982.
75. **Lin, D. and Lin, S.,** Actin polymerization induced by a motility-related high-affinity cytochalasin binding complex from human erythrocyte membrane, *Proc. Natl. Acad. Sci. U.S.A.*, 76, 2345—2349, 1979.
76. **Cohen, C. and Foley, S.,** Spectrin-dependent and -independent association of F-actin with the erythrocyte membrane, *J. Cell. Biol.*, 86, 694—698, 1980.
77. **Fowler, V. and Taylor, D.,** Spectrin plus band 4.1 cross-link actin, *J. Cell. Biol.*, 85, 361—376, 1980.
78. **Wolf, L., Lux, S., and Ohanian, V.,** Regulation of spectrin-actin binding by protein 4.1 and polyphosphates, *J. Cell. Biol.*, 87, 203a, 1980.
79. **Cohen, C. and Foley, S.,** The role of band 4.1 in the association of actin with erythrocyte membranes, *Biochim. Biophys. Acta*, 698, 691—701, 1982.
80. **Cohen, C. M., Tyler, J. M., and Branton, D.,** Spectrin-actin associations studied by electron microscopy of shadowed preparations, *Cell*, 21, 875—883, 1980.
81. **Ungewickell, E., Bennett, P., and Calvert, R.,** In vitro formation of a complex between cytoskeletal proteins of the human erythrocyte, *Nature (London)*, 280, 811—814, 1979.
82. **Yu, J. and Goodman, S.,** The spectrin-binding proteins(s) of the human erythrocyte membrane, *Proc. Natl. Acad. Sci. U.S.A.*, 76, 2340—2344, 1979.
83. **Siegel, D. and Branton, D.,** Human erythrocyte band 4.9, *J. Cell. Biol.*, 95, 265a, 1982.
84. **Leblond, P. F., de Boisfleury, A., and Bessis, M.,** Erythrocyte shape in hereditary spherocytosis. A scanning electron microscopic study and relationship to deformability, *Nouv. Rev. Fr. Hematol.*, 13, 873—883, 1973.
85. **Agre, P., Orringer, E. P., and Bennett, V.,** Deficient red cell spectrin in severe, recessively inherited spherocytosis, *N. Engl. J. Med.*, 306, 1155—1161, 1982.
86. **Wolfe, L. C., John, K. M., Falcone, B. A., et al.,** A genetic defect in the binding of protein 4.1 to spectrin in a kindred with hereditary spherocytosis, *N. Engl. J. Med.*, 307, 1367—1374, 1982.
87. **Goodman, S. R., Shiffer, K. A., Casoria, L. A., et al.,** Identification of the molecular defect in the erythrocyte membrane skeleton of some kindreds with hereditary spherocytosis, *Blood*, 60, 772—784, 1982.
88. **Liu, S. C., Palek, J., Prchal, J., et al.,** Altered spectrin dimer-dimer associations and instability of erythrocyte membrane skeletons in hereditary pyropoikilocytosis, *J. Clin. Invest.*, 68, 597—605, 1981.
89. **Palek, J., Liu, S. C., Liu, P. Y., et al.,** Altered assembly of spectrin in red cell membranes in hereditary pyropoikilocytosis, *Blood*, 57, 130—139, 1981.
90. **Lawler, J., Liu, S. C., Palek, J., et al.,** A molecular defect of spectrin in hereditary pyropoikilocytosis: alterations in the trypsin-resistant domain involved in spectrin self-association, *J. Clin. Invest.*, 70, 1019—1030, 1982.
91. **Mentzer, W. C., Turetski, T., Mohandas, N., et al.,** Identification of the hereditary pyropoikilocytosis carrier state, *Blood*, 63, 1439—1446, 1984.
92. **Zarkowsky, H. S., Mohandas, N., Speaker, C. B., and Shohet, S. B.,** A congenital hemolytic anemia with thermal sensitivity of the erythrocyte membrane, *Br. J. Haematol.*, 29, 537—543, 1975.
93. **Mohandas, N., Clark, M. R., Jacobs, M. S., et al.,** Analysis of factors regulating erythrocyte deformability, *J. Clin. Invest.*, 66, 563—573, 1980.

94. **Chang, K., Williamson, J., and Zarkowsky, H.,** Effects of heat on the circular dichroism of spectrin in hereditary pyropoikilocytosis, *J. Clin. Invest.,* 64, 326—328, 1979.
95. **Mohandas, N., Clark, M. R., and Heath, B. P.,** A technique to detect reduced mechanical stability of red cell membranes: relevance to elliptocytic disorders, *Blood,* 59, 768—774, 1982.
96. **Coetzer, T. and Zail, S.,** Spectrin tetramer-dimer equilibrium in hereditary elliptocytosis, *Blood,* 59, 900—905, 1982.
97. **Liu, S. C., Palek, J., and Prchal, J.,** Defective spectrin dimer-dimer association in hereditary elliptocytosis, *Proc. Natl. Acad. Sci. U.S.A.,* 79, 2072—2076, 1982.
98. **Lawler, J., Liu, S. C., and Palek, J.,** A molecular defect of spectrin in a subset of patients with hereditary elliptocytosis. Alterations in the α subunit domain involved in spectrin self-association, *J. Clin. Invest.,* 73, 1688—1695, 1984.
99. **Agre, P., Orringer, E. P., Chiu, D. H. K., and Bennett, V.,** A molecular defect in two families with hemolytic poikilocytic anemia. Reduction of high affinity membrane binding sites for ankyrin, *J. Clin. Invest.,* 68, 1566—1576, 1981.
100. **Feo, C. J., Fischer, S., Piau, J. P., et al.,** Premiere observation de l'absence d'une proteine de la membrane erythrocytaire (band 4_1) dans un cas anemie elliptocytaire familiale, *Nouv. Rev. Fr. Hematol.,* 22, 315—325, 1980.
101. **Tchernia, G., Mohandas, N., and Shohet, S. B.,** Deficiency of skeletal membrane protein band 4.1 in homozygous hereditary elliptocytosis, *J. Clin. Invest.,* 68, 454—460, 1981.
102. **Ways, P. and Hanahan, D. J.,** Characterization and quantification of red cell lipids in normal man, *J. Lipid Res.,* 5, 318—328, 1964.
103. **van Deenen, L. L. M. and de Gier, J.,** Chemical composition and metabolism of lipids in red cells of various animal species, in *The Red Blood Cell: A Comprehensive Treatise,* Bishop, C. and Surgenor, D. M., Eds., Academic Press, New York, 1964, 243—307.
104. **Nelson, G. J.,** Composition of neutral lipids from erythrocytes of common mammals, *J. Lipid Res.,* 8, 374—379, 1967.
105. **Shohet, S. B., Nathan, D. G., and Karnovsky, M. L.,** Stages in the incorporation of fatty acids into red blood cells, *J. Clin. Invest.,* 47, 1096—1108, 1968.
106. **Sweeley, C. C. and Dawson, G.,** *Lipids of the Erythrocyte Red Cell Membrane: Structure and Function,* Jamieson, G. A. and Greenwalt, T. J., Eds., J. B. Lippincott, Philadelphia, 1969, 172—232.
107. **Dodge, J. T. and Phillips, G. B.,** Composition of phospholipids and of phospholipid fatty acids and aldehydes in human red cells, *J. Lipid Res.,* 8, 667—675, 1967.
108. **Cooper, R. A.,** Lipids of human red cell membrane: normal composition and variability in disease, *Semin. Hematol.,* 7, 296—322, 1970.
109. **van Deenen, L. L. M.,** Topology and dynamics of phospholipids in membranes, *FEBS Lett.,* 123, 3—15, 1981.
110. **Verkleij, A. J., Zwaal, R. F. A., Roelofsen, B., et al.,** The asymmetric distribution of phospholipids in the human red cell membrane, *Biochim. Biophys. Acta,* 323, 178—193, 1973.
111. **Gortner, E. and Grendel, F.,** On biomolecular layer or lipoids on the chromocytes of the blood, *J. Exp. Med.,* 41, 439—443, 1925.
112. **Danielli, J. F. and Davson, H.,** A contribution to the theory of permeability of thin films, *J. Cell. Comp. Physiol.,* 5, 495—508, 1935.
113. **Op den Kamp, J. A. F.,** Lipid asymmetry in membranes, *Annu. Rev. Biochem.,* 48, 47—71, 1979.
114. **Etemadi, A. H.,** Membrane asymmetry. A survey and critical appraisal of the methodology, *Biochim. Biophys. Acta,* 604, 423—475, 1980.
115. **Zwaal, R. F. A., Roelofsen, B., and Colley, C. M.,** Localization of red cell membrane constituents, *Biochim. Biophys. Acta,* 300, 159—182, 1973.
116. **Marinetti, G. V. and Crain, R. C.,** Topology of amino-phospholipids in the red cell membrane, *J. Supramol. Struct.,* 8, 191—213, 1978.
117. **Williams, J. H., Kuchmak, M., and Witter, R.,** Fatty acids in phospholipids isolated from human red cells, *Lipids,* 1, 391—398, 1966.
118. **Williamson, P., Bateman, K. K., et al.,** Involvement of spectrin in the maintenance of phase-state asymmetry in the erythrocyte membrane, *Cell,* 30, 725—733, 1982.
119. **Haest, C. W. M., Plasa, G., Kamp, D., and Deuticke, B.,** Spectrin as a stabilizer of the phospholipid asymmetry in the human erythrocyte membrane, *Biochim. Biophys. Acta,* 509, 21—32, 1978.
120. **Mombers, C., Verkleij, A. J., de Gier, J., and van Deenen, L. L. M.,** The interaction of spectrin-actin and synthetic phospholipids, *Biochim. Biophys. Acta,* 551, 271—281, 1979.
121. **Mombers, C., de Gier, J., Demel, R. A., and van Deenen, L. L. M.,** Spectrin-phospholipid interaction, a monolayer study, *Biochim. Biophys. Acta,* 603, 52—62, 1980.
122. **Franck, P. F. H., Chiu, D. T.-Y., op den Kamp, J. A. F., et al.,** Accelerated transbilayer movement of phosphatidylcholine in sickled erythrocytes, *J. Biol. Chem.,* 258, 8435—8442, 1983.

123. **Chiu, D., Lubin, B., and Shohet, S. B.**, Erythrocyte membrane lipid reorganization during the sickling process, *Br. J. Haematol.*, 41, 223—234, 1979.
124. **Lubin, B., Chiu, D., Bastacky, J., et al.**, Abnormalities in membrane phospholipid organization in sickled erythrocytes, *J. Clin. Invest.*, 67, 1643—1649, 1981.
125. **Lux, S. E., John, K. M., and Karnovsky, J.**, Irreversible deformation of the spectrin-actin lattice in irreversibly sickled cells, *J. Clin. Invest.*, 58, 955—963, 1976.
126. **de Gier, J. and van Deenen, L. L. M.**, A dietary investigation on the variations in phospholipid characteristics of red-cell membranes, *Biochim. Biophys. Acta*, 84, 294—304, 1964.
127. **Mulder, E., van den Berg, J. W. O., and van Deenen, L. L. M.**, Metabolism of red-cell lipids. II. Conversion of lysophosphoglycerides, *Biochim. Biophys. Acta*, 106, 118—127, 1965.
128. **Shohet, S. B.**, Release of phospholipid fatty acid from human erythrocytes, *J. Clin. Invest.*, 49, 1668—1678, 1970.
129. **Renooy, W., van Golde, L. M. G., Zwaal, R. F. A., et al.**, Topological asymmetry of phospholipid metabolism in rat erythrocyte membranes, *Eur. J. Biochem.*, 61, 53—58, 1976.
130. **Mohandas, N., Wyatt, J., Mel, S. F., et al.**, Lipid translocation across the human erythrocyte membrane, *J. Biol. Chem.*, 257, 6537—6543, 1982.
131. **Hirata, F. and Axelrod, J.**, Phospholipid methylation and biological signal transmission, *Science*, 209, 1082—1090, 1980.
132. **Kahelenberg, A., Walker, C., and Rothrlick, R.**, Evidence for an asymmetric distribution of phospholipids in the human erythrocyte membrane, *Can. J. Biochem.*, 52, 803—806, 1974.
133. **Hirata, F. and Axelrod, J.**, Enzymatic synthesis and rapid translocation of phosphatidylcholine by two methyltransferases in erythrocyte membranes, *Proc. Natl. Acad. Sci. U.S.A.*, 75, 2348—2352, 1978.
134. **Hirata, F. and Axelrod, J.**, Enzymatic methylation of phosphatidylethanolamine increases erythrocyte membrane fluidity, *Nature (London)*, 275, 219—220, 1978.
135. **Bilezikian, J. P., Spiegel, A. M., Gammon, D. E., and Aurbach, G. D.**, The role of guanyl nucleotides in the expression of catecholamine-responsive adenylate cyclase during maturation of the rat reticulocyte, *Mol. Pharmacol.*, 13, 786—795, 1977.
136. **Rimon, G., Hanski, E., Braun, S., and Levitzki, A.**, Mode of coupling between hormone receptors and adenylate cyclase elucidated by modulation of membrane fluidity, *Nature (London)*, 276, 394—396, 1978.
137. **Strittmatter, W. J., Hirata, F., and Axelrod, J.**, Increased Ca^{2+}-ATPase activity associated with methylation of phospholipids in human erythrocytes, *Biochem. Biophys. Res. Commun.*, 88, 147—153, 1979.
138. **Shohet, S. B.**, Hemolysis and changes in erythrocyte membrane lipids, *N. Engl. J. Med.*, 286, 577—583, 638—644, 1972.
139. **Sheetz, M. P. and Singer, S. J.**, Biological membranes as bilayer couples, a mechanism of drug-erythrocyte interactions, *Proc. Natl. Acad. Sci. U.S.A.*, 72, 4457—4461, 1974.
140. **Deuticke, B.**, Transformation and restoration of biconcave shape of human erythrocytes induced by amphiphilic agents and changes of ionic environment, *Biochem. Biophys. Acta*, 163, 494—500, 1968.
141. **Ways, P. and Song, D.**, Etiology of the RBC phospholipid abnormalities in abetalipoproteinemia, *Clin. Res.*, 13, 283, 1965.
142. **Oski, F. A. and Barness, L. A.**, Hemolytic anemia in vitamin E deficiency, *Am. J. Clin. Nutr.*, 21, 45—56, 1968.
143. **Ritchie, J. H., Fish, M. B., McMasters, V., and Grossman, M.**, Edema and hemolytic anemia in premature infants: vitamin E deficiency, *N. Engl. J. Med.*, 279, 1185—1190, 1968.
144. **Farrell, P. M., Bieri, J. G., Fratantoni, J. F., et al.**, The occurrence and effects of vitamin E deficiency: a study in patients with cystic fibrosis, *J. Clin. Invest.*, 60, 233—241, 1977.
145. **Spielberg, S. P., Boxer, L. A., Corash, L. M., and Schulman, J. D.**, Improved erythrocyte survival with high-dose vitamin E in chronic hemolyzing G6PD and glutathione synthetase deficiencies, *Ann. Intern. Med.*, 90, 53—54, 1979.
146. **Corash, L. M., Spielberg, S., Bartsocas, C., et al.**, Reduced chronic hemolysis during high-dose vitamin E administration in Mediterranean-type glucose-6-phosphate dehydrogenase deficiency, *N. Engl. J. Med.*, 303, 416—420, 1980.
147. **Rachmilewitz, E. A., Kahane, I., Lubin, B. H., and Shohet, S. B.**, Peroxidation of red blood cell membranes in beta thalassemia and effects of oral vitamin E, *Blood*, 46, 1027, 1975.
148. **Jaffé, E. R. and Gottfried, E. L.**, Hereditary non-spherocytic hemolytic disease associated with an altered phospholipid composition of the erythrocytes, *J. Clin. Invest.*, 47, 1375—1388, 1968.
149. **Yawata, Y., Sugihara, T., Mori, M., et al.**, Lipid analyses and fluidity studies by electron spin resonance of red cell membranes in hereditary high red cell membrane phosphatidylcholine hemolytic anemia, *Blood*, 64, 1129, 1984.
150. **Shohet, S. B., Livermore, B. M., Nathan, D. G., and Jaffé, E. R.**, Hereditary hemolytic anemia associated with abnormal membrane lipids: mechanism of accumulation of phosphatidyl choline, *Blood*, 38, 445—456, 1971.

INDEX

A

B

C

D

E

F

G

H

I

J

K

L

M

N

O

P

Q

R

S

T

U

V

W

X

Z